Principles and Practice of Herbal Medicine

Principles and Practice of Herbal Medicine

Editor: George Moore

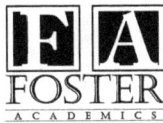

FA FOSTER
ACADEMICS

www.fosteracademics.com

www.fosteracademics.com

FA
FOSTER
ACADEMICS

Cataloging-in-Publication Data

Principles and practice of herbal medicine / edited by George Moore.
   p. cm.
Includes bibliographical references and index.
ISBN 978-1-63242-608-6
1. Herbs--Therapeutic use. 2. Botany, Medical. 3. Materia medica, Vegetable.
4. Medicinal plants. I. Moore, George.
RM666.H33 P75 2019
615.321--dc23

Foster Academics,
118-35 Queens Blvd., Suite 400,
Forest Hills, NY 11375, USA

ISBN 978-1-63242-608-6 (Hardback)

Contents

Preface

The study of botany and the use of medicinal plants fall under the science of herbalism. Throughout human history, plants have been used for the treatment of diseases and ailments. Many of the pharmaceuticals used today have a history of use as herbal remedies, such as quinine, aspirin, digitalis and opium. Modern medicine uses plant-derived compounds for the development of evidence-based pharmaceutical drugs. The scope of herbal medicine may extend to incorporate fungal and bee products, shells, animal parts and minerals. Herbal remedies are prevalently used in patients with chronic diseases like diabetes, cancer, end-stage renal disease and asthma. Prescription drugs are used along with herbal extracts, herbal teas and essential oils. This book traces the progress of herbal medicine and highlights some of its key principles and practices. It includes some of the vital pieces of work being conducted across the world, on various herbal medicines. Those in search of information to further their knowledge will be greatly assisted by this book.

This book is a result of research of several months to collate the most relevant data in the field.

When I was approached with the idea of this book and the proposal to edit it, I was overwhelmed. It gave me an opportunity to reach out to all those who share a common interest with me in this field. I had 3 main parameters for editing this text:

1. Accuracy – The data and information provided in this book should be up-to-date and valuable to the readers.

2. Structure – The data must be presented in a structured format for easy understanding and better grasping of the readers.

3. Universal Approach – This book not only targets students but also experts and innovators in the field, thus my aim was to present topics which are of use to all.

Thus, it took me a couple of months to finish the editing of this book.

I would like to make a special mention of my publisher who considered me worthy of this opportunity and also supported me throughout the editing process. I would also like to thank the editing team at the back-end who extended their help whenever required.

Editor

Herbal formula Xinshuitong capsule exerts its cardioprotective effects via mitochondria in the hypoxia-reoxygenated human cardiomyocytes

Chunjiang Tan[*][†], Jianwei Zeng, Yanbin Wu, Jiahui Zhang and Wenlie Chen[†]

Abstract

Background: The collapse of mitochondrial membrane potential ($\Delta\Psi m$) resulted in the cell apoptosis and heart failure. Xinshuitong Capsule (XST) could ameliorate left ventricular ejection fraction (LVEF), New York Heart Association (NYHA) classes and the quality of life in patients with chronic heart failure in our clinical study, however, its cardioprotective mechanisms remain unclear.

Methods: Primary human cardiomyocytes were subjected to hypoxia-reoxygenation and treated with XST200, 400 and 600 μg/ml. The model group was free of XST and the control group was cultured in normal conditions. Cell viability, $\Delta\Psi m$, the activity of mitochondrial respiratory chain complexes, ATPase activity, reactive oxygen species (ROS) and apoptosis cells were determined in all the groups.

Results: The cell viability in the XST-treated groups was significantly higher than that in the model group ($P < 0.05$). Coupled with the restoration of the $\Delta\Psi m$, the number of polarized cells increased dose dependently in the XST-treated groups. XST also restored the lost activities of mitochondrial respiratory chain complexes I-IV induced by the oxidative stress. The total of mitochondrial ATPase activity was significantly elevated at XST400 and 600 μg/ml compared to the model group ($P < 0.05$). The levels of mitochondrial ROS and the number of apoptosis cells declined in the XST-treated groups compared to those in the model group ($P < 0.05$).

Conclusions: XST, via restoration of $\Delta\Psi m$ and the mitochondrial respiratory chain complexes I-IV activities, and suppression of mitochondrial ROS generation and the apoptosis cells, maintained the integrity of the mitochondrial membrane to exert its cardioprotective effects in the hypoxia-reoxygenated human cardiomyocytes.

Keywords: Xinshuitong capsule, Mitochondrial potential, Hypoxia-reoxygenated human cardiomyocytes

Background

Mitochondria, as the power house of the heart, are highly packed in the cardiomyocytes. Cardiac cells under prolonged hypoxia condition have been shown with the opening of mitochondrial permeability transition pore (MPTP) [1]. Due to the opening of MPTP causes a transient hyperpolarization, followed by depolarization, and subsequently the collapse of the mitochondrial membrane potential ($\Delta\Psi m$), which is characterized by mitochondrial swelling and uncoupling. Thus, MPTP opening and mitochondrial $\Delta\Psi m$ collapse have been regarded as a primary mediator of apoptosis in the ischemia-reperfusion heart injury [2, 3].

The mitochondrial electron transport chain (ETC) is found in the inner membrane, where it serves as the site of oxidative phosphorylation through the use of ATP synthase. During this chemical process, ROS can be formed as a byproduct of normal cellular aerobic metabolism in the heart [4, 5]. Thus, the major process from which the heart derives sufficient energy can also result in the production of ROS [5]. On the other hand, ROS can depress the activity of mitochondrial ETC and alter

---
* Correspondence: tchunj@126.com; chen.wl@163.com
[†]Chunjiang Tan and Wenlie Chen contributed equally to this work.
Fujian Academy of Integrative Medicine, Fujian University of Traditional Chinese Medicine, Fuzhou, Fujian, China

ion pump function in heart [6]. Mounting evidence has strongly implicated ROS signaling in the genesis of cardiac hypertrophy [7–9]. Therefore, maintaining the integrity of the mitochondrial membrane, enhancing antioxidant defense may be a therapeutic method for the protection of cardiomyocytes against the injury of ischemia or hypoxia.

Xinshuitong Capsule (XST, awarded the Invention Patent of the People's Republic of China, No.ZL201210197892.X), a Chinese herbal medicine formula for chronic heart failure (CHF), which consists of Astragali radix, Pseudostellariae radix and Salviae miltiorrhizae radix et al., has the effects of benefiting Qi and Yang, activating blood and eliminating stasis, and inducing diuresis to alleviate edema. Our previous clinical study showed that the CHF patients, who received XST treatment (3 capsules, tid.), were significantly ameliorated in left ventricular ejection fraction (LVEF), New York Heart Association (NYHA) classes, the symptoms and the quality of life compared to the control group [10]. In vitro, XST-treated hypoxia-reoxygenated human cardiomyocytes showed more tolerant to hypoxia stress. The cells exhibited more regular shape and size than the control [11]. However, the drug's cardioprotective mechanisms remain elusive, especially, its actions on MPTP and mitochondrial apoptosis pathway. Thus, in current experiments, mitochondrial $\Delta\Psi m$ and mitochondrial mass, the activities of the mitochondrial ETC and the mitochondrial ATPase, and their associations with ROS levels and apoptosis cells will be studied in the hypoxia-reoxygenated cardiomyocytes.

Methods
Hypoxia-reoxygenated cell model
Primary human cardiomyocyte (HCM) was purchased from American Science Cell Research Laboratories (San Diego. USA). When the cells reached 80–90% confluence, they ere placed on a 96-well plate or a petri dish at a density of 0.75×10^5 cells/ml in a hypoxia chamber ($80\%N_2, 10\%H_2, 10\%CO_2$ and $0.2\%O_2$) for 12 h,11 following by 2 h reoxygenation. During the process of hypoxia and reoxygenation, the study group were exposed to the water-extract of XST (200, 400 and 600 µg/ml, respectively), while the model group was cultured in the identical conditions free of XST treatment, and the control group was cultured in normal conditions. The drug's low and high concentrations used in the current experiment were comparable to the human serum levels in the previous clinical study.

Cell viability assay
As described before [12], cell viability was estimated by the assay of 3-[4,5-dimethylthiazol-2-yl]-diphenyl-tetrazolium bromide (MTT, Sigma-Aldrich). Briefly, after treatment, the cells were washed twice with phosphate-buffered saline (PBS, pH 7.4), and then added 100ul MTT in PBS (0.5 mg/

ml) and incubated for 4 h at 37 °C. Followed by removing MTT and oscillating for 10 min, cell viability was estimated at absorbance 570 nm by a Tecan Infinite M200 Pro microplate reader (Tecan, Mannedorf, Swizerland).

Mitochondrial $\Delta\Psi m$ detected by JC-1 staining
As JC-1 (5,5′,6,6′-tetrachloro-1,1′,3,3′-tetraethylbenzimidazolyl-carbocyanine iodide, Beyotime, China) is a lipophilic fluorescent cation that is incorporated into the mitochondrial membrane, where it can form aggregates due to the state of the mitochondrial $\Delta\Psi m$. This aggregation changes the fluorescence properties of JC-1 from green to orange fluorescence as the $\Delta\Psi m$ increased. After treatment, cells were harvested, re-suspended and incubated with 10 µg/ml JC-1 at 37 °C for 30 min as before [13, 14]. The cells were then washed and centrifuged, the intact living cells stained the mitochondria with JC-1 would exhibit a pronounced orange fluorescence, however, the cells with a breakdown of $\Delta\Psi m$ showed a decrease of the orange fluorescence (or a increase of the green fluorescence). Thus, the intact and injured cells could be distinguished, and the cell populations will be counted according to the different fluorescence by the flow cytometry (BD Biosciences, CA) (JC-1 green: Ex/Em = 485/525 nm; JC-1 red: Ex/Em =535/590 nm).

Similarly, the fluorescence intensity of JC-1 as the index of $\Delta\Psi m$ alterations could be detected by a confocal microscope (Carl Zeiss AG, Oberkochen, Germany), and the ratio of red/green fluorescence intensity is indicated as the alterations of mitochondrial $\Delta\Psi m$.

For quantification of mitochondrial mass, we used Mitotracker Green probe (Molecular Probes), which preferentially accumulates in mitochondria regardless of the mitochondrial membrane potential and provides an accurate assessment of mitochondrial mass. Firstly, the cells were washed with PBS and incubated at 37 °C for 30 min with 100 nM MitoTracker Green FM (Molecular Probes) and then harvested using trypsin/EDTA and re-suspended in PBS. Fluorescence intensity was detected with excitation and emission wavelengths of 490 and 516 nm, respectively, and values were corrected for total protein (mg/ml).

Determination of the activities of mitochondrial respiratory chain complexes
According to manufacturer's instructions, mitochondrial isolation was performed at 4 °C using a Kit for cultured mammal cell (Thermo Scientific Rockford. USA).

The activities of mitochondrial respiratory chain complexes were analyzed by spectrophotometer (Secomam, Domont,France) as described before [13]. Briefly, complex I (NADH dehydrogenase, EC 1.6.5.3) enzyme activity was measured as a decline in absorbance from NADH oxidation by decylubiquinone before and after adding rotenone (St. Louis, MO, USA). Complex II (succinate dehydrogenase, EC 1.3.5.1) activity was

Herbal formula Xinshuitong capsule exerts its cardioprotective effects via mitochondria...

3

determined as a function of the decrease in absorbance from 2, 6-dichloroindophenol reduction. Complex III (ubiquinone cytochrome c oxidoreductase, EC 1.10.2.2) activity was calculated as a function of increase in absorbance from cytochrome c reduction. And complex IV (cytochrome c oxidoreductase, EC 1.9.3.1) activity was measured as a function of the decrease in absorbance from cytochrome c oxidation. Mitochondrial complexes activities were normalized to whole mitochondrial protein content and expressed as arbitrary units.

Determination of mitochondrial total ATPase activity

Cell mitochondria and submitochondrial particles were prepared as described before [14]. Briefly, the mitochondrial particles were incubated at 37 °C for 60 min in a 0.5 ml medium containing 2 mmol/l ATP, 100 mmol/l NaCl, 20 mmol/l KCL, 5 mmol/l MgCl$_2$, 1 mmol/l EDTA in 50 mmol/l Tris–HCl (pH = 7.0). The tubes were chilled immediately and centrifuged at 200×g for 10 min. Inorganic phosphate liberated in the supernatant was calculated as an indication of ATPase activity according to Fiske and Subbarow [15]. Protein determination was carried out in accordance with Lowry [16] with crystalline bovine serum albumin as a standard.

Determination of mitochondrial ROS

As described before [13], mitochondrial ROS production was determined using Amplex Red (Molecular Probes, Eugene, OR, USA). Briefly, superoxide dismutase (SOD) was added at 40 units/ml to convert all superoxide into H$_2$O$_2$. Resorufin formation (Amplex Red oxidation by H$_2$O$_2$) was detected at an excitation/emission wavelength of 545/590 nm using a spectrophotometer (Secomam, Domont, France). Readings of resorufin formation were recorded every 5 min for 30 min, and a slope (i.e., rate of formation) was produced. The slope obtained was converted into the rate of H$_2$O$_2$ production with a standard curve. The assay was done at 37 °C in 96-well plates using succinate. The data was converted to nmol/mg protein/minute.

Quantitative assessment of apoptosis cells by flow cytometry

As described before [17], Annexin V-APC/7-AAD Apoptosis Detection Kits (Becton-Dickinson Biosciences) were used to detect apoptosis cells. The cells stained with annexinV+/7-AAD- were considered apoptosis cells, and the percentage of apoptosis cells was determined by flow cytometry.

Statistical analysis

Software of SPSS Version 19.0 was used for statistical analysis. Numerical data are expressed as means ± SD. The significance of differences was examined using the ANOVA method. Results with $P<0.05$ were considered to be significant.

Results

XST increased the viability of hypoxia-reoxygenated HCM

As shown in Fig. 1, the cell viability in the XST-treated 200, 400 and 600 μg/ml group were 77, 81 and 84%,

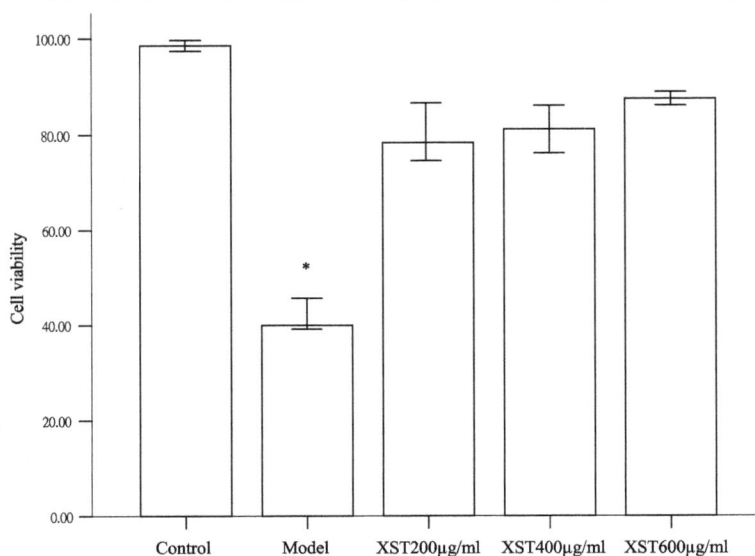

Fig. 1 Bar graphs showed the cell viability in the three XST-treated groups were significantly increased compared with the model group. No difference was found between the XST-treated groups or the XST-treated groups compared to the control group. All samples were checked in three independent experiments with three replicates each. Data are represented as the mean ± SD (*$P<0.05$ vs. each of the three XST-treated groups or the control group)

respectively, which showed a significant difference than the model group (42.20%, $P < 0.05$). However, the cell viability exhibited no difference between the three dosages of XST ($P > 0.05$). Under the light microscope, cells in the three XST-treated groups and the control group grew similarly well, and the cells were like in size and shape. By contrast, most of the cells in the model group showed swelling and was out of the regular shape and size (figures not shown). The data indicated that XST could protect the cells against hypoxia-induced injury.

XST dose-dependently increased the number of polarized cells

JC-1 is capable of entering selectively into mitochondria, and the color of the dye changes reversibly from green to orange as the mitochondrial membrane becomes more polarized. Based upon the specific fluorescent characteristics, the cells could be classified into two groups of cells by the flow cytometer, and the two kinds of fluorescence were indicated as the two populations of cells. Quantitative assessment was reflected by the dot plots as indicated in Fig. 2 The ratio of red/green fluorescence, as

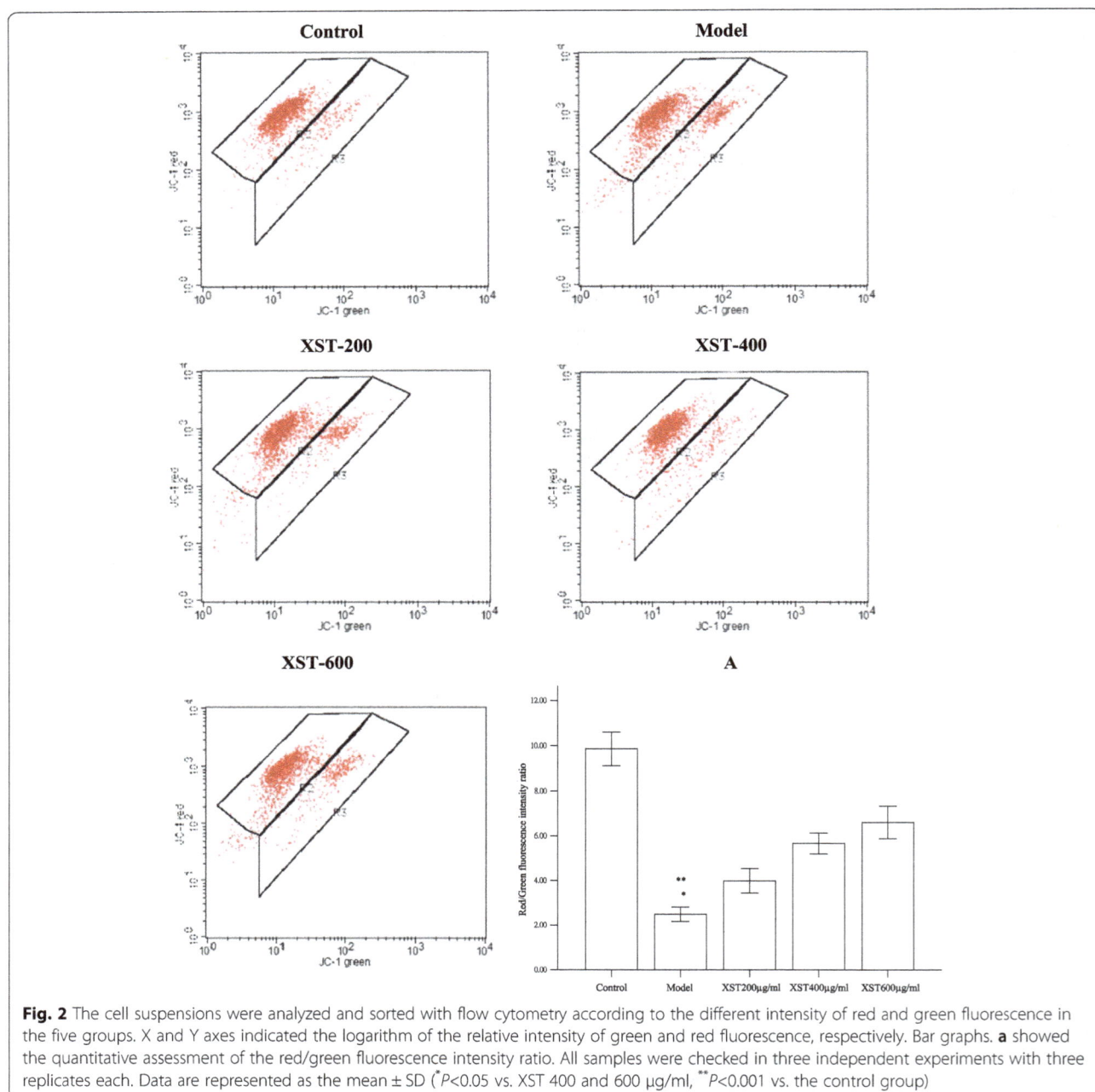

Fig. 2 The cell suspensions were analyzed and sorted with flow cytometry according to the different intensity of red and green fluorescence in the five groups. X and Y axes indicated the logarithm of the relative intensity of green and red fluorescence, respectively. Bar graphs. **a** showed the quantitative assessment of the red/green fluorescence intensity ratio. All samples were checked in three independent experiments with three replicates each. Data are represented as the mean ± SD (*$P<0.05$ vs. XST 400 and 600 µg/ml, **$P<0.001$ vs. the control group)

the index of cell populations, showed a dose-dependent increase in the three XST-treated groups. A significant difference was noted at XST400 and XST600ug/ml compared to the model group ($P < 0.05$), suggesting that XST could increase the polarized cell populations (Fig. 2a).

XST dose dependently restored the loss of ΔΨm and mitochondrial mass induced by hypoxia

The intensity of red fluorescence of JC-1 aggregates detected by confocal laser scanning microscopy decreased in the model group, however, XST could dose dependently increase the fluorescence, indicating that the drug could restore the loss of Δψm induced by hypoxia as showed in Fig. 3. Further, the red/green fluorescence ratio in XST-treated 200, 400 and 600μg/ml groups was 55, 81 and 85%, respectively, a significant difference was found in the XST-treated groups compared to the model group (18%). However, no difference was found between XST400, XST600 ug/ml and the control ($P > 0.05$) as indicated by the bar graph Fig. 3a.

Further, an accurate assessment of mitochondrial mass was conducted, showing the green fluorescence increased in the XST-treated groups (Fig. 4). A significant elevation was noted in XST-400 and 600μg/ml groups compared to that in the model group, suggesting the drug prevented the loss of mitochondria in the hypoxia cells. The data was in line with the status of mitochondrial Δψm detected in above experiments. Additionally, morphological observations showed the cells in the XST-treated groups were more uniform in shape and size compared to those in the model group.

XST restored the mitochondrial electron transport chain complexes activities

The activities of mitochondria complexes I, II, III, and IV were assessed by spectrophotometric methods. As showed in Fig. 5, the activities of complexes I- IV were reduced in varying degrees in the model group. XST could dose dependently restore the activities of complexes I, II and III, but the activity of complex IV showed no difference among XST 200, 400 and 600 μg/ml groups. Complexes I-IV activities were significantly elevated in XST 200 and 400 μg/ml groups than those in the model group ($P < 0.05$); in the XST 600 μg/ml group, the activities of complexes I-IV restored nearly to the normal levels. The data indicated that the drug could dose dependently restore the activities of the mitochondrial electron transport chain complexes I-IV.

XST increased mitochondrial total ATPase activity in the hypoxia-reoxygenated HCM

Mitochondrial total ATPase activity was determined by estimating the amount of ATP hydrolyzed in terms of inorganic phosphorus (Pi) liberated in the cell supernatant. As shown in Fig. 6, the ATPase activity in the model group

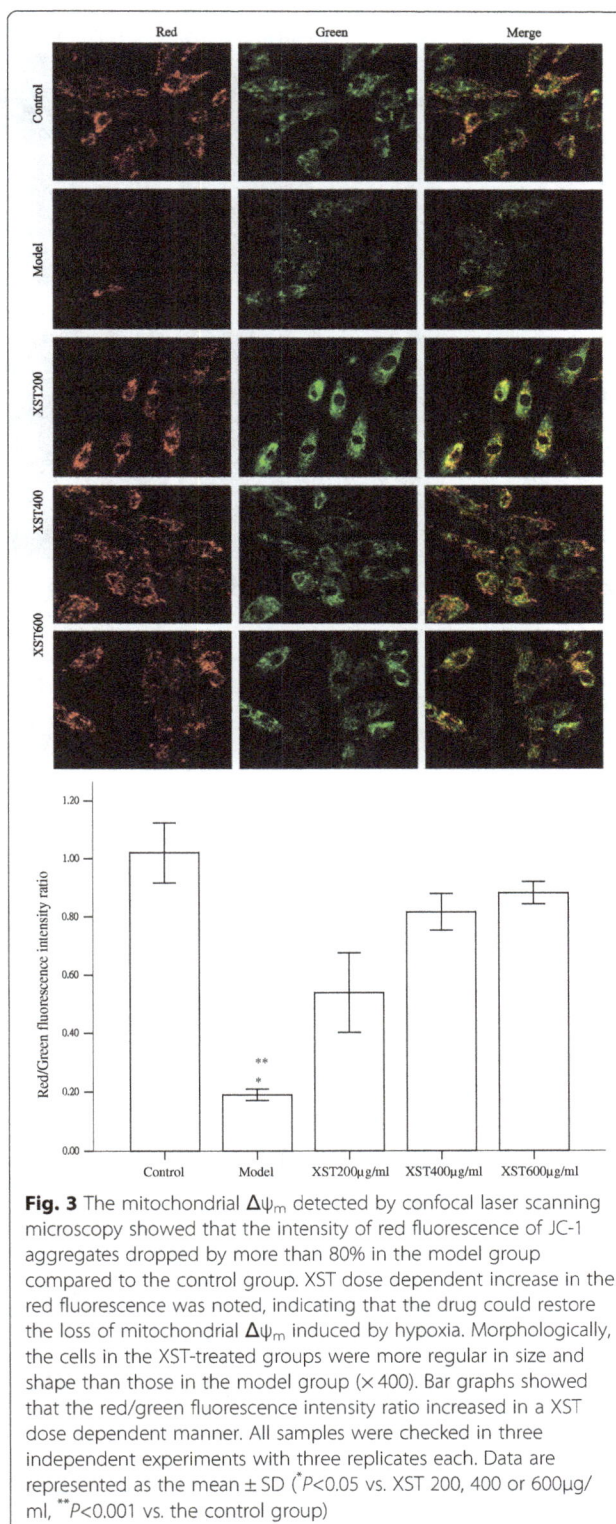

Fig. 3 The mitochondrial Δψ$_m$ detected by confocal laser scanning microscopy showed that the intensity of red fluorescence of JC-1 aggregates dropped by more than 80% in the model group compared to the control group. XST dose dependent increase in the red fluorescence was noted, indicating that the drug could restore the loss of mitochondrial Δψ$_m$ induced by hypoxia. Morphologically, the cells in the XST-treated groups were more regular in size and shape than those in the model group (× 400). Bar graphs showed that the red/green fluorescence intensity ratio increased in a XST dose dependent manner. All samples were checked in three independent experiments with three replicates each. Data are represented as the mean ± SD ($^*P<0.05$ vs. XST 200, 400 or 600μg/ml, $^{**}P<0.001$ vs. the control group)

decreased about 70% compared to the control ($P < 0.05$), however, the activity increased about 40, 52 and 60% in the XST-treated 200, 400 and 600 μg/ml groups compared to

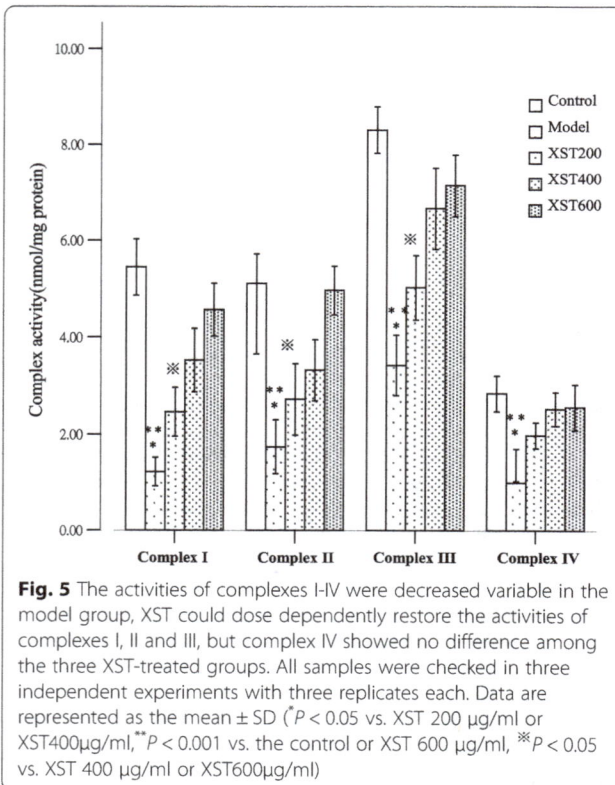

Fig. 4 Mitochondrial content (using MitoTracker Green) was detected in the five groups, showing the green fluorescence increased in a XST dose dependent manner. Quantitative assessment showed that XST-treated groups were significantly greater than that in the control (bar graphs (**a**). All samples were checked in three independent experiments with three replicates each. Data are represented as the mean ± SD ($^{*}P$<0.05 vs. XST 400 and 600 µg/ml, $^{**}P$<0.001 vs. the control group)

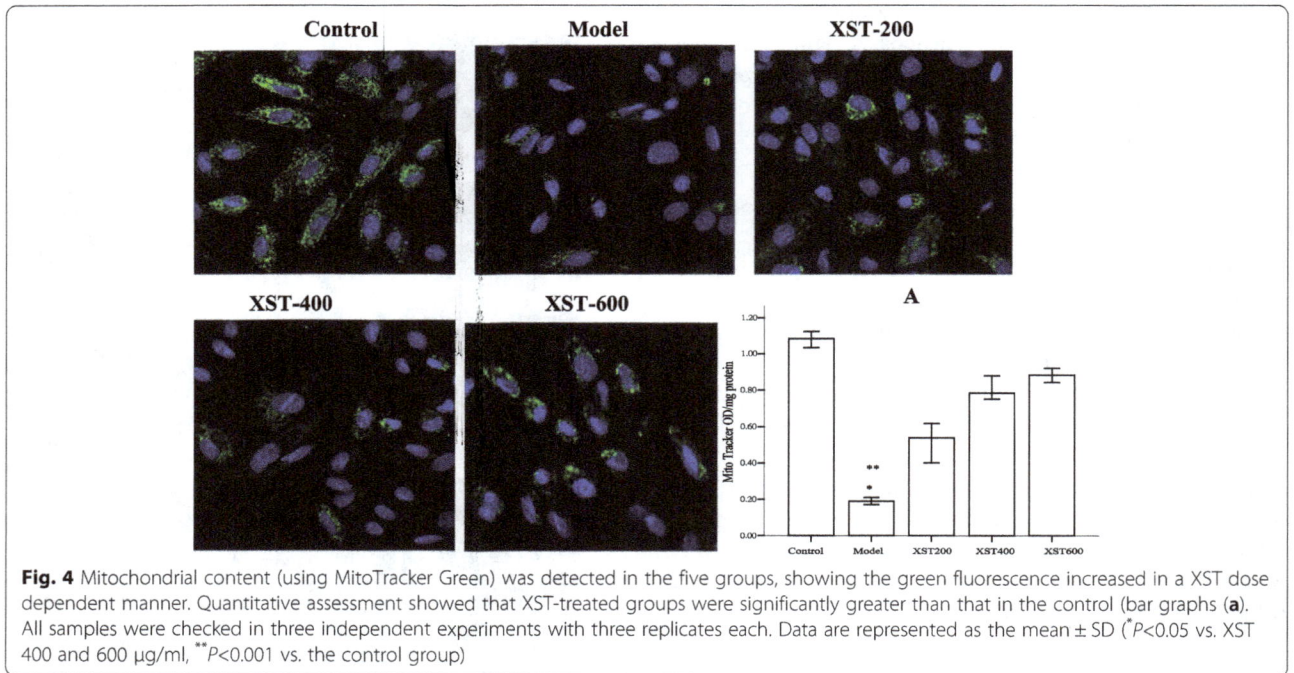

Fig. 5 The activities of complexes I-IV were decreased variable in the model group, XST could dose dependently restore the activities of complexes I, II and III, but complex IV showed no difference among the three XST-treated groups. All samples were checked in three independent experiments with three replicates each. Data are represented as the mean ± SD ($^{*}P$ < 0.05 vs. XST 200 µg/ml or XST400µg/ml,$^{**}P$ < 0.001 vs. the control or XST 600 µg/ml, $^{※}P$ < 0.05 vs. XST 400 µg/ml or XST600µg/ml)

the model group (P < 0.05), which indicated that XST dose dependently increased the mitochondrial ATPase activity induced by hypoxia. The XST-induced elevation of ATPase activity was correlated with the increase in mitochondrial $\Delta\psi$m and the activities of mitochondrial complexes I-IV in the XST-treated groups (Figs. 3 and 5).

XST decreasedmitochondrial ROS production in the hypoxia-reoxygenated HCM

As shown in Fig. 7, the mitochondrial ROS in the model group was about three times higher than that in the control group (P<0.05), however, all the three XST-treated groups exhibited a significant decrease in ROS levels compared to the model group (P<0.05), no difference was noted between the three dosages of XST-treated groups (P > 0.05). Previous studies reported that the increase in mitochondrial $\Delta\psi$m and ATPase activity led to the decrease in mitochondrial ROS production [18]. Here, we confirmed that the XST-induced increase in $\Delta\psi$m and ATPase activity was coupled with a decrease in ROS. The data suggested that the three dosages of XST had the similar inhibitory effects on the production of mitochondrial ROS in hypoxia-reoxygenated HCM.

XST decreased the apoptosis cells in the hypoxia-reoxygenated HCM

As detected by flow cytometry, apoptosis cells, which stained with annexinV+/7-AAD-, were significantly increased in the model group than those in the control group (P < 0.05) (Fig. 8). XST treatment could significantly decrease the apoptosis cells; however, no

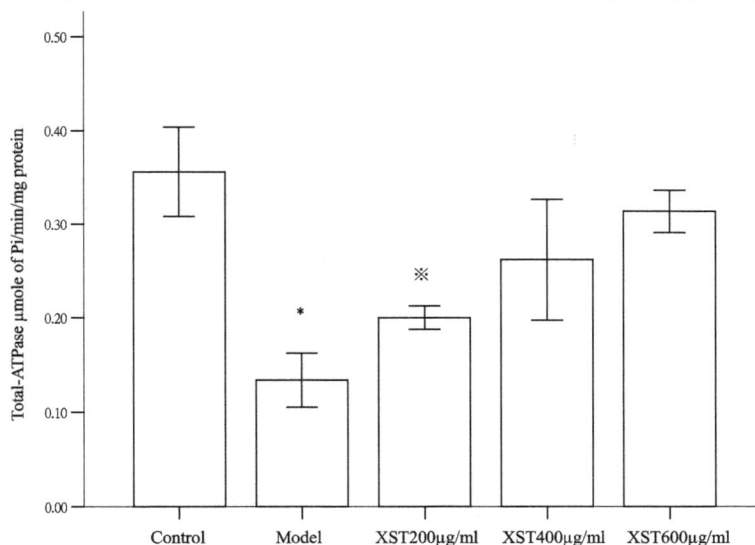

Fig. 6 Mitochondrial ATPase activity in cardiomyocytes was determined by estimating the amount of ATP hydrolysis in terms of inorganic phosphorus (Pi) liberated in the cell supernatant. A significant decrease was found in the model group compared to that in the control. Three XST-treated groups exhibited a dose-dependent increase in the activity as showed in bar graphs. All samples were checked in three independent experiments with three replicates each. Data are represented as the mean ± SD (*$P < 0.05$ vs.XST 400 and 600 μg/ml, ※$P < 0.05$ vs. 600 μg/ml)

difference was noted between the three XST-treated groups ($P > 0.05$). The quantitative assessment of the apoptosis cells was indicated by bar graphs Fig. 8a.

Discussion

Mitochondria, as the dominant source of heart ATP, represent approximately one-third of the mass of the heart and play a critical role in maintaining cellular function. The mitochondrion is very susceptible to damage mediated by ischemia or ischemia/reperfusion. The damaged mitochondria cause a depletion in ATP and a release of cytochrome c, which leads to activation of caspases and onset of apoptosis [19–21]. As such, maintaining mitochondrial homeostasis is critical to cell survival.

Current experiments showed that XST could maintain the activities of mitochondrial electron transport chain

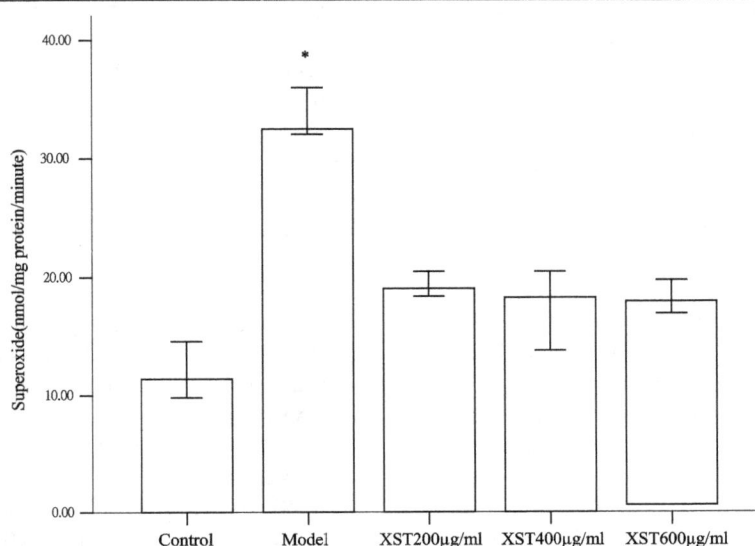

Fig. 7 Mitochondrial ROS in the model group showed significantly higher than that in the control group, however, ROS levels exhibited a significant decrease in the XST-treated groups compared to those in the model group. No difference was noted between the three XST-treated groups. All samples were tested in three independent experiments with three replicates each. Data are represented as the mean ± SD. (*$P<0.05$ vs. each XST-treated group or the control group)

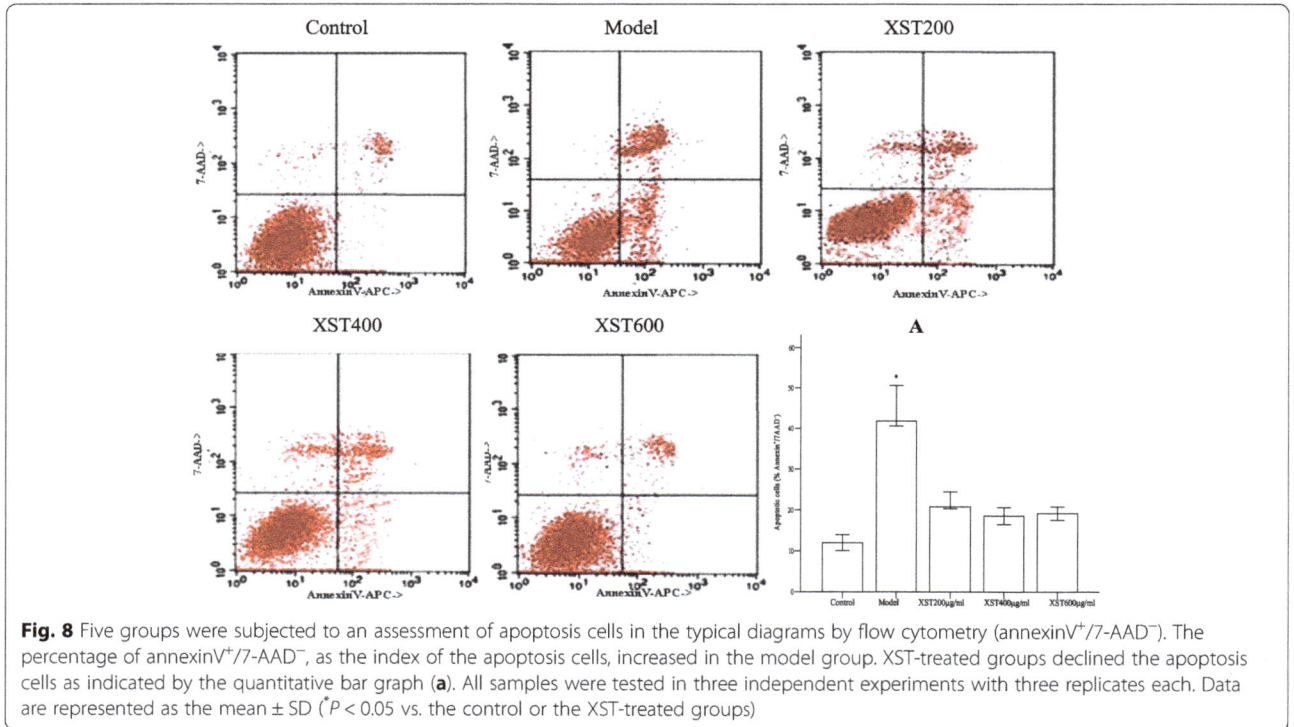

Fig. 8 Five groups were subjected to an assessment of apoptosis cells in the typical diagrams by flow cytometry (annexinV$^+$/7-AAD$^-$). The percentage of annexinV$^+$/7-AAD$^-$, as the index of the apoptosis cells, increased in the model group. XST-treated groups declined the apoptosis cells as indicated by the quantitative bar graph (**a**). All samples were tested in three independent experiments with three replicates each. Data are represented as the mean ± SD ($^*P < 0.05$ vs. the control or the XST-treated groups)

complexes I-IV, and restore the mitochondrial $\Delta\psi$m and mitochondria mass induced by oxidative stress in the cardiomyocytes. Further, the drug could activate mitochondrial total ATPase to supply cells energy to raise the cell viability in the anoxic conditions. On the other hand, XST could suppress the mitochondrial ROS generation and attenuate the ROS-induced damage to the cells, which may partly account for this drug's inhibition of apoptosis and the increase in cell viability. The current data suggested that XST exerted its cardioprotective effects via maintaining the integrity of mitochondria in the hypoxia-reoxygenated HCM.

Our previous clinical study showed that the CHF patients treated with XST (0.3 g each capsule, three capsules each time, tid.) showed significant improvement in LVEF, NYHA classes, as well as the symptoms (dyspnea, edema and etc.) and the patients' quality of life [22]. Further, in vitro experiments verified that dosages 200-600 μg/ml had the optimal cell protective effects in the oxidative stress conditions [11]. Based on the previous data, we used these dosages in the current study, which confirmed that XST could restore the $\Delta\Psi$m and mitochondria mass to elevate the polarized cell populations. Treated at XST600μg/ml, the activities of respiratory chain complexes I-IV regained their activities nearly to the normal levels, and the total of mitochondrial ATPase activity was raised by XST. On the other hand, XST suppressed the generation of mitochondrial ROS and

cell apoptosis. The data may partly shed a light on the drug's therapeutic effects on the CHF patients.

Previous studies showed that an elevated $\Delta\Psi$m was associated with the enhanced mitochondrial ROS formation [18, 23], and a slight decrease in $\Delta\Psi$m could prevent ROS formation without seriously compromising cellular energetics [18, 24, 25]. However, in the isolated energized cardiac mitochondria, which were induced by hypoxia, caused the inhibition of the activity of the electron transport chain, and this mild decrease in $\Delta\Psi$m led to ROS formation during reoxygenation [26]. The collapse of mitochondrial $\Delta\Psi$m, regarded as an index of mitochondrial inner integrity, would go hand in hand with the dysfunctions of the mitochondrial respiratory chain and a decline of ATPase activity, which led to the elevation of mitochondrial ROS formation and cell apoptosis. The phenomena were supported in the current experiments as showed in Figs. 3, 5 and 7. XST treatment could restore the loss of $\Delta\Psi$m and repaired the dysfunctions of the mitochondrial respiratory chain. Additionally, XST could activate ATPase and suppress ROS formation, resulted in the decline in apoptosis cells in the hypoxia-reoxygenated HCM. These data suggested that XST possibly exerted its cardioprotective effects partly through mitochondria. Mitochondrial respiratory chain, especially, complex I, III and III, were seen as the prime source of ROS [27–30]. ROS generations are decreased when the available electrons are limited and potential energy for the transfer is low [30].

Recent study found that when the electron transport chain functions of complexes I, III and III are at the sub optimal level, the rate of mitochondrial free radical production is inversely increasing proportional to the rate of electron transport [31], suggesting that the elevated ROS levels found under these conditions may originate extra-mitochondrially or are attributed to the defective antioxidant defense. Our experiments showed that XST-induced elevation of mitochondrial respiratory chain complexes activities was inversely correlated with the levels of mitochondria-derived ROS in the XST-treated groups (Figs. 5 and 7). Possibly, the drug suppressed ROS generation extra-mitochondrially, or through the antioxidant defense or other mechanisms. For example, other powerful sources of mitochondrial ROS production are represented by the mitochondrial NO synthase [32, 33], and the byproducts of several cellular enzymes including NADPH oxidases, xanthine oxidase [22, 23, 34]. Nevertheless, further studies should be taken to investigate the XST's specific mechanisms on inhibition of ROS generation.

Impaired $\Delta\Psi m$, a sign of the early stage of cell apoptosis [35], occurred before nucleus apoptosis characteristics (chromatin condensed and DNA rupture). Once the mitochondrial transmembrane potential collapse, apoptosis procedure is irreversible [36]. In this experiment, we confirmed that the decreased $\Delta\Psi m$ was associated with the increase in the apoptosis cells (Figs. 5 and 6). XST, via elevation of $\Delta\Psi m$ and inhibition of mitochondrial ROS generation, exerted its anti-apoptotic effects in the hypoxia-reoxygenated HCM. Conclusively, the drug, via ensuring the integrity of the mitochondrial membrane, exerted its cardioprotective effects in the hypoxia-reoxygenated HCM.

Abbreviations
CHF: Chronic heart failure; ETC: Mitochondrial electron transport chain; HCM: Primary human cardiomyocyte; LVEF: Left ventricular ejection fraction; MPTP: Mitochondrial permeability transition pore; MTT: 3-[4,5-dimethylthiazol-2-yl]-diphenyl-tetrazolium bromide; NYHA: New York Heart Association; PBS: Phosphate-buffered saline; Pi: Inorganic phosphorus; ROS: Reactive oxygen species; SOD: Superoxide dismutase; XST: Xinshuitong Capsule; $\Delta\Psi m$: Mitochondrial membrane potential

Acknowledgments
Thanks for the Molecular Biology Centre Laboratory of Fujian Academy of Integrative Medicine, Fujian Key Laboratory of Integrative Medicine on Geriatrics for the experiments.

Funding
This study is supported by the projects from Fujian Natural Science Foundation of China (No. 2013 J01334) Fujian Natural Science Foundation of Chinese-foreign cooperation Key Projects (No.2014I0012), Fujian Province Health and Family Planning Council (No.wzzy201313),Fujian University of TCM Supported Project (No.X2014137) and Fujian province health and family planning commission Foundation(No. 2017-CX-39).

Authors' contributions
CT Data collection and writing the paper, JZ and YW Drug quality inspection, JZH Cell experiments Cell viability assay, $\Delta\Psi m$ detection, mitochondrial respiratory chain complexes, total ATPase activity, mitochondrial ROS, apoptosis cells, WC Study design and experimental director, All authors have read and approved the final manuscript to submitted to this journal.

Competing interests
The authors declare that they have no competing interests.

References
1. Weiss JN, Korge P, Honda HM, Ping P. Role of the mitochondrial permeability transition in myocardial disease. Circ Res. 2003;93:292–301.
2. Crompton M. The mitochondrial permeability transition pore and its role in cell death. Biochem J. 1999;341:233–49.
3. Duchen MR, McGuinness O, Brown LA, Crompton M. On the involvement of a cyclosporin a sensitive mitochondrial pore in types are beyond the experimental reach of this study. A myocardial reperfusion injuryCardiovasc Res. 1993;27:1790–4.
4. Davies KJ. Oxidative stress: the paradox of aerobic life. Biochem Soc Symp. 1995;61:1–31.
5. Ide T, Tsutsui H, Kinugawa S, Utsumi H, Kang D, Hattori N, Uchida K, Arimura KI, Egashira K, Takeshita A. Mitochondrial electron transport complex I is a potential source of oxygen free radicals in the failing myocardium. Circ Res. 1999;85:357–63.
6. Giordano FJ. Oxygen, oxidative stress, hypoxia, and heart failure. J Clin Invest. 2005;115:500–8.
7. Kwon SH, Pimentel DR, Remondino A, Sawyer DB, Colucci WS. H_2O_2 regulates regulates cardiac myocyte phenotype via concentration dependent activation of distinct kinase pathways. J Mol Cell Cardiol. 2003;35:615–21.
8. Li JM, Gall NP, Grieve DJ, Chen M, Shah AM. Activation of NADPH oxidase during progression of cardiac hypertrophy to failure. Hypertension. 2002;40:477–84.
9. Li PC, Yang YC, Hwang GY, Kao LS, Lin CY. Inhibition of reverse-mode sodium-calcium exchanger activity and apoptosis by Levosimendan in human cardiomyocyte progenitor cell-derived cardiomyocytes after anoxia and reoxygenation. PLoS One. 2014;9:e85909.
10. Tan CJ, Chen WL, Lin JM, Lin RH, Tan LF. Clinical research of Xinshuitong capsule on chronic heart failure in patients with diuretic resistance. Chin Arch Tradit Chin Med. 2011;29:837–9.
11. Tan CJ, Wu YB, Chen WL, Lin RH. Xinshuitong capsule ameliorates hypertrophy of cardiomyocytes via aquaporin pathway in the ischemia-reperfusion rat hearts. Int J Cardiol. 2011;152:S54.
12. Xu L, Deng Y, Feng L, Li D, Chen X, Ma C, Liu X, Yin J, Yang M, Teng F, Wu W, Guan S, Jiang B, Guo D. Cardio-protection of salvianolic acid B through inhibition of apoptosis network. PLoS One. 2011;6:e24036.
13. Kavazis AN, Talbert EE, Smuder AJ, Hudson MB, Nelson WB, Powers SK. Mechanical ventilation induces diaphragmatic mitochondrial dysfunction and increased oxidant production. Free Radic Biol Med. 2009;46:842–50.
14. Alexander T. Assembly of the mitochondrial membrane system. I. Characterization of some enzymes of the inner membrane of yeast mitochondria. J Biol Chem. 1969;244:5020–6.
15. Fiske CH, Subbarow Y. The colorimetric determination of phosphorus. J Biol Chem. 1925;66:375–400.
16. Lowry OH, Rosebrough NJ, Farr AL, Randall RJ. Protein measurement with the folin phenol reagent. J Biol Chem. 1951;193:265–75.
17. Almeida A, Moncada S, Bolaños JP. Nitric oxide switches on glycolysis through the AMP protein kinase and 6-phosphofructo-2-kinase pathway. Nat Cell Biol. 2004;6:45–51.
18. Korshunov SS, Skulachev VP, Starkov AA. High protonic potential actuates a mechanism of production of reactive oxygen species in mitochondria. FEBS Lett. 1997;416:15–8.
19. Aluri HS, Simpson DC, Allegood JC, Hu Y, Szczepanek K, Gronert S, Chen Q, Lesnefsky EJ. Electron flow into cytochrome c coupled with reactive oxygen species from the electron transport chain converts cytochrome c to a cardiolipin peroxidase: role during ischemia-reperfusion. Biochim Biophys Acta. 2014;1840:9–18.
20. Lesnefsky EJ, Moghaddas S, Tandler B, Kerner J, Hoppel CL. Mitochondrial

dys-function in cardiac disease: ischemia–reperfusion,aging,and heart failure. J Mol Cell Cardiol. 2001;33:1065–89.

21. Chen Q, Moghaddas S, Hoppel CL, Lesnefsky EJ. Reversible blockade of electron transport during ischemia protects mitochondria and decreases myocardial injury following reperfusion. J Pharmaco Exp Ther. 2006;319:1405–12.

22. Liu Y, Fiskum G, Schubert D. Generation of reactive oxygen species by the mitochondrial electron transport chain. J Neurochemistry. 2002;80:780–7.

23. Skulachev VP. Uncoupling: new approaches to an old problem of bioenergetics. Biochim Biophys Acta. 1998;1363:100–24.

24. Brand MD, Buckingham JA, Esteves TC, Green K, Lambert AJ, Miwa S, Murphy MP, Pakay JL, Talbot DA, Echtay KS. Mitochondrial superoxide and aging: uncoupling-protein activity and superoxide production. Biochem Soc Symp. 2004;71:203–13.

25. Brookes PS. Mitochondrial H(+) leak and ROS generation: an odd couple. Free Radic Biol Med. 2005;38:12–23.

26. Korge P, Ping P, Weiss JN. Reactive oxygen species production in energized cardiac mitochondria during hypoxia/reoxygenation: modulation by nitric oxide. Circ Res. 2008;103:873–80.

27. Petrosillo G, Ruggiero F, Di Venosa N, Paradies G. Decreased complex III activity in mitochondria isolated from rat heart subjected to ischemia and reperfusion: role of reactive oxygen species and cardiolipin. FASEB J. 2003;17:714–6.

28. Zhang J, Piantadosi CA. Mitochondrial oxidative stress after carbon monoxide hypoxia in the rat brain. J Clin Invest. 1992;90:1193–9.

29. Rustin P, Chretien D, Bourgeron T, Gerard B, Rotig A, Saudubray JM, Munnich A. Biochemical and molecular investigations in respiratory chain deficiencies. Clin Chim Acta. 1994;228:35–51.

30. Cadenas E, Davies KJ. Mitochondrial free radical generation, oxidative stress, and aging. Free Radic Biol Med. 2000;29:222–30.

31. Vinogradov AD, Grivennikova VG. Generation of superoxide-radical by the NADH: ubiquinone oxidoreductase of heart mitochondria. Biochemistry. 2005;70:120–7.

32. Poderoso JJ, Carreras MC, Lisdero C, Riobó N, Schöpfer F, Boveris A. Nitric oxide inhibits electron transfer and increases superoxide radical production in rat heart mitochondria and submitochondrial particles. Arch Biochem Biophys. 1996;328:85–92.

33. Dröge W. Free radicals in the physiological control of cell function. Physiol Rev. 2002;82:47–95.

34. Turrens JF. Mitochondrial formation of reactive oxygen species. J Physiol. 2003;552:335–44.

35. Mathur A, Hong Y, Kemp BK. Evaluation of fluorescent dyes for the detection of mitochondrial membrane potential changes in cultured cardiomyocytes. Cardiovasc Res. 2000;46:126–38.

36. Suh DH, Kim MK, Kim HS. Mitochondrial permeability transition pore as a selective target for anti-cancer therapy. Front Oncol. 2013;3:41.

2

Inhibitory effects of *Euphorbia supina* on *Propionibacterium acnes*-induced skin inflammation in vitro and in vivo

Hyeon-Ji Lim[1†], Yong-Deok Jeon[1†] 🔾, Sa-Haeng Kang[2], Min-Kyoung Shin[1], Ki-Min Lee[1], Se-Eun Jung[1], Ji-Yun Cha[2], Hoon-Yoen Lee[2], Bo-Ram Kim[2], Sung-Woo Hwang[2], Jong-Hyun Lee[3], Takashi Sugita[4], Otomi Cho[4], Hyun Myung[5], Jong-Sik Jin[1*] and Young-Mi Lee[2*]

Abstract

Background: *Euphorbia supina* (ES) plant has been used as treatment for inflammatory conditions. The antibacterial effect and the anti-inflammatory mechanism of ES for *Propionibacterium* (*P.*) *acnes*-induced inflammation in THP-1 cells and acne animal model remain unclear. Therefore, the objective of the present study was to determine the antibacterial and anti-inflammatory activities of ES against *P. acnes*, the etiologic agent of skin inflammation.

Method: The antibacterial activities of ES were tested with disc diffusion and broth dilution methods. Cytotoxicity of ES at different doses was evaluated by the MTT assay. THP-1 cells were stimulated by heat-killed *P. acnes* in the presence of ES. The pro-inflammatory cytokines and mRNA levels were measured by ELISA and real-time-PCR. MAPK expression was analyzed by Western blot. The living *P. acnes* was intradermally injected into the ear of BLBC/c mice. Subsequently, chemical composition of ES was analyzed by liquids chromatography-mass spectrometry (LC-MS).

Result: ES had stronger antibacterial activity against *P. acnes* and inhibitory activity on lipase. ES had no significant cytotoxicity on THP-1 cells. ES suppressed the mRNA levels and production of IL-8, TNF-a, IL-1β in vitro. ES inhibited the expression levels of pro-inflammatory cytokines and the MAPK signaling pathway. Ear thickness and inflammatory cells were markedly reduced by ES treatment. Protocatechuic acid, gallic acid, quercetin, and kaempferol were detected by LC-MS analysis in ES.

Conclusions: Our results demonstrate antibacterial and anti-inflammatory activities of ES extract against *P. acnes*. It is suggested that ES extract might be used to treatment anti-inflammatory skin disease.

Background

Acne, one of the most common skin diseases, affects more than 80% of all adolescents [1]. Acne is an inflammatory disorder of the pilosebaceous unit characterized by excessive sebum production, follicular hyperkeratinization, and colonization of *Propionibacterium* (*P.*) *acnes* [2], a Gram-positive anaerobic bacterium. It has been reported that *P. acnes* is a major factor in acne inflammatory reaction by

activating toll-like receptors TLR2 and TLR4 [3]. During acne inflammatory reaction, *P. acnes* induces the production of pro-inflammatory cytokines such as interleukin (IL)-1β, IL-6, IL-8, and tumor necrosis factor (TNF)-α in monocytes and keratinocytes [4, 5]. IL-8, a CXC chemokine, is a strong proinflammatory chemotactic factor for lymphocytes, basophils, and neutrophils. It is increased in keratinocytes by *P. acnes* stimulation [6]. Therefore, suppression of *P. acnes*-induced inflammatory cytokine is one of the major targets for treating acne inflammation.

Euphorbia supina (ES) plant has been used for traditional formulations of herbal medications. It has various pharmacological effects, including anti-oxidant, anti-arthritic, detoxification, diuretic, and hemostatic effects in various cell types [7]. ES contains a number of biologically organic

---

* Correspondence: jongsik.jin@jbnu.ac.kr; ymlee@wku.ac.kr
†Hyeon-Ji Lim and Yong-Deok Jeon contributed equally to this work.
[1]Department of Oriental Medicine Resources, Chonbuk National University, 79 Gobongro, Iksan, Jeollabuk-do 54596, South Korea
[2]Department of Oriental Pharmacy, College of Pharmacy, Wonkwang-Oriental Medicine Research Institute, Wonkwang University, Iksan, Jeollabuk-do 54538, South Korea
Full list of author information is available at the end of the article

substances including tannins, terpenoids, and polyphenols [8]. Recent studies have shown that ES possesses antibacterial activity against *Staphylococcus aureus* [9]. It can also inhibit cancer cell proliferation of U937 human leukemic cells [10]. However, the antibacterial effect and anti-inflammatory mechanism of ES in *P. acnes*-induced inflammation in vitro and in vivo remain unclear. Therefore, the objective of this study was to determine the antibacterial and anti-inflammatory effects of ES in an in vitro model using heat-killed *P. acnes* and living *P. acnes*-induced acne skin disease model.

Methods

ES preparation

The dried ES was purchased from Wonkwang PHARMACEUTICAL CORPORATION (Iksan, Korea). ES was washed twice with distilled water followed by drying, then extracted with 70% ethanol at room temperature for 3 days. The extract was concentrated with a vacuum evaporator and stored at 4 °C before experiments. The yield of ES extract was 6.14%. A voucher specimen (JUHES-1660) has been deposited at Department of Oriental Medicine Resources, Chonbuk National University (Iksan, Korea).

Preparation of *P.acnes*

P. acnes (KCTC 3315, Daejeon, Korea) was obtained from the Korean Collection for Type Culture (KCTC, Daejeon, Korea) and grown under anaerobic condition in 10 ml of GAM (Nissui Pharmaceutical, Japan) liquid medium at 37 °C for OD600 = 1.0 (logarithmic growth phase). A total cell count of 10 ml of *P.acnes* suspension was approximately 1.34×10^9 colony forming unit (CFU). *P. acnes* were harvested by centrifugation at 4000 rpm for 15 min at 4 °C to remove supernatant. Bacterial pellets were washed three times with 10 ml of PBS and finally suspended in 1 ml of PBS. The *P. acnes* suspension was incubated at 80 °C for 30 min for heat-killing reaction. To use cell stimulation heat-killed *P. acnes* suspension was stored at 4 °C until use. To use in vivo experiment living *P. acnes* suspension was stored at – 80 °C until use.

Antibacterial assay

ES was dissolved in dimethyl sulfoxide (DMSO) at different concentrations (100, 200 mg/ml). Each concentration of ES was then impregnated onto a paper disc (8 mm in diameter) and placed on the top of GAM agar plate containing 100 μl of bacterial solution containing *P. acnes*. These plates were incubated at 37 °C for 48 h under anaerobic condition. Tetracycline was employed as a positive control. Minimum inhibitory concentration (MIC) test was performed in sterile 96-well plates using broth dilution method. Briefly, bacteria were cultured to

stationary phase for 48 h at 37 °C. The turbidity and cell numbers were measured 0.418 at 620 nm and 1.64×10^7 CFU, respectively. The cultivated bacteria was added into microplate at 0.5% of total volume (200 μl). ES extract was adjusted to concentrations through serial dilution in culture medium into 0 to 9 mg/ml. After incubating at 37 °C in an anaerobic jar for 48 h, the turbidity was obtained on a microplate ELISA reader as an indicator of bacterial growth.

To test minimum bactericidal concentration (MBC), 1 μl of various concentrations of the ES extract mixed with diluted solution of *P. acnes* for 48 h, 37 °C. And then MBC was performed by sub culturing the MIC dilutions on the sterile GAM agar broth. The lowest concentration of the extract in which bacteria failed to grow (99% no growth) was reported as MBC.

Lipase activity

P.acnes was grown in brain heart infusion (BHI) broth, and 100 μl amounts of cell suspensions (5.0×10^8 cells/mL) in BHI broth with final concentrations of 0.01, 0.1, 1, 10, 100 μg/mL ES were added to wells of 96well plates. The plates were anaerobically incubated at 37 °C for 24 h. Fifty microliter amounts of supernatants were centrifuged and the supernatants mixed with 50 μl of 10 mM 4-methyl umbelliferyl oleate (4-MUO) (Sigma Aldrich, St. Louis, USA) dissolved in 13 mM Tris-HCL, 0.15 M NaCl, and 1.3 mM $CaCl_2$ (pH 8.0). The mixtures were incubated for 30 min at 25 °C under light illumination. Enzymatic reactions were terminated by adding 100 μl of 0.1 M sodium citrate (pH 4.2). The levels of 4-methylumbelliferone released by the lipase were measured using a fluorometric microplate reader (Fluoroskan Ascent™; Thermo Fisher Scientific, MA, USA); the excitation wavelength was 355 nm and the emission wavelength was 460 nm.

Cell viability assay

Human monocyte THP-1 cells were maintained in RPMI 1640 (Gibco, Carlsbad, CA, USA) supplemented with 10% fetal bovine serum (FBS, WELGENE, South Korea) and 1% penicillin (Gibco, USA) at 37 °C in an atmosphere with 5% CO_2.

MTT assay was performed to measure cell viability. Briefly, THP-1 cells (3.0×10^4 cells/well) was incubated with various concentration of ES (0.1–10 μg/ml) for 24 h. MTT solution (500 μg/ml) was then added to each well and incubated at 37 °C for 8 h. Formazan crystal produced by living cell was dissolved in DMSO. The absorbance of each well was measured at wavelength of 540 nm on a microplate ELISA reader.

Enzyme-linked immunosorbent assay (ELISA)

THP-1 cells (3.0×10^5 cells/well) were pre-treated with indicated concentrations of ES (0.1–10 μg/ml) for 1 h followed by stimulation with heat-killed *P. acnes* for 18 h.

The levels of IL-1β, IL-8, and TNF-α in culture media were measured with an ELISA kit (BD Pharmingen, San Diego, CA, USA). The absorbance of the ELISA plate was measured at wavelength of 405 nm using an automated microplate ELISA reader.

RNA isolation and real- time RT PCR

Total cellular RNA was isolated from human monocyte THP-1 cells using easy-BLUE reagent Kit (iNtRON Biotechnology, Seoul, South Korea). Total RNA was used as template for first-strand cDNA synthesis using a Power cDNA Synthesis Kit (iNtRON Biotechnology, Seoul, South Korea) according to the manufacturer's instructions. The transcription levels of genes were determined with a StepOnePlus Real-time PCR System (Applied Biosystems, Foster City, CA, USA). The relative gene expression was calculated using the comparative CT method with StepOne Software v2.1 (Applied Biosystems, Foster City, CA, USA). The expression of β-actin mRNA was used as an endogenous control. We used TNF-Forward primer 5'-TTACGCCTT TGAAGTTAGCAG-3' and TNF-Reverse primer 5'-CGTC CAAATACATCGCAAC-3' for TNF-α, 5'- TCTTTGAAG AAGAGCCCGTCCTC- 3' /5'-GGATCCACACTCTCCA GCTGCA- 3' for IL-1β, and 5'- GAATACTCTATTGC CGATGGT-3'/5'-CGATGGGTTTGCGTTTG-3' primers for β-Actin as an internal control.

Western blot analysis

Stimulated cells were rinsed with ice-cold PBS and lysed using lysis buffer (iNtRon Biotech, Seoul, South Korea) for 1 h. Total cell lysates were centrifuged at 12,000×g at 4 °C for 10 min to obtain supernatants. After bicinchoninic acid (BCA, Sigma) protein quantification assay, the supernatant was mixed with 2× sample buffer, boiled at 95 °C for 5 min, separated by 10% SDS-polyacrylamide gel electrophoresis, and transferred to nitrocellulose membrane (Roche Diagnostics, IL, US). These membranes were blocked with 5% skim milk in PBS-Tween-20 (PBST) for 1 h at room temperature followed by overnight incubation with anti-phospho-JNK, anti-p38, and anti-ERK antibodies at 4 °C. After washing three times with PBST, these membranes were incubated with secondary antibodies for 1 h at room temperature followed by three times of washes with PBST. The protein-antibody complexes were visualized with ECL Western blotting Luminol Reagent (Santa Cruz Biotech, CA, USA). Images were recorded with an LAS-4000 image reader (Fujifilm Life Sciences, Tokyo, Japan).

Experimental animal model

All experimental protocols (CBNU2016–085) were approved by the Committee on the Care of Laboratory Animal Resources, Chonbuk National University and were conducted in accordance with the Guide for the Care and Use of Laboratory Animals. Male BALB/c mice (6 weeks old) were obtained from SAMTAKO (Osan, South Korea). They were individually housed in polycarbonate cages and maintained under constant temperature (25–27 °C) with a 12 h light-dark cycle. They were provided free access to standard diet and tap water. These animals were allowed to acclimate to these conditions for at least 7 days before the experiment.

These mice were randomly divided into 4 different groups (4 mice/group) as follows: B: non-treatment, PA: Live *P. acnes* (1.34×10^9 CFU/ 20 μl PBS) was intradermally injected into the left ear. The right ear was received an equal amount of PBS. PA/ES 1 mg and PA/ES 10 mg with live *P. acnes* were intradermal injected into both the left and right ears. At 24 h after the injection, ES (1 or 10 mg/ml in PBS) was applied to the surface of the right ear skin of each group. At the end of each treatment period, these animals were sacrificed by cervical dislocation and their ears were measured using a micro-caliper (Mitutoyo, Kanagawa, Japan).

Histological analysis

Ear section sample was fixed with 10% formaldehyde, embedded in paraffin wax, routinely processed and sectioned into 4-μm-thick slices. These ear sections were stained with hematoxylin and eosin (H&E) followed by examination with a light microscope to determine the presence of edema and inflammatory cell accumulation.

HPLC-MS

The extract of ES was dissolved in MeOH into 0.1 mg/ml. Gallic acid (Sigma aldrich chemie GmbH, Germany), protocatechuic acid (Hwi analytik GmbH, Germany), quercetin

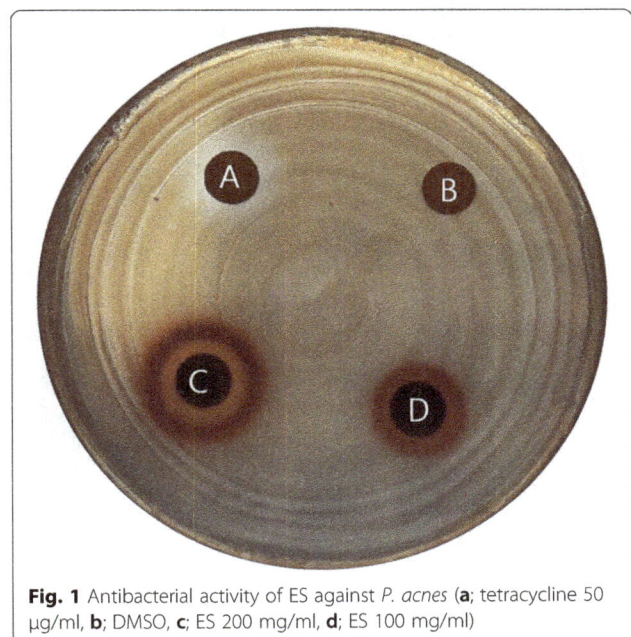

Fig. 1 Antibacterial activity of ES against *P. acnes* (**a**; tetracycline 50 μg/ml, **b**; DMSO, **c**; ES 200 mg/ml, **d**; ES 100 mg/ml)

Table 1 The inhibitory effect of ES on lipase activity. P.acnes (5.0×108 cells/ ml) and 0.01 –.100 µg/ml of ES were added to 96 well plates. 24 h later, 50 µl of supernatants were mixed with 50 µl of 4-MUO. 30 min later, 100 µl of 0.1 M sodium citrate was added. Then lipase.activity was measured using fluorometric microplate reader. Values represent mean ± SD ($n =.4$). Data were analyzed by Tukey post hoc test (*$P < 0.05$ versus P.acnes alone)

		Inhibition (%)	SD
P.acnes (5×108 CFU)	ES 100 µg/ml	59.88	6.52*
P.acnes (5×108 CFU)	ES 10 µg/ml	2.20	5.38
P.acnes (5×108 CFU)	ES 1 µg/ml	5.00	8.38
P.acnes (5×108 CFU)	ES 0.1 µg/ml	0.53	2.34
P.acnes (5×108 CFU)	ES 0.01 µg/ml	0.75	3.34
P.acnes (5×108 CFU)	ES 0 µg/ml		

(Tokyo Chemical Industry, Tokyo, Japan) and kaempferol (Santa Cruz Biotechnology Inc., USA) were dissolved in MeOH for analysis, either. HPLC was performed on an Agilent 1100 system (Agilent Technologies, Waldbronn, Germany) with a photodiode array detector DAD (G1315D)

and Agilent 1100 series quard pump (G1311A), and an Agilent 6410 Triple Quadrupole LC/MS mass spectrometer (Agilent Technologies, Waldbronn, Germany) coupled with an ESI (electrospray ionization) interface and an ion trap mass analyzer. The ESI (electrospray ionization) source was operated in negative ionization modes. Analysis of included compounds were performed under the following conditions: column, TSK-gel ODS-80Ts (Tosoh Co., Tokyo, Japan 4.6 mm X 150 mm); mobile phase, 0.1% formic acid (solvent system A) and CH_3CN (solvent system B) in a gradient mode (B from 20 to 80% in 30 min); sample injection, 5 µl; flow rate, 0.5 ml/min; temperature, 30 °C, UV wavelength, 254 nm and 350 nm. High-purity nitrogen was used as dry gas at a flow rate at 10 L/min, gas temperature at 300 °C; fragmentor voltage 150 V. Nitrogen was used as nebulizer at 30 psi and capillary voltage, ±4000 V.

Statistical analysis

All results are presented as mean ± S.E.M. Results were analyzed using Graph Pad Prism version 5.0 program (Graph Pad Software, Inc., La Jolla, CA, USA). One-way

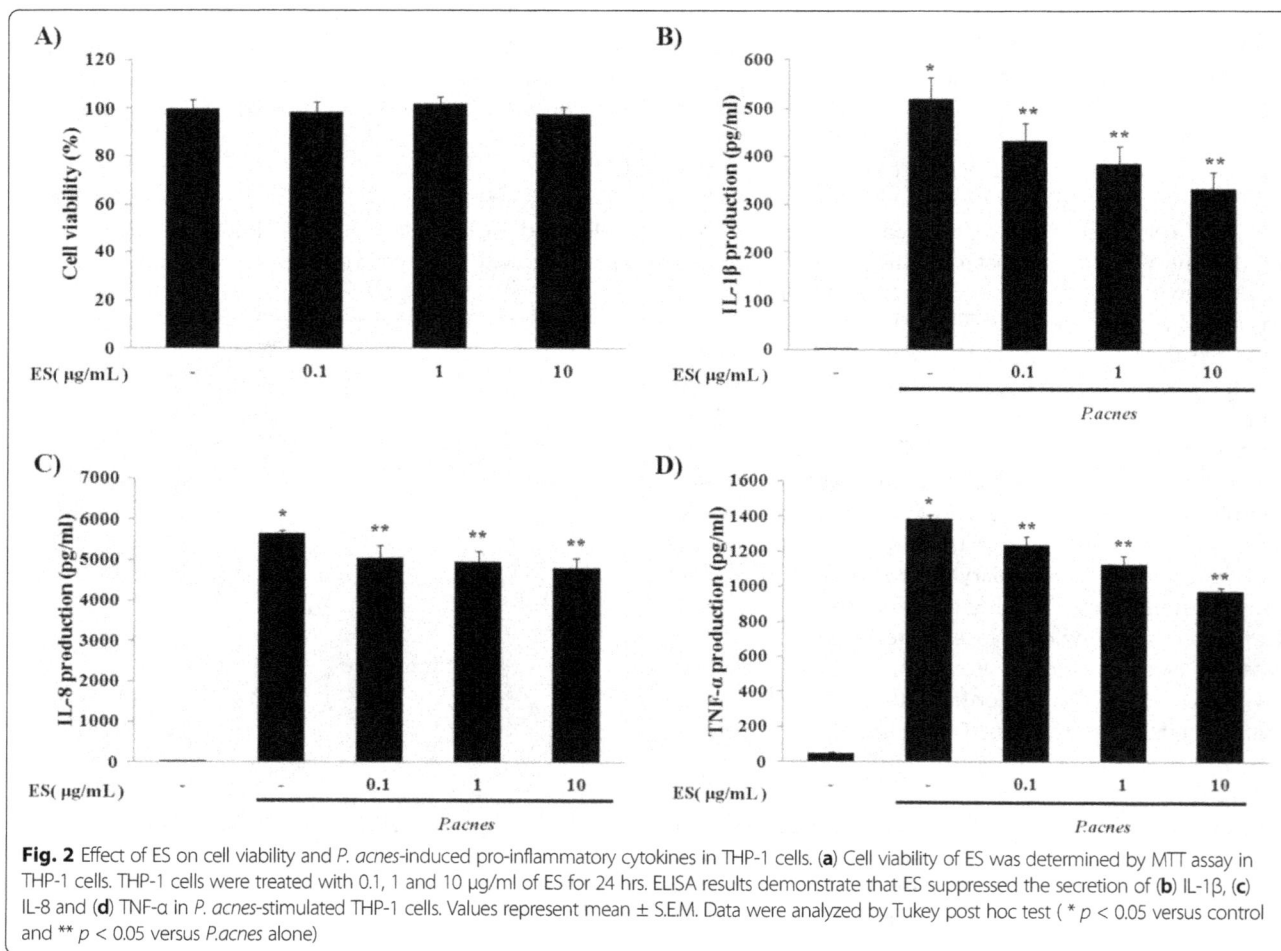

Fig. 2 Effect of ES on cell viability and *P. acnes*-induced pro-inflammatory cytokines in THP-1 cells. (**a**) Cell viability of ES was determined by MTT assay in THP-1 cells. THP-1 cells were treated with 0.1, 1 and 10 µg/ml of ES for 24 hrs. ELISA results demonstrate that ES suppressed the secretion of (**b**) IL-1β, (**c**) IL-8 and (**d**) TNF-α in *P. acnes*-stimulated THP-1 cells. Values represent mean ± S.E.M. Data were analyzed by Tukey post hoc test (* $p < 0.05$ versus control and ** $p < 0.05$ versus *P.acnes* alone)

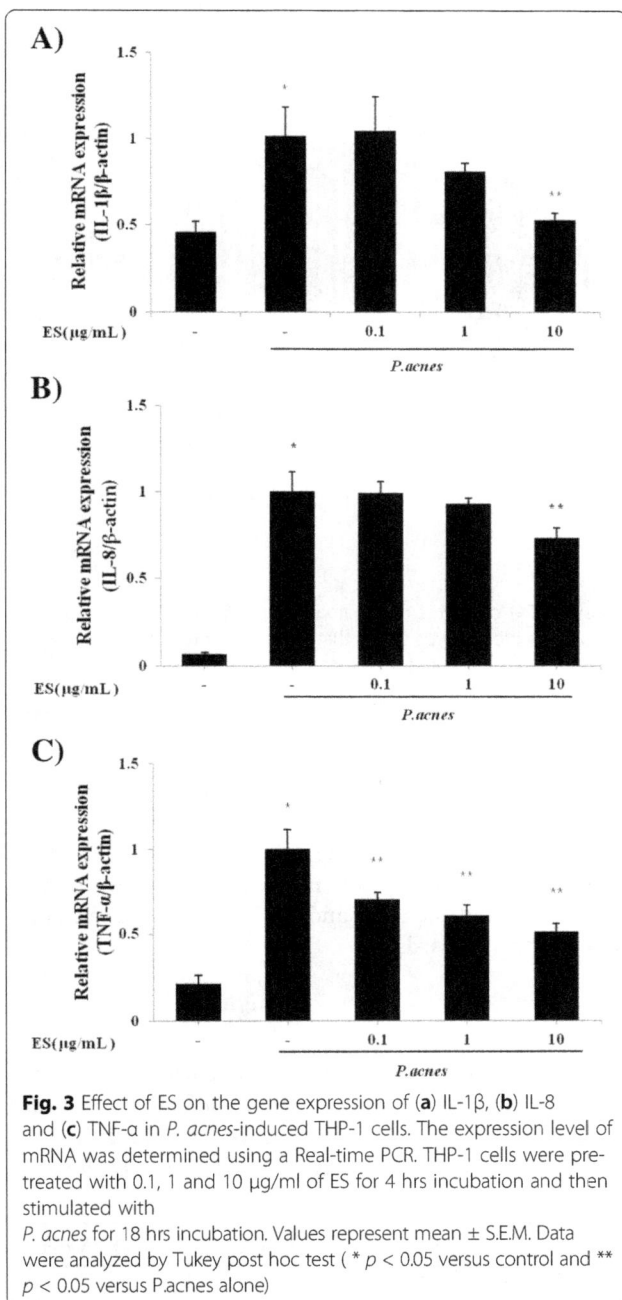

Fig. 3 Effect of ES on the gene expression of (**a**) IL-1β, (**b**) IL-8 and (**c**) TNF-α in *P. acnes*-induced THP-1 cells. The expression level of mRNA was determined using a Real-time PCR. THP-1 cells were pre-treated with 0.1, 1 and 10 μg/ml of ES for 4 hrs incubation and then stimulated with *P. acnes* for 18 hrs incubation. Values represent mean ± S.E.M. Data were analyzed by Tukey post hoc test (* $p < 0.05$ versus control and ** $p < 0.05$ versus P.acnes alone)

analysis of variance with Tukey hoc post test was used to determine the differences. Statistical significance was considered when P value was less than 0.05.

Result

Anti-bacterial activity of ES against *P. acnes*

To evaluate the antibacterial activity of ES extract against *P. acnes* growth, bacteria was co-cultured with various concentrations of ES for 48 h. The MIC value of ES was determined to be 3.0 mg/ml. The MBC value of ES was found to be 7.0 mg/ml. We further performed disc diffusion assay using DMSO as a negative control and tetracycline as a positive control. ES ethanol extracts at concentrations of 100 mg/ml, 200 mg/ml, resulted in clear zones of 9.0 mm, 14.0 mm diameter, respectively (Fig. 1). However the lower concentration of ES (50 mg/ml, 20 mg/ml, and 10 mg/ml) had no antibacterial activity against *P. acnes* (data was not shown). In addition, ES had antibacterial activity against other skin microbes such as *Propionibacterium granulosum* (*P. granulosum*), *Staphylococcus aureus* (*S. aureus*), and *Staphylococcus epidermis* (*S. epidermis*) in concentration of 200 mg/ml (Additional file 1: Figure S1). In addition, ES has effect of lipase inhibition on *P.acnes*. The production of lipase on *P.acnes* was reduced by ES treatment (59.88 ± 6.52% on ES 100 μg/ml treatment) (Table 1.).

Effects of ES on heat-killed *P. acnes*-induced pro-inflammatory cytokines in THP-1 cells

Cell viability of THP-1 cells was determined by MTT assay. THP-1 cells were treated with various concentrations of ES (0.1, 1, or 10 μg/ml) for 24 h. ES had no significant cytotoxicity on THP-1 cells (Fig. 2a). After treatment with ES, the suppressive effect of ES on heat-killed *P. acnes*-stimulated inflammatory cytokine secretion was determined. ES suppressed the secretion of TNF-α, IL-1β, and IL-8 in THP-1 cells treated with heat-killed *P. acnes*. These results suggest that ES could effectively inhibit pro-inflammatory cytokine secretion in *P. acnes*-stimulated THP-1 cells (Fig. 2b, c, d).

We also determined the mRNA expression levels of cytokines after ES treatment by real time RT PCR. Our results showed that ES suppressed the mRNA expression levels of TNF-α, IL-1β, and IL-8 in *P. acnes* induced THP-1 cells (Fig. 3).

Regulatory effects of ES on activated MAPK signaling pathway in heat-killed *P.acnes*-treated THP-1 cells

To determine the influence of anti-inflammatory properties of ES on MAPK signaling pathway, the levels of MAPK activation were examined by Western blotting analysis. As shown in Fig. 4, the phosphorylation levels of p38, JNK, and ERK were markedly increased in THP-1 cells treated with heat-killed *P.acnes*. However, ES treatment decreased *P. acnes*-induced phosphorylation of MAPKs such as p38, JNK, and ERK.

Effects of ES on *P. acnes*-induced inflammation in vivo

To investigate the anti-inflammatory effects of ES on mice ears, live *P. acnes* were intradermally injected into mice ear. At 24 h post injection of live *P. acnes*, ES (1 mg/ml or 10 mg/ml) was injected into mice ears. At 24 h post ES injection, mice were sacrificed and ear

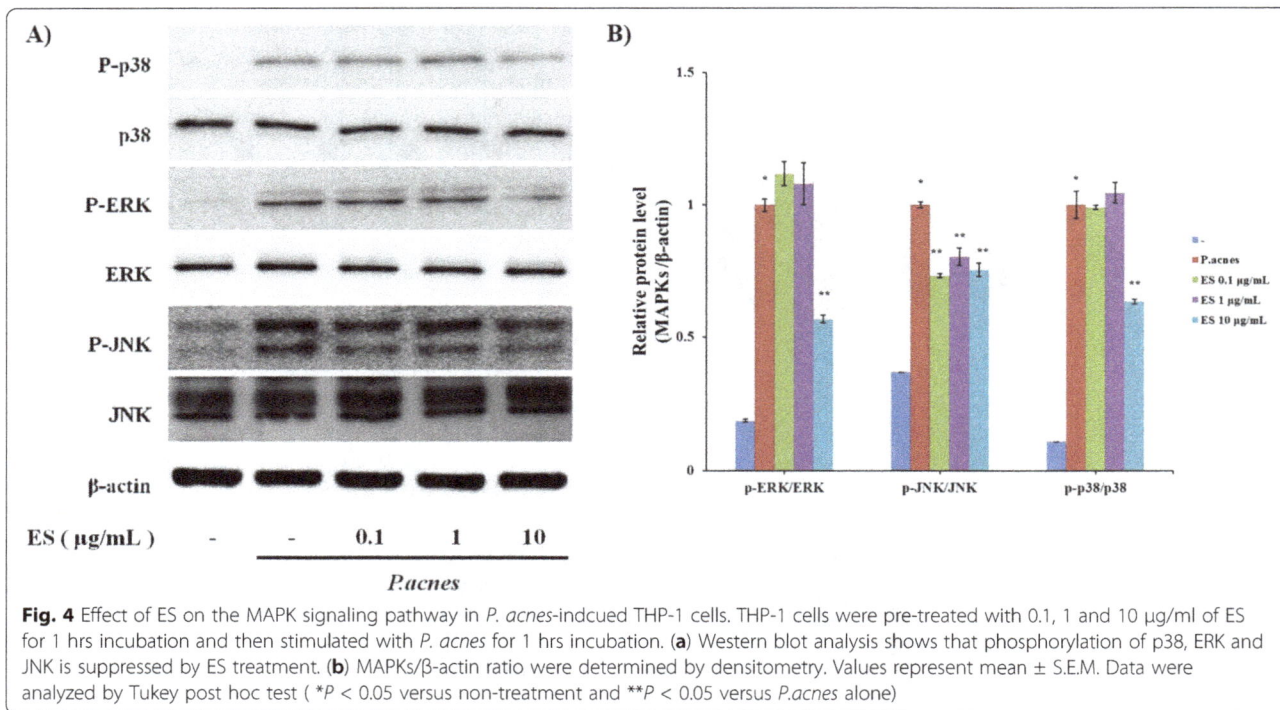

Fig. 4 Effect of ES on the MAPK signaling pathway in *P. acnes*-indcued THP-1 cells. THP-1 cells were pre-treated with 0.1, 1 and 10 μg/ml of ES for 1 hrs incubation and then stimulated with *P. acnes* for 1 hrs incubation. (**a**) Western blot analysis shows that phosphorylation of p38, ERK and JNK is suppressed by ES treatment. (**b**) MAPKs/β-actin ratio were determined by densitometry. Values represent mean ± S.E.M. Data were analyzed by Tukey post hoc test (*$P < 0.05$ versus non-treatment and **$P < 0.05$ versus *P.acnes* alone)

thickness was measured by micro-caliper. The ear thickness of the *P. acnes*-treated group was increased 1.7 fold compared to that of non-treated group. Co-injection of 10 mg/ml of ES significantly reduced ear thickness (Fig. 5a). Inflammatory cells and thickness of epidermis were observed in H&E-stained section of *P. acnes*-injected ears. Intradermal injection with ES at 1 or 10 mg/ml significantly reduced the number of inflammatory cells and thickness of epidermis in a dose dependent manner (Fig. 5b).

Chemical composition of ES

When analyzed with LC/MS system, the retention times of gallic acid, protocatechuic acid, quercetin and kaempferol were 4.5, 5.6, 17.0 and 19.8 min, respectively (Fig. 6). Quantitative analysis of quercetin and kaempferol gave a concentration of 4.480 mg/ml and 0.538 mg/ml in the extract. All of compounds mentioned above, were identified by retention time and molecular ion peak compared with standards.

Discussion

P. acnes is one of the most abundant bacterium on the skin [2]. Although acnes is not an infectious disorder, the role of *P. acnes*, a Gram-positive bacterium that colonizes on the pilosebaceous unit, has been outlined in

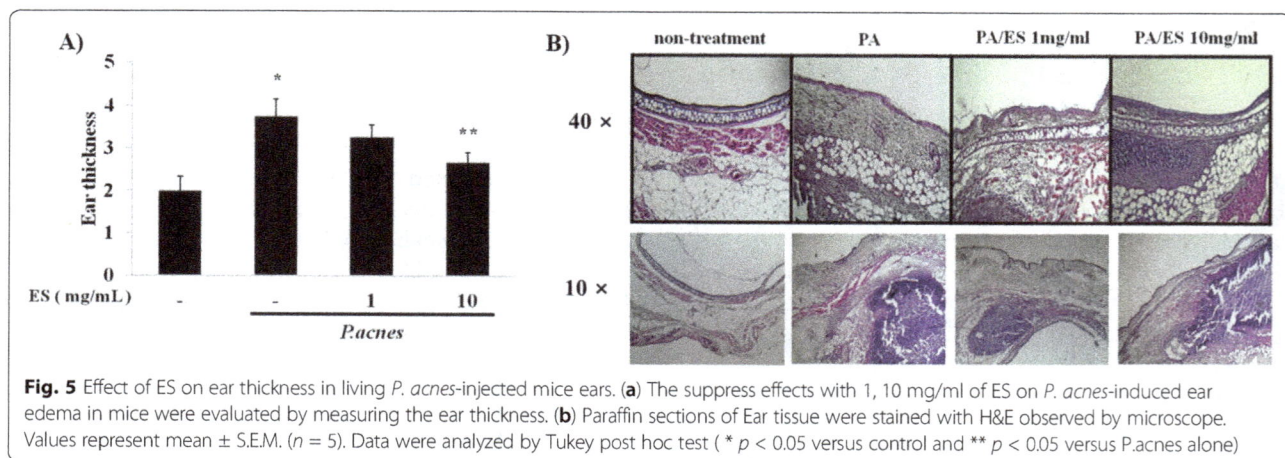

Fig. 5 Effect of ES on ear thickness in living *P. acnes*-injected mice ears. (**a**) The suppress effects with 1, 10 mg/ml of ES on *P. acnes*-induced ear edema in mice were evaluated by measuring the ear thickness. (**b**) Paraffin sections of Ear tissue were stained with H&E observed by microscope. Values represent mean ± S.E.M. (*n* = 5). Data were analyzed by Tukey post hoc test (* $p < 0.05$ versus control and ** $p < 0.05$ versus P.acnes alone)

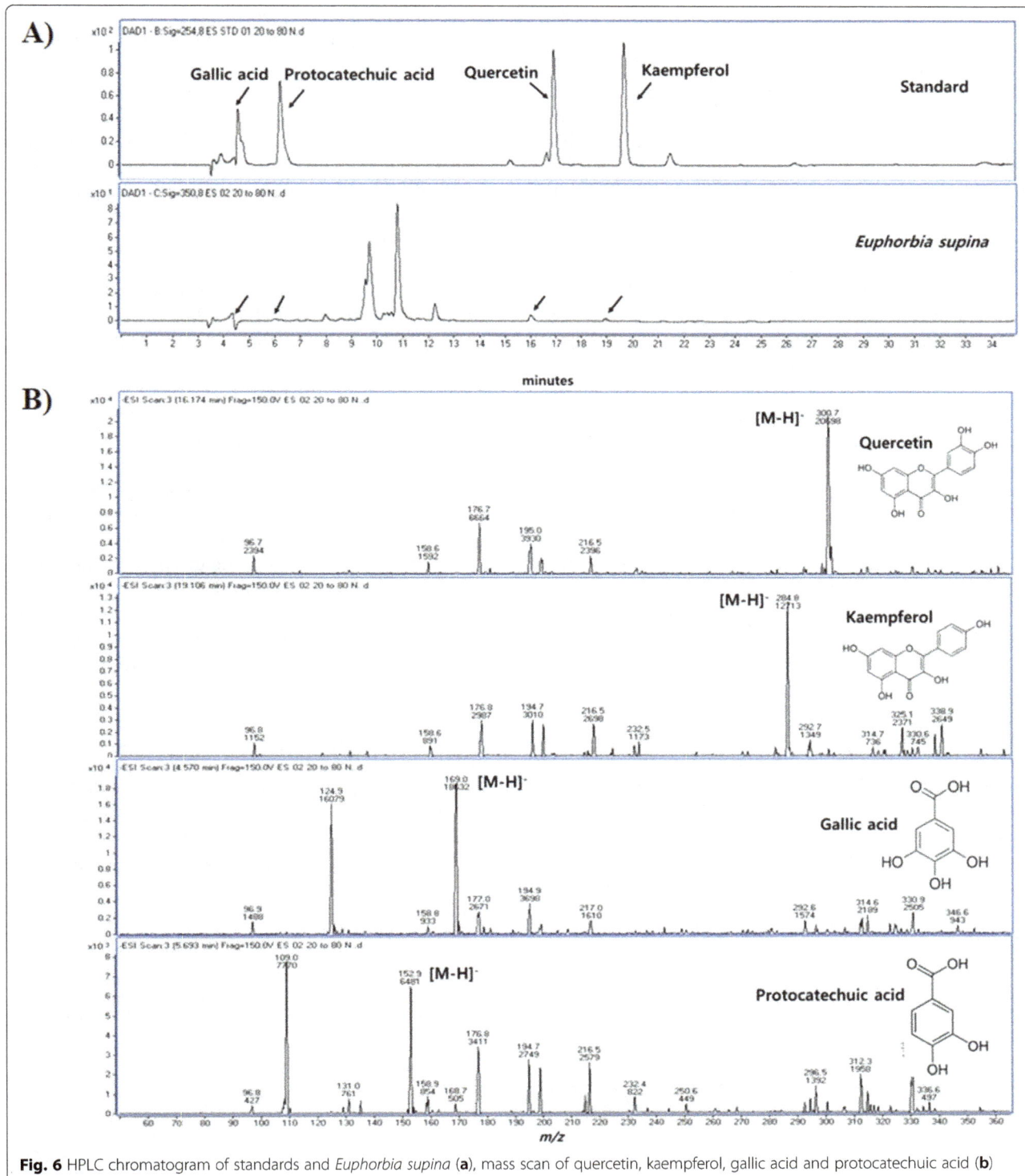

Fig. 6 HPLC chromatogram of standards and *Euphorbia supina* (**a**), mass scan of quercetin, kaempferol, gallic acid and protocatechuic acid (**b**)

previous studies [11]. Injection of *P. acnes* into sterile keratinous cysts can lead to their rupture with consequent inflammation [12], thus providing evidence of inflammatory properties of *P. acnes*. In addition, heat-killed *P.acnes* can induce inflammatory response. Heat-killed

P.acnes induced nitric oxide (NO) and IL-8 production in keratinocyte. Also, heat-killed *P.acnes* influenced activation of p38 MAP kinase [13]. In this study, *P.acnes* was used to induce inflammatory response including production of pro-inflammatory cytokines in THP-1 cells.

ES is a species of Euphorbiaceae traditionally used in eastern Asia for medicinal purposes [14]. ES is known to possess biologically active compounds. ES extract has compounds such as gallic acid, protocatechuic acid, nodakenin, quercetin, and kaemferol [8]. Especially, protocatechuic acid, gallic acid, quercetin, and laempferol were found as ingredients of ES (Fig. 6). Protocatechuic acid is known as having suppressive effect on TNBS-induced colitis [15], preventive effect on LPS-induced inflammatory response in fibroblast [16], and anti-oxidative effect [17]. In addition, gallic acid has several effects on allergic reaction [18], type 2 diabetes symptoms [19], oxidative stress, and hypertension [20]. These constituents (protocatetuic acid and gallic acid) might influence the regulatory effect of ES on P.acnes-induced ear inflammation.

Thus, this study investigated the potential of ES as an antibacterial agent for the treatment of acne vulgaris. However, ES has strong antibacterial activity. We observed that ES was nearly equally active against skin flora such as *Streptococcus aures* (JCM20624), *Propionibacterium granulosum* (KCTC5747), and *Staphylococcus epidermidis* (KCTC1917) (Additional file 1: Figure S1). Furthermore, the lipase activity of *P.acnes* is presented to have role of hydrolysis of sebum triglyceride to free fatty acids. In this process, acnes and skin inflammation is deepen [21]. For this reason, inhibition of lipase is can be a strategy to reduce skin inflammation. ES extract inhibited lipase activity of *P. acnes* (Table 1).

Several studies have reported that the anti-inflammatory effects of ES. ES extract has been reported to be able to reduce the levels of inflammatory mediators such as nitric oxide, IL-6, leukotrienes, and β-hexosaminidase [7]. Recent studies have declared that TNF-a and IL-8 can modulate inflammatory responses in monocytes [22, 23]. Our results showed that *P. acnes* induced secretion of TNF-a, IL-1β, and IL-8 in monocytic THP-1 cells. Moreover, ES treatments effectively inhibited the expression of these cytokines.

The fact that IL-1β is secreted in acne skin condition has proposed valuable effects of IL-1β-targeted therapy in patients suffering from anti-inflammatory acne-lesions [24, 26]. *P. acnes* is able to induce the secretion of chemokine CXCL8 in monocytes and keratinocyte [25, 26]. We also observed that the mRNA expression levels of cytokines in *P. acnes*-induced THP-1 cells were decreased by ES treatment. Our results showed that ES could reduce the expression levels of *P. acnes*-induced TNF-a, IL-8, and IL-1β at transcriptional level.

MAPK and NF-kB pathways have been proposed to be associated with *P. acnes*-induced inflammatory cytokine production [5]. MAPK signaling pathways can adjust cellular reaction to diffusion, differentiation, apoptosis, and inflammation in humans [27]. Previously studies have reported that melitin can suppress MAPK pathway in *P. acnes*-stimulated HaCaT keratinocytes [28]. We observed that *P. acnes* activated the phosphorylation of

MAPK in THP-1 cells. Treatment with *ES* suppressed the phosphorylation levels of p38, JNK, and ERK induced by *P. acnes*.

Based on our in vivo results, we observed the anti-inflammatory effects of ES in *P. acnes*-treated animal model. Several studies have described that injection of live *P. acnes* can lead to the development of inflammatory skin disease in ear-inflammation model [26]. These studies have demonstrated that live *P. acnes* treated group has roughly 2 fold increase in ear thickness compared to PBS treated ear [26]. *P.acnes* can lead to accumulate immune cells such as neutrophil, monocyte, and eosinophil. Also, *P.acnes*-injected ear secrets IL-1β, MMP-2 and 9, and integrin α6 [29]. Our results also showed that injection of ES (10 mg/ml) significantly reduced ear thickness and the number of inflammatory cells.

In summary, our results demonstrated the antibacterial and anti-inflammatory effect of ES against *P. acnes* both in vitro and in vivo. ES significantly decreased the expression levels of various inflammatory cytokines in heat-killed *P. acnes*-treated THP-1 monocytic cells. In addition, *P. acnes*-induced inflammatory responses were inhibited by ES treatment through suppressing MAPK phosphorylation. Our results also showed that ES could inhibit *P. acnes*-induced inflammatory response in animal model. Our data suggested that ES extract could be used to treatment anti-inflammatory skin disease.

Conclusions
ES extract has shown strong antibacterial activity against *P. acnes*. ES extract suppressed pro-inflammatory cytokines and MAPK signaling pathway. ES extract inhibited dermatitis in a mice model of acnes induced by intradermal injection of *P. acnes*. This study provides that ES extract might be used to treatment anti-inflammatory skin disease.

Funding
This research was financially supported by the Ministry of Trade, Industry & Energy (MOTIE), Korea Institute for Advancement of Technology (KIAT) through the Encouragement Program for The Industries of Economic Cooperation Region (R0004536).

Authors' contributions
HJL and YDJ performed the in vivo mouse model experiment and analyzed data. SHK, JYC, HYL, JHL, BRK, and SWH supported the in vitro experiment and collected data. KML, TS and OC provided technical and material support about microbial experiments. MKS performed analysis of extract constituent. HM provided detail and botanic information of ES. HJL and YDJ collected the data, undertook the statistical analyses, and wrote the manuscript. YML and JSJ designed and supervised the study, including editing of the manuscript. All authors shared the raw data of this experimental study. Also, all authors contributed to and have approved the final manuscript.

Competing interests

The authors declare that there are no conflicts of interest.

Author details

[1]Department of Oriental Medicine Resources, Chonbuk National University, 79 Gobongro, Iksan, Jeollabuk-do 54596, South Korea. [2]Department of Oriental Pharmacy, College of Pharmacy, Wonkwang-Oriental Medicine Research Institute, Wonkwang University, Iksan, Jeollabuk-do 54538, South Korea. [3]Department of Pharmacy, College of Pharmacy, Dongduk Woman's University, 23-1 Wolgok-Dong, SungBuk-Gu, Seoul 02748, South Korea. [4]Department of Microbiology, Meiji Pharmaceutical University, 2-522-1 Noshio, Kiyose, Tokyo 204-8588, Japan. [5]Department of Ecology Landscape Architecture-Design, College of Environmental and Bioresource Sciences, Chonbuk National University, Iksan, South Korea.

References

1. Grange PA, et al. Production of superoxide anions by keratinocytes initiates P. acnes-induced inflammation of the skin. PLoS Pathog. 2009;5(7):e1000527.
2. Williams HC, Dellavalle RP, Garner S, Sarah. Acne vulgaris. Lancet. 2012; 379(9813):361–72.
3. Jugeau S, et al. Induction of toll-like receptors by Propionibacterium acnes. Br J Dermatol. 2005;153(6):1105–13.
4. Vowels BR, YANG S, LEYDEN, James J. Induction of proinflammatory cytokines by a soluble factor of Propionibacterium acnes: implications for chronic inflammatory acne. Infect Immun. 1995;63(8):3158–65.
5. Huang W-C, et al. Anti-bacterial and anti-inflammatory properties of capric acid against Propionibacterium acnes: a comparative study with lauric acid. J Dermatol Sci. 2014;73(3):232–40.
6. Pretsch A, et al. Antimicrobial and anti-inflammatory activities of endophytic fungi Talaromyces wortmannii extracts against acne-inducing bacteria. PLoS One. 2014;9(6):e97929.
7. Chae H-S, et al. Euphorbia supina inhibits inflammatory mediators in mouse bone marrow-derived mast cells and macrophages. Int Immunopharmacol. 2015;29(2):966–73.
8. Song Y, et al. Determination of polyphenol components of Korean prostrate spurge (Euphorbia supina) by using liquid chromatography—tandem mass spectrometry: overall contribution to antioxidant activity. J Anal Methods Chem. 2014;2014.
9. Joung D-K, et al. Antibacterial effect of Euphorbia supina extracts against methicillin-resistant Staphylococcus aureus under dark and light intensity. Afr J Pharm Pharmacol. 2011;5(18):2056–61.
10. Han M-H, et al. Polyphenols from Korean prostrate spurge Euphorbia supina induce apoptosis through the Fas-associated extrinsic pathway and activation of ERK in human leukemic U937 cells. Oncol Rep. 2016;36(1):99–107.
11. Mouser PE, et al. Propionibacterium acnes-reactive T helper-1 cells in the skin of patients with acne vulgaris. J Investig Dermatol. 2003;121(5):1226–8.
12. Leyden JJ. Therapy for acne vulgaris. N Engl J Med. 1997;336(16):1156–62.
13. Lyte P, Sur R, Nigam A, Southall MD. Heat-killed Propionibacterium acnes is capable of inducing inflammatory responses in skin. Exp Dermatol. 2009; 18(12):1070–2.
14. Luyen BTT, et al. Anti-inflammatory components of Euphorbia humifusa Willd. Bioorg Med Chem Lett. 2014;24(8):1895–900.
15. Crespo I, San-Miguel B, Mauriz JL, Ortiz de Urbina JJ, Almar M, Tunon MJ, Gonzalez-Gallego J. Protective effect of protocatechuic acid on TNBS-induced colitis in mice is associated with modulation of the Sphk/S1P signaling pathway. Nutrients. 2017;16, 9(3).
16. Wang Y, Zhou J, Fu S, Wang C, Zhou B. Preventive effects of protocatechuic acid on LPS-induced inflammatory response in human gingival fibroblasts via activating PPAR-γ. Inflammation. 2015;38(3):1080–4.
17. Fei X, Je IG, Shin TY, Kim SH, Seo SY. Synthesis of gallic acid analogs as histamine and pro-inflammatory cytokine inhibitors for treatment of mact cell-mediated allergic inflammation. Molecules. 2017;29(22):6.
18. Ferk F, Kundi M, Brath H, Szekers T, Al-Serori H, Misik M, Saiko P, Marculescu R, Wagner KH, Knasmueller S. Gallic acid improves health-associated biochemical parameters and prevents oxidative damage of DNA in type 2 diabetes patients: Results of a placebo-controlled pilot study. Mol Nutr Food Res 2018, 62.4. https://doi.org/10.1002/mnfr.201700482.
19. Jin L, Piao ZH, Sun S Liu B, Kim GR, Seok YM, Lin MQ, Ryu Y, Choi SY, Kee HJ, Jeong MH. Gallic acid reduces blood pressure and attenuates oxidative stress and cardiac hypertrophy in spontaneously hypertensive rats. Sci Rep. 2017;7(1):15607.
20. Olafsdottir A, et al. A heteroglycan from the cyanobacterium Nostoc commune modulates LPS-induced inflammatory cytokine secretion by THP-1 monocytes through phosphorylation of ERK1/2 and Akt. Phytomedicine. 2014;21(11):1451–7.
21. Lee WL, Shalita AR, Suntharalingam KS, Fikrig SM. Neutrophil chemotaxis by Propionibacterium acnes lipase and its inhibition. Infect Immun. 1982;53(1):71–6.
22. Lee W-R, et al. Protective effect of melittin against inflammation and apoptosis on Propionibacterium acnes-induced human THP-1 monocytic cell. Eur J Pharmacol. 2014;740:218–26.
23. Kistowska M, et al. IL-1β drives inflammatory responses to Propionibacterium acnes in vitro and in vivo. J Investig Dermatol. 2014;134(3):677–85.
24. Grange PA, et al. Nicotinamide inhibits Propionibacterium acnes-induced IL-8 production in keratinocytes through the NF-κB and MAPK pathways. J Dermatol Sci. 2009;56(2):106–12.
25. Rottboell L, et al. Exploring Valrubicin's effect on Propionibacterium acnes-induced skin inflammation in vitro and in vivo. Derm Rep. 2015;7(3).
26. Lin Z-C, et al. Eupafolin nanoparticles protect HaCaT keratinocytes from particulate matter-induced inflammation and oxidative stress. Int J Nanomedicine. 2016;11:3907.
27. Lee W-R, et al. The protective effects of Melittin on Propionibacterium acnes–induced inflammatory responses in vitro and in vivo. J Investig Dermatol. 2014;134(7):1922–30.
28. Lee WJ, Lee KC, Kim MJ, Jang YH, Lee SJ, Kim DW. Efficacy of red or infrared light-emitting diodes in a mouse model of Propionibacterium acnes-induced inflammation. Ann Dermatol. 2016;28(2):186–91.

3

Water extract of *Clinacanthus nutans* leaves exhibits in vitro, ex vivo and in vivo anti-angiogenic activities in endothelial cell via suppression of cell proliferation

Chin Theng Ng[1,7], Lai Yen Fong[2], Jun Jie Tan[3], Nor Fadilah Rajab[4], Faridah Abas[5], Khozirah Shaari[6], Kok Meng Chan[4], Fariza Juliana[4] and Yoke Keong Yong[7*]

Abstract

Background: *Clinacanthus nutans* (Burm. f.) Lindau. has traditionally been using in South East Asia countries to manage cancer. However, scientific evidence is generally lacking to support this traditional claim. This study aims to investigate the in vitro, ex-vivo and in vivo effects of *C. nutans* extracts on angiogenesis.

Methods: *C. nutans* leaves was extracted with 50–100% ethanol or deionised water at 1% (*w/v*). Human umbilical veins endothelial cell (HUVEC) proliferation was examined using MTT assay. The in vitro anti-angiogenic effects of *C. nutans* were assessed using wound scratch, tube formation and transwell migration assays. The VEGF levels secreted by human oral squamous cell carcinoma (HSC-4) cell and HUVEC permeability were also measured. Besides, the rat aortic ring and chick embryo chorioallantoic membrane (CAM) assays, representing ex vivo and in vivo models, respectively, were performed.

Results: The MTT assay revealed that water extract of *C. nutans* leaves exhibited the highest activity, compared to the ethanol extracts. Therefore, the water extract was chosen for subsequent experiments. *C. nutans* leaf extract significantly suppressed endothelial cell proliferation and migration in both absence and presence of VEGF. However, the water extract failed to suppress HUVEC transmigration, differentiation and permeability. *C. nutans* water extract also did not suppress HSC-4 cell-induced VEGF production. Importantly, *C. nutans* water extract significantly abolished the sprouting of vessels in aortic rings as well as in chick embryo CAM.

Conclusion: In conclusion, these findings reveal potential anti-angiogenic effects of *C. nutans*, providing new evidence for its potential application as an anti-angiogenic agent.

Keywords: *Clinacanthus nutans*, Acanthaceae, Angiogenesis, Chick embryo choriollantoic membrane, Aortic ring

Background

Angiogenesis is the main contributor to the transition of pre-invasive and dormant tumour cells to a more invasive and malignant cells, through establishing additional blood vessel network from pre-existing vasculature to enable more efficient oxygen and nutrient delivery for growth. Such pathologic event is orchestrated by overexpression of vascular endothelial growth factor (VEGF) secreted by tumour cells, the known factor that promotes endothelial cell proliferation, invasion, migration and capillary tube formation [1]. Hence, inhibition of tumour angiogenesis by targeting VEGF pathway has emerged as an important strategy in combating cancers [2].

However, the new blood vessels formed are unlike normal blood vessels; they exhibit increased permeability, and cause diminished blood flow and create hypoxic microenvironment within the tumour [3]. To date, not more than 15 identified anti-cancer drugs that target tumour angiogenesis are granted approval from US Food and Drug Administration. In addition to undesirable side

* Correspondence: yoke_keong@upm.edu.my
[7]Department of Human Anatomy, Faculty of Medicine and Health Sciences, Universiti Putra Malaysia, 43400 UPM Serdang, Selangor, Malaysia
Full list of author information is available at the end of the article

effects and low patient survival, those agents often couple with low therapeutic efficacy and high risk of drug resistance after long-term treatment, as reported in trials involving small cell lung cancer patients treated with bevacizumab and sunitinib [4]. The current anti-angiogenic drugs are single-target based agents which often could not achieve desired outcomes from inhibiting angiogenesis, mainly because of the redundancy in the angiogenic pathways.

Traditional plant extracts are source of multi-targeted therapeutic agents as they contain various medicinal phytochemicals. The production cost is usually low due to their abundance in nature. Plant extracts may also reduce the risk of adaptive resistance that is commonly seen in therapy with single agent [3]. *Clinacanthus nutans* (Burm. f.) Lindau. is locally known as Sabah Snake Grass, belonging to the Acanthaceae family. *C. nutans* has been used traditionally as a medicinal herb in tropical Asia to treat various diseases such as insect bites, diabetes mellitus, diuretics and fever [5]. Previous studies have reported that *C. nutans* possesses cytotoxicity [6], anti-proliferative, anti-oxidant [7] and anti-inflammatory [8] activities. Ethanol extract of *C. nutans* has been shown to impede hepatoma in mice through induction of apoptosis and enhancement of immune response [9]. Researchers have also demonstrated that *C. nutans* methanol extract induces human melanoma cell apoptosis [10]. Despite claims regarding the use of *C. nutans* in treating various cancers, the anti-angiogenic potential of *C. nutans* has never been carefully examined. Here we showed that *C. nutans* is a potential anti-cancer agent that possesses inhibitory effects on VEGF-mediated angiogenic events, based on in vitro findings using human umbilical vein endothelial cells (HUVECs), ex vivo test using rat aortic ring and in vivo investigation using chick embryo chorioallantoic membrane (CAM) assays.

Methods
Chemicals and reagents
HUVECs, EndoGRO culture media, human $VEGF_{165}$, Millicell cell culture inserts with pore size of 8.0 μm, in vitro vascular permeability assay kit and EndoGRO-LS complete culture media kit were purchased from Milipore. Growth factor-reduced matrigel was purchased from BD Bioscience. Human oral squamous cell carcinoma (HSC-4) cells and Dulbecco's Modified Eagle's Medium (DMEM) were purchased from American Type Culture Collection (ATCC). Human VEGF Quantikine ELISA kit was purchased from R&D Systems. Suramin (purity> 99% by TLC) was purchased from Sigma-Aldrich.

Plant material
Whole plant of *Clinacanthus nutans* (Burm. f.) Lindau was harvested from the Sendayan Commodities Development Centre in Seremban, Negeri Sembilan, Malaysia. The plant

was verified by Dr. Shamsul Khamis, botanist at Institute of Bioscience, Universiti Putra Malaysia. The specimen of *C. nutans* has been deposited at the herbarium of the Institute of Bioscience, Universiti Putra Malaysia (voucher number: SK 2883/15).

C. nutans leaf extraction
C. nutans leaf extracts were obtained from our previous work [11]. Briefly, the plant was harvested, cleaned with water, dried and separated into leaves and stems. The leaves were then dried at room temperature under the shade in a well-ventilated room and ground to fine powder. Next, the ground powder was extracted by sonicating in 50, 70, and 100% ethanol or deionised water at 1% (*w/v*) for 1 h without heating. The extraction was repeated thrice for each sample, followed by filtered-sterilization and vacuum evaporation to dry and freeze-dry the extracted samples prior to storing at 4 °C until further analysis.

Cell culture
HUVECs were purchased from Merck, Malaysia, and grown in T-25 cell culture flasks with EndoGRO culture media. HUVECs between passage three to six were used in the experiments. Human oral squamous cell carcinoma (HSC-4) cells from American Type Culture Collection (ATCC) were maintained in Dulbecco-modified Eagle Medium (DMEM) supplemented with 10% FBS and 4 mM L-glutamine. All the cells were incubated at 37 °C in an incubator with 95% humidified air and 5% CO_2.

Cell proliferation assay
Cell proliferation assay was performed as described previously by Mosmann [12], with some modifications. HUVECs were plated onto 96-well plates at a cell density of 1.0×10^4 cells per well. After 24 h, cells were treated with different *C. nutans* extracts and subsequently incubated for 24, 48 and 72 h in separate well plates. After indicated times, 10 μl of MTT (5 mg/ml stock concentration) was added into each well and incubated in an incubator for additional 4 h. Then, MTT solution was removed and the purple formazan was dissolved in 100 μl of dimethyl sulfoxide (DMSO). The absorbance was measured using a microplate reader (Tecan M200 Infinite) at a wavelength of 570 nm with a reference wavelength of 650 nm.

Wound healing assay
The assay was carried out according to Kavitha et al. [13] with some modifications. HUVECs were plated onto 6-well plates and allowed to grow until confluence. Then, a defined scratch gap was created using a 100–200 μl-pipette tip. All detached/dead cells were removed by several washes with media. Then, cells were

co-treated with human $VEGF_{165}$ and *C. nutans* extracts. Images were captured at 40× magnification, at 0 h (baseline) and 12 h as soon as the gap in VEGF-treated groups was completely covered by cells, using an inverted microscope (Olympus CKX31). The cell migration was quantified using the formula: Initial wound distance minus final wound distance divided by two [13].

Tube formation assay

Tube formation method was performed according to Arnaoutova and Kleinman [14]. Briefly, growth factor-reduced Matrigel™ was pipetted into pre-chilled 96-well plates and polymerized at 37 °C for 30mins. HUVECs (1.5×10^4 cells per well) were seeded onto the Matrigel-coated plates. *C. nutans* extract at 50 to 1000 μg/ml were added at plating. After 3 h, the tubular structure was visualized and the images were captured using an inverted microscope at 40× magnification. The tube length was quantified using an Image J with integrated angiogenesis analyser plugin (Gilles Carpentier, Faculté des Sciences et. Technolo-gie, Université Paris Est, Creteil Val de Marne, France).

Transwell migration assay

Transmigration of HUVECs was studied as described previously by Kavitha et al. [13] with slight modifications. Briefly, HUVECs (3×10^4 cells per well) were cultured on Millicell cell culture inserts with pore size of 8.0 μm, and treated with 50 to 1000 μg/ml *C. nutans* extract dissolved in EndoGRO media supplemented with 0.5% FBS. Bottom wells were filled with 750 μl of Endo-GRO media containing 10 ng/ml human $VEGF_{165}$ and extract similar to that of the inserts. After 6 h, non-migrated cells on the insert membrane were removed by cotton swabs, and migrated cells were fixed with 4% paraformaldehyde and stained with 0.1% crystal violet. The dyes were extracted using 10% acetic acid and the absorbance was measured by a microplate reader at 590 nm.

In vitro vascular permeability assay

The in vitro vascular permeability assay was performed according to manufacturer's protocol. Briefly, HUVECs were grown to confluence on collagen-coated inserts. Next, the monolayers were treated with different concentrations of *C. nutans* extract. After 24 h, FITC-dextran solution was added onto the cultured HUVEC monolayer for 20 min, and the fluorescence intensity of FITC-dextran that crossed the cell layer were measured using Tecan Infinite M200 fluorescence plate reader at 485/530 nm (Excitation/Emission), as described previously by Ng et al. [15].

VEGF levels

HSC-4 cells were seeded onto 96-well plates at a cell density of 1×10^4 cells per well. Then, cells were treated with 50 to 1000 μg/ml of *C. nutans* extract for 72 h. VEGF levels in HSC-4 were quantified using Human VEGF Quantikine ELISA kit. Absorbance were read at 450 nm and corrected to 570 nm.

Experimental animal

Healthy male Spradue Dawley rats (aged 6–8 weeks old) from the Faculty of Medicine and Health Sciences, Universiti Putra Malaysia, were acclimatized for 7 days under standard environmental conditions. The rats were free access to standard laboratory chow and water ad libitum, and were kept in a room with 12 h day/night cycle.

Ex-vivo aortic ring assay

The animals were euthanized by CO_2 exposure and aortas were isolated from male *Sprague Dawley* rats (UPM/IACUC/AUP-R071/2015) according to Bellacen and Lewis [16]. Pre-chilled 48-well plates were filled with 150 μl of Matrigel™ and allowed to polymerise for 30 mins at 37 °C. Rat aortas were rinsed with cold sterile phosphate-buffered saline and cut into 1 mm-long cross sections. Aortic rings were placed on Matrigel and covered with an additional 150 μl of Matrigel. The aortic rings were fed with 500 μl of complete culture media, or supplemented with *C. nutan* at 50 to 1000 μg/ml. The treatments were replaced daily. Growing sprouts, at day 8, were photographed with an inverted microscope (Olympus), and the sprout length was analysed by Image J NIH software program.

In vivo chick embryo chorioallantoic membrane (CAM) assay

Fertilized chicken eggs were purchased from a poultry farm (Hing Hong Sdn. Bhd) and incubated in a 38 °C oven with 60% humidified air for 72 h. The CAM assay was performed according to West et al. [17]. Briefly, the shell of eggs was gently cleaned and wiped with 70% ethanol. With caution, a small hole was created with an 18-gauge needle on the narrow end of the eggs and 3 ml of albumin was removed. The needle hole was then sealed with clear tapes. Subsequently, a small window was carefully created on the top-most surface of the eggshells. The windows were then covered by sterile parafilm and the eggs were placed back into the oven. After 8 days, 500, 1000 and 2000 μg/ml of *C. nutans* were applied onto sterile filter disks and dried before grafting on the CAM. After that, the windows were sealed by a sterile parafilm and the eggs were placed back into the oven. After 48 h, the CAMs were fixed with 4% paraformaldehyde at 4 °C, overnight. Angiogenesis levels were determined by counting the number of vessels contacted to *C. nutans* disks.

Statistical analysis

The data were expressed as the mean ± SEM. Statistical analysis was performed using IBM SPSS 20.0. One-way analysis of variance (ANOVA) followed by Tukey's test was used to compare means for the multiple groups. p values less than 0.05 ($p < 0.05$) were considered to be statistically significant.

Results

C. nutans water extract suppresses endothelial cell growth

Extraction of *C. nutans* using 50, 70 and 100% ethanol did not affect HUVEC viability regardless of its concentrations up to 100 μg/ml. Such effect remains unaltered even with prolonged treatment time from 24 to 72 h (Fig. 1). On the contrary, 50 and 100 μg/ml of *C. nutans* in water extract showed significant reduction of HUVEC viability to 80.20 ± 5.82 and 79.33 ± 4.81%, respectively, after 48 and 72 h as compared to untreated control. At a lower *C. nutans* concentration of 25 μg/ml, such significant difference was only observed after 72 h (Fig. 1). These data suggest that the water soluble compounds within the *C. nutans* water extract could suppress endothelial cell growth. We then tested the *C. nutans* water extract at higher concentrations ranging from 50 to 1000 μg/ml to see if the anti-proliferative effect can be seen within 24 h without causing significant cytotoxicity.

However, water extract of *C. nutans* neither suppressed HUVEC growth, nor caused cell death after 24 h (data not shown).

VEGF is the known driver of endothelial cell proliferation within tumour microenvironment condition [18]. To better mimic the pathologic conditions, we treated the HUVEC with the water extract of *C. nutans* in the presence of VEGF for 24, 48 and 72 h. As expected, with increasing concentration of *C. nutans* from 50 to 1000 μg/ml, the water extract significantly suppressed VEGF-induced HUVECs proliferation from 80.72 ± 0.42% to 67.25 ± 1.42% ($p < 0.05$) in 48 h, and 78.37 ± 2.09 to 48.88 ± 0.93% in 72 h ($p < 0.05$) as compared to VEGF alone (Fig. 2). These findings suggest the water extract could suppress endothelial growth in dose-dependent manner.

C. nutans water extract suppresses endothelial cell migration

Next, we examined the effects of ethanol and water extract of *C. nutans* on endothelial cell migration based on wound-healing assay. Again, no inhibitory effect was observed in ethanol extract-treated group. However, when HUVECs were treated with the *C. nutans* water extract with increasing concentrations from 12.5 μg/ml to 100 μg/ml, the migration distance was reduced from 83.21 ± 4.24% to 81.50 ± 5.29% ($p < 0.05$) (Fig. 3).

In contrast, HUVECs were also found less migratory when tested with *C. nutans* water extracts at high concentrations from 50 μg/ml to 1000 μg/ml, with the measured cell migration distance value significantly reduced

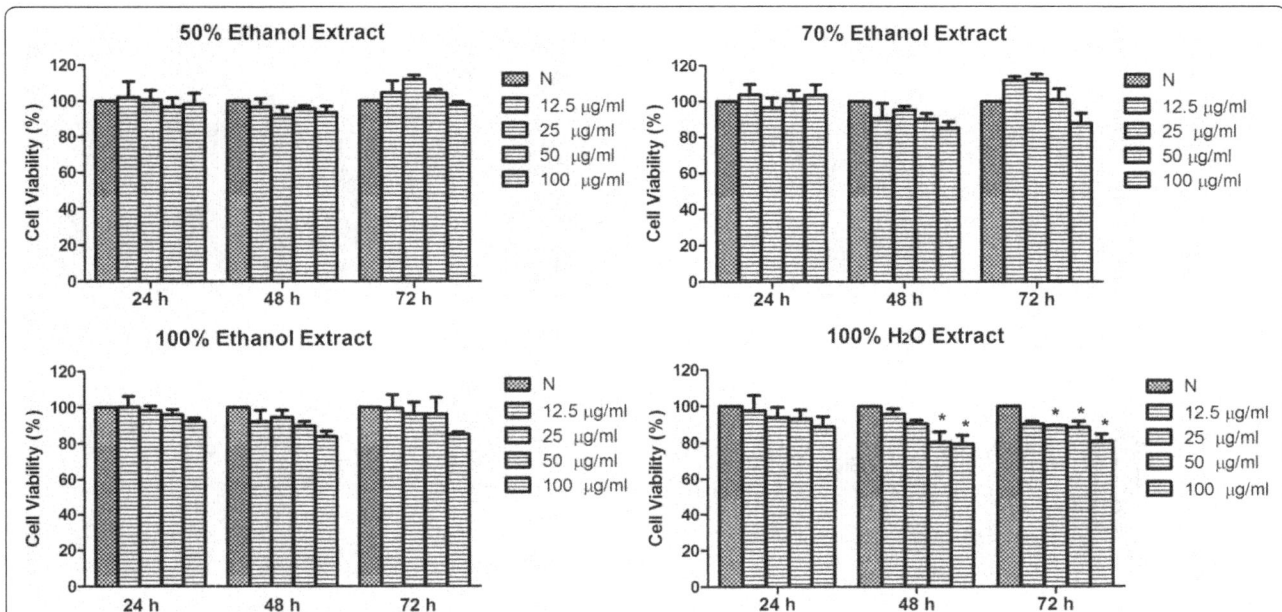

Fig. 1 Effects of 50, 70, 100% ethanol extracts and 100% water extract of *C. nutans* leaves on endothelial cell proliferation at 24, 48 and 72 h. The water extract of *C. nutans* leaves was chosen for subsequent experiments. The values presented are the mean ± SEM of three independent experiments and compared against normal control (N). *$p < 0.05$ were considered significant

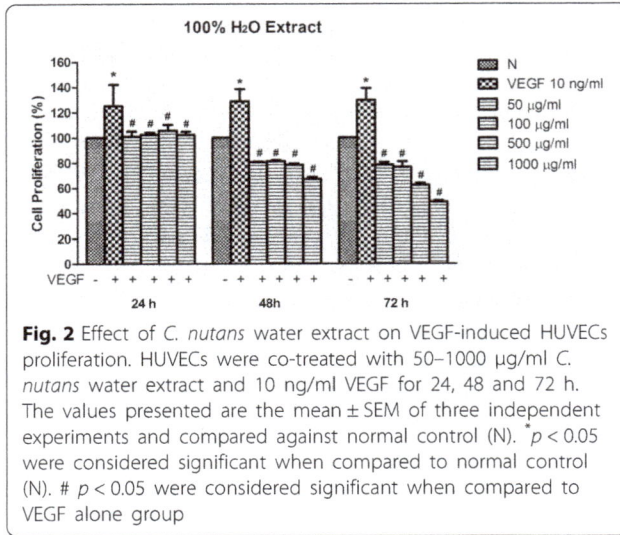

Fig. 2 Effect of *C. nutans* water extract on VEGF-induced HUVECs proliferation. HUVECs were co-treated with 50–1000 µg/ml *C. nutans* water extract and 10 ng/ml VEGF for 24, 48 and 72 h. The values presented are the mean ± SEM of three independent experiments and compared against normal control (N). $^*p < 0.05$ were considered significant when compared to normal control (N). # $p < 0.05$ were considered significant when compared to VEGF alone group

from $82.04 \pm 0.92\%$ to $77.16 \pm 4.33\%$ ($p < 0.05$) (Fig. 4) in the presence of VEGF. These results suggest that water extract of *C. nutans* disrupts VEGF-stimulated HUVEC migration.

C. nutans water extract does not suppress VEGF-induced HUVECs transmigration

Endothelial cell migration is known to be driven by VEGF gradient [19]. A Boyden chamber assay, which creates VEGF gradient between the upper and lower chambers, was used to investigate effect of *C. nutans* water extract on HUVEC-transmembrane cell migration. As shown in Fig. 5, VEGF induced HUVEC-transmembrane migration by 1.71 ± 0.07 fold as compared to the untreated control. However, this event was not reversed by *C. nutans* water extract, confirming the inability of *C. nutans* water extract in altering HUVEC chemotaxis in response to VEGF.

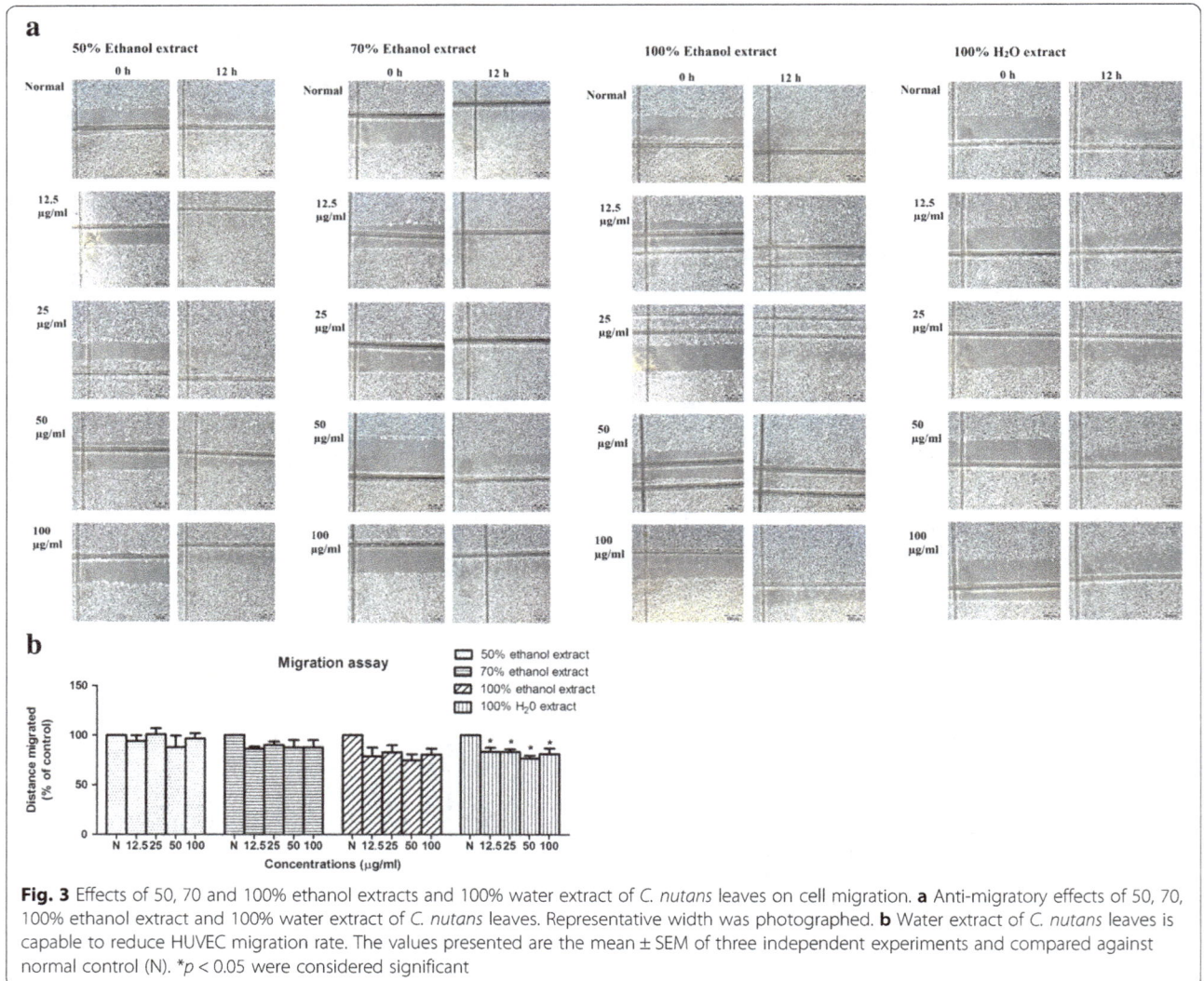

Fig. 3 Effects of 50, 70 and 100% ethanol extracts and 100% water extract of *C. nutans* leaves on cell migration. **a** Anti-migratory effects of 50, 70, 100% ethanol extract and 100% water extract of *C. nutans* leaves. Representative width was photographed. **b** Water extract of *C. nutans* leaves is capable to reduce HUVEC migration rate. The values presented are the mean ± SEM of three independent experiments and compared against normal control (N). $^*p < 0.05$ were considered significant

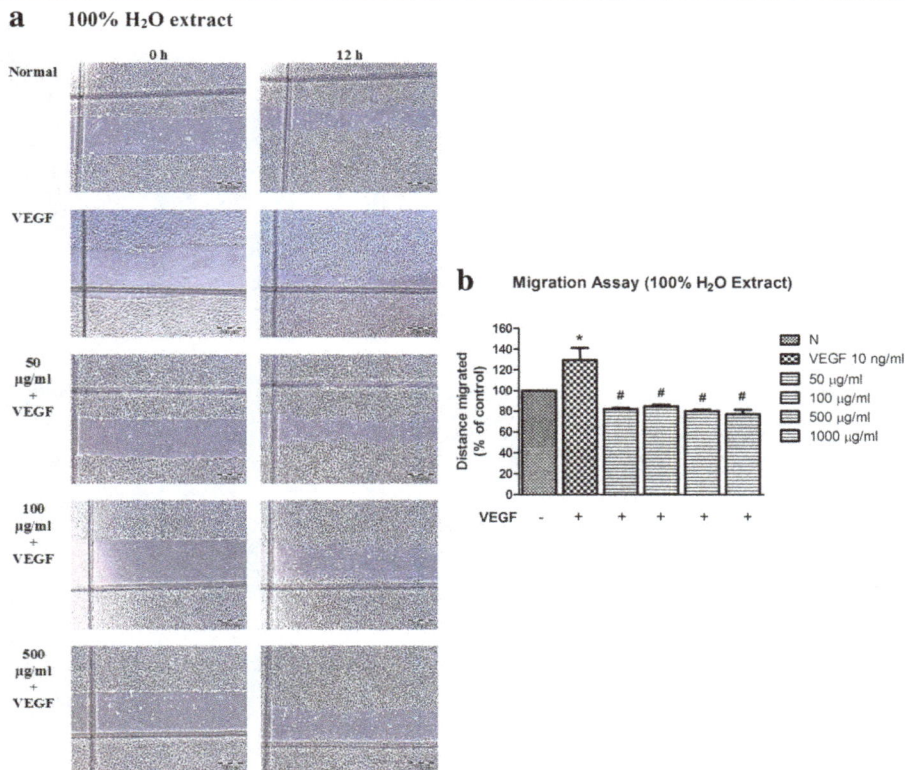

Fig. 4 Effect of *C. nutans* water extract on VEGF-induced cell migration. **a** Anti-migratory effect of 100% water extract of *C. nutans* leaves. Representative width were photographed. **b** HUVECs treated with water extract of *C. nutans* leaves showed reduction in migration rate. The values presented are the mean ± SEM of three independent experiments. *$p < 0.05$ were considered significant when compared to normal control (N); #$p < 0.05$ were considered significant when compared to VEGF alone group

C. nutans water extract does not suppress VEGF-induced capillary tube formation

It is known that a complex endothelial tubular network can be formed when endothelial cells were cultured in three dimensions Matrigel bed in the presence of VEGF [20], and such event can be disrupted by Suramin, a drug which is commonly used in treating sleeping sickness and river blindness [21]. Here we showed that VEGF induced HUVEC capillary tube formation in Matrigel after 3 h, with the measured tube length of 126.30 ± 5.64% as compared to untreated control; whereas Suramin treated-HUVECs lost its tube formation capability completely (Fig. 6). To examine if the water extract of *C. nutans* could suppress VEGF-induced endothelial tube formation, we tested the extract at high concentrations from 50 to 1000 µg/ml. However, no suppressive effect was observed in all *C. nutans* treated group.

C. nutans water extract increases endothelial permeability

The endothelial permeability, measured by fluorescent unit relative to the amount of fluorescein isothiocyanate (FITC)-dextran which passes through the cell monolayer, showed that *C. nutans* water extract significantly increased endothelial permeability levels to 211.80 ± 22.03, 228.10 ± 5.23, 223.20 ± 11.80 and 226.80 ± 43.67% when treated at 50, 100, 500 and 1000 µg/ml, respectively (Fig. 7). VEGF was used as a reference whereby VEGF increased HUVEC permeability to 202.27 ± 9.90% of control.

As VEGF secreted by tumor cells plays a crucial role in neoangiogenesis, we also investigate *C. nutans* water extract if it is capable of inhibiting VEGF secretion by human oral squamous cell carcinoma, HSC-4 cells [22]. Nonetheless, all doses of *C. nutans* water extract failed to reduce the VEGF level at 72 h post-treatment (data not shown). These data indicate that *C. nutans* does not attenuate VEGF production by cancer cells.

C. nutans water extract suppresses VEGF-induced aortic ring sprouting and angiogenesis in CAM model

To investigate the effect of *C. nutans* water extract on the VEGF-induced vascular sprouting, a rat aortic ring assay was performed. In the control, the non-stimulated aortic rings exhibited a sprout area of 1.14 ± 0.09 mm^2 (Fig. 8). Similar to the tube formation assay, the aortic ring sprouting effect was improved to 1.74 ± 0.28 mm^2

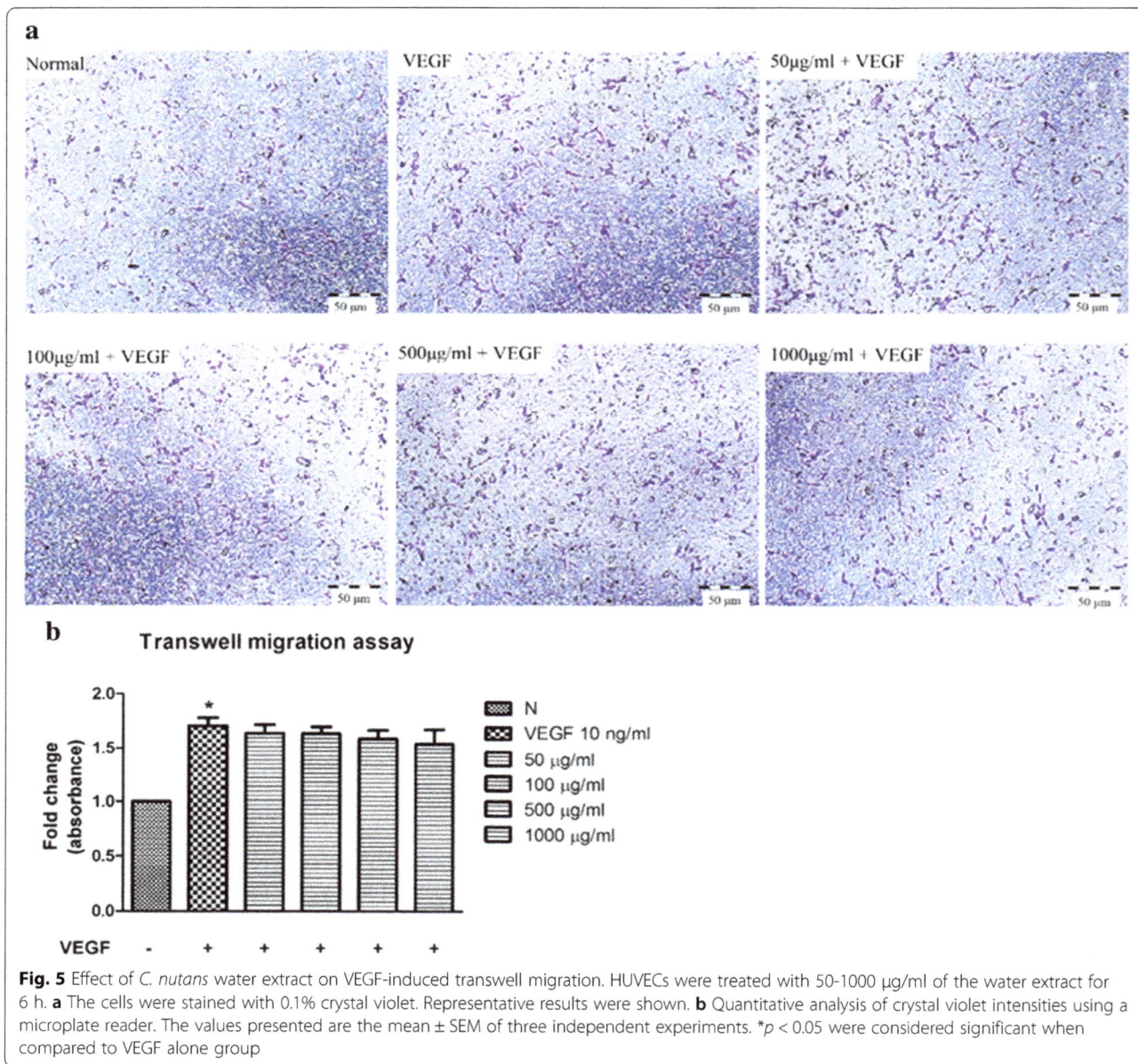

Fig. 5 Effect of *C. nutans* water extract on VEGF-induced transwell migration. HUVECs were treated with 50-1000 μg/ml of the water extract for 6 h. **a** The cells were stained with 0.1% crystal violet. Representative results were shown. **b** Quantitative analysis of crystal violet intensities using a microplate reader. The values presented are the mean ± SEM of three independent experiments. *$p < 0.05$ were considered significant when compared to VEGF alone group

in the presence of VEGF, but was completed abolished by 50 μM Suramin. When the rings were treated with 100, 500 and 1000 μg/ml of *C. nutans* water extracts, sprout area was significantly reduced to 0.71 ± 0.05, 0.33 ± 0.03 and 0.03 ± 0.03 mm^2, respectively. These data indicate that *C. nutans* water extract inhibits vascular sprouting and fusion of neovessels ex vivo. We then tested this effect in an in vivo CAM model, and observed the similar capability in *C. nutans* water extract, of which successfully diminish microvessel counts to 14.90 ± 1.40 and 13.40 ± 1.49 at 1000 and 2000 μg respectively, as compared to VEGF treated (23.50 ± 1.94) and water-treated control group (15.90 ± 1.34) (Fig. 9).

These results suggest that *C. nutans* water extract inhibits angiogenesis in vivo.

Discussion

Tumour angiogenesis is one the main contributing factors that promotes tumour progression. Thus, targeting the blood supply may limit its growth and progression [23]. However, simultaneous targeting of multiple aspects may be required to achieve robust antiangiogenic response. This multi-targeted effect can be achieved by using combinations of drugs, or from natural medicinal herb extracts which possess various active ingredients. *C. nutans* has emerged as a potential regimen for cancer

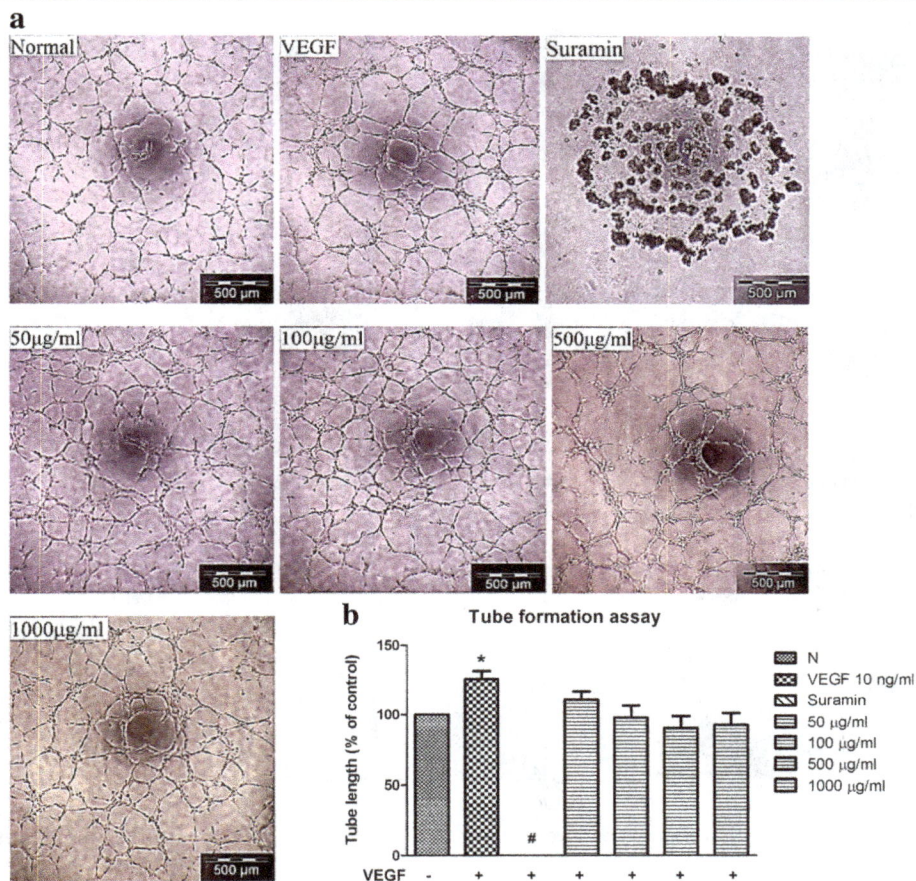

Fig. 6 Effect of *C. nutans* water extract on VEGF-induced capillary-like endothelial tube formation. **a** Microscopic examination demonstrated *C. nutans* extract does not suppressed VEGF-induced capillary-tube like formation in comparison with VEGF group. **b** Capillary-tube like vessel density was calculated and compared. The values presented are the mean ± SEM of three independent experiments. *$p < 0.05$ were considered significant when compared to normal control (N); #$p < 0.05$ were considered significant when compared to VEGF alone group

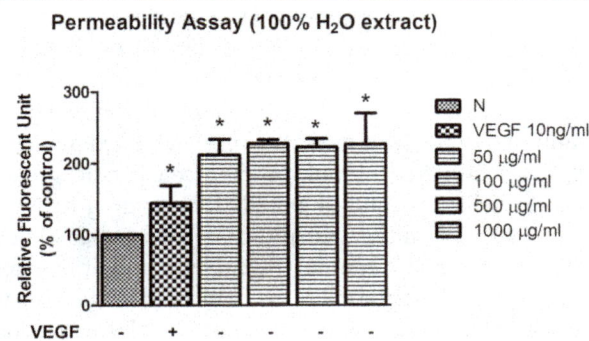

Fig. 7 Effect of *C. nutans* leaf extract on endothelial permeability. The values presented are the mean ± SEM of three independent experiments. *$p < 0.05$ were considered significant when compared to normal control (N)

patients as accumulating lay testimonies claimed that *C. nutans* leaves capable to treat various cancer diseases [7]. Whilst more scientific evidence is needed to conclude its therapeutic use, our previous study has also shown that the *C. nutans* leaves exhibiting anti-proliferative and cytotoxicity effect against numbers of cancer cell lines [7]. Here, we demonstrated the potential of *C. nutans* extracts as being the antiangiogenic agent in cancer treatment.

Under physiological conditions, endothelial cell migration is coordinated by cytoskeleton reorganization where protrusions formed by lamellipodia direct the migrating cells, and this is followed by contraction of stress fibres which allows the cell body to move forward [24]. This dynamic and tightly regulated process, however, is disrupted during tumour angiogenesis, resulting in excessive cell migration and proliferation, the pivotal processes that eventually leads to structure tube and microvessel morphogenesis. In this study, we showed that these processes can be inhibited by *C. nutans*,

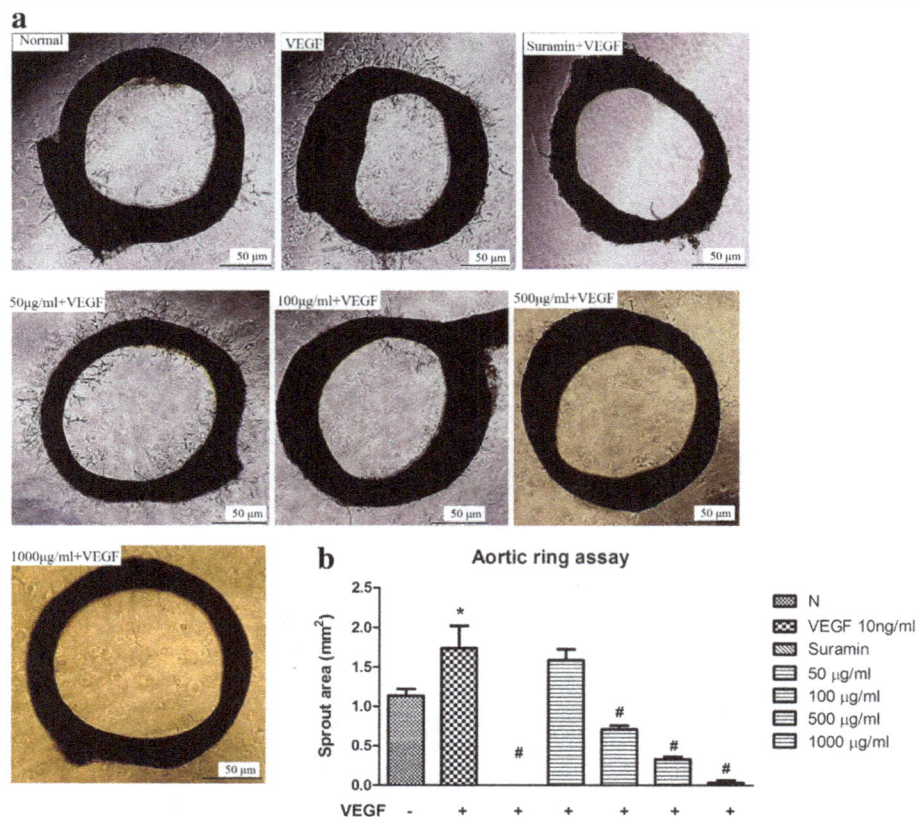

Fig. 8 Effect of *C. nutans* leaf extract on VEGF-induced microvessel sprouting of rat aortic ring. Suramin at a dose of 50 µM was used as a positive control. **a** *C. nutans* water extract inhibited vessel sprouting in rat aorta ring induced by VEGF. Representative results were shown. **b** The sprout length was quantified. The values presented are the mean ± SEM of three independent experiments. *$p < 0.05$ were considered significant when compared to normal control (N); #$p < 0.05$ were considered significant when compared to VEGF alone group. ($n = 3$)

particularly the extracts from the water soluble fraction. We also tested the effect of the extracts and confirmed their efficacy even in the presence of human $VEGF_{165}$, the most abundant and active isoform of VEGF-A monomer [24], which mediates angiogenesis within tumour microenvironment [25]. Taken together, our data support the notion that the water extract of *C. nutans* is capable of inhibiting VEGF-stimulated angiogenesis by targeting endothelial cell proliferation, structure tubes and microvessel formation, but not endothelial migration. Endothelial cell migration also depends on the existence of a VEGF gradient, which serves as an attractant and regulates the motion of the endothelial tip cell [19]. The Boyden chamber assay demonstrated that *C. nutans* water extract does not prevent HUVEC migration towards a chemotatic gradient, indicating that *C. nutans* does not inhibit VEGF-induced chemotaxis (Fig. 5). "Wound healing" and Boyden chamber both are type of assay to determine the migration rate of the endothelial cells, interestingly, "wound healing" assay was inhibited by the extract but Boyden chamber model failed to be inhibited by the extract. Previously reported that "wound repair" model is a multi-step process involving spreading, proliferation and migration events [26, 27], and our data showed that extract significantly suppressed proliferation. This again confirmed that extract inhibits "wound repair" model may via suppression of proliferation process. However, Boyden chamber model is mainly involved in migration process, thus, this indicate extracts not be able to suppress endothelial migration.

Vascular hyperpermeability is a hallmark of acute inflammation, a pathologic event that responsible for oedema and coronary heart diseases [28]. In cancers, chronic vessel hyperpermeability may facilitate leukocyte infiltration into the tumour, promote metastatic spread of cancer cells [29], and impaired efficient drug delivery due to increased interstitial pressure [30]. Drugs which capable to normalize tumour vasculature and attenuates the exaggerated permeability has emerged to be a new concept in anti-angiogenic therapy [31]. Normalization of abnormal vasculature able to increase the efficacy of conventional therapies and decrease the rate of metastasis even though it makes the vasculature to be more efficient for oxygen delivery towards the tumour [31].

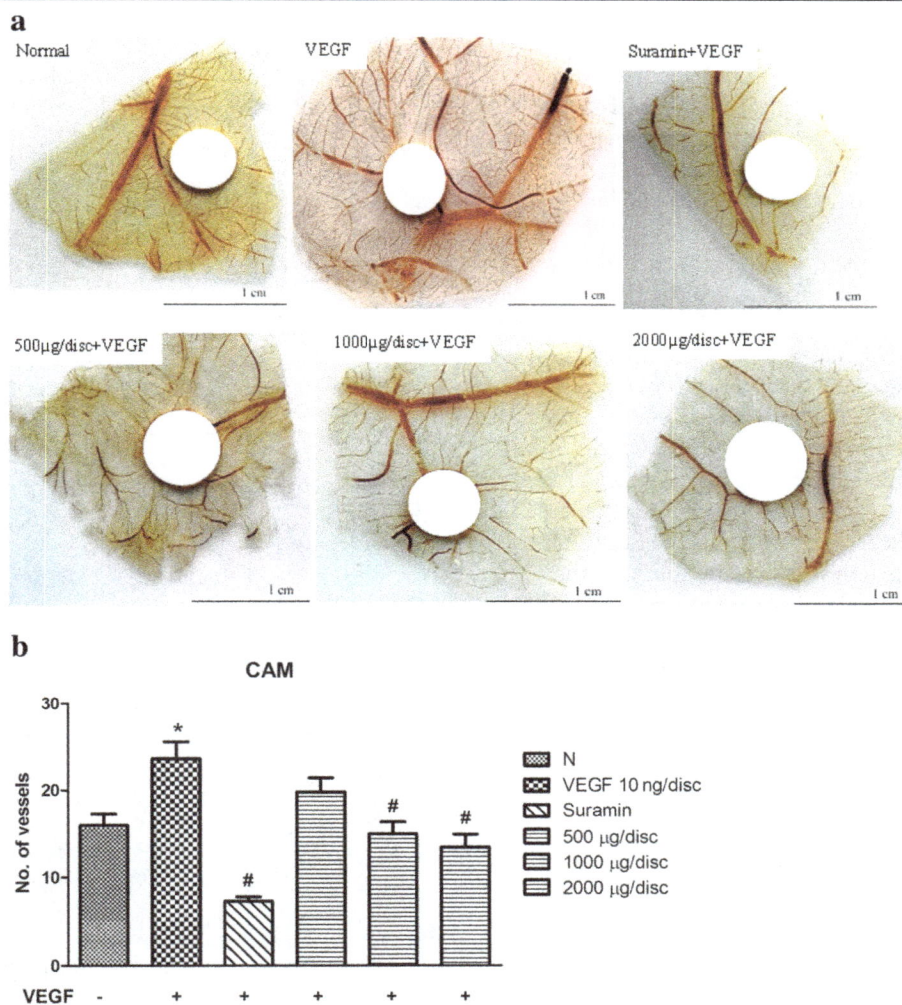

Fig. 9 Effect of *C. nutans* water extract on VEGF-induced angiogenesis. Suramin at a dose of 1000 μg/disc was used as a positive control. **a** *C. nutans* extract inhibited vessel sprouting in CAM model induced by VEGF. Representative results were shown. **b** The histogram shows the number of blood vessels contacting the discs. The values presented are the mean ± SEM of three independent experiments. *$p < 0.05$ were considered significant when compared to normal control (N); #$p < 0.05$ were considered significant when compared to VEGF alone group

Noteworthy, our findings suggest that *C. nutans* water extract could cause an increase in HUVEC permeability without addition of VEGF. The underlying mechanism is unknown; however, this data discouraged further study and development of *C. nutans* water extract as a potential therapeutic agent.

Apart from the cellular systems, we also examined the beneficial effects of *C. nutans* water extract using both ex vivo and in vivo models. In comparison to isolated cell culture, these models are more physiologically relevant because they allow complex cellular interactions to occur. The aortic ring assay is a type of organ culture that permits the interactions of endothelial cells with their surrounding heterotypic cells. In this assay, the endothelial cells are in a quiescent and non-proliferative state at the time of explantation. In response to pro-angiogenic agents, the cells proliferate, migrate and differentiate into tubular networks, resembling the in vivo condition [32]. In the present study, we found that *C. nutans* water extract significantly inhibits the microvessel outgrowth triggered by VEGF (Fig. 8), suggesting that the water extract of *C. nutans* leaves also possesses potential anti-angiogenic properties in isolated aortic tissues. The CAM model was used due to easy accessibility and highly vascularized nature of the system [33]. We demonstrated that *C. nutans* water extract prevents new blood vessel formation in the CAM model (Fig. 9). This finding is in line with the inhibitory effects of *C. nutans* on cell proliferation and migration observed in vitro, implying that the anti-angiogenic effects of *C. nutans* in HUVECs can be translated to in vivo models as well. GC-MS, chemical, ^{1}H NMR and ^{13}C NMR, HPLC with tandem mass spectrometry (LC/MS/MS) showed that vitexin, isovitexin and betulin [34] were among the phytochemicals that present in *C. nutans* extract which had previously demonstrated anti-angiogenesis activities [35–37]. Thus, the observed angiogenic activities in this study were likely the effect of, but not limited to, these active compounds, albeit further in-depth investigation is needed.

Number of angiogenic growth factors are known to be involved in the process of angiogenesis, this including VEGF, fibroblast growth factors, and the platelet-derived endothelial cell growth factor [38]. Binding of these angiogenic growth factors to its corresponding receptors on the surface of normal endothelial cell promote the activation of endothelial cells [39]. As a result, new blood vessels sprout from the pre-existing blood vessels. Anti-angiogenic therapies targeting various steps in this process. For instance, bevacizumab specifically binds to VEGF and thus inactivate VEGF [40]. On the other hand, Sunitinib malate has been shown to be a potent inhibitor of VEGF receptors [41]. In the current data, *C. nutans* water extract does not inhibit VEGF secretion by cancer cells. This may indicate that *C. nutans* water extract is specific to inhibit the action of VEGF on endothelial cells but not the production of VEGF from the cancer cells. Further investigation is needed in order to confirm whether *C. nutans* water extract is acting through the VEGF receptor.

Conclusion

In conclusion, we showed that *C. nutans* is capable of impeding VEGF-induced blood vessel formation by targeting on endothelial cell proliferation, aortic vessel sprouting and the growth of micro-vessels in CAM. For the first time, we demonstrate the anti-angiogenic potential of *C. nutans* in water extract and this activity may be associated with the active compounds such as vitexin, isovitexin and betulin. However, more in-depth investigations to identify the molecular target for therapeutic intervention and to evaluate the efficacy and safety of *C. nutans* water extract in diseased animal models are required to warrant translation to therapeutics for clinical use.

Abbreviations
CAM: Chorioallantoic membrane; FITC: Fluorescein isothiocyanate; HUVECs: Human umbilical vein endothelial cells; VEGF: Vascular endothelial growth factor

Acknowledgements
This study was completed in the support by the funding from NKEA Research Grant Scheme (NRGS) No.NH1014D071, Herbal Development Office (HDO), Ministry of Agriculture and Agro-based Industry, Malaysia.

Funding
Research funding from NKEA Research Grant Scheme (NRGS) No.NH1014D071, Herbal Development Office (HDO), Ministry of Agriculture and Agro-based Industry, Malaysia.

Authors' contributions
CTN, LYF, JJT, NFR and YKY participated in the design of the research; YKY and JJT guided the group of researchers. FA, KS and FJ contributed to plant collection, identification and extraction; CTN and LYF carried out the experiments and analysed the data under supervision of YKY. CTN and YKY wrote the paper; JJT, NFR and KMC critically revised the manuscript. All authors read and approved the final manuscript.

Competing interests
The authors declare that they have no competing interests.

Author details
[1]Physiology Unit, Faculty of Medicine, AIMST University, 08100 Bedong, Kedah, Malaysia. [2]Department of Pre-clinical Sciences, Faculty of Medicine and Health Sciences, Universiti Tunku Abdul Rahman, 43000 Kajang, Selangor, Malaysia. [3]Advance Medical and Dental Institute, Universiti Sains Malaysia, Penang, Malaysia. [4]Faculty of Health Sciences, Universiti Kebangsaan Malaysia, 50300 Kuala Lumpur, Malaysia. [5]Department of Food Science, Faculty of Food Science and Technology, Universiti Putra Malaysia, 43400 UPM Serdang, Malaysia. [6]Faculty of Science, Universiti Putra Malaysia, 43400 UPM Serdang, Malaysia. [7]Department of Human Anatomy, Faculty of Medicine and Health Sciences, Universiti Putra Malaysia, 43400 UPM Serdang, Selangor, Malaysia.

References
1. Shibuya M. Vascular endothelial growth factor (VEGF) and its receptor (VEGFR) signaling in angiogenesis: a crucial target for anti- and pro-angiogenic therapies. Genes Cancer. 2011;2:1097–105.
2. Casey SC, Amedei A, Aquilano K, Azmi AS, Benencia F, Bhakta D, et al. Cancer prevention and therapy through the modulation of the tumor microenvironment. Semin Cancer Biol. 2015;35:S199–223.
3. Wang Z, Dabrosin C, Yin X, Fuster MM, Arreola A, Rathmell WK, et al. Broad targeting of angiogenesis for cancer prevention and therapy. Semin Cancer Biol. 2015;35:S224–43.
4. Roviello G, Zanotti L, Cappelletti MR, Gobbi A, Senti C, Bottini A, et al. No advantage in survival with targeted therapies as maintenance in patients with limited and extensive-stage small cell lung cancer: a literature-based meta-analysis of randomized trials. Clin Lung Cancer. 2016;17:334–40.
5. Alam A, Ferdosh S, Ghafoor K, Hakim A, Juraimi AS, Khatib A, et al. *Clinacanthus nutans*: a review of the medicinal uses, pharmacology and phytochemistry. Asian Pac J Trop Med. 2016;9:402–9.
6. Teoh PL, Cheng AYF, Liau M, Lem FF, Kaling GP, Chua FN, et al. Chemical composition and cytotoxic properties of *Clinacanthus nutans* root extracts. Pharm Biol. 2017;55:394–401.
7. Yong YK, Tan JJ, Teh SS, Mah SH, Ee GCL, Chiong HS, et al. *Clinacanthus nutans* extracts are antioxidant with antiproliferative effect on cultured human cancer cell lines. Evid Based Complement Alternat Med. 2013;2013: 462751.
8. Mai CW, Yap KS, Kho MT, Ismail NH, Yusoff K, Shaari K, et al. Mechanisms underlying the anti-inflammatory effects of *Clinacanthus nutans* Lindau extracts: inhibition of cytokine production and toll-like receptor-4 activation. Front Pharmacol. 2016;7:7.
9. Huang D, Guo W, Gao J, Chen J, Olatunji JO. *Clinacanthus nutans* (Burm. f.) Lindau ethanol extract inhibits hepatoma in mice through upregulation of the immune response. Molecules. 2015;20:17405–28.
10. Fong SY, Piva T, Dekiwadia C, Urban S, Huynh T. Comparison of cytotoxicity between extracts of *Clinacanthus nutans* (Burm. f.) Lindau leaves from different locations and the induction of apoptosis by the crude methanol leaf extract in D24 human melanoma cells. BMC Complement Altern Med. 2016;16:368.
11. Khoo LW, Mediani A, Zolkeflee NKZ, Leong SW, Ismail IS, Khatib A, et al. Phytochemical diversity of Clinacanthus nutans extracts and their bioactivity correlations elucidated by NMR based metabolomics. Phytochem Lett. 2015; 14:123–33.
12. Mosmann T. Rapid colorimetric assay for cellular growth and survival: application to proliferation and cytotoxicity assays. J Immunol Methods. 1983;65:55–63.

13. Kavitha CV, Agarwal C, Agarwal R, Deep G. Asiatic acid inhibits pro-angiogenic effects of VEGF and human gliomas in endothelial cell culture models. PLoS One. 2011;6:e22745.

14. Arnaoutova I, Kleinman HK. In vitro angiogenesis: endothelial cell tube formation on gelled basement membrane extract. Nat Protoc. 2010;5:628–35.

15. Ng CT, Fong LY, Sulaiman MR, Moklas MAM, Yong YK, Hakim MN, et al. Interferon-gamma increases endothelial permeability by causing activation of p38 MAP kinase and actin cytoskeleton alteration. J Interf Cytokine Res. 2015;35:513–22.

16. Bellacen K, Lewis EC. Aortic ring assay. J Vis Exp. 2009;33:e1564.

17. West DC, Thompson WD, Sells PG, Burbridge MF. Angiogenesis assays using chick chorioallantoic membrane. Methods Mol Med. 2001;46:107–29.

18. Simons M, Gordon E, Claesson-Welsh L. Mechanisms and regulation of endothelial VEGF receptor signalling. Nat Rev Mol Cell Biol. 2016;17:611–25.

19. Norton KA, Popel AS. Effects of endothelial cell proliferation and migration rates in a computational model of sprouting angiogenesis. Sci Rep. 2016;6:36992.

20. Des Rieux A, Ucakar B, Mupendwa BPK, Colau D, Feron O, Carmeliet P, et al. 3D systems delivering VEGF to promote angiogenesis for tissue engineering. J Control Release. 2011;150:272–8.

21. Margolles-Clark E, Jacques-Silva MC, Ganesan L, Umland O, Kenyon NS, Ricordi C, et al. Suramin inhibits the CD40–CD154 costimulatory interaction: a possible mechanism for immunosuppressive effects. Biochem Pharmacol. 2009;77:1236–45.

22. Michi Y, Morita I, Amagasa T, Murota S. Human oral squamous cell carcinoma cell lines promote angiogenesis via expression of vascular endothelial growth factor and upregulation of KDR/flk-1 expression in endothelial cells. Oral Oncol. 2000;36:81–8.

23. Linkous AG, Yazlovitskaya EM. Novel therapeutic approaches for targeting tumor angiogenesis. Anticancer Res. 2012;32:1–12.

24. Lamalice L, Le Boeuf F, Huot J. Endothelial cell migration during angiogenesis. Circ Res. 2007;100:782–94.

25. Hoeben A, Landuyt B, Highley MS, Wildiers H, Van Oosterom AT, De Bruijn EA. Vascular endothelial growth factor and angiogenesis. Pharmacol Rev. 2004;56:549–80.

26. Wong MK, Gotlieb AI. The reorganization of microfilaments, centrosomes, and microtubules during in vitro small wound reendothelialization. J Cell Biol. 1988;107:1777–83.

27. Coomber BL, Gotlieb AI. In vitro endothelial wound repair. Interaction of cell migration and proliferation. Arteriosclerosis. 1990;10:215–22.

28. Weis SM. Vascular permeability in cardiovascular disease and cancer. Curr Opin Hematol. 2008;15:243–9.

29. Claesson-Welsh L. Vascular permeability—the essentials. Ups J Med Sci. 2015;120:135–43.

30. Azzi S, Hebda JK, Gavard J. Vascular permeability and drug delivery in cancers. Front Oncol. 2013;3:211.

31. Jain RK. Normalization of tumor vasculature: an emerging concept in antiangiogenic therapy. Science. 2005;307:58–62.

32. Staton CA, Reed MW, Brown NJ. A critical analysis of current in vitro and in vivo angiogenesis assays. Int J Exp Pathol. 2009;90:195–221.

33. Ribatti D. Chicken chorioallantoic membrane angiogenesis model. Methods Mol Biol. 2012;843:47–57.

34. Zulkipli IN, Rajabalaya R, Idris A, Sulaiman NA, David SR. Clinacanthus nutans: a review on ethnomedical uses, chemical constituents and pharmacological properties. Pharm Biol. 2017;55:1093–113.

35. Wang J, Zheng X, Zeng G, , Zhou Y, Yuan H. Purified vitexin compound 1 inhibits growth and angiogenesis through activation of FOXO3a by inactivation of Akt in hepatocellular carcinoma. Int J Mol Med 2014; 33:441–448.

36. Abu Bakar AR, Ripen AM, Merican AF, Mohamad SB. Enzymatic inhibitory activity of Ficus deltoidea leaf extract on matrix metalloproteinase-2, 8 and 9. Nat Prod Res. 2018; https://doi.org/10.1080/14786419.2018.1434631

37. Dehelean CA, Feflea S, Gheorgheosu D, Cimpean AM, Muntean D, Amiji MM. Anti-angiogenic and anti-cancer evaluation of betulin nanoemulsion in chicken chorioallantoic membrane and skin carcinoma in Balb/c mice. J Biomed Nanotechnol. 2013;9:577–89.

38. Nguyen M. Angiogenic factors as tumor markers. Investig New Drugs. 1997; 15:29–37.

39. Nor JE, Christensen J, Mooney DJ, Polverini PJ. Vascular endothelial growth factor (VEGF)-mediated angiogenesis is associated with enhanced endothelial cell survival and induction of Bcl-2 expression. Am J Pathol. 1999;154:375–84.

40. Shih T, Lindley C. Bevacizumab: an angiogenesis inhibitor for the treatment of solid malignancies. Clin Ther. 2006;28:1779–802.

41. Faivre S, Delbaldo C, Vera K, Robert C, Lozahic S, Lassau N, et al. Safety, pharmacokinetic, and antitumor activity of SU11248, a novel oral multitarget tyrosine kinase inhibitor, in patients with cancer. J Clin Oncol. 2006;24:25–35.

4

Induction of programmed cell death in *Trypanosoma cruzi* by *Lippia alba* essential oils and their major and synergistic terpenes (citral, limonene and caryophyllene oxide)

Érika Marcela Moreno[1], Sandra Milena Leal[1,2], Elena E. Stashenko[3] and Liliana Torcoroma García[1*] (ID)

Abstract

Background: Chagas Disease caused by *Trypanosoma cruzi* infection, is one of the most important neglected tropical diseases (NTD), without an effective therapy for the successful parasite eradication or for the blocking of the disease's progression, in its advanced stages. Due to their low toxicity, wide pharmacologic spectrum, and potential synergies, medicinal plants as *Lippia alba*, offer a promising reserve of bioactive molecules. The principal goal of this work is to characterize the inhibitory properties and cellular effects of the Citral and Carvone *L. alba* chemotype essential oils (EOs) and their main bioactive terpenes (and the synergies among them) on *T. cruzi* forms.

Methods: Twelve *L. alba* EOs, produced under diverse environmental conditions, were extracted by microwave assisted hydrodistillation, and chemically characterized using gas chromatography coupled mass spectrometry. Trypanocidal activity and cytotoxicity were determined for each oil, and their major compounds, on epimastigotes (Epi), trypomastigotes (Tryp), amastigotes (Amas), and Vero cells. Pharmacologic interactions were defined by a matrix of combinations among the most trypanocidal terpenes (limonene, carvone; citral and caryophyllene oxide). The treated cell phenotype was assessed by fluorescent and optic microscopy, flow cytometry, and DNA electrophoresis assays.

Results: The *L. alba* EOs displayed significant differences in their chemical composition and trypanocidal performance ($p = 0.0001$). Citral chemotype oils were more trypanocidal than Carvone EOs, with Inhibitory Concentration 50 (IC_{50}) of 14 ± 1.5 μg/mL, 22 ± 1.4 μg/mL and 74 ± 4.4 μg/mL, on Epi, Tryp and Amas, respectively. Limonene exhibited synergistic interaction with citral, caryophyllene oxide and Benznidazole (decreasing by 17 times its IC_{50}) and was the most effective and selective treatment. The cellular analysis suggested that these oils or their bioactive terpenes (citral, caryophyllene oxide and limonene) could be inducing *T. cruzi* cell death by an apoptotic-like mechanism.

Conclusions: EOs extracted from *L. alba* Citral chemotype demonstrated significant trypanocidal activity on the three forms of *T. cruzi* studied, and their composition and trypanocidal performance were influenced by production parameters. Citral, caryophyllene oxide, and limonene showed a possible induction of an apoptotic-like phenotype. The best selective anti-*T. cruzi* activity was achieved by limonene, the effects of which were also synergic with citral, caryophyllene oxide and benznidazole.

Keywords: *Lippia alba*, Essential oils, Citral, Caryophyllene oxide, Limonene, Synergy, *Trypanosoma cruzi*

---

* Correspondence: l.torcoroma@udes.edu.co
[1]Infectious Disease Research Program, Universidad de Santander, 680006 Bucaramanga, Colombia
Full list of author information is available at the end of the article

Background

Chagas Disease is one of the most important Neglected Tropical Diseases (NTDs) worldwide, and is one of the most relevant public health problems in Latin America. This infection, caused by the hemoflagellated protozoan *Trypanosoma cruzi*, currently affects an estimated 7 million people in the world, with around 99% of all registered cases occurring in Central and South American countries [1]. The global costs of this disease are calculated at approximately USD $7.19 billion per year [2], with regional economic losses of almost US $1.2 billion, annually [3]. In Colombia, the prevalence of this trypanosomiasis is estimated to be within a range of 700,000 – 1,200,000 cases, with more than 8,000,000 persons at risk [4].

In regions where the condition is endemic, disease-control efforts principally centered on preventing or reducing the *T. cruzi* transmission cycle by vector eradication and massive blood donation screening [5]. However, bigger challenges remain; in particular, those associated with the changing epidemiological profile of the infection (diversity of vectors, reservoirs, and modes of transmission), being the most significant problem, the lack of effective therapies to cure the *T. cruzi* infection or to prevent the progression of the disease, principally in advanced stages.

At present, the conventional Chagas Disease treatments are etiologic, and are comprised of only two possible options, Nifurtimox (NFX) (Lampit®, Bayer) and Benznidazole (BNZ) (Rochagan® in Brazil and Radanil® in Argentina, Roche). These two treatments have remained the standard since their introduction into clinical therapy more than 40 years ago [6]. As disadvantages, these treatments are highly toxic (often accompanied by serious side effects like digestive intolerance, severe anorexia and neurological disorders) [7]; involve prolonged treatment times; and demonstrate variable trypanocidal effectiveness in acute stage (with about 80% being associated with natural resistance). They also display limited efficacy in the late phase of the infection (in which the benefits of these therapies have not clearly defined) [8, 9].

In general, these conventional therapies do not take into account the complex cascade of cellular events leading to Chagasic cardiomyopathy, which are not only associated with the parasite's presence, but also involve exacerbated and persistent immune response (with cellular and neuronal damage) [10, 11]. These latter factors are those which govern the microvasculopathy and cardiac failure associated with the condition [10, 11].

In this regard, the research and development of new alternative therapies for Chagas Disease remain pressing concerns. New pharmacological approaches should be more efficient and selective, seeking complete parasite elimination, but with adequate modulation of the host immune response and limitation of cellular damage [11]. To this end, in the last two decades, intensive research has been focused on the study of the properties of whole extracts or compounds isolated from plants or synthesized based on natural prototypes, which have shown promising results against parasite infections [12, 13].

Essential oils (EOs) extracted from aromatic plants and their main components have been described as broad-spectrum antimicrobial agents [14], with significant anthelmintic and antiprotozoal activity [15, 16]. Some terpenes of these oils such as citral (*Lippia alba* and *Cymbopogon citratus*), caryophyllene oxide (*Aframomum sceptrum*, *Achillea millefolium*, and *Piper var brachypodon*), and limonene (*L. origanoides* and *L. pedunculosa*) have demonstrated efficient trypanocidal activity on extra and intracellular forms of *T. cruzi* [17–20]. In addition, these terpenes have been found to exhibit other interesting biological properties, such as being anti-inflammatory immunomodulators, selective antioxidants, and cytoprotectors [21–24]. The presence of citral, caryophyllene and limonene has been identified in EOs isolated from two chemotypes (Citral and Carvone) of the aromatic shrub *Lippia alba* (Miller) N.E. Brown (Verbenaceae), that grows in the Colombian province of Santander [21, 25]. *L. alba* represents the seventh species most cited in traditional Brazilian medicine [26]. The "healers" use their leaves as an infusion to treat health problems such as hypertension, digestive, colds and local wound healing [27, 28]. In the state of Boyacá, Colombia, it is frequently used as an analgesic, for digestive (diarrhea, stomach pain) and respiratory problems (flu and cough) [29]. Previous screening studies with these oils evidenced selective inhibition and cytotoxicity against trypanosomatid parasites, in vitro [30]. Taking into consideration their numerous functions, *L. alba* EOs and their bioactive terpenes are a promising platform for development of holistic therapies to combat Chagas Disease. This kind of approach could allow for a selective eradication of the parasite, with less toxicity (even with chemoprotection), and for controlling the host immune response, through a possible synergistic interaction of the compounds involved [22, 31, 32].

The principal goal of this work is to characterize the inhibitory properties and cellular effects of the Citral and Carvone *L. alba* chemotype EOs and their main bioactive terpenes on *T. cruzi* epimastigotes, trypomastigotes, and amastigotes cyclic forms. The IC_{50} was determined for each of these compounds, and possible pharmacologic interactions were defined by a matrix of combinations of the trypanocidal compounds (from Carvone chemotype: limonene and carvone; and from Citral chemotype: citral and caryophyllene oxide). The phenotype of the parasites and mammal cells treated with EOs or terpenes was followed by fluorescent and optic microscopy, flow cytometry, and DNA electrophoresis assays.

Methods

Plant material

In this study, specimens of the Citral and Carvone chemotypes of *Lippia alba* (Miller) N. E. Brown (Verbenaceae) were planted in the National Research Center for Agroindustrialization of Aromatic Medical and Tropical species (CENIVAM, in Spanish) located in Bucaramanga, Santander, Colombia, at an altitude of 960 m above sea level. The formal identification of the plant specimens used in this study was provided by Prof. Jorge Luis Fernández Alonso and the vouchers were deposited at the Colombian National Herbarium (Universidad Nacional de Colombia) under Herbarium Codes COL480750 and COL512077, for Carvone and Citral chemotypes of *L. alba*, respectively. A range of environmental and production conditions were used in order to produce 76 EOs with possible diversity in their main compounds. In this regard, the vegetal material was grown, collected, and extracted under the following factors. 1) season: defined as dry (January to March, 26.3 °C temperature, with 68.9% relative humidity, and 1.05 mm/day precipitation) and rainy (April to November, mean temperature of 24.5 °C, relative humidity of 81.3%, and 4.13 mm of daily precipitation); 2) *L. alba* chemotypes (53 from Carvone and 23 from Citral); 3) part of plant harvested (root, stem, fresh and mature leaves, and flowers); 4) vegetal material conditions (fresh and dry); and 5) extraction time (from 30 to 90 min).

Essential oils extraction and characterization

The oil extraction was performed by microwave-assisted hydrodistillation (MWHD), as described elsewhere [25, 29]. Briefly, a domestic microwave oven (Kendo, 2.45 GHz, 800 W) was modified with a side orifice through which an external Dean-Stark trap joined a round flask that contained the plant material (100 g) and water (0.5 L), inside the oven. Three 15 min heating periods at full power were used to perform the hydrodistillation. The Dean-Stark trap permitted to decant the essential oil from the condensate. A gas chromatograph GC 7890 (Agilent Technologies, AT, Palo Alto, CA, U.S.A.) coupled to a mass selective detector MSD 5975C (AT, Palo Alto, CA, U.S.A.), using electron impact ionization (EI, 70 eV) was used for essential oil characterization. This system included a split/splitless injector (1:30 split ratio), and a MS-ChemStation G1701-DA data system, with the WILEY, NIST and QUADLIB 2007 spectral libraries. For their GC-MS assays, individual essential oil samples (50 μL) were mixed with *n*-tetradecane (2 μL, internal standard) and diluted with dichloromethane to a final volume of 1.0 mL. Helium (99.9995%) was used as the carrier gas, with 155 kPa column head pressure and 27 cm s^{-1} linear velocity (1 mL minute-1, at constant flow), in two columns of different polarities (DB-5MS and DB-WAX from J&W Scientific, USA). The GC oven

temperature was programmed from 50 °C (5 min) to 150 °C (2 min) at 5 °C min^{-1}, then to 230 °C (10 min) at 5 °C min^{-1}. When the DB-5MS column was used, a final heating to 275 °C (15 min) at 10 °C min^{-1} was added. The temperatures of the injection port, ionization chamber and of the transfer line were set at 250, 230 and 285 °C, respectively. For the polar DB-WAX column, the transfer line temperature was set at 230 °C. Mass spectra and reconstructed (total) ion chromatograms were obtained by automatic scanning in the mass range *m/z* 30–400 at 4.5 scan s^{-1}. Compound relative abundances were calculated from the chromatographic area of profiles obtained with an AT 7890 gas chromatograph provided with flame ionization detection (FID, 250 °C). The chromatographic columns, carrier gas and oven temperature programs employed in GC-FID analysis were the same as described previously for the GC-MS system. The EO compounds were identified using mass spectra and linear retention indices relative to C_8-C_{32} n-alkanes [33]. Several terpenoid standard compounds, such as limonene, carvone, geranial, geraniol, β-caryophyllene, and β-caryophyllene oxide, obtained from Sigma-Aldrich (St. Louis, MO, U.S.A., with purities above 98%) were used. The extracted EOs were preserved at 4 °C and protected from light before GC-MS and cellular analysis. Finally, the 76 EOs were arranged into 12 groups, according to the significant differences in the percentages of their major terpenes and one oil of each group was arbitrarily selected for further biological analysis, comprising six EOs from Citral chemotype (A13, A20, A23, A24, A25, and A28), and six from the Carvone chemotype (B7, B16, B37, 2B8, 2B18, and 2B19).

Terpenes and drugs

The terpenes S (+) carvone, D (+) limonene, (–) caryophyllene oxide, and citral were purchased from Sigma-Aldrich (St. Louis, MO). The reference medication BNZ (Radanil®, Roche) was donated by Santander's State Secretary of Health, and purified by Dr. Leonor Yamile Vargas, from the Environmental Chemistry Program at Universidad Santo Tomás de Aquino (Bucaramanga). Concentrations ranging from 1.85 to 50 μg/mL were used for epimastigote (Epi) and amastigote (Amas) assays and 0.39 to 3.12 μg/mL for trypomastigote (Tryp) assays. The oils (at a density of 0.9 g/mL) and terpene stock solutions were prepared in dimethyl-sulfoxide (DMSO, Sigma-Aldrich (St. Louis, MO)), to get a 10% (*v/v*) solution, without exceeding a DMSO final concentration of 0.1%, in any solution. Working solutions (3.7 to 300 μg/mL) were diluted immediately prior to use with Liver Infusion Tryptose (LIT, Becton Dickinson, FL, USA) media and Dulbecco's Modified Eagle's Medium (DMEM, Life Technology, CA, USA) for *T. cruzi* cells and Vero lineage, respectively.

Cell cultures

Vero lineage derived from African Green Monkey Kidney (Vero, ATCC CCL-81) was used for selectivity index determination and for Tryp and Amas production. These cells were grown on DMEM (Life Technology, CA, USA) media, pH: 7.4; supplemented with 10% of inactivated Fetal Bovine Serum (FBSi), 1000 U/mL of penicillin, and 100 µg/mL of streptomycin; and incubated at 37 °C with 90% humidity and a 5% CO_2 atmosphere. Epi of *T. cruzi* I (TcI) SYLVIO-X10 strain, were donated by Dr. Marcos López-Casillas, from Fundación Cardiovascular de Colombia and grown in LIT medium (Merck) supplemented with 10% FBSi, and incubated at 28 °C. The Trypomastigotes Derived from Cells (TDC) were obtained by infection of a confluent monolayer of Vero cells with 12 day-old stationary growth phase Epi and incubated under the same conditions described above for Vero cells.

Cytotoxic activity on Vero cells

Vero cells (3×10^5 cel/mL) were incubated at 37 °C in a 5% CO_2 atmosphere and at 95% humidity for 24 h to ensure the formation of a confluent monolayer. After this time, the cells were treated with the EOs or their terpenes in four different concentrations (11.1, 33.3, 100, and 300 µg/mL). Thereafter, the lineages were incubated for 70 h at 37 °C in a 5% CO_2 atmosphere and re-incubated 2 more hours with WST-1 (Roche, Mannheim, Germany), after which Optical Density (OD) measurements were analyzed by spectrophotometry. The cytotoxicity percentage was calculated using [(OD_{450nm} Control − OD_{450nm} treatment) / OD_{450nm} treatment)] × 100. The results were expressed as Cytotoxic Concentration 50 (CC_{50}).

Anti-parasitic activity on *T. cruzi*

T. cruzi Epi (5×10^5 Epi/mL) and TDC (5×10^5 cells/mL) in the exponential growth phase were plated in a 96-well standard microplate in LIT medium (at 28 °C) and in D-MEM medium (at 37 °C in a 5% CO_2 atmosphere), respectively. Both cultures were supplemented with 10% FBSi. For the trypanocidal assays, the EOs or their terpenes were added at varying concentrations (3.7 to 100 µg/mL) and incubated at the same culture conditions for 72 (Epi) or 24 h (Tryp). The growth inhibition was estimated by light microscopy through a differential count using the Trypan Blue (Gibco) dye exclusion technique. The results were expressed in terms of Inhibitory Concentration 50 (IC_{50}) or the concentration at which parasite growth is inhibited by 50%. For Amas assays, a monolayer of Vero cells (3×10^5 cel/mL) was infected with TDC in a 1:3 cell:parasite ratio and incubated for 24 h until Amas development occurred. Then, these intracellular forms were exposed for 120 h to EOs or terpenes in a treatment applied in two doses (at 0 and 48 h), under the same conditions described above. Growth inhibition analysis was

assessed in Giemsa-stained films using light microscopy to determine the infected and uninfected cell percentage in a total of 300 cells. Cells without treatment and those treated with BNZ were used as negative and positive controls, respectively.

Pharmacological interaction among terpenes on *T. cruzi*

A matrix of pharmacological interactions between limonene (the most selective terpene) and the other major EO terpenes was created for the three cyclic forms of *T. cruzi*, using the fixed-ratio isobologram method, as described previously by Fivelman et al. [34] with some modifications (Table 1). In the interaction matrix, the estimated IC_{50} for each terpene was used as fixed-value for the combinations. In addition, a mixture of limonene and BNZ was also evaluated.

The susceptibility evaluation was performed following the protocol described above for in vitro anti-parasitic activity. The Fractional Inhibitory Concentration (FIC) was calculated by: (Compound X (FIC) = Compound X (IC_{50}) in combination) / (Compound X (IC_{50}) alone); and the sum of FIC (ΣFIC) was determined by: ΣFIC = Compound X (FIC) + Compound Y (FIC). In this manner, synergistic, antagonist, or additive interactions were defined by $\overline{X}\Sigma CIF < 1$, $\overline{X}\Sigma CIF > 1$ or $\overline{X}\Sigma CIF = 1$, respectively [31].

Analysis of cell death

The death phenotype was analyzed by optical and fluorescent microscopy using phase contrast (fluorescence microscopy, Nikon Eclipse Ni). The cell morphology in Epi treated with two doses of the IC_{50} ($2xIC_{50}$), was examined by the 4 ',6diamidino-2, phenylindole probe (DAPI, 1 µg/mL, Sigma Aldrich) and a TUNEL assay (Molecular Probes, Invitrogen) for DNA fragmentation using a Terminal desoxynucleotidyl Transferase (TdT) label with d-UTP fluorescein. Determination of an oligonucleosomal-DNA ladder in treated parasites was also evaluated through DNA gel electrophoresis. Evaluation of the mitochondrial potential membrane in living parasites was performed with MitoTracker Red CMXRos (579 nm/599 nm emission/excitation wavelength) [35]. As a positive and negative apoptosis control, a 15 day-old

Table 1 Interaction matrix among terpenes

Combination ID Number	Limonene (Compound X)	Compound Y
1	0.0	8× IC_{50}
2	½ IC_{50}	4× IC_{50}
3	IC_{50}	2× IC_{50}
4	2× IC_{50}	IC_{50}
5	4× IC_{50}	½ IC_{50}
6	8× IC_{50}	0.0

IC_{50} Inhibitory Concentration 50, *x* Number of times

Epi culture and an untreated fresh parasite culture were used, respectively.

Flow cytometry analysis

For cell death characterization, an Annexin V/Dead with SYTOX® Green (Molecular Probes, Invitrogen) kit was used following the procedure specified in the manufacturer's instructions. The phosphatidylserine externalization was determined by employing a recombinant Annexin V conjugated to the Orange Fluorescent phycobiliprotein R-PE, and to the necrotic cells using SYTOX™ Green nucleic acid stain. Briefly, 1×10^6 Epi per mL were treated with $2xIC_{50}$ for 48 h, washed, and suspended in 1X Annexin-Binding Buffer. Next, R-PE Annexin V and SYTOX® Green Stain were added and incubated at 37 °C, 5% CO_2, and 95% humidity, and analyzed in a FACSCanto II Flow Cytometer (provided by Dr. Marcos López from Fundación Cardiovascular de Colombia), with 488 nm/575 nm Excitation/Emission filters for R-PE and 503 nm/524 nm Excitation/Emission filters for SYTOX.

Statistical analysis

Each treatment was tested in triplicate in three independent assays. The IC_{50} and CC_{50} were calculated by sigmoidal regression using the statistical software Msxlfit™ (ID Business Solution). The cytotoxicity analysis and statistically-significant difference determinations were performed using a Welch's test for analysis of variances using SPSS 15.0 Software (IBM). Multiple comparison analysis was accomplished using a Tukey test with a 95% confidence level.

Results

Chemical composition and trypanocidal activity of *L. alba* EOs
This work studied the trypanocidal properties of 12 EOs isolated from Citral and Carvone *L. alba* chemotypes produced under an array of standardized conditions for planting, collecting and extracting of the vegetal material. A typical chromatographic profile for each chemotype essential oil, obtained by mass spectra and linear retention indices, is showed in Fig. 1a and b, for Carvone and Citral oils, respectively. The corresponding peak assignment of these chromatograms are listed in Table 2.

All the EOs presented diversity in their chemical composition, and this variety also appeared as significant differences in their trypanocidal performance on the three cyclic forms of the parasite (Epi: F = 1320.080; $p = 0.000$; Tryp: F = 628.786; $p = 0.000$; Amas: F = 853.422; $p = 0.000$) (Tables 3 and 4, Fig. 2a).

The best trypanocidal performance was observed in oils isolated from Citral chemotype plants, with IC_{50} values of 14 ± 1.5, 22 ± 1.4, and 74 ± 4.4 μg/mL on Epi, Tryp, and Amas, respectively ($p < 0.05$). Among these, the two lowest IC_{50} achieved were by A20 (9 ± 1.2 and 13.9 ± 0.9 μg/mL, on Epi and Tryp, respectively, $p < 0.05$)

and A23 (8 ± 1.3 and 17 ± 1.3 μg/mL, on Epi and Tryp, respectively, $p < 0.05$) (Table 3, Fig. 2a). However, these oils also displayed a low selectivity, with high toxicity levels on Vero cells (A20: $CC_{50=}$ 66 ± 5.9 μg/mL; A23: $CC_{50=}$ 51 ± 6.2 μg/mL). Alternatively, oil A13 exhibited a significant level of anti-*T. cruzi* activity on the three cyclic forms (with IC_{50} of 17 ± 1.7 μg/mL, (SI = 7); IC_{50} 21 ± 1.6 μg/mL, (SI = 5.7); and IC_{50} 88 ± 5.4 μg/mL (SI = 1.4), on Epi, Tryp, and Amas, respectively); high cell death percentages (CDP) (Epi = 85 ± 1.7%; Tryp = 100%; Amas = 57 ± 3.1%; $p < 0.05$), at 100 μg/mL; and low toxic effect on mammal cells (CC_{50} 120 ± 10 μg/mL) (Table 3, Fig. 2a).

In contrast, EOs extracted from Carvone chemotype plants showed higher mean IC_{50} values (88 ± 3.7, 45 ± 2.5, and > 150 μg/mL on Epi, Tryp, and Amas, respectively (Table 4)), with a CDP under 60%, even at high concentrations (100 μg/mL), in both Epi (mean CDP of 56 ± 2.3%) and Tryp (mean CDP of 81 ± 3.1%) forms (Table 4). Among Carvone chemotype oils, the best trypanocidal activity was demonstrated by B7 with IC_{50} 81 ± 2.4 μg/mL, SI = 2.5, and a CDP of 60.1% on Epi forms; and IC_{50} 37 ± 2.1 μg/mL, SI = 5.5, and a CDP of 84.5%, on Tryp stages ($p < 0.05$) (Table 4, Fig. 2a). On *T. cruzi* replicative intracellular forms, none of the Carvone oils demonstrated significant activity (mean $IC_{50} >$ 150 μg/mL; mean CDP 21 ± 4.4%). Nevertheless, on host cells (Vero) these EOs exhibited lower cytotoxicity (mean CC_{50} of 200 ± 11 μg/mL) than Citral oils (mean CC_{50} of 87 ± 8.3 μg/mL) (Table 4, Fig. 2a).

Trypanocidal activity of *L. alba* Terpenes
For further studies using individual compounds, four of the major terpenes were selected from the *L. alba* EOs from both chemotypes, Citral (citral and (–) caryophyllene oxide) and Carvone (D (+) limonene and S (+) carvone). Table 5 presents the IC_{50} values obtained on the three studied parasitic forms and the CC_{50} values estimated on Vero cells.

Among the studied terpenes, D (+) limonene exhibited the best IC_{50} on Tryp (IC_{50} 9 ± 0.8 μg/mL, SI = 32.8, $p < 0.05$), and Amas (IC_{50} 29 ± 0.7 μg/mL, SI = 10.3, $p < 0.05$) forms, (Table 5, Fig. 2b), with the most selective and the least toxic performance on mammal cells (CC_{50} 297 ± 2.4 μg/mL, and SI = 7.1, $p < 0.05$), with a CC_{50} even lower than the reference drug (BNZ: CC_{50} 139 ± 2.3 μg/mL). At the other end of the spectrum, S (+) carvone constituted the terpene with the worst trypanocidal activity on all evolutionary *T. cruzi* forms (Epi: IC_{50} 177 ± 7.9 μg/mL, and SI = 1.4; Tryp: IC_{50} 124 ± 7.8 μg/mL, and SI = 1.9; Amas: $IC_{50} >$ 100 μg/mL) (Table 5). It is worth pointing out that all the terpenoid fractions, except carvone, were able to induce significant cell death on extracellular forms of the parasite at 50 μg/mL (Epi: CDP = 66 ± 1.9%; Tryp: CDP = 90 ± 1.2%, $p < 0.05$) with caryophyllene oxide being the terpene with the highest rate of death on Epi (78 ± 2.3%), and Tryp (98 ± 0.5%, $p < 0.05$).

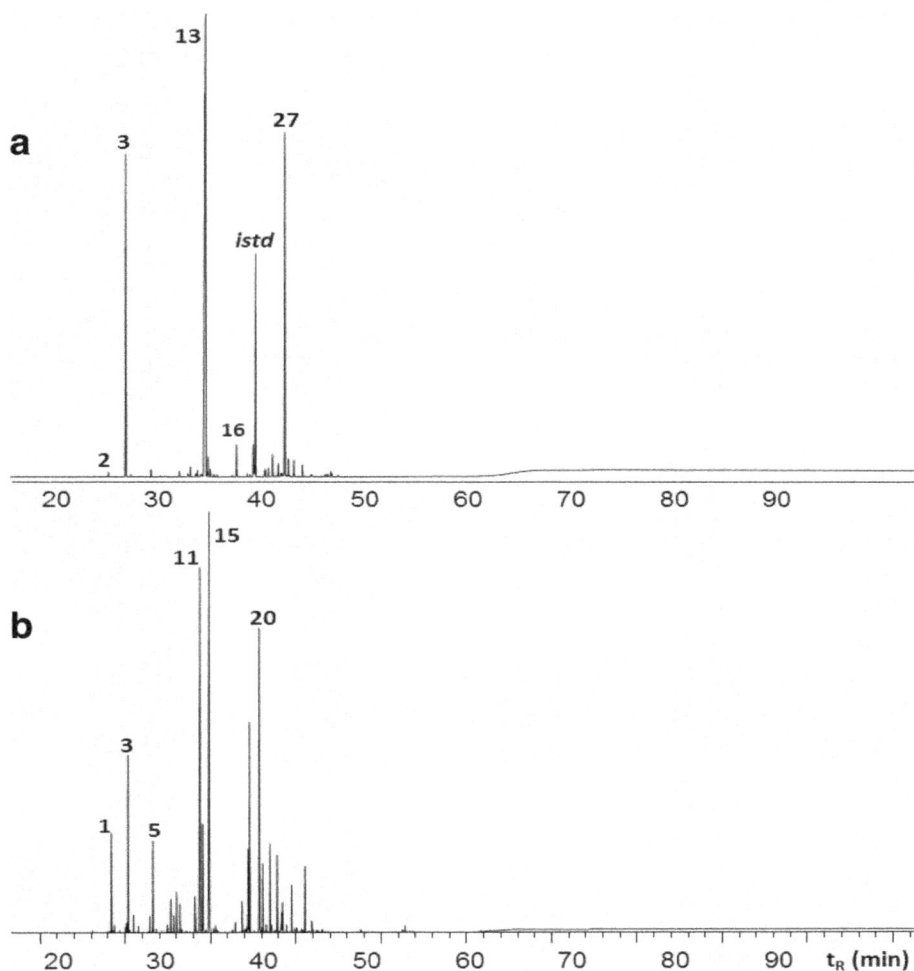

Fig. 1 Typical gas chromatography-mass spectrometry (GC-MS) profiles, in a DB-5 (60 m) column with a mass selective detector (EI. 70 eV), of essential oils obtained from *Lippia alba* Carvone (**a**) and Citral (**b**) chemotypes by microwave-assisted hydrodistillation (MWHD). The corresponding peak identification is showed in Table 2

Terpene pharmacological interactions on *T. cruzi*

Because D (+) limonene demonstrated the best performance as a selective trypanocidal agent on all the evolutionary forms of *T. cruzi*, this monoterpene was selected as a fixed-compound of a pharmacological interaction matrix among terpenes and BNZ. This matrix was assembled taking the IC_{50} values determined previously (Table 5). Following the FIC value interpretation described by Azeredo and Soares, (2013) [31], all the evaluated interactions were found to be synergic on both extra and intracellular forms of the parasite (except limonene with carvone, with $\Sigma FIC = 1.10$ and 1.04, on Epi and Tryp, respectively) (Table 6). Figure 3 shows these pharmacological relations as isobolograms of the mean FIC of each combination. The highest synergy was exhibited by limonene/BNZ combinations (Epi: $\Sigma FIC = 0.44$; Tryp: $\Sigma FIC = 0.42$; Amas: $\Sigma FIC = 0.58$) (Table 6, Fig. 3), with the best trypanocidal performance achieved by the

$4xIC_{50}$ limonene:$\frac{1}{2}IC_{50}$ BNZ mixture (4 times IC_{50} limonene plus one half of the IC_{50} of BNZ), which reduced by 14, 16, and 17 times the BNZ IC_{50} on Amas, Epi, and Tryp, respectively. Despite its good performance, this combination also resulted in an increased cytotoxicity on Vero cells ($\Sigma FIC = 0.54$). On the other hand, limonene with caryophyllene oxide represented the second-best combination by anti-parasitic efficacy (Epi Σ FIC = 0.49; Tryp Σ FIC = 0.45; and Amas Σ FIC = 0.71), while offering an additional advantage of reduction of the individual cytotoxicity of each terpene on Vero cells ($\Sigma FIC = 1.22$) (Table 6, Fig. 3).

Morphological analysis on *T. cruzi* forms

The morphological changes induced by the treatments studied (EOs, terpenes, or BNZ, and their combinations) were analyzed by optical and fluorescent microscopy using phase contrast, and nuclear specific (DAPI) and

Table 2 Peak assignment for GC-MS profiles of essential oils extracted by microwave-assisted hydrodistillation (MWHD) from *Lippia alba* Carvone (A) and Citral (B) chemotypes plants growing in Bucaramanga (Colombia)

Peak	Compound	LRI		Relative Quantity, %	
		DB-5MS[a]	DB-WAX[b]	Carvone (A)	Citral (B)
1	6-Methyl-5-hepten-2-one	986	1241	–	3.3
2	β-Myrcene	991	1064	0.8	–
3	Limonene	1034	1105	29.1	6.6
4	*trans*-β-Ocimene	1047	1153	0.7	0.2
5	Linalool	1100	1453	0.6	1.9
6	Citronellal	1154	1381	–	1.1
7	Borneol	1181	1613	0.8	–
8	*cis*-Dihydrocarvone	1203	1517	0.2	–
9	*trans*-Dihydrocarvone	1211	1537	0.2	–
10	Nerol	1231	1708	–	0.8
11	Neral	1248	1589	–	21.5
12	Geraniol	1252	1755	–	5.6
13	Carvone	1258	1653	35.0	–
14	Piperitone	1264	1641	2.4	–
15	Geranial	1275	1643	–	28.7
16	Piperitenone	1349	1842	4.0	–
17	Geranyl Acetate	1379	1662	–	1.5
18	β-Bourboneno	1396	1428	1.2	–
19	β-Elemene	1397	1496	1.0	3.0
20	*trans*-β-Caryophyllene	1436	1506	0.2	12.1
21	β-Gurjunene	1444	1447	0.2	–
22	α-Guaiene	1447	1498	–	1.8
23	*trans*-β-Farnesene	1456	1570	0.7	–
24	α-Humulene	1471	1580	0.1	2.7
25	γ-Gurjunene	1475	1587	0.4	–
26	Germacrene D	1486	1552	0.1	2.6
27	Bicyclosesquiphellandrene	1496	1624	8.2	–
28	Bicyclogermacrene	1509	1608	0.5	–
29	α-Bulnesene	1515	1627	–	1.4
30	Cubebol	1528	1855	0.5	–
31	Germacrene-4-ol	1591	1967	0.6	–
32	Caryophyllene Oxide	1600	1909	–	2.3

LRI Linear retention index
[a]Linear Retention Index experimentally determined in DB-5MS (60 m) column
[b]Linear Retention Index experimentally determined in DB-WAX (60 m) column

mitochondrial membrane potential (Mitotracker Red CMXRos [35]) stains. As shown in Fig. 4, some of the tested treatments induced significant changes on parasitic morphology such as: spherical cell conformation, reduced cytoplasmic volume (Fig. 4a, DIC), mitochondrial membrane potential depletion (Fig. 4a, MitoTracker), and formation of a nuclear speckled/condensation pattern (Fig. 4a, DAPI). In one unique finding, the caryophyllene oxide treatment also caused a flagellum to be lost. Conversely, *T.*

cruzi cells treated with BNZ displayed cellular edema and loss of cellular membrane integrity, but with conserved mitochondrial energetic potential (Fig. 4a). Under the same conditions, Vero host cells did not present visible morphological alterations (data not shown).

DNA fragmentation

A possible endonuclease activation triggered by studied compounds (oils, terpenes or their combinations) was

Table 3 Relative chemical composition and anti-proliferative effect on *T. cruzi* of EOs extracted from the Citral chemotype of *L. alba*

Season	Material	EO[a]	Extra[b] Time min[c]	Part Plant	Chemical Composition					Epi[f]		Tryp[j]		Amas[k]		Vero
					Neral %	Geraniol %	Geranial %	Caryop[d] %	CarOx[e] %	IC$_{50}$[g] ± SD[h] µg/mL	SI[i]	IC$_{50}$[g] SD[h] µg/mL	SI[i]	IC$_{50}$[g] ± SD[h] µg/mL	SI[i]	CC$_{50}$[l] ± SD[h] µg/mL
Dry	Dry	A28	45	Infl[m]	19.3	31.5	31.3	2.3	–	14 ± 2.6	7.1	31 ± 1.9	3.1	66 ± 4.8	1.5	97 ± 11
Rainy	Fresh	A25	45	AL[n]	22.8	5.3	27.5	4.6	2.8	18 ± 0.7	5.3	19.4 ± 0.9	4.9	> 33.3	ND[r]	95 ± 9.2
	Dry	A13	30	YL[o]	30.6	–	54.5	2.9	–	17 ± 1.7	7.0	21 ± 1.6	5.7	88 ± 5.4	1.4	121 ± 10.1
		A20	30	ML[p]	32.1	–	54	4	2.4	9 ± 1.2	7.8	14 ± 0.9	4.7	> 33.3	ND	66 ± 5.9
		A23	90	ML	28	–	37.8	6.8	2.9	8 ± 1.3	6.2	17 ± 1.3	3.0	> 33.3	ND	51 ± 6.2
		A24	90	ML	24	–	34.3	2	5.7	16 ± 1.6	5.7	29 ± 1.8	3.1	69 ± 3.0	1.3	91 ± 7.1
		BNZ[q]	–	–	–	–	–	–	–	17 ± 0.9	8.2	1.2 ± 0.1	116.3	6 ± 0.9	22.4	139 ± 2.3

[a]*EO* Essential oil, [b]*Extra* Extraction, [c]*min* Minutes, [d]*Caryop* Caryophyllene, [e]*CarOx* Caryophyllene oxide, [f]*Epi* Epimastigote, [g]*IC$_{50}$* Inhibitory concentration 50, [i]*SD* Standard deviation, [i]*SI* Selectivity index (CC$_{50}$/IC$_{50}$), [j]*Tryp* Trypomastigote, [k]*Amas* Amastigote, [l]*CC$_{50}$* Cytotoxic concentration 50, [m]*Infl* Inflorescences, [n]*AL* All leaves, [o]*YL* Young leaves, [p]*ML* Mature leaves, [q]*BNZ* Benznidazole, [r]*ND* Not determined

assessed through agarose gel DNA electrophoresis and TUNEL analyses. DNA degradation was observed by band disappearance in agarose gel (data not shown) and confirmed through green fluorescence on nuclei and kinetoplasts from Epi forms treated for 48 h with double doses at IC$_{50}$ (2xIC$_{50}$) of limonene, caryophyllene oxide, and the mix limonene:BNZ; with percentages of 94, 99, and 98, respectively (Fig. 4b). Non-significant fragmentation was observed on untreated Epi (Fig. 4b).

Phosphatidylserine externalization

A flow cytometry analysis was carried out to determine the general mechanism of cell death. As expected, untreated Epi showed high viability rates (99.7%) (Fig. 5a), whereas the various terpene treatments (48 h at 2xIC$_{50}$) caused high percentages of cell death, with 95.7, 89.2, 78.4, and 95.9% for cayophyllene oxide, limonene, citral, and the combination limonene:BNZ, respectively ($p = 0.0001$). No treatment showed statistically significant levels of negative SYTOX + positive Annexin V ($p > 0.05$), except the apoptosis positive control (15 day-old parasite culture) (13.6%) (Fig. 5f). On the other hand, all the treated cultures displayed high percentages of positive SYTOX and positive Annexin V. These results suggest a possible trigger of a late apoptosis mechanism (Fig. 5).

Discussion

In Chagas Disease, the pathogen-specific treatments – such as BNZ – should be prescribed for acute cases and for younger patients with little or no evidence of established cardiomyopathy [36, 37]. On the other hand, recent results from global trials have questioned the benefit of these therapies in chronic patients [8, 36]. In the case of BNZ, the drug demonstrated a significant decrease of the circulating parasite load, but no substantial effect in the prevention of the clinical decline [8, 36]. Therefore, most patients with advanced *T. cruzi* disease receive only symptomatic treatment for cardiomyopathy or digestive symptoms. This absence of an association between parasite clearance by BNZ and the clinical progression of heart disease has been ascribed to both the restricted activity of the treatment in the inflammatory and fibrotic cardiomyopathy lesions, as well as the irreversibility of this damage [36]. Thus, alternative

Table 4 Relative chemical composition and anti-proliferative effect on *T. cruzi* of EOs extracted from the Carvone chemotype of *L. alba*

Season	Material	EO[a]	Extra[b] Time min[c]	Part Plant	Chemical Composition				Epi[f]		Tryp[j]		Amas[k]		Vero
					Limonene %	Carvone %	Piper[d] %	BCE[e] %	IC$_{50}$[g] ± SD[h] µg/mL	SI[i]	IC$_{50}$[g] SD[h] µg/mL	SI[i]	IC$_{50}$[g] ± SD[h] µg/mL	SI[i]	CC$_{50}$[l] ± SD[h] µg/mL
Dry	Fresh	B7	30	AL[m]	19.3	31.5	31.3	2.3	81 ± 2.4	2.5	37 ± 2.1	5.5	> 150	ND[o]	203 ± 7.5
Rainy	Dry	2B8	90	YL[n]	22.8	5.3	27.5	4.6	96 ± 4.4	1.9	47 ± 3.8	4.0	> 150	ND	186 ± 11.7
	Fresh	B16	90	AL	30.6	–	54.5	2.9	97 ± 3.2	2.2	57 ± 3.0	3.8	> 150	ND	216 ± 9.6
	Dry	B37	30	YL	32.1	–	54	4	92 ± 3.9	2.1	43 ± 1.8	4.5	> 150	ND	196 ± 18.2
	Dry	2B18	45	AL	28	–	37.8	6.8	86 ± 4.8	1.9	34 ± 3.1	4.9	> 150	ND	165 ± 10.2
	Dry	2B19	90	AL	24	–	34.3	2	78 ± 3.5	2.9	51 ± 1.4	4.4	> 150	ND	226 ± 8.5

[a]*EO* Essential oil, [b]*Extra* Extraction, [c]*min* Minutes, [d]*Piper* Piperitenone, [e]*BCE* Bicyclosesquiphellandrene, [f]*Epi* Epimastigote, [g]*IC$_{50}$* Inhibitory concentration 50; [h]*SD* Standard deviation, [i]*SI* Selectivity index (CC$_{50}$/IC$_{50}$), [j]*Tryp* Trypomastigote, [k]*Amas* Amastigote, [l]*CC$_{50}$* Cytotoxic concentration 50, [m]*AL* All leaves, [n]*YL* Young leaves, [o]*ND* Not determined

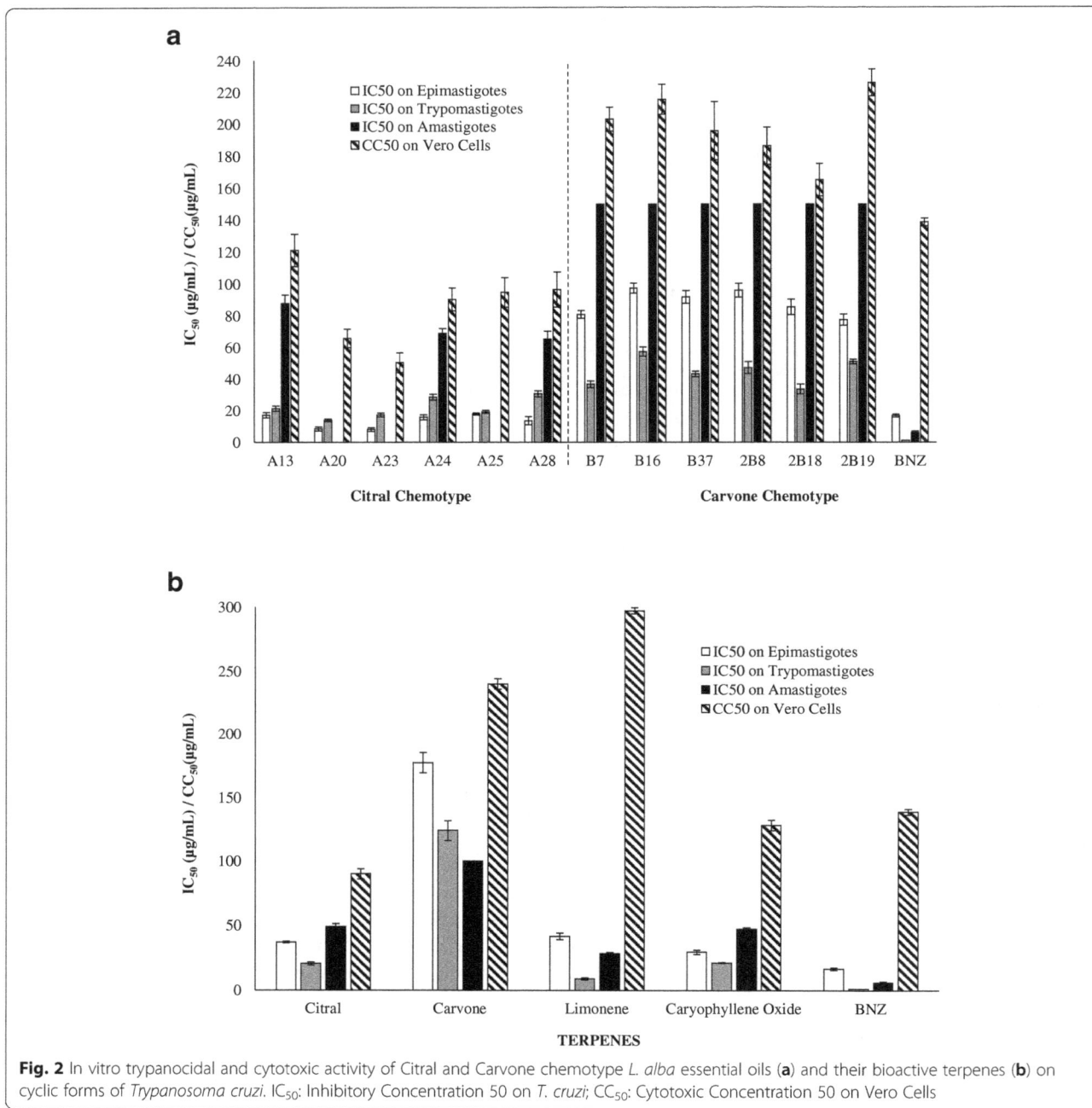

Fig. 2 In vitro trypanocidal and cytotoxic activity of Citral and Carvone chemotype *L. alba* essential oils (**a**) and their bioactive terpenes (**b**) on cyclic forms of *Trypanosoma cruzi*. IC$_{50}$: Inhibitory Concentration 50 on *T. cruzi*; CC$_{50}$: Cytotoxic Concentration 50 on Vero Cells

Table 5 Anti-parasitic effect on *Trypanosoma cruzi* of the major terpenes of Citral and Carvone chemotype *L. alba* essential oils

Terpenes	Epi[a] IC$_{50}$[b] ± SD[c] (µg/mL)	SI[d]	Tryp[e] IC$_{50}$[b] ± SD[c] (µg/mL)	SI[d]	Amas[h] IC$_{50}$[b] ± SD[c] (µg/mL)	SI[d]	Vero CC$_{50}$[i] ± SD[c] (µg/mL)
CarOx[j]	30 ± 1.7	4.3	22 ± 0.3	5.9	47 ± 1.0	2.7	128 ± 4.2
Limonene	42 ± 2.5	7.1	9 ± 0.8	32.8	29 ± 0.7	10.3	297 ± 2.4
Citral	37 ± 0.7	2.4	21 ± 1	4.3	49 ± 2.3	1.8	90 ± 3.9
Carvone	177 ± 7.9	1.4	124 ± 8	1.9	> 100	ND[i]	240 ± 4.1
BNZ[k]	17 ± 0.9	8.2	1.2 ± 0.1	116.3	6.2 ± 0.9	22.4	139 ± 2.3

[a]*Epi* Epimastigote, [b]*IC$_{50}$* Inhibitory concentration 50, [c]*SD* Standard deviation, [d]*SI* Selectivity index (CC$_{50}$/IC$_{50}$), [g]*Tryp* Trypomastigote, [h]*Amas* Amastigote, [i]*CC$_{50}$* Cytotoxic concentration 50, [j]*CarOx* Caryophyllene oxide, [k]*BNZ* Benznidazole, [l]*ND* Not determinated

Table 6 Pharmacological interactions among terpenes derived from *L. alba*

Parasitic Form	Limonene + Compound	ΣFIC[f] µg/mL ± SD[g]	Pharmacological interaction
Epi[a]	CarOx[d]	0.5 ± 0.13	Synergism
	Carvone	1.1 ± 0.08	Antagonism
	Citral	0.7 ± 0.13	Synergism
	BNZ[e]	0.4 ± 0.13	Synergism
Tryp[b]	CarOx[d]	0.4 ± 0.10	Synergism
	Carvone	1.04 ± 0.04	Antagonism
	Citral	0.6 ± 0.10	Synergism
	BNZ[e]	0.4 ± 0.10	Synergism
Amas[c]	CarOx[d]	0.7 ± 0.23	Synergism
	Carvone	ND[h]	ND[h]
	Citral	0.8 ± 0.15	Synergism
	BNZ[e]	0.6 ± 0.13	Synergism
Vero	CarOx[d]	1.2 ± 0.16	Antagonism
	Carvone	1.0 ± 0.07	Additive
	Citral	1.0 ± 0.07	Antagonism
	BNZ[e]	0.5 ± 0.18	Synergism

[a]*Epi* Epimastigote, [b]*Tryp* Trypomastigote, [c]*Amas* Amastigote, [d]*CarOx* Caryophyllene oxide, [e]*BNZ* Benznidazole, [f]*FIC* Fractional inhibitory concentration, [g]*SD* Standard deviation, [h]*ND* Not determinated

approaches for Chagas infection management should aim to control not only the parasite load, but also all the factors associated with cardiomyopathy progression (oxidative stress and immune effectors, among others) [36, 38].

Since parasitic protozoa are very sensitive to oxidative stress [39], the most common trypanocidal and anti-chagasic drugs like Nitroimidazoles derived (BNZ) and Nitrofurans (NFX) were developed based on their capability to induce Reactive Oxygen Species (ROS) production [40]. However, the clinical use of both medicines has been limited due to their high toxicity [41], mutagenic potential [42], the severity of their side effects [38, 41], and the lack of significant effects on clinical disease progression in the late stages of *T. cruzi* infection [8, 37].

In general, the development of new trypanocidal agents has been focused on the use of molecules that alter the cellular redox potential and take advantage of the scarce antioxidant defenses of the parasite [39, 40]. A similar anti-protozoal effect has been described for essential oils rich in terpenes extracted from aromatic plants [43]. In this regard, EOs derived from *Cymbopogon citratus* showed promising results, with low IC$_{50}$ values against *T. cruzi* (15.5 µg/mL for Epi and Tryp; and 5.1 µg/mL for Amas) [17]. These trypanocidal effects were attributed to the high levels of the oxygenated monoterpene citral (a mixture of neral and geranial) [17]. Similar outcomes were obtained with oils extracted from a Colombian (Santander) variant of *L. alba* (Citral chemotype), which were rich in such terpenes as citral, geraniol, timol, and caryophyllene oxide [30].

In this work, we tested the trypanocidal and cytotoxic activity of 12 EOs, derived from two different plant chemotypes (Citral and Carvone) of *L. alba,* which were produced under controlled conditions of growth (geographic location, cultivation environment, and soil), plant parameters (age and part), material state (fresh or dry) and extraction conditions (time). These standardized procedures were prepared taking into consideration the recognized high phenotypical plasticity of the plant in response to genetic, environmental, and production parameters [25], which can induce significant variations in its EO constituents, as well as in their biological activities [25, 44].

In this regard, our results also confirmed significant differences in the major chemical compounds (terpenes), and trypanocidal activity of the *L. alba* oils produced under varying parameters (Tables 3 and 4, and Fig. 2a). While mixtures rich in citral and caryophyllene oxide (Citral chemotype EOs) achieved good performance on extracellular forms of *T. cruzi* (mean IC$_{50}$ values of 13.6 and 21.9 µg/mL on Epi and Tryp, respectively) (Table 3); EOs of the same plant but rich in carvone and limonene (Carvone chemotype), displayed poor inhibitory results (mean IC$_{50}$ values of 88.2 and 44.9 µg/mL for Epi and Tryp, respectively) (Table 4). Individual assays with a solution of citral consistently found that this compound caused an efficient arrest of the parasite's growth with IC$_{50}$ values of 37.2 and 20.8 µg/mL on Epi and Tryp, respectively (Table 5).

With respect to citral, several studies on cancer and immune cell line models have demonstrated its interesting

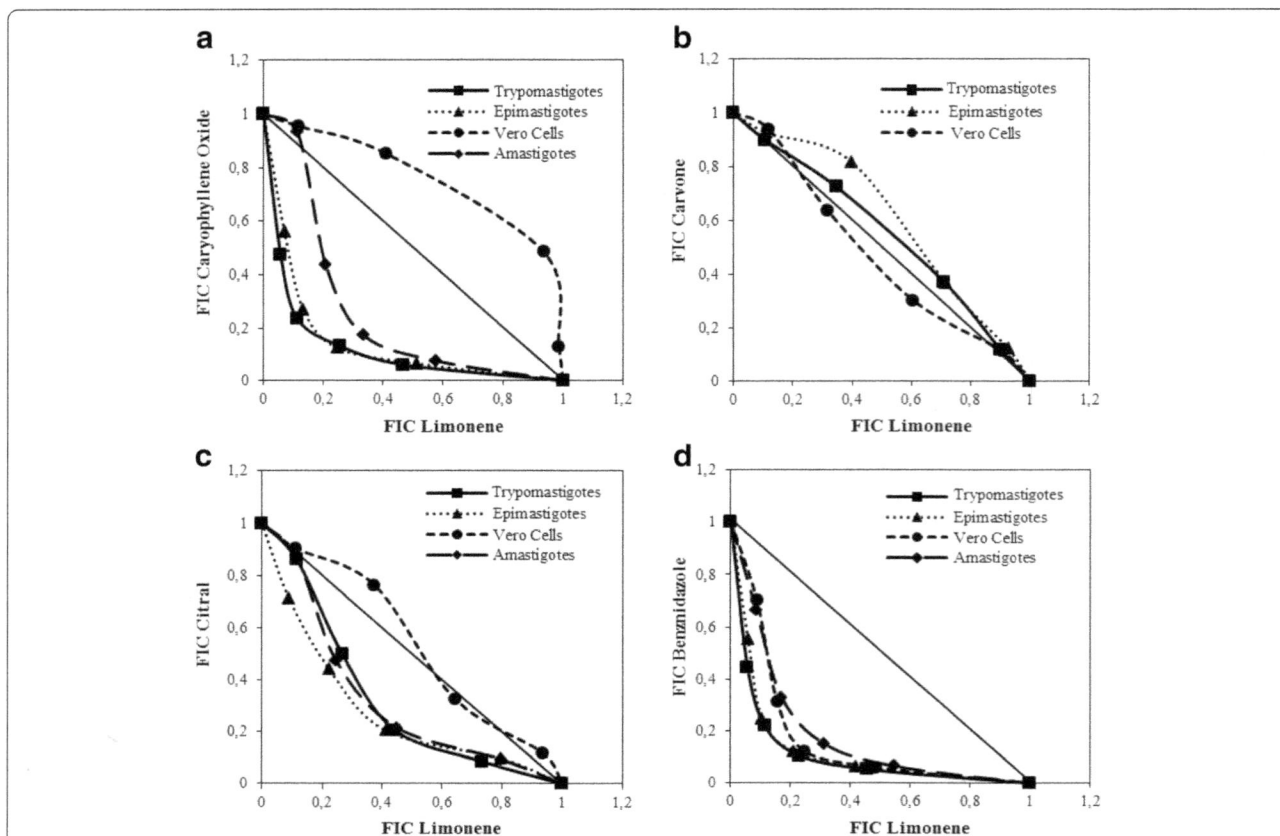

Fig. 3 Pharmacological interaction isobolograms among major terpenes of the Citral and Carvone chemotype *L. alba* essential oils: **a** limonene with caryophyllene oxide; **b** limonene with carvone; **c** limonene with citral; and **d** limonene with Benznidazole (BNZ). The interaction tests were performed on Epimastigotes, Trypomastigotes and Amastigotes of *T. cruzi* and Vero cells. Dotted lines correspond to an additive effect; points below, on, and above line indicate a synergistic, additive, and antagonistic effect, respectively

biological properties. As an anti-tumoral, this monoterpene exhibited significant anti-proliferative effects, in vitro and in vivo [45–48] and this cell growth inhibition was ascribed to the induction of mitochondrial apoptosis pathways (through p53 activation triggered by an ROS increase) [45]. In addition, citral has also been described as anti-inflammatory agent. In lipopolysaccharide (LPS)-stimulated macrophages, this terpene was found to suppress the expression of pro-inflammatory markers such as NLRP2 (NLR Family Pyrin Domain Containing 2), Interleukin (IL) 6 and IL-1β [24], Tumoral Necrosis Factor (TNF) α [49], as well as to activate the Peroxisome Proliferator-Activated Receptor (PPAR) γ dependent-Cyclooxygenase 2 (COX2) promotor [50]. It is worth mentioning that over a range of different cells, the expression of COX2 is regulated in a variety of ways; playing an important role in tumoral genesis, inflammation, development, and circulatory homeostasis. In these activated macrophages, citral also blocks the genic expression of the LPS-induced Nitric Oxide Synthase (iNOS) [51] and, consequently, the production of Nitric Oxide (NO). It is thought that this inhibition could suppress transcriptional activation and the translocation of the nuclear factor-kappa

B (NF-κB). These results suggest that citral is an anti-inflammatory agent whose effects could be associated with NF-κB suppression [51], indicating that this compound may be a promising candidate for the treatment of inflammatory conditions like Chagas Disease.

Similarly, anticancer and anti-inflammatory properties have also been attributed to caryophyllene oxide, another major and bioactive constituent of Citral chemotype *L. alba* EOs. On human prostate and breast cancer cells, this sesquiterpene isolated from the EOs of medicinal plants such as guava (*Psidium guajava*), oregano (*Origanum vulgare* L.), cinnamon (*Cinnamomum spp.*), clove (*Eugenia caryophyllata*), and black pepper (*Piper nigrum* L.), inhibited constitutive survival pathways (PI3K/AKT/mTOR/S6 K1) and ROS-dependent MAPK activation during tumorigenesis; triggering apoptosis on tumoral lineages and preventing inflammation, angiogenesis, and metastasis [52]. Furthermore, on stimulated primary splenocytes, caryophyllene oxide significantly increases the Th2/Th1 coefficient [22].

In our work, caryophyllene oxide was correlated with a trypanocidal effect, being found to be one of the major

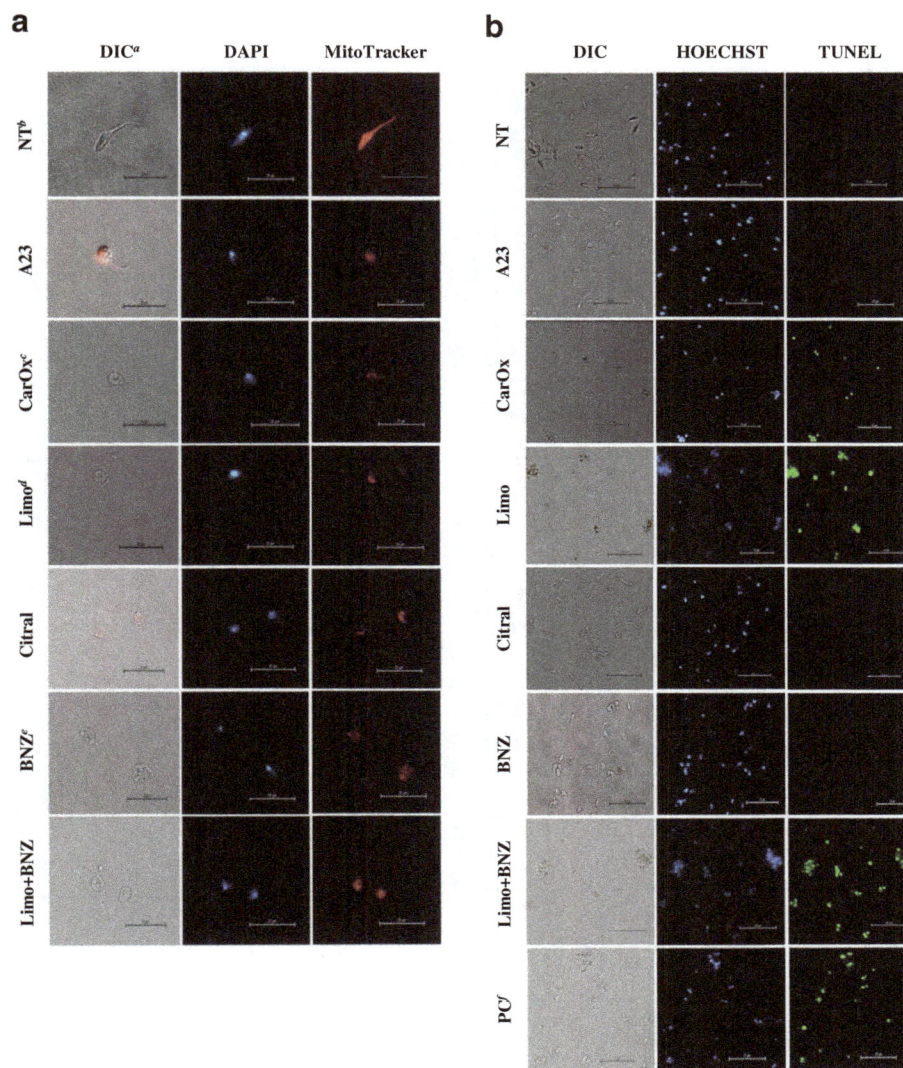

Fig. 4 Cell morphology changes of *Trypanosoma cruzi* by fluorescent and optical microscopy. **a** Cell morphology, mitochondrial membrane potential, nuclear and kinetoplast DNA of *T. cruzi* epimastigotes after treatment with essential oils, terpenes, or BNZ. **b** DNA fragmentation analysis by TUNEL assay on *T.cruzi* epimastigotes treated with terpenes. The preserved parasitic DNA was visualized with a blue HOECHST fluorescent probe (negative TUNEL) and the free DNA strands were observed in green (positive TUNEL). [a]DIC: Differential Interference Contrast Microscopy; [b]NT: No Treatment; [c]CarOx: caryophyllene oxide; [d]Limo: limonene; [e]BNZ: Benznidazole; [f]PC: Positive control: DAPI: cells stained with DAPI nuclear fluorescent stain observed in UV filter. MitoTracker: cells stained with MitoTracker Red CMXRos stain observed in an Excitation/Emission 579/599 (nm) filter. Photographs are representative of 10 observed fields

components of the most trypanocidal EOs studied: A23 and A20 (*L. alba* citral chemotype). Similarly, Cheikh Ali et al., [18], found a minimal lethal concentration of 0.1 µg/mL for EOs extracted from *Aframomum sceptrum* on cyclic forms of *T. brucei*; this trypanocidal action being associated with the presence of caryophyllene oxide. In the present study, this compound demonstrated a significant anti-proliferative effect against *T. cruzi* Epi (IC$_{50}$ = 29.8 µg/mL), Tryp (IC$_{50}$ = 21.6 µg/mL), and Amas (IC$_{50}$ = 47.4 µg/mL) (Table 5).

Another major *L. alba* terpene studied herein was limonene. This monoterpene is one of the main components of

the Carvone chemotype oils. Due its beneficial pharmacological characteristics such as: low toxicity (used as food additive for decades) [53], high bioavailability [54], and selective anti-tumoral effect on a variety of cancer cell lines (leukemia, lymphoma, prostate, hepatic, colorectal, pancreatic, gastric, and breast, among others [54–57]); several research efforts have been undertaken with respect to this monoterpene. Interestingly, on a prostate cancer model, limonene caused apoptotic programmed cell death by the induction of a selective oxidative stress on tumoral cells [57]. As for protozoa, cancer cells are highly vulnerable to cell death induced by pro-oxidant agents (such as

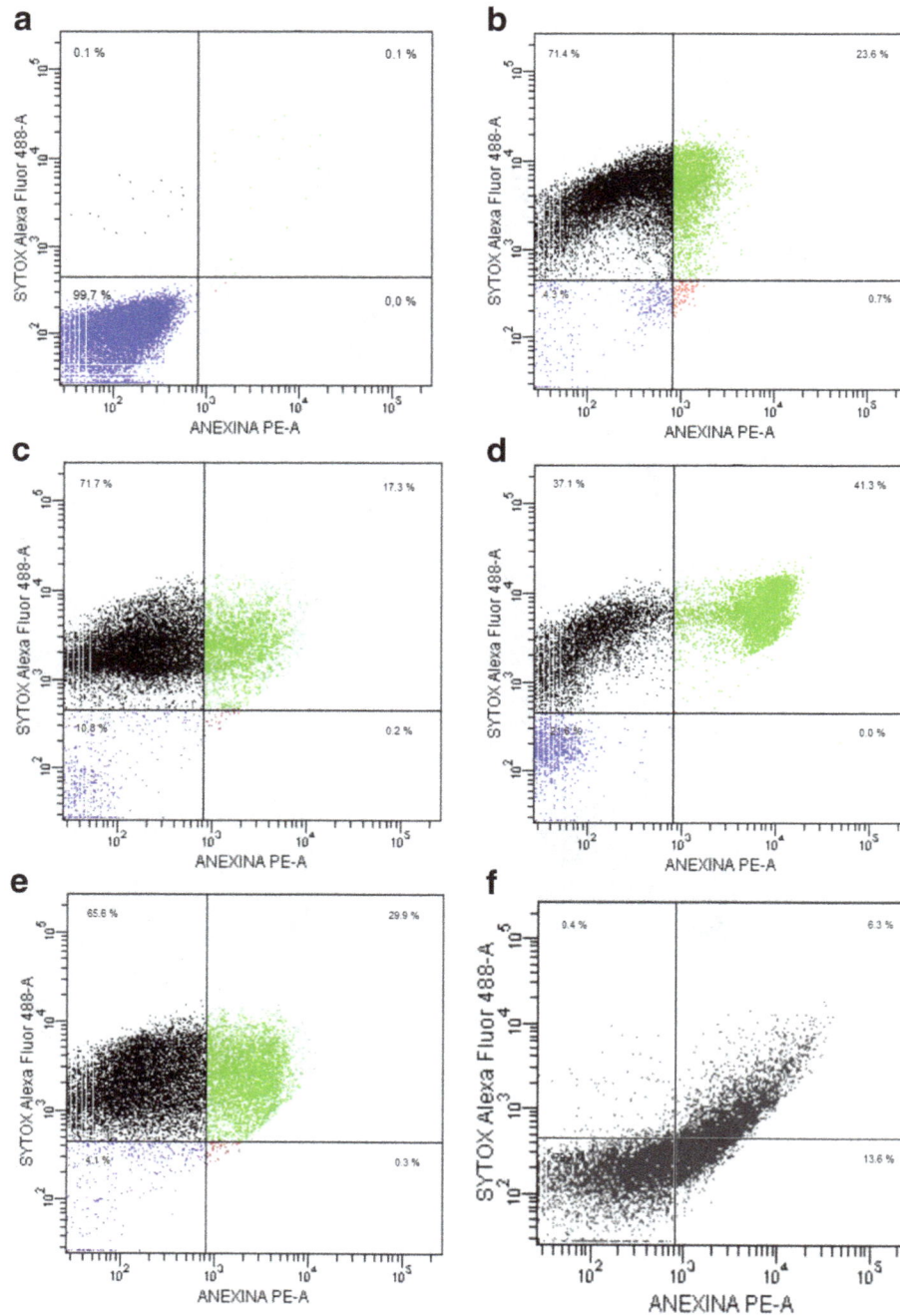

Fig. 5 Flow cytometry analysis of phosphatidylserine externalization of *T. cruzi* epimastigotes treated with terpenes or Benznidazole. **a** Negative control (untreated culture). **b** caryophyllene oxide; **c** limonene; **d** citral; **e** limonene:BNZ; and **f** apoptosis positive control (15 day-old parasite culture). The flow cytometry histograms are representative of two independent experiments

limonene) due their high metabolism and their deficient antioxidant mechanisms [58]. In this study, limonene was the best trypanocidal and most selective terpene with the lowest inhibitory doses (IC$_{50}$ of 9.0, 28.7, and 41.8 μg/mL on Tryp, Amas, and Epi, respectively). However, this good performance was not replicated when *T. cruzi* forms were treated with oils rich in carvone and limonene (*L. alba* Carvone chemotype EOs displayed higher IC$_{50}$ levels on Epi = 88.2 μg/mL, Tryp = 44.9 μg/mL, and Amas > 150 μg/mL) (Table 5). Interestingly, carvone was the least effective trypanocidal terpene, with the lowest values of cell death percentage induction and highest IC_{50} results (Table 5). These results were associated with the strong antioxidant capability previously ascribed to this monoterpene [59]. Accordingly, a possible antagonism seems likely between limonene and carvone (which was present in the oil mixture in levels close to 42%) (Table 4). Pharmacological interaction tests confirmed that the presence of carvone in the *L. alba* Carvone chemotype oils, impaired the limonene's trypanocidal performance on *T. cruzi* Tryp (ΣCIF: 1.04 µg/mL) and Epi (ΣCIF: 1.10 µg/mL) forms (Table 6). In further assays, limonene presented a synergistic pharmacological interaction with the other bioactive *L. alba* terpenes (citral and caryophyllene oxide), and with BNZ, exhibiting ΣFIC values < 0.8 µg/mL on the three parasite forms analyzed (Table 6). In combination with BNZ, limonene caused a significant decrease of the BNZ-IC_{50}, by 14, 16, and 17 times on Amas, Epi, and Tryp, respectively (Table 6).

These positive interactions could have been due to the simultaneal action of these compounds on diverse and additive mechanisms that lead to cell death in susceptible lineages. Such mechanisms may include: a) polymerization microtubules disruption (citral) [60]; b) endoplasmic reticulum stress induction (citral) [60]; c) PIP3/AKT survival pathway inhibition (limonene, citral, and caryophyllene oxide) [52, 61, 62]; d) oxidative stress stimulation (limonene, citral, and caryophyllene oxide) [52, 57, 63]; and e) apoptosis by caspases activation (citral and limonene) [61–63], among others.

It is important to add that the parasite cells treated for 48 h with some of the studied compounds (A23 oil, citral, caryophyllene oxide, limonene, and the mixture of limonene and BNZ) evidenced typical characteristics of apoptosis, such as cytoplasmic blebbing, cell shrinkage, flagellum absence, loss of mitochondrial membrane potential, condensation of the nuclear chromatin, and DNA fragmentation (Fig. 4a). Also, the treatment of parasites with caryophyllene oxide or limonene (alone, in combination, or with BNZ) led to positive results in TUNEL assays (Fig. 4b). Correspondingly, an impairment of membrane potential (Fig. 4) and the externalization of phosphatidylserine (Fig. 5) were observed on *T. cruzi* cells treated with citral, limonene, and caryophyllene oxide. These results suggest a possible activation of an early apoptosis mechanism that rapidly progresses to late apoptosis (positive SYTOX plus positive Annexin V) accompanied by DNA fragmentation. In trypanosomatids like *Leishmania donovani*, *T. brucei*, and *T. cruzi*, these same characteristics have been reported in parasites suffering calcium imbalance and oxidative stress (by ROS) [64], mitochondrial enzyme knockdown [65], or treatment with sterols [66]. In these studies, the previously mentioned features were associated with a possible programmed cell death such as apoptosis or autophagy [67].

In an illness with a complex pathogenesis like Chagas Disease (which involves the parasitic persistence that triggers and sustains an anti-inflammatory immune response), the use of synergic drugs (like limonene/caryophyllene oxide) with several biological advantages (significant trypanocidal activity [32], low toxicity on mammal tissues [53]; and anti-genotoxic [68], chemoprotective [23], and anti-inflammatory activity [22]) could be an interesting platform for the development of an adjuvant therapy that enhances the therapeutic effects of the conventional treatments, principally in advanced stage of the infection (probably improving trypanocidal action, reducing therapeutic doses, increasing tolerance, or retarding resistance development) [69].

Conclusions

In this work, a range of growth, plant, and extraction parameters were found to significantly influence the chemical composition and trypanocidal activity of essential oils isolated from *L. alba* Citral and Carvone chemotypes. *L. alba* Citral chemotype oils, extracted under known and controlled conditions, presented significant trypanocidal activity on three cyclic *T. cruzi* forms: epimastigotes, trypomastigotes, and amastigotes. Assays using pure solutions of the main terpenes that constitute *L. alba* EOs, confirmed an association among parasitological activity and the presence of citral and caryophyllene oxide. Tests using EOs extracted from Carvone chemotype (rich in carvone and limonene), and their most important components, established an antagonistic relationship between carvone and limonene in their trypanocidal performance. Nevertheless, in this study, the best anti-*T. cruzi*, and most selective, activity was achieved by limonene. Citral, caryophyllene oxide, and limonene exhibited the induction of a possible apoptotic-like phenotype. In the synergistic interaction tests, limonene also improved the trypanocidal performance of citral, caryophyllene oxide, and even BNZ, on the three parasitic forms studied. The best synergic terpene activity was displayed by the limonene and caryophyllene oxide combination. These results should be confirmed by further pre-clinical studies and could be of interest for the development of alternative and adjuvant treatments improving the tolerance and parasitological efficacy, and broadening the spectrum of the effects, of the current conventional therapies for late phases of Chagas Disease. In such research, *L. alba* EOs represent a renewable source for commercial exploitation of these terpenes.

Abbreviations
ΣFIC: Sum FIC; AL: All Leaves; Amas: Amastigote; ANOVA: Analysis of variance; BCE: Bicyclosesquiphellandrene; BNZ: Benznidazole; CarOx: Caryophyllene oxide; Caryop: Caryophyllene; CC_{50}: Cytotoxic Concentration 50; CDP: Cell death percentages; CENIVAM: National Research Center for Agroindustrialization of Aromatic Medical and Tropical Species; COX2: Cyclooxygenase 2; DAPI: 4',6-diamidino-2-phenylindole; DMEM: Dulbecco's Modified Eagle's Medium; DMSO: Dimethyl sulfoxide;

DNA: Deoxyribonucleic acid; EO: Essential oil; Epi: Epimastigotes; FBS$_i$: Inactivated Fetal Bovine Serum; FIC: Fractional Inhibitory Concentration; GC-MS: Gas chromatography coupled mass spectrometry; IC$_{50}$: Inhibitory Concentration 50; IL: Interleukin; Inf: Inflorescences; iNOS: Induced Nitric Oxide Synthase; *L. alba*: *Lippia alba*; LIT: Liver Infusion Tryptose; LPS: Lipopolysaccharide; Min: Minutes; ML: Mature leaves; mm: Millimeter; MWHD: Microwave-Assisted Hydrodistillation; ND: Not determined; NF-kB: Nuclear factor-kappa B; NFX: Nifurtimox; NLRP2: NLR Family Pyrin Domain Containing 2; nm: Nanometer; NO: Nitric Oxide; NTD: Neglected Tropical Disease; OD: Optical Density; PBS: Phosphate Buffered Saline; Piper: Piperitenone; PPAR: Peroxisome Proliferator-Activated Receptor; ROS: Reactive species of oxygen; RPMI: Roswell Park Memorial Institute; SD: Standard deviation; SI: Selectivity index; *T. brucei*: *Trypanosoma brucei*; *T. cruzi*: *Trypanosoma cruzi*; TDC: Trypomastigotes Derived from Cells; TdT: Terminal desoxynucleotidyl Transferase; TNF: Tumor Necrosis Factor; Tryp: Trypomastigote; UTP: Uridine Triphosphate; YL: Young leaves

Acknowledgements

This study was supported by the Vicerrectoría de Investigaciones – Universidad de Santander, under grant 005-14; and the Vicerrectoría de Investigación y Extensión – Universidad Industrial de Santander, under grant 5658. The authors would like to express their appreciation to Dr. Marcos López Casillas and to Dr. Wendy Grey Nieto Pérez for their support in flow cytometry assays; to Dr. Yamile Leonor Vargas for Benznidazole purification, and to Dr. Camilo Durán, Qm. Carlos Ramírez, and Qm. Yaride Pérez for their support during the collection and characterization of EO samples. We are grateful to Mr. Emile Blanchette for assistance in the proofreading of this study.

Funding

This research was supported by the Vicerrectoría de Investigaciones – Universidad de Santander, under grant 005–14; and the Vicerrectoría de Investigación y Extensión – Universidad Industrial de Santander, under grant 5658.

Authors' contributions

LTG conceived the study, designed all the experiments, and reviewed all the results and findings. EMM performed and analyzed all the trypanocidal, cytotoxic, and cell death assays, carried out data collection and analysis, and wrote the manuscript. EES collected the plants, and extracted and chemically characterized the essential oils. SML participated in the trypanocidal, cytotoxic, and synergistic tests. All authors read, revised, and approved the final manuscript.

Competing interests

The authors declare that they have no competing interests.

Author details

[1]Infectious Disease Research Program, Universidad de Santander, 680006 Bucaramanga, Colombia. [2]Bacteriology and Clinical Laboratory Program, Universidad de Santander, 680006 Bucaramanga, Colombia. [3]National Research Center for Agroindustrialization of Aromatic Medical and Tropical Species (CENIVAM), Universidad Industrial de Santander, 680002 Bucaramanga, Colombia.

References

1. World Health Organization. Investing to Overcome the Global Impact of Neglected Tropical Diseases: 3rd WHO Rep Neglect Trop D. 2015.
2. Robertson LJ, Devleesschauwer B, De Noya BA, González ON, Torgerson PR. *Trypanosoma cruzi*: time for international recognition as a foodborne parasite. PLoS Neglect Trop D. 2016;10(6):e0004656.
3. Hotez PJ, Dumonteil E, Heffernan MJ, Bottazzi ME. Innovation for the 'bottom 100 million': eliminating neglected tropical diseases in the Americas. In: Curtis N, Finn A, Pollard A, editors. Hot topics in infection and immunity in children IX advances in experimental medicine and biology. Springer: New York; 2013. p. 1–12.
4. Cruz Bermúdez HF, Moreno Collazos JE. Seroprevalencia de tamizaje de Chagas y factores asociados a coinfección en un banco de sangre de Colombia durante 2006-2011. Rev Med Risaralda. 2015;21(1):26–30.
5. Coura JR. The main sceneries of Chagas disease transmission. The vectors, blood and oral transmissions-a comprehensive review. Mem Inst Oswaldo Cruz. 2015;110(3):277–82.
6. Bustamante JM, Tarleton RL. Potential new clinical therapies for Chagas disease. Expert Rev Clin Pharmacol. 2014;7(3):317–25.
7. Bern C. Chagas' disease. N Engl J Med. 2015;373(5):456–66.
8. Morillo CA, Marin-Neto JA, Avezum A, Sosa-Estani S, Rassi A Jr, Rosas F, Guhl F. Randomized trial of benznidazole for chronic Chagas' cardiomyopathy. N Engl J Med. 2015;373(14):1295–306.
9. Rassi A, De Rezende JM. American trypanosomiasis (Chagas disease). Infect Dis Clin N Am. 2012;26(2):275–91.
10. Bonney KM, Engman DM. Autoimmune pathogenesis of Chagas heart disease: looking back, looking ahead. Am J Pathol. 2015;185(6):1537–47.
11. Rassi A Jr, Neto M, Antonio J, Rassi A. Chronic Chagas cardiomyopathy: a review of the main pathogenic mechanisms and the efficacy of aetiological treatment following the Benznidazole evaluation for interrupting Trypanosomiasis (BENEFIT) trial. Mem Inst Oswaldo Cruz. 2017;112(3):224–35.
12. Schmidt TJ, Khalid S, Romanha AJ, Alves T, Biavatti M, Brun R, et al. The potential of secondary metabolites from plants as drugs or leads against protozoan neglected diseases-part II. Curr Med Chem. 2012;19(14):2176–228.
13. Al-Snafi AE. Antiparasitic effects of medicinal plants (part 1)-a review. IOSR PHR. 2016a;6(10):51–66.
14. Raut JS, Karuppayil SM. A status review on the medicinal properties of essential oils. Ind Crop Prod J. 2014;62:250–64.
15. Borges AR, De Albuquerque Aires JR, Higino TMM, De Medeiros MDGF, Citó AMDGL, Lopes JAD, De Figueiredo RCBQ. Trypanocidal and cytotoxic activities of essential oils from medicinal plants of northeast of Brazil. Exp Parasitol. 2012;132(2):123–8.
16. Al-Snafi AE. Antiparasitic, antiprotozoal, molluscicidal and insecticidal activity of medicinal plants (part 2)–plant based review. Sch Acad J Pharm. 2016b;5(6):194–207.
17. Santoro GF, Cardoso MG, Guimarães LGL, Freire JM, Soares MJ. Anti-proliferative effect of the essential oil of *Cymbopogon citratus* (DC) Stapf (lemongrass) on intracellular amastigotes, bloodstream trypomastigotes and culture epimastigotes of *Trypanosoma cruzi* (Protozoa: Kinetoplastida). Parasitology. 2007;134(11):1649–56.
18. Cheikh Ali Z, Adiko M, Bouttier S, Bories C, Okpekon T, Poupon E, Champy P. Composition, and antimicrobial and remarkable antiprotozoal activities of the essential oil of rhizomes of *Aframomum sceptrum* K. Schum. (Zingiberaceae). Chem Biodivers. 2011;8(4):658–67.
19. Santos NN, Menezes LR, Dos Santos JA, Meira CS, Guimarhes ET, Soares MB, Costa EV. A new source of (R)-limonene and rotundifolone from leaves of *Lippia pedunculosa* (verbenaceae) and their trypanocidal properties. Nat Prod Commun. 2014;9(6):737–9.
20. Villamizar LH, Cardoso MDG, Andrade JD, Teixeira ML, Soares MJ. Linalool, a Piper aduncum essential oil component, has selective activity against *Trypanosoma cruzi* trypomastigote forms at 4° C. Mem Inst Oswaldo Cruz. 2017;112(2):131–9.
21. Stashenko EE, Martínez JR, Durán DC, Córdoba Y, Caballero D. Estudio comparativo de la composición química y la actividad antioxidante de los aceites esenciales de algunas plantas del género *Lippia* (Verbenaceae) cultivadas en Colombia. Rev Acad Colomb Ci Exact Fís Nat. 2014;38:89–105.
22. Ku CM, Lin JY. Anti-inflammatory effects of 27 selected terpenoid compounds tested through modulating Th1/Th2 cytokine secretion profiles using murine primary splenocytes. Food Chem. 2013;141(2):1104–13.

23. Bai J, Zheng Y, Wang G, Liu P. Protective effect of D-limonene against oxidative stress-induced cell damage in human lens epithelial cells via the p38 pathway. Oxidative Med Cell Longev. 2015;2016:1–12.

24. Liao PC, Yang TS, Chou JC, Chen J, Lee SC, Kuo YH, Ho LC, Chao LKP. Anti-inflammatory activity of neral and geranial isolated from fruits of Litsea cubeba Lour. J Funct Foods. 2015;19:248–58.

25. García LT, Leal AF, Moreno ÉM, Stashenko EE, Arteaga HJ. Differential anti-proliferative effect on K562 leukemia cells of Lippia alba (Verbenaceae) essential oils produced under diverse growing, collection and extraction conditions. Ind Crop Prod J. 2017;96:140–8.

26. Hennebelle T, Sahpaz S, Joseph H, Bailleul F. Ethnopharmacology of Lippia alba. J Ethnopharmacol. 2008;116(2):211–22.

27. Di Stasi LC, Oliveira GP, Carvalhaes MA, Queiroz-Junior M, Tien OS, Kakinami SH, Reis MS. Medicinal plants popularly used in the Brazilian tropical Atlantic Forest. Fitoterapia. 2002;73(1):69–91.

28. Pinto EDPP, Amorozo MCDM, Furlan A. Conhecimento popular sobre plantas medicinais em comunidades rurais de mata atlântica–Itacaré, BA. Brasil Acta bot bras. 2006;20(4):751–62.

29. Toscano GJ. Uso tradicional de plantas medicinales en la vereda San Isidro, municipio de San José de Pare-Boyacá: un estudio preliminar usando técnicas cuantitativas. Acta biol Colomb. 2006;11(2):1137–46.

30. Escobar P, Milena Leal S, Herrera LV, Martinez JR, Stashenko E. Chemical composition and antiprotozoal activities of Colombian Lippia spp essential oils and their major components. Mem Inst Oswaldo Cruz. 2010;105(2):184–90.

31. Azeredo CM, Soares MJ. Combination of the essential oils constituents citral, eugenol and thymol enhance their inhibitory effect on Crithidia fasciculata and Trypanosoma cruzi growth. Rev Bras Farmacogn. 2013;23(5):762–8.

32. Polanco-Hernández G, Escalante-Erosa F, García-Sosa K, Rosado ME, Guzmán-Marín E, Acosta-Viana KY, Giménez-Turba A, Salamanca E, Peña-Rodríguez LM. Synergistic effect of lupenone and caryophyllene oxide against Trypanosoma cruzi. J Evid Based Complementary Altern Med. 2013;2013.

33. Adams R. Identification of essential oil components by gas chromatography / mass spectrometry. fourth ed. Illinois: Carol Stream; 2007. p. 804.

34. Fivelman QL, Adagu IS, Warhurst DC. Modified fixed-ratio isobologram method for studying in vitro interactions between atovaquone and proguanil or dihydroartemisinin against drug-resistant strains of Plasmodium falciparum. Antimicrob Agents Chemother. 2004;48(11):4097–102.

35. Pendergrass W, Wolf N, Poot M. Efficacy of MitoTracker green™ and CMXrosamine to measure changes in mitochondrial membrane potentials in living cells and tissues. Cytom Part A. 2004;61(2):162–9.

36. Urbina JA. Recent clinical trials for the etiological treatment of chronic Chagas disease: advances, challenges and perspectives. J Eukariot Microbiol. 2015;62(1):149–56.

37. Malik LH, Singh GD, Amsterdam EA. The epidemiology, clinical manifestations, and management of chagas heart disease. Clin Cardiol. 2015;38(9):565–9.

38. Viotti R, De Noya BA, Araujo-Jorge T, Grijalva MJ, Guhl F, López MC, Torrico F. Towards a paradigm shift in the treatment of chronic Chagas disease. Antimicrob Agents Chemother. 2014;58(2):635–9.

39. Turrens JF. Oxidative stress and antioxidant defenses: a target for the treatment of diseases caused by parasitic protozoa. Mol Asp Med. 2004;25(1):211–20.

40. Wilkinson SR, Kelly JM. Trypanocidal drugs: mechanisms, resistance and new targets. Expert Rev Mol Med. 2009;11:e31.

41. Molina I, Salvador F, Sanchez-Montalva A, Treviño B, Serre N, Sao Avilés A, Almirante B. Toxic profile of benznidazole in patients with chronic Chagas disease: risk factors and comparison of the product from two different manufacturers. Antimicrob Agents Chemother. 2015;59(10):6125–31.

42. Rajao MA, Furtado C, Alves CL, Passos Silva DG, Moura MB, Schamber Reis BL, Mendes IC. Unveiling Benznidazole's mechanism of action through overexpression of DNA repair proteins in Trypanosoma cruzi. Environ Mol Mutagen. 2014;55(4):309–21.

43. Kpoviessi S, Bero J, Agbani P, Gbaguidi F, Kpadonou-Kpoviessi B, Sinsin B, Quetin-Leclercq J. Chemical composition, cytotoxicity and in vitro antitrypanosomal and antiplasmodial activity of the essential oils of four Cymbopogon species from Benin. J Ethnopharmacol. 2014;151(1):652–9.

44. Teles S, Pereira JA, Santos CH, Menezes RV, Malheiro R, Lucchese AM, Silva F. Geographical origin and drying methodology may affect the essential oil of Lippia alba (mill) NE Brown. Ind Crop Prod. 2012;37(1):247–52.

45. Liu Y, Whelan RJ, Pattnaik BR, Ludwig K, Subudhi E, Rowland H, Felder M. Terpenoids from Zingiber officinale (ginger) induce apoptosis in endometrial cancer cells through the activation of p53. PLoS One. 2012;7(12):e53178.

46. Dudai N, Weinstein Y, Krup M, Rabinski T, Ofir R. Citral is a new inducer of caspase-3 in tumor cell lines. Planta Med. 2005;71(05):484–8.

47. Zeng S, Kapur A, Patankar MS, Xiong MP. Formulation, characterization, and antitumor properties of trans-and cis-citral in the 4T1 breast cancer xenograft mouse model. Pharm Res. 2015;32(8):2548–58.

48. Mesa-Arango AC, Montiel-Ramos J, Zapata B, Durán C, Betancur-Galvis L, Stashenko E. Citral and carvone chemotypes from the essential oils of Colombian Lippia alba (mill.) NE Brown: composition, cytotoxicity and antifungal activity. Mem Inst Oswaldo Cruz. 2009;104(6):878–84.

49. De Paula PM, Da Silva GN, Luperini BCO, Bachiega TF, De Castro Marcondes JP, Sforcin JM, Salvadori DMF. Citral and eugenol modulate DNA damage and pro-inflammatory mediator genes in murine peritoneal macrophages. Mol Biol Rep. 2014;41(11):7043–51.

50. Katsukawa M, Nakata R, Takizawa Y, Hori K, Takahashi S, Inoue H. Citral, a component of lemongrass oil, activates PPARα and γ and suppresses COX-2 expression. BBA-Mol Cell Biol Lipid. 2010;1801(11):1214–20.

51. Lee HJ, Jeong HS, Kim DJ, Noh YH, Yuk DY, Hong JT. Inhibitory effect of citral on NO production by suppression of iNOS expression and NF-κB activation in RAW264. 7 cells. Arch Pharm Res. 2008;31(3):342–9.

52. Park KR, Nam D, Yun HM, Lee SG, Jang HJ, Sethi G, Ahn KS. β-Caryophyllene oxide inhibits growth and induces apoptosis through the suppression of PI3K/AKT/mTOR/S6K1 pathways and ROS-mediated MAPKs activation. Cancer Lett. 2011;312(2):178–88.

53. Sun J. D-limonene: safety and clinical applications. Altern Med Rev. 2007;12(3):259.

54. Xiu-zhen WLZ. Growth inhibition effects of D-limonene on human gastric carcinoma MGC803 cells. Life Sci Instrum. 2009;1:012.

55. Kapoor S. D-limonene: an emerging antineoplastic agent. Hum Exp Toxicol. 2013;32(11):1228.

56. Miller JA, Lang JE, Ley M, Nagle R, Hsu CH, Thompson PA, Chow HS. Human breast tissue disposition and bioactivity of limonene in women with early-stage breast cancer. Cancer Prev Res. 2013;6(6):577–84.

57. Rabi T, Bishayee A. D-limonene sensitizes docetaxel-induced cytotoxicity in human prostate cancer cells: generation of reactive oxygen species and induction of apoptosis. J Carcinog. 2009;8:9.

58. Trachootham D, Zhou Y, Zhang H, Demizu Y, Chen Z, Pelicano H, et al. Selective killing of oncogenically transformed cells through a ROS-mediated mechanism by β-phenylethyl isothiocyanate. Cancer Cell. 2006;10(3):241–52.

59. Stashenko EE, Jaramillo BE, Martínez JR. Comparison of different extraction methods for the analysis of volatile secondary metabolites of Lippia alba (mill.) NE Brown, grown in Colombia, and evaluation of its in vitro antioxidant activity. J Chromatogr A. 2004;1025(1):93–103.

60. Chaimovitsh D, Altshuler O, Belausov E, Abu Abied M, Rubin B, Sadot E, Dudai N. The relative effect of citral on mitotic microtubules in wheat roots and BY2 cells. Plant Biol. 2012;14(2):354–64.

61. Jia SS, Xi GP, Zhang M, Chen YB, Lei B, Dong XS, Yang YM. Induction of apoptosis by D-limonene is mediated by inactivation of Akt in LS174T human colon cancer cells. Oncol Rep. 2013;29(1):349–54.

62. Xia H, Liang W, Song Q, Chen X, Chen X, Hong J. The in vitro study of apoptosis in NB4 cell induced by citral. Cytotechnology. 2013;65(1):49–57.

63. Kapur A, Felder M, Fass L, Kaur J, Czarnecki A, Rathi K, Patankar M. The monoterpene, citral, increases intracellular oxygen radicals and inhibits cancer cell proliferation by inducing apoptosis and endoplasmic reticulum stress. Clin Cancer Res. 2016;615(22):19106–4404.

64. Das R, Roy A, Dutta N, Majumder HK. Reactive oxygen species and imbalance of calcium homeostasis contributes to curcumin induced programmed cell death in Leishmania donovani. Apoptosis. 2008;13(7):867–82.

65. García LT, Leite NR, Alfonzo JD, Thiemann OH. Effects of Trypanosoma brucei tryptophanyl-tRNA synthetases silencing by RNA interference. Mem Inst Oswaldo Cruz. 2007;102(6):757–62.

66. Menna-Barreto RF, Salomão K, Dantas AP, Santa-Rita RM, Soares MJ, Barbosa HS, De Castro SL. Different cell death pathways induced by drugs in Trypanosoma cruzi: an ultrastructural study. Micron. 2009;40(2):157–68.

67. Jimenez V, Paredes R, Sosa MA, Galanti N. Natural programmed cell death in T. cruzi epimastigotes maintained in axenic cultures. J Cell Biochem. 2008;105(3):688–98.

68. López M, Stashenko EE, Fuentes JL. Chemical composition and antigenotoxic properties of Lippia alba essential oils. Genet Biol Mol. 2011;34(3):479–88.

69. Chou TC. Theoretical basis, experimental design, and computerized simulation of synergism and antagonism in drug combination studies. Pharmacol Rev. 2006;58(3):621–81.

5

Astragalus membranaceus (Fisch.) Bunge repairs intestinal mucosal injury induced by LPS in mice

Yizhe Cui[†] , Qiuju Wang[†], Rui Sun, Li Guo, Mengzhu Wang, Junfeng Jia, Chuang Xu[*] and Rui Wu[*]

Abstract

Background: Astragalus membranaceus (Fisch.) Bunge is one of the most widely used traditional Chinese herbal medicines. It is used as immune stimulant, tonic, antioxidant, hepatoprotectant, diuretic, antidiabetic, anticancer, and expectorant. The purpose of the study was to investigate the curative effects of the decoction obtained from Astragalus membranaceus root in intestinal mucosal injury induced by LPS in mice. An LPS-induced intestinal mucosal injury mice model was applied in the study.

Methods: The mice were post-treated with Astragalus membranaceus decoction (AMD) for 4 days after 3 days LPS induction. ELISA kit was used to detect the content of tumor necrosis factor (TNF)-α, interleukin (IL)-1β, IL-4,IL-6 and IL-8 in the serum of each group mice. The morphological changes in intestinal mucosa at the end of the experiments were observed. Both VH (villus height) and CD (crypt depth) were measured using H&E-stained sections.

Results: There were significant differences in IL-1β, IL-4,IL-6, IL-8 and TNF-α levels in AMD-treated group on the 7th day compared to the controls group. The VH was lower in duodenum, jejunum and the ileum in LPS-treated mice compared to the control animals. Similarly, there was also decrease in V/C. Compared to the control mice, for AMD-treated mice, VH and CD had no significantly differences.

Conclusions: Astragalus membranaceus reduced intestinal mucosal damage and promoted tissue repair by inhibiting the expression of inflammatory cytokine.

Keywords: Astragalus membranaceus (Fisch.) Bunge, Decoction, Mice, Lipopolysaccharide

Background

Intestinal mucosa is a natural barrier against bacteria. It prevents viruses and other harmful bacteria from entering the blood [1]. Endotoxin is the lipopolysaccharide (LPS) in the cell wall of Gram-negative bacteria, which has a variety of biological activity and is decomposed and released in the process of bacterial metabolism or after death. LPS can stimulate the release of inflammatory mediators from macrophages and neutrophils and eventually lead to the imbalance of inflammatory and anti-inflammatory reactions and the occurrence of excessive systemic inflammation [2].

Astragalus membranaceus (Fisch.) Bunge (syn. Astragalus propinquus Schischkin) (AM), also known as Huangqi or milk vetch root in China, is an important medicine in traditional Chinese medicine. [3]. This herb possesses many common pharmacological activities, such as multiple organ protection [4, 5], antioxidant [6], hypoglycemic [7], antiviral [8] and so on, and has their own pharmacological properties and mechanisms. Studies have shown that A. membranaceus can enhance the contraction of the right ventricular myocardium in rats in a dose-dependent manner [9] and has recently been reported to be a potential promote tissue wound repair. The water extract of A. membranaceus is one of the main active preparations obtained from the root of this specie. However, there are not so many reports studies focusing on the decoction of AM. Some studies showed that gastric mucosa and atrophic pathological damage

* Correspondence: xuchuang7175@163.com; fuhewu@126.com
†Yizhe Cui and Qiuju Wang contributed equally to this work.
College of Animal Science and Veterinary Medicine, Heilongjiang Bayi Agricultural University, 2# Xinyang Road, New Development District, Daqing 163319, Heilongjiang, China

significantly reduced in rats after Huangqi intervention [10]. However, it is still not elucidated whether oral administration of *Astragalus membranaceus* decoction (AMD) could provide a repair effect during intestinal mucosal injury and what is the underlying mechanism. In this study, we explored the repair effect of AMD in LPS induced experimental intestinal mucosal injury in mice.

Methods

Drugs and reagents

LPS (*Escherichia coli* O55:B5) and all other chemicals were obtained from Sigma-Aldrich (St. Louis, MO, USA). Distilled water was filtered through a Milli-Q system from EMD Millipore Corporation (Billerica, MA, USA). LPS was suspended in physiological saline and stored as a 20 mg/ml stock. Dilutions prior to injection were into physiological saline. Animals were weighed prior to injection of LPS and stock LPS was diluted to the appropriate dose for each animal.

Plant material

Astragalus membranaceus was purchased from Fu Rui Bang Chinese Medicine Co., Ltd. (Daqing, China), then it was authenticated by Dr. Pengyu Jia and also deposited in Veterinary drug research and Development Center, Heilongjiang Bayi Agricultural University, Heilongjiang, China) according to Chinese Pharmacopoeia (The Pharmacopoeia Commission of PRC, 2010).

Animals

Male ICR mice weighing 22–25 g were purchased from the Animal Experiment Center of HARBIN MEDICAL UNIVERSITY (DAQING) [Certification no. SYXK (HEI) 2,014,005]. Mice were maintained on a standard light/dark cycle under controlled temperature (22 ± 2 °C) and humidity (50 ± 10%) with certified standard diet and water adlibitum. Mice were habituated to animal facilities for 1 week before the experiment. All the experimental procedures were approved by, and conducted in accordance with Principles of Laboratory Animal Care and according to the rules and ethics set forth by the Ethical Committee of Heilongjiang Bayi Agricultural University.

Extraction procedure

The general preparation procedure of *Astragalus membranaceus* decoction (AMD) is as follows [11]. Briefly, 100 g the root of *Astragalus membranaceus* was extracted by refluxing with water (1:8, *w/v*) for 1.5 h following sonicating for 30 min, then the extraction solutions were combined to be filtered and concentrated to 100 mL under reduced pressure. The concentrations of the residues were 1 g/mL for *Astragalus membranaceus*. Finally, the concentration be adjusted to the required with distilled water for

intragastrical administration. After being autoclaved at 100 °C for 20 min, the stock solution was stored at 4 °C.

Grouping and treatment

In experiments, animals were randomized into three groups of ten individuals (Fig. 1). The control group, LPS-treated group and AMD-treated group. Mice in the LPS groups and the AMD group, were intraperitoneally injected with LPS (*Escherichia coli* 055:B5, 5 mg/kg; Sigma) for 3 days. The chosen dose of LPS was based on Die Dai's study and preliminary experiments [12]. AMD-treated groups were given *Astragalus membranaceus* decoction by intragastric administration once daily and treatments lasted for 4 days after 3 days LPS induction. Briefly, 1 ml syringe with No. 12 gavage needle was used in intragastric administration. The volume of gavage was usually 0.1 ml/10 g body weight. Mice in control group were received physiological saline for 7 days. After euthanizing the mice by carbon dioxide, blood was obtained by cardiac puncture on the 7th day. On collection, blood samples were centrifuged at 5000 rpm for 10 min, and were subsequently stored at − 80 °C before metabolomics analysis. Survivals were recorded for 72 h.

Determination of inflammatory cytokine levels

Cytokine levels in serum were determined by ELISA by using commercially available kits (Endogen, Cambridge,MA). For each assay, serum was serially diluted to ensure that values obtained were within the linear range of the standards provided with each kit. Each sample was done in duplicate, and data from individual mice were averaged.

Histopathology

Specimens of the intestinal wall of the duodenum, jejunum and ileum were prepared for histological examination by fixing in 4% formaldehyde-buffered solution, embedding in paraffin, and sectioning. Paraffin sections were cut into slices of 4 μm and stained with H&E staining solution. Finally, the stained sections were observed and photographed under a light microscope (with 100× magnification). Villous height and the associated crypt depth were evaluated using the Image Pro plus 4 analysis software (Media Cybernetics, Baltimore, MD, USA) processing and analysis system. For each intestinal sample, at least 10 well-oriented were measured and the mean value was calculated. The method was the same as described by Nabuurs et al. [13].

Data analysis

Data were presented as mean and standard deviation (SD). One-way ANOVA showed significant differences among groups. A level of $P < 0.05$ was considered statistically significant. Analysis was performed with the software SPSS version 16.0 (SPSS Inc., USA).

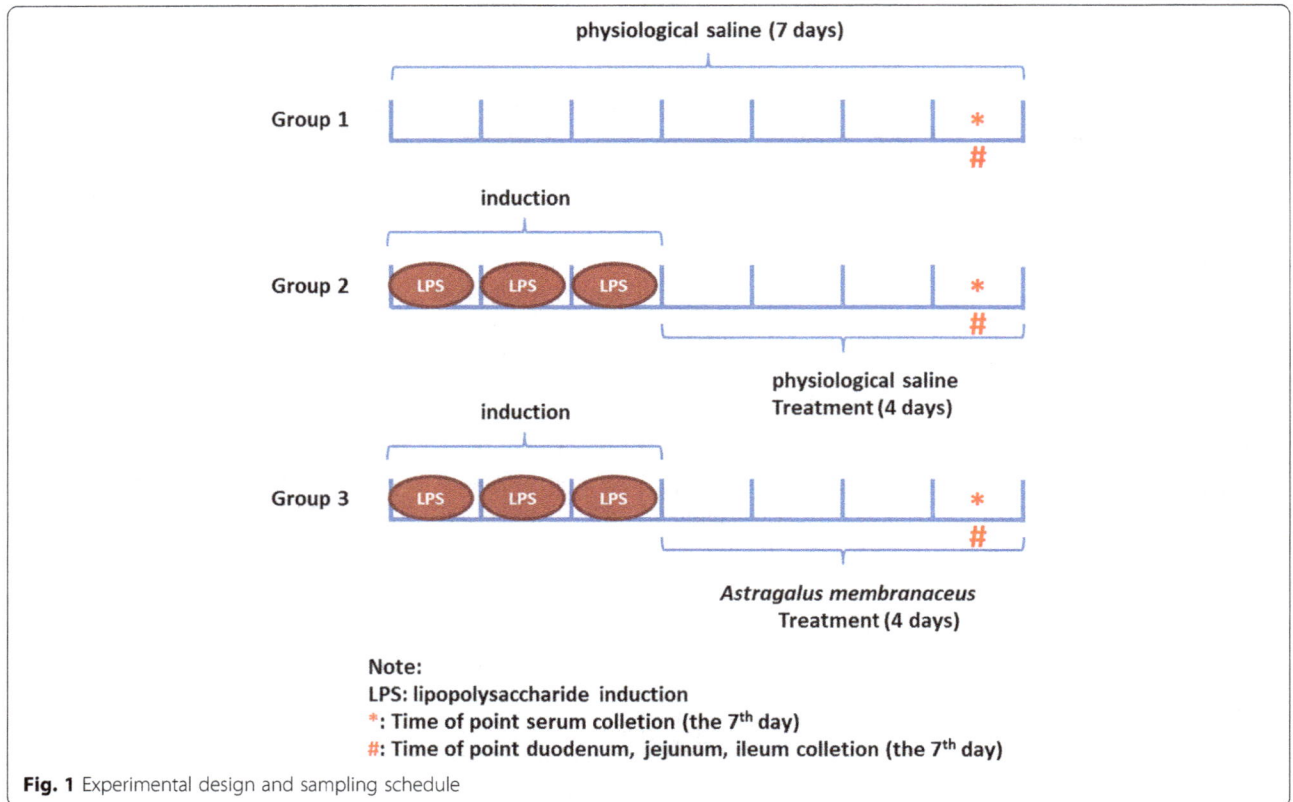

Fig. 1 Experimental design and sampling schedule

Results

Serum concentrations of cytokine

The serum levels of IL-1β, IL-4,IL-6, IL-8 and TNF-α are important biochemical markers for evaluating intestinal mucosal structure and function [14]. In this experiment, the induction of LSP caused significantly higher levels ($P < 0.05$) of IL-1β, IL-4,IL-6, IL-8 and TNF-α in model group on the 7th day compared to the control group (Table 1). Compared with LPS group, the level of inflammatory cytokines decreased significantly ($P < 0.05$) in AMD group. Meanwhile, there were no significant differences of IL-1β, IL-4,IL-6, IL-8 and TNF-α levels in AMD-treated group on the 7th day compared to control group, though the level of IL-4 and IL-1β was higher in AMD group than that in control group, there was no

Table 1 Serum levels of cytokines in LPS- and AMD-treated mice

Parameters	Controls	LPS	AMD
TNF-α (pg/mL)	15.64 ± 1.04	50.30 ± 8.26[*]	7.29 ± 1.12
IL-1β (pg/mL)	6.21 ± 0.45	9.36 ± 0.71[*]	7.26 ± 0.45
IL-4 (pg/mL)	3.47 ± 0.33	11.81 ± 0.39[*]	3.65 ± 0.43
IL-6 (pg/mL)	11.34 ± 0.21	14.25 ± 0.36[*]	8.96 ± 0.63
IL-8 (pg/mL)	9.51 ± 1.07	11.86 ± 0.66[*]	7.93 ± 1.13

The data are expressed as the mean ± SD ($n = 10$ per treatment group).
[*]Statistically different from the control group; [*]$P < 0.05$. Tumor necrosis factor (TNF)-α, interleukin (IL) IL-1β, IL-4,IL-6 and IL-8

significant differences. The results suggested that AMD had no effect on the immunity of the body, moreover curative treated AMD was effective in ameliorating LPS-induced intestinal mucosal damage.

Histopathological changes in intestinal tissue

Pathological examinations of the intestinal mucosal injury were carried out and the LPS-treatment and AMD-treatment are shown in Fig. 2. Compared with the control animals, the pathological changes were obvious, LPS-treated groups caused significant mucosal damage, that is, epithelial shedding, villi fracturing, mucosal atrophy, edema and the villus had shortened on the 7th day after LPS injection (Fig. 2). However, as time goes on, the intestinal mucosa damage begins to recover slowly in the AMD-treated groups on the 7th day. These observations showed that AMD has obvious beneficial effects against intestinal mucosal damage.

Histomorphological analyses

The VH and CD, which indicated intestinal villus's absorptive functions, were measured. The experiments showed that the VH was lower in duodenum, jejunum and the ileum in LPS-treated mice compared to the control animals. Similarly, there was decrease in V/C. Compared to the control mice, for AMD-treated mice, VH and CD had no significantly differences (Fig. 3).

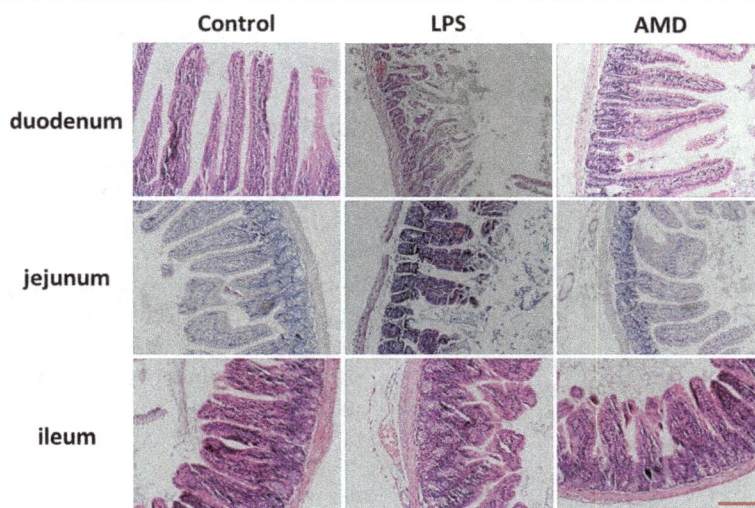

Fig. 2 Histomorphometric analyses of intestinal mucosa time changes. Histological appearance of mice intestinal mucosa after haematoxylin and eosin (H&E) stain (original magnification 100×). Scale bars: 50 μm

Discussion

Intestinal mucosal injury is associated with intestinal inflammation [15]. We investigated whether AMD could ameliorate the inflammatory response in mice induced by LPS. A large number of studies suggest that the intestinal ischemia/reperfusion injury, LPS challenge, and intestinal inflammatory diseases can induce the expression of inflammatory cytokines in humans and animals [16]. Both in vitro and in vivo studies show that over-secretory of inflammatory cytokines can have a negative effects on intestinal mucosal integrity, permeability and epithelial function of the intestinal mucosa [17]. The imbalance of cytokine and chemokine secretion plays an important role in mucosal defense. IL-8 is produced by macrophages and epithelial cells. It can chemotaxis and activate neutrophils, which leads to mucous edema, leukocyte infiltration, increased vascular damage and permeability, resulting in immune inflammatory lesions [18]. IL-4 can play a role in pro-inflammatory factors alone in the gut of mice, which can trigger inflammation [19]. The study showed that LPS was identified by Toll like receptor 4 (TLR4) to release TNF-α, IL-1 beta and IL-6 and other cytokines, which mediate and promote the occurrence of inflammatory bowel disease (IBD) [20]. Intraperitoneal injection of LPS can cause intestinal mucosal inflammation, which is characterized by increased inflammatory and anti-inflammatory cytokines. TNF-α plays a major role in causing intestinal inflammation, and its role is to accumulate inflammatory cells to the local tissues of the inflammation, cause edema, activate coagulation cascade, and form granuloma [21]. The common way to treat IBD in clinic is to inhibit TNF-α by using TNF-α antagonist to improve and alleviate IBD symptoms. In this experiment, the mice were intraperitoneally injected with LPS to establish a model of intestinal injury in mice. LPS challenge increased the level of TNF-α, IL-1β, IL-4, IL-6 and IL-8 in the serum (Table 1). Importantly, AMD reduced the concentrations of TNF-α, IL-1β, IL-4, IL-6 and IL-8 in the serum, compared to LPS-challenged mice. These findings indicate that the AMD has beneficial effects in reducing intestinal mucosal inflammation. AMD may inhibit intestinal immune damage, reduce intestinal mucosal edema and promote intestinal mucosal repair by downregulating the expression of cytokine.

The structural characteristics of the small intestinal mucosa are circular folds, intestinal villi and microvilli. These characteristics greatly expand the surface area of the small intestine and make the nutrients fully digested and absorbed in the small intestine. The complete structure of the small intestine is the physiological basis of its digestion and absorption function, and its morphological and structural changes directly affect the surface area of villi, thereby affecting the body's ability to absorb nutrients [22]. The integrity and height of the intestinal villi determine the absorption area of the small intestine, the absorption of nutrients and the growth of the animals [23]. Therefore, the increase of the villi height, the ratio of the villi/crypt or the decrease of the depth of the recess is related to the improvement of the digestion and absorption of nutrients [24]. Compared with the LPS group, AMD increased the villus height and villus/crypt ratio of the duodenum, as well as the villus height and chorionic ratio of the jejunum and ileum. Crypt depth was significantly reduced in the duodenum and the jejunum, compared with the LPS group. The expression of inflammatory cytokines was consistent with the

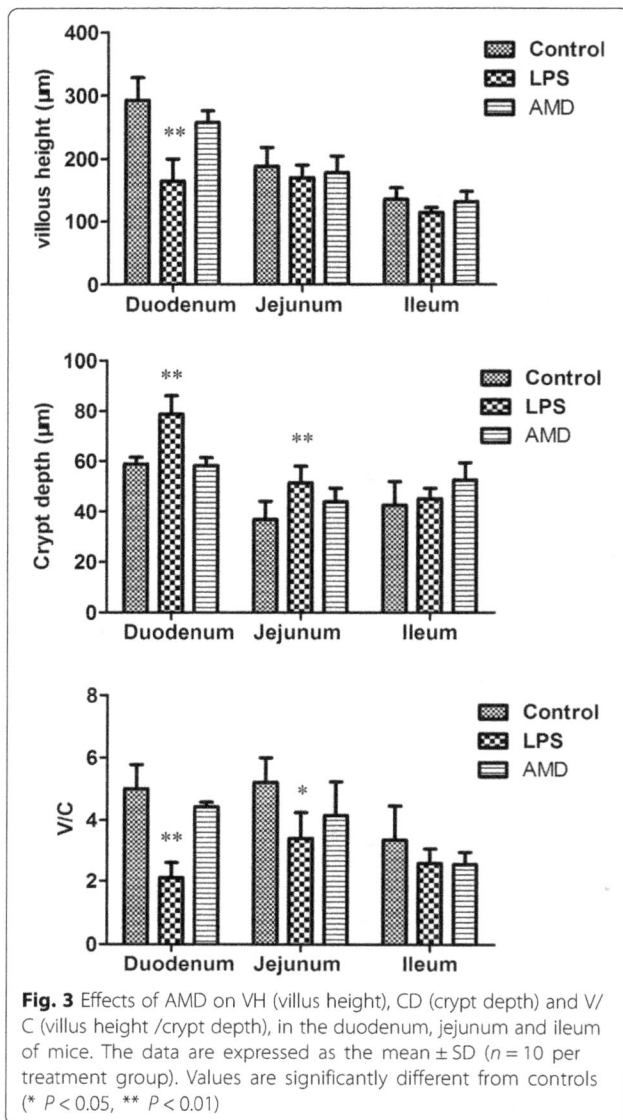

Fig. 3 Effects of AMD on VH (villus height), CD (crypt depth) and V/C (villus height /crypt depth), in the duodenum, jejunum and ileum of mice. The data are expressed as the mean ± SD (*n* = 10 per treatment group). Values are significantly different from controls (* *P* < 0.05, ** *P* < 0.01)

colon weight index, and reducing macroscopically and histological scores [32], which is similar to the results of this experiment.

Conclusions

Astragalus membranaceus treatment can protect small intestinal mucosa against LPS injury. Also, *A. membranaceus* promotes tissue repair by inhibiting the expression of inflammatory cytokine. These findings indicate that *A. membranaceus* can partly reduce small intestinal mucosa injury induced by LPS. Further studies of *A. membranaceus* are necessary to develop a new effective plant-derived therapeutic modality for intestinal mucosal injury.

Abbreviations
AM: *Astragalus membranaceus* (Fisch.) Bunge (syn. *Astragalus propinquus* Schischkin); AMD: *Astragalus membranaceus* decoction; CD: Crypt depth; H&E: Haematoxylin and eosin; IBD: Inflammatory bowel disease; IL: Interleukin; LPS: Lipopolysaccharide; SD: Standard deviation; TNF: Tumor necrosis factor; V/C: Villus height /Crypt depth; VH: Villus height

Funding
This work was supported by Natural Science Foundation of Heilongjiang Province (C201444), China Scholarship council (201508230118), Postdoctoral Program Foundation of Heilongjiang Bayi Agricultural University of China (601038), Doctoral Program Foundation of Heilongjiang Bayi Agricultural University of China (XDB-2016-10) and China Postdoctoral Science Foundation (2017 M620124; 2018 T110320).

Authors' contributions
YC and QW contributed equally to this work. YC, QW, CX and RW designed the research; YC, RS, LG, YC performed the research; MW, JJ analyzed the data; and YC and QW wrote the paper. All authors read and approved the final manuscript.

Competing interests
The authors declare that they have no competing interests.

alteration in the structure of intestinal villi (Table 1 Based on these results, we concluded that AMD protected the intestinal mucosa from the LPS-induced injury.

AM is a well-known medicinal herb for reinforcing Qi (the vital energy) in traditional Chinese medicine [25]. *Astragalus* polysaccharides has the characteristics of antioxidation [26], immunomodulation [27], antiviral, antitumor activities [28] and cardiovascular protection [29]. AM and its active components have been proved to be effective in the treatment of a variety of diseases, such as diabetes mellitus [30] and cardiovascular disorders [31]. In recent years, astragal's polysaccharides effectively reduced the mucosal damage of experimental colitis in mice by shortening colonic length, reducing

References
1. Vancamelbeke M, Vermeire S. The intestinal barrier: a fundamental role in health and disease. Expert Rev Gastroenterol Hepatol. 2017;11(9):821–34.
2. Waseem T, Duxbury M, Ito H, Ashley SW, Robinson MK. Exogenous ghrelin modulates release of pro-inflammatory and anti-inflammatory cytokines in LPS-stimulated macrophages through distinct signaling pathways. Surgery. 2008;143(3):334–42.
3. Guo K, He X, Lu D, Zhang Y, Li X, Yan Z, Qin B. Cycloartane-type triterpenoids from Astragalus hoantchy French. Nat Prod Res. 2017;31(3):314–9.
4. Wang XQ, Wang L, Tu YC, Zhang YC. Traditional Chinese medicine for refractory nephrotic syndrome: strategies and promising treatments. Evid Based Complement Alternat Med. 2018;2018:8746349.
5. Kim GD, Oh J, Park HJ, Bae K, Lee SK. Magnolol inhibits angiogenesis by regulating ROS-mediated apoptosis and the PI3K/AKT/mTOR signaling pathway in mES/EB-derived endothelial-like cells. Int J Oncol. 2013;43(2):600–10.
6. Li H, Wang P, Huang F, Jin J, Wu H, Zhang B, Wang Z, Shi H, Wu X. Astragaloside IV protects blood-brain barrier integrity from LPS-induced

disruption via activating Nrf2 antioxidant signaling pathway in mice. Toxicol Appl Pharmacol. 2018;340:58–66.

7. Cui K, Zhang S, Jiang X, Xie W. Novel synergic antidiabetic effects of Astragalus polysaccharides combined with Crataegus flavonoids via improvement of islet function and liver metabolism. Mol Med Rep. 2016; 13(6):4737–44.

8. Wang Y, Chen Y, Du H, Yang J, Ming K, Song M, Liu J. Comparison of the anti-duck hepatitis a virus activities of phosphorylated and sulfated Astragalus polysaccharides. Exp Biol Med. 2017;242(3):344–53.

9. Cao Y, Shen T, Huang X, Lin Y, Chen B, Pang J, Li G, Wang Q, Zohrabian S, Duan C, et al. Astragalus polysaccharide restores autophagic flux and improves cardiomyocyte function in doxorubicin-induced cardiotoxicity. Oncotarget. 2017;8(3):4837–48.

10. Zhu X, Liu S, Zhou J, Wang H, Fu R, Wu X, Wang J, Lu F. Effect of Astragalus polysaccharides on chronic atrophic gastritis induced by N-methyl-N'-nitro-N-nitrosoguanidine in rats. Drug Res. 2013;63(11):597–602.

11. Cho CH, Mei QB, Shang P, Lee SS, So HL, Guo X, Li Y. Study of the gastrointestinal protective effects of polysaccharides from Angelica sinensis in rats. Planta Med. 2000;66(4):348–51.

12. Dai D, Gao Y, Chen J, Huang Y, Zhang Z, Xu F. Time-resolved metabolomics analysis of individual differences during the early stage of lipopolysaccharide-treated rats. Sci Rep. 2016;6:34136.

13. Nabuurs MJ, Hoogendoorn A, van der Molen EJ, van Osta AL. Villus height and crypt depth in weaned and unweaned pigs, reared under various circumstances in the Netherlands. Res Vet Sci. 1993;55(1):78–84.

14. Xiao K, Cao ST, Ie F J, Lin FH, Wang L, Hu CH. Anemonin improves intestinal barrier restoration and influences TGF-beta1 and EGFR signaling pathways in LPS-challenged piglets. Innate Immun. 2016;22(5):344–52.

15. Blikslager AT, Moeser AJ, Gookin JL, Jones SL, Odle J. Restoration of barrier function in injured intestinal mucosa. Physiol Rev. 2007;87(2):545–64.

16. Liu Y, Huang J, Hou Y, Zhu H, Zhao S, Ding B, Yin Y, Yi G, Shi J, Fan W. Dietary arginine supplementation alleviates intestinal mucosal disruption induced by Escherichia coli lipopolysaccharide in weaned pigs. Br J Nutr. 2008;100(3):552–60.

17. Oswald IP, Dozois CM, Barlagne R, Fournout S, Johansen MV, Bogh HO. Cytokine mRNA expression in pigs infected with Schistosoma japonicum. Parasitology. 2001;122(Pt 3):299–307.

18. Reddy KP, Markowitz JE, Ruchelli ED, Baldassano RN, Brown KA. Lamina propria and circulating interleukin-8 in newly and previously diagnosed pediatric inflammatory bowel disease patients. Dig Dis Sci. 2007;52(2):365–72.

19. Chen J, Gong C, Mao H, Li Z, Fang Z, Chen Q, Lin M, Jiang X, Hu Y, Wang W et al: E2F1/SP3/STAT6 axis is required for IL-4-induced epithelial-mesenchymal transition of colorectal cancer cells. Int J Oncol 2018;53(2): 567–78.

20. Liu HM, Liao JF, Lee TY. Farnesoid X receptor agonist GW4064 ameliorates lipopolysaccharide-induced ileocolitis through TLR4/MyD88 pathway related mitochondrial dysfunction in mice. Biochem Biophys Res Commun. 2017; 490(3):841–8.

21. Allocca M, Bonifacio C, Fiorino G, Spinelli A, Furfaro F, Balzarini L, Bonovas S, Danese S. Efficacy of tumour necrosis factor antagonists in stricturing Crohn's disease: a tertiary center real-life experience. Dig Liver Dis. 2017; 49(8):872–7.

22. Collins JT, Bhimji SS: Anatomy, Abdomen, Small Intestine. In: StatPearls. edn. Treasure Island (FL); 2017.

23. Greig CJ, Cowles RA. Muscarinic acetylcholine receptors participate in small intestinal mucosal homeostasis. J Pediatr Surg. 2017;52(6):1031–4.

24. Hou Y, Wang L, Yi D, Ding B, Yang Z, Li J, Chen X, Qiu Y, Wu G. N-acetylcysteine reduces inflammation in the small intestine by regulating redox, EGF and TLR4 signaling. Amino Acids. 2013;45(3):513–22.

25. Lin HQ, Gong AG, Wang HY, Duan R, Dong TT, Zhao KJ, Tsim KW. Danggui Buxue tang (Astragali Radix and Angelicae Sinensis Radix) for menopausal symptoms: a review. J Ethnopharmacol. 2017;199:205–10.

26. Huang WM, Liang YQ, Tang LJ, Ding Y, Wang XH. Antioxidant and anti-inflammatory effects of Astragalus polysaccharide on EA.hy926 cells. Exp Ther Med. 2013;6(1):199–203.

27. Du X, Zhao B, Li J, Cao X, Diao M, Feng H, Chen X, Chen Z, Zeng X. Astragalus polysaccharides enhance immune responses of HBV DNA vaccination via promoting the dendritic cell maturation and suppressing Treg frequency in mice. Int Immunopharmacol. 2012;14(4):463–70.

28. Dang SS, Jia XL, Song P, Cheng YA, Zhang X, Sun MZ, Liu EQ. Inhibitory effect of emodin and Astragalus polysaccharide on the replication of HBV. World J Gastroenterol. 2009;15(45):5669–73.

29. Yang M, Lin HB, Gong S, Chen PY, Geng LL, Zeng YM, Li DY. Effect of Astragalus polysaccharides on expression of TNF-alpha, IL-1beta and NFATc4 in a rat model of experimental colitis. Cytokine. 2014;70(2):81–6.

30. Zhang K, Pugliese M, Pugliese A, Passantino A. Biological active ingredients of traditional Chinese herb Astragalus membranaceus on treatment of diabetes: a systematic review. Mini Rev Med Chem. 2015;15(4):315–29.

31. Sun S, Yang S, Dai M, Jia X, Wang Q, Zhang Z, Mao Y. The effect of Astragalus polysaccharides on attenuation of diabetic cardiomyopathy through inhibiting the extrinsic and intrinsic apoptotic pathways in high glucose -stimulated H9C2 cells. BMC Complement Altern Med. 2017;17(1):310.

32. Zhao HM, Wang Y, Huang XY, Huang MF, Xu R, Yue HY, Zhou BG, Huang HY, Sun QM, Liu DY. Astragalus polysaccharide attenuates rat experimental colitis by inducing regulatory T cells in intestinal Peyer's patches. World J Gastroenterol. 2016;22(11):3175–85.

6

Concurrent regulation of LKB1 and CaMKK2 in the activation of AMPK in castrate-resistant prostate cancer by a well-defined polyherbal mixture with anticancer properties

Amber F. MacDonald[1], Ahmed Bettaieb[1], Dallas R. Donohoe[1], Dina S. Alani[1], Anna Han[1,5], Yi Zhao[1,4] and Jay Whelan[1,2,3]* (iD)

Abstract

Background: Zyflamend, a blend of herbal extracts, effectively inhibits tumor growth using preclinical models of castrate-resistant prostate cancer mediated in part by 5′-adenosine monophosphate-activated protein kinase (AMPK), a master energy sensor of the cell. Clinically, treatment with Zyflamend and/or metformin (activators of AMPK) had benefits in castrate-resistant prostate cancer patients who no longer responded to treatment. Two predominant upstream kinases are known to activate AMPK: liver kinase B1 (LKB1), a tumor suppressor, and calcium-calmodulin kinase kinase-2 (CaMKK2), a tumor promotor over-expressed in many cancers. The objective was to interrogate how Zyflamend activates AMPK by determining the roles of LKB1 and CaMKK2.

Methods: AMPK activation was determined in CWR22Rv1 cells treated with a variety of inhibitors of LKB1 and CaMKK2 in the presence and absence of Zyflamend, and in LKB1-null HeLa cells that constitutively express CaMKK2, following transfection with wild type LKB1 or catalytically-dead mutants. Upstream regulation by Zyflamend of LKB1 and CaMKK2 was investigated targeting protein kinase C-zeta (PKCζ) and death-associated protein kinase (DAPK), respectively.

Results: Zyflamend's activation of AMPK appears to be LKB1 dependent, while simultaneously inhibiting CaMKK2 activity. Zyflamend failed to rescue the activation of AMPK in the presence of pharmacological and molecular inhibitors of LKB1, an effect not observed in the presence of inhibitors of CaMKK2. Using LKB1-null and catalytically-dead LKB1-transfected HeLa cells that constitutively express CaMKK2, ionomycin (activator of CaMKK2) increased phosphorylation of AMPK, but Zyflamend only had an effect in cells transfected with wild type LKB1. Zyflamend appears to inhibit CaMKK2 by DAPK-mediated phosphorylation of CaMKK2 at Ser511, an effect prevented by a DAPK inhibitor. Alternatively, Zyflamend mediates LKB1 activation via increased phosphorylation of PKCζ, where it induced translocation of PKCζ and LKB1 to their respective active compartments in HeLa cells following treatment. Altering the catalytic activity of LKB1 did not alter this translocation.

(Continued on next page)

* Correspondence: jwhelan@utk.edu
[1]Department of Nutrition, University of Tennessee, 1215 West Cumberland Avenue, 229 Jessie Harris Building, Knoxville, TN 37996, USA
[2]Tennessee Agricultural Experiment Station, University of Tennessee, Knoxville, TN 37996, USA
Full list of author information is available at the end of the article

(Continued from previous page)

Discussion: Zyflamend's activation of AMPK is mediated by LKB1, possibly via PKCζ, but independent of CaMKK2 by a mechanism that appears to involve DAPK.

Conclusions: Therefore, this is the first evidence that natural products simultaneously and antithetically regulate upstream kinases, known to be involved in cancer, via the activation of AMPK.

Keywords: Zyflamend, AMPK, LKB1, CaMKK2, CWR22Rv1, HeLa, DAPK, PKC-zeta, Prostate cancer, Castrate-resistant

Background

Prostate cancer is the second leading cause of death for men in the United States [1]. While early stages of the disease are treatable, with 5-year survival rates near 100%, prognosis for advanced forms are less promising [2]. Initially, prostate cancer cells rely on androgens for growth, and chemically-mediated deprivation (hormone deprivation therapy) is a common therapy that results in cancer regression [3]. Relapse in the absence of androgens (castrate-resistant prostate cancer) is inevitable for most individuals and is associated with increased expression and activation of the androgen receptor, a major determinant in survival [4, 5]. Due to the poor prognosis of castrate-resistant prostate cancer, concomitant use of natural products to enhance effectiveness is being explored clinically and experimentally [3, 6–10].

Zyflamend (New Chapter, Inc. Brattleboro, VT) is a poly-herbal supplement derived from the extracts of ten different herbs: rosemary, turmeric, holy basil, ginger, green tea, hu zhang, barberry, oregano, Chinese goldthread, and baikal skullcap. Most research using Zyflamend has focused its effects on a variety of cancer models, including oral [11], mammary [12], bone [13], pancreas [14, 15], skin [11, 16], colorectal [15], with an emphasis on prostate [6–9, 17–21], and its beneficial effects appear to be related to the synergy of action of its components [22]. The effects of Zyflamend

and its mechanisms on prostate cancer has been reviewed elsewhere and can be summarized in Fig. 1 [3]. Zyflamend inhibits signaling pathways of inflammation, affects cell survival by enhancing apoptotic and tumor suppressor genes, epigenetically modifies histones, down regulates the androgen receptor and influences the energetics of the cell. The latter pathways are critically important in cancer as rapidly dividing cells rely on the increased synthesis of macromolecules (lipids, proteins, nucleotides, etc) (as reviewed in [23]).

5′-adenosine monophosphate-activated protein kinase (AMPK) is a key regulator of energy in the cell and responds to deficits in adenosine triphosphate (ATP). The protein contains a catalytic subunit (α-subunit), and two regulatory subunits, β and γ-subunits. Under conditions of energy stress the following occurs, (i) increased levels of AMP or ADP bind to the γ-subunit causing allosteric activation of the protein (ATP is a competitive inhibitor), (ii) increased affinity for upstream kinases that target phosphorylation at Thr172 of the α-subunit (increasing catalytic activity > 100 fold), and (iii) reduced affinity for phosphatases that are involved in dephosphorylation at Thr172 [24]. When activated, AMPK is instrumental in inhibiting anabolic pathways that consume ATP, such as lipogenesis and protein synthesis, and enhances

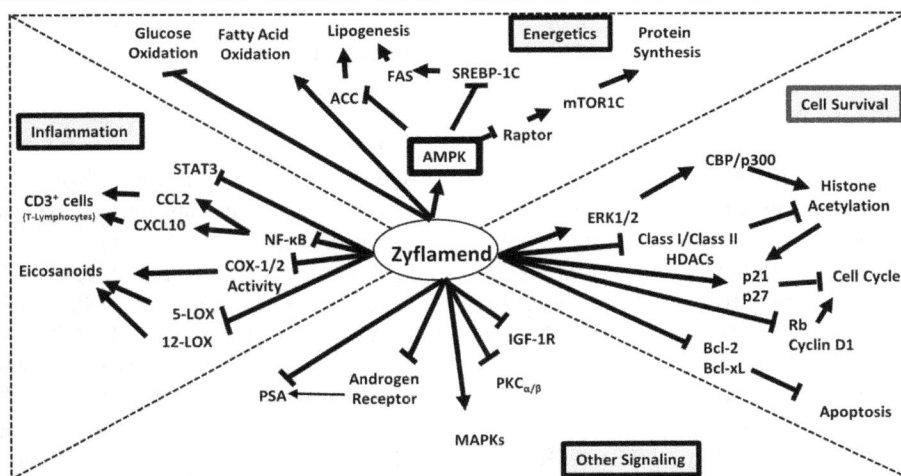

Fig. 1 Summary of the effects of Zyflamend on prostate cancer (with permission from reference [3])

catabolic pathways that generate ATP, such as fatty acid oxidation [23].

Clinically, treatment with Zyflamend and/or metformin (activator of AMPK) had benefits in castrate-resistant prostate cancer patients who no longer responded to a variety of treatments (e.g., hormone ablation, immune-, chemo-, and radiation therapy). Recently, it was determined that tumor suppressor properties of Zyflamend are associated with the activation of AMPK and its downstream signaling, where siRNA knockdown, pharmacological inhibition and over expression of AMPK confirmed Zyflamend's involvement [10]. This involves inhibiting the mammalian target of rapamycin complex-1 (mTORC1) and protein synthesis, lipogenesis by targeting the expression of *(i)* fatty acid synthase, *(ii)* the sterol regulatory element-binding transcription factor-1c, and *(iii)* inhibiting the activity of acetyl CoA carboxylase (ACC). What is not known is how Zyflamend upregulates AMPK. Four kinases have been identified that activate AMPK at Thr172, liver kinases B1 (LKB1), calcium-calmodulin kinase kinase-2 (CaMKK2), transforming growth factor-β activated protein kinase-1 (TAK1) and mixed lineage kinase 3 (MLK3) [25–28]. LKB1 and CaMKK2 are important in a number of cancers, including castrate-resistant prostate cancer (as reviewed in [29]), while the involvement of TAK1 and MLK3 has yet to be determined. LKB1 responds to increases in AMP and ADP, while increases in intracellular calcium is needed for activation of CaMKK2 without requiring elevation in AMP or ADP.

Interestingly, while both LKB1 and CaMKK2 are involved in activating AMPK, their effects on cancer appear to be quite different. LKB1 has anticancer properties because its mutation/deletion is associated with a variety of cancers [30]. CaMKK2, on the other hand, is overexpressed in a number of cancers, including castrate-resistant prostate cancer [31, 32]. Therefore, the overall objective of this paper was to interrogate how Zyflamend activates AMPK in a model of castrate-resistant prostate cancer and the roles LKB1 and CaMKK2 play in that activation.

The major findings of this research revealed that although LKB1 and CaMMK2 are upstream kinases that can activate AMPK, Zyflamend inhibits CaMMK2, a protein overexpressed in many cancers, while simultaneously upregulates LKB1, a reported tumor suppressor. This is the first report linking the simultaneous antagonistic regulation of these two proteins. Upstream regulation of CaMKK2 appears to be mediated by the antitumorigenic death associated protein kinase (DAPK) [33–36], not epigenetically, but via phosphorylation at Ser511 [37]. This is only the second paper to link DAPK activity with the negative regulation of CaMKK2 via phosphorylation at Ser511, and the only one involving cancer cells.

Methods

Zyflamend (New Chapter, Inc. Brattleboro, VT), purchased from Earth Fare Supermarket (Knoxville, TN), is composed of extracts from the following herbs (w/w): rosemary (*Rosmarinus officinalis* 19.2%), turmeric (*Curcuma longa* 14.1%), holy basil (*Ocimum sanctum* 12.8%), ginger (*Zingiber officinale* 12.8%), green tea (*Camellia sinensis* 12.8%), hu zhang (*Polygonum cuspidatum* 10.2%), barberry (*Berberis vulgaris* 5.1%), oregano (*Origanum vulgare* 5.1%), Chinese goldthread (*Coptis chinensis* 5.1%), and baikal skullcap (*Scutellaria baicalensis* 2.5%). Detailed description and characterization of the preparation of Zyflamend and quality assurance of the mixture has been described previously in detail [7]. This description includes rigorously generated verifiable quality control of its constituents via multiple independent laboratories whose biological effects have been duplicated using different lots, at different times, under different experimental conditions, in different laboratories across the United States.

Dulbecco's Modified Eagle Medium (DMEM), G418, penicillin/streptomycin, puromycin, fetal bovine serum (FBS) and trypsin were purchased from Invitrogen (Carlsbad, CA). Cloning vectors were purchased from Addgene (Cambridge, MA). Antibodies for PKC-zeta (PKCζ), LKB1, phospho-LKB1, green fluorescent protein (GFP), Histone B, Flag, and Tubulin were from Santa Cruz Biotechnology (Santa Cruz, CA). AMPK and phospho-AMPK were from Cell Signaling Technology (Beverly, MA). The following chemical reagents were purchased: 5-aminoimidazole-4-carboxamide ribonucleotide (AICAR) (AdipoGen Life Sciences, San Diego, CA); 1,2-<u>bis</u>(o-aminophenoxy)ethane-*N,N,N′,N′*-tetraacetic acid acetoxymethyl ester (BAPTA-AM) and ethylene glycol-bis(β-aminoethyl ether)-N,N,N′,N′-tetraacetic acid (EGTA) (Thermo Scientific, Rockville, IL); STO-609, radicicol, and PKCζ Pseudo-substrate Inhibitor (Santa Cruz Biotechnology, Dallas, TX); ionomycin (Sigma-Aldrich, St. Louis, MO); and Death Associated Protein Kinase Inhibitor (DAPKi) (Merck Millipore, Billerica, MA).

Cell culture

CWR22Rv1 cells (American Type Culture Collection, Rockville, MD), a human-derived castrate-resistant prostate cancer cell line, were cultured in RPMI 1640 media, supplemented with 10% FBS. To mimic an androgen-depleted state, the cells were incubated overnight with 0.5% FBS. HeLa cells (ATCC, Rockville, MD), a human-derived cervical cancer cell line that do not express LKB1, and HCT116 cells (ATCC, Rockville, MD), a human derived colorectal cancer cell line, were cultured in DMEM media supplemented with 10% FBS and 25 mM glucose. All cells were incubated under an atmosphere of 5% CO_2, at 37 °C. For activation of AMPK via

LKB1-dependent or CaMKK2-dependent pathways, cells were treated with AICAR (a cell permeable analog of AMP) (1 mM, 1 h) or ionomycin (calcium ionophore) (1 μM, 1 h), respectively. For experiments using inhibitors of CaMKK2, cells were pre-treated with the selective CaMKK2 inhibitor STO-609 (10 μM, 30 min) or the calcium chelators BAPTA-AM (30 μM, 30 min) or EGTA (2 mM, 30 min). For inhibition of LKB1 or DAPK, cells were pre-treated with radicicol (5 μM, 24 h) or DAPKi (20 μM, 24 h), respectively. For inhibition of PKCζ, cells were pre-treated with the selective PKCζ pseudo-substrate inhibitor (5 μM, 30 min). For all experiments involving Zyflamend, cells were treated with Zyflamend at 200 μg/mL for 30 min unless otherwise indicated.

Down regulation of LKB1 by small interfering RNA

CWR22Rv1 cells were seeded in RPMI medium containing 10% FBS and incubated overnight before media was replaced with RNA transfection medium containing 0.5% FBS. Cells were transfected with 20 nmol of siRNA targeting LKB1 (Thermo Scientific/Dharmacon #L-005035-00) and a siRNA non-targeting control (Thermo Scientific/Dharmacon #D-001810-10-05). Western blot analysis confirmed the efficiency of knockdown to be 76% 48 h after transfection, at which time cells were treated with a vehicle or Zyflamend (200 μg/mL) for 30 min.

Overexpression of LKB1 in HeLa cells

Human WT or catalytically dead (KD) mutants of LKB1 were transfected into HeLa cells using Lipofectamine 3000 (Invitrogen, Carlsbad, CA) following manufacturer's guidelines. Cells were cultured for additional 48 h prior experiments. For total protein lysates, cells were lysed in radio-immunoprecipitation assay buffer (RIPA: 10 M Tris-HCl, pH 7.4, 150 mM NaCl, 0.1% sodium dodecyl sulfate [SDS], 1% Triton X-100, 1% sodium deoxycholate, 5 mM EDTA, 1 mM NaF, 1 mM sodium orthovanadate and protease inhibitors). Lysates were clarified by centrifugation at 13,000 rpm for 10 min, and protein concentrations were determined using a bicinchoninic acid assay kit (Pierce Chemical). Proteins (10 μg) were separated by SDS-polyacrylamide gel electrophoresis (SDS-PAGE) (8–12%) [38], transferred to polyvinylidene difluoride (PVDF) membranes and immunodetected using the indicated antibodies. Proteins were detected using enhanced chemiluminescence (Amersham Biosciences). Resulting immunoreactive bands were quantified using FluorChem Q Imaging software (Alpha Innotech).

Subcellular fractionation

Following Zyflamend treatment, fractionation was performed in HeLa cells as described previously with modifications [39, 40]. Briefly, cells were washed with cold buffer A (100 mM sucrose, 1 mM EGTA, 20 mM 3-(N-morpholino)propanesulfonic acid (MOPS), pH 7.4) and resuspended in lysis buffer B (100 mM sucrose, 1 mM EGTA, 20 mM MOPS, 0.1 dithiothreitol (DTT), 5% freshly added percoll, 0.01% digitonin, 1 mM phenylmethylsulfonyl fluoride (PMSF) and cocktail of protease inhibitors, pH 7,4). Membranes were broken using a dounce homogenizer (200 strokes/sample). Debris and unbroken cells were removed by centrifugation (500 g for 10 min) and supernatants were then centrifuged (2500 g, 5 min) to separate nuclei (pellet). Supernatants were centrifuged again (15,000 g, 15 min) to separate mitochondria. Nuclear fraction was resuspended in radioimmunoprecipitation assay (RIPA) buffer containing proteases inhibitors. Cellular distribution and translocation of the indicated proteins were analyzed by SDS-PAGE and Western blot as described above. Purity of nuclear and cytoplasmic fractions was verified using antibodies against histone B and tubulin (Santa Cruz Biotechnology, Dallas, TX), respectively.

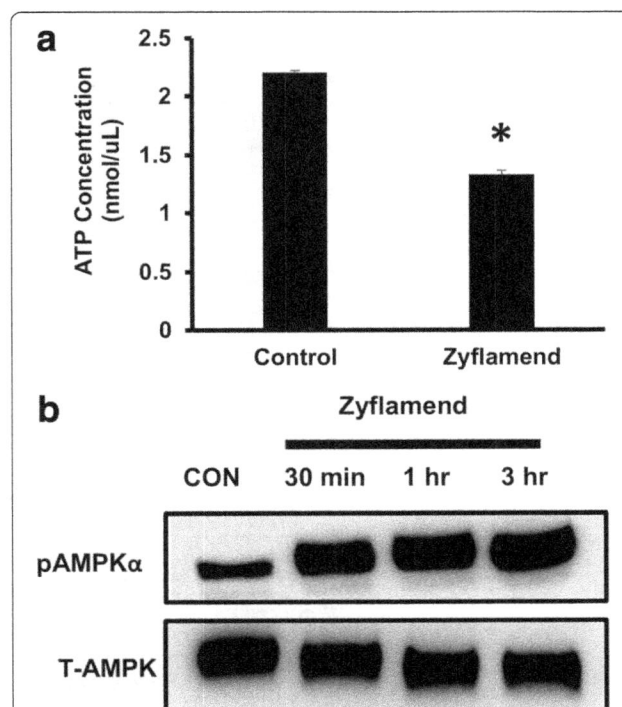

Fig. 2 The effects of Zyflamend on cellular ATP levels and phosphorylation of AMPKα (at Thr172) in CWR22Rv1 cells. **a** ATP levels of CWR22Rv1 cells treated in the presence or absence of Zyflamend (200 μg/mL, 30 min). **b** The effects of Zyflamend (200 μg/mL, 30 min – 3 h) on phosphorylation of AMPKα in CWR22Rv1 cells. Data is presented as mean ± SEM, $n = 4$. Abbreviations: Con, Control

Western blotting

Cells were lysed in RIPA lysis buffer (Thermo Scientific, Rockford, IL). Protein concentration was measured using a Bradford protein assay (Thermo Scientific, Rockford, IL). Equal amount of protein (30 μg) were separated by 8% SDS-PAGE and transferred to a PVDF membrane by electroblotting. Membranes were blocked by 5% non-fat dry milk (LabScientific, Highlands, NJ) or bovine serum albumin (Santa Cruz Biotechnology, Dallas, TX) in 0.1% Tris-buffered saline-Tween-20 (TBST) for 1 h at room temperature and incubated in TBST containing primary antibodies overnight at 4 °C. Membranes were incubated with anti-rabbit or anti-mouse secondary antibody conjugated with horseradish peroxidase (HRP) (Cell Signaling Technology, Danver, MA) for 1 h at room temperature. Protein expression was detected with Super Signal West Pico Chemiluminescent Substrate (Thermo Scientific, Rockford, IL) and membranes were exposed and analyzed via *Li-Cor Odyssey FC* imaging system (Li-Cor, Lincoln, NE). Antibodies against p-AMPKα (Thr172), AMPKα, p-ACC (Ser79), ACC, p-LKB1 (Ser428), LKB1, p- PKCζ (Thr410), PKCζ, and p-CaMKKβ (Ser511) were used to detect target protein level at 1:1000. β-Actin or glyceraldehyde 3-phosphate dehydrogenase (GAPDH) (Santa Cruz Biotechnology, Dallas, TX) was used as the loading control.

ATP assay

Cellular ATP concentration was determined using a fluorometric ATP assay kit (BioRad, Milpitas, CA) following the manufacturer's instructions, and fluorescence

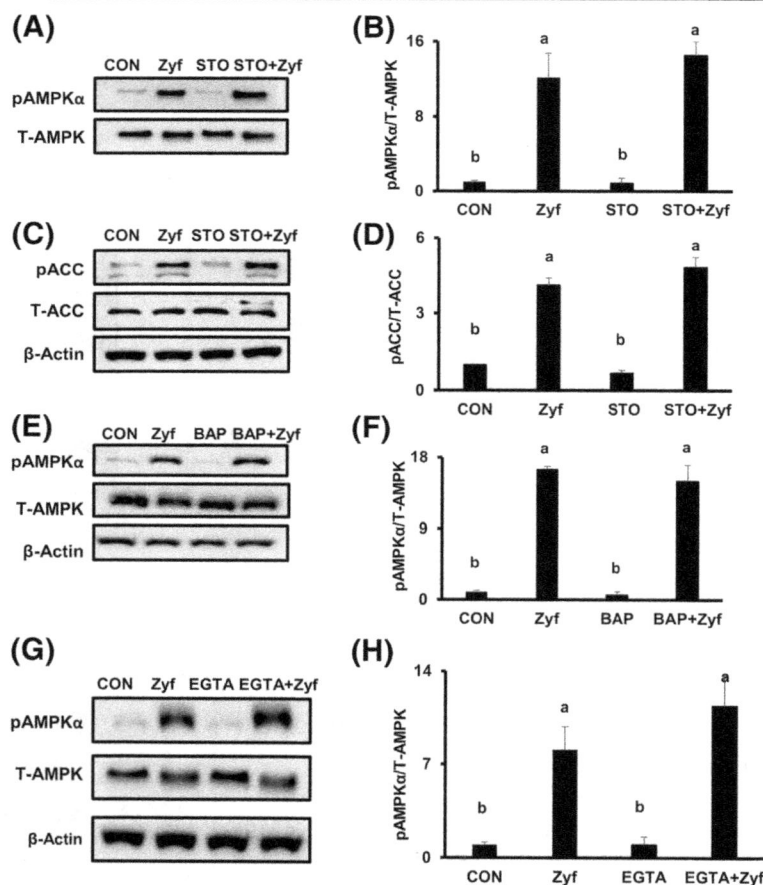

Fig. 3 The effects of CaMKK2 inhibition by STO-609, BAPTA-AM and EGTA on pAMPKα (at Thr172) and pACC (at Ser79), ± Zyflamend in CWR22Rv1 cells. (**A-D**) Western blot of pAMPKα and pACC following treatment of STO-609 (10 μM, 30 min) ± Zyflamend (200 μg/mL, 30 min). (**E, F**) Western blot of pAMPKα following treatment of BAPTA-AM (30 μM, 30 min) ± Zyflamend (200 μg/mL, 30 min). (**G, H**) Western blot of pAMPKα following treatment of EGTA (2 mM, 30 min) ± Zyflamend (200 μg/mL, 30 min). Data are presented as mean ± SEM, n = 3. Bars with different letters are statistically different at p < 0.05. Abbreviations: BAP, BAPTA-AM (1, 2-bis(o-aminophenoxy)ethane-N,N,N',N'-tetraacetic acid acetoxymethyl ester); CON, Control; EGTA, ethylene glycol-bis (β-aminoethyl ether)-N, N, N',N'-tetraacetic acid; STO, STO-609; Zyf, Zyflamend

was read at 525 nm on a Glowmax Multi Detection System (Promega Corporation, Madison, WI).

Statistics

For Western blot, protein was analyzed from 3 independent samples and presented as mean ± SEM. For ATP concentration, results are presented as mean ± SEM. For multiple comparisons, data was analyzed using IBM SPSS Statistics 24 and tested by one-way analysis of variance (ANOVA) followed by a Tukey's post-hoc test. Two-group comparisons were analyzed by two-tailed Student's T-test. Results were considered statistically significant at $p < 0.05$.

Results

Effect of Zyflamend on cell proliferation, ATP levels and AMPK phosphorylation in CWR22Rv1 cells

Zyflamend (200 µg/mL) inhibited cell proliferation in CWR22Rv1 cells in a concentration and time dependent manner (Additional file 1: Figure S1, replicating previously published results [6, 8]). Similar results were replicated in a variety of immortalized prostate-derived cells lines [8] and in the HCT116 colorectal cell line (Additional file 2: Figure S2). Because Zyflamend has been shown to change the energetics of CWR22Rv1 cells [3, 10], levels of ATP were determined. In the presence of Zyflamend, ATP levels were reduced by ~ 40% (Fig. 2a) and AMPK phosphorylation (Thr172) was significantly increased (Fig. 2b). These results were replicated in the HCT116 colorectal cell line to demonstrate that these effects are not specific for prostate cancer cells (Additional file 2: Figure S2).

AMPK activation by CaMKK2 in the presence and absence of Zyflamend in CWR22Rv1 cells

Zyflamend significantly increased the phosphorylation of AMPK (Thr172) (Fig. 3A and B) and its downstream target ACC (Ser79) (Fig. 3C and D), results unaffected by pretreatment with the CaMKK2 inhibitor STO-609 (Fig. 3A-D, lane 4/bar 4). To confirm that the activation of AMPK by Zyflamend is independent of CaMKK2, cells were pre-treated with the calcium chelators BAPTA-AM and EGTA, as CaMKK2 activation is dependent upon intracellular calcium. Pretreatment with BAPTA-AM (Fig. 3E and F) and EGTA (Fig. 3G and H) failed to prevent phosphorylation of AMPK in the presence of Zyflamend. Zyflamend increased the phosphorylation of CaMKK2 at Ser511 (Fig. 4A), a phosphorylation site that results in its inhibition and reported to be mediated by DAPK [37]. Pretreatment with a DAPK inhibitor attenuated Zyflamend's ability to increase phosphorylation of CaMKK2 at Ser511 in a time-dependent manner (Fig. 4A-C), suggesting phosphorylation of CaMKK2 in the presence of Zyflamend is mediated by DAPK. Pretreatment of cells with DAPKi failed to prevent phosphorylation of AMPK in the presence of Zyflamend, further confirming that the activation of AMPK by Zyflamend is independent of CaMKK2 (Fig. 4D and E).

AMPK activation by LKB1 in the presence and absence of Zyflamend in CWR22Rv1 cells

Zyflamend significantly increased the phosphorylation of LKB1 (Ser428) (Fig. 5A), AMPK (Thr172) (Fig. 5C) and ACC (Ser79) (Fig. 5E). In the presence of radicicol, a

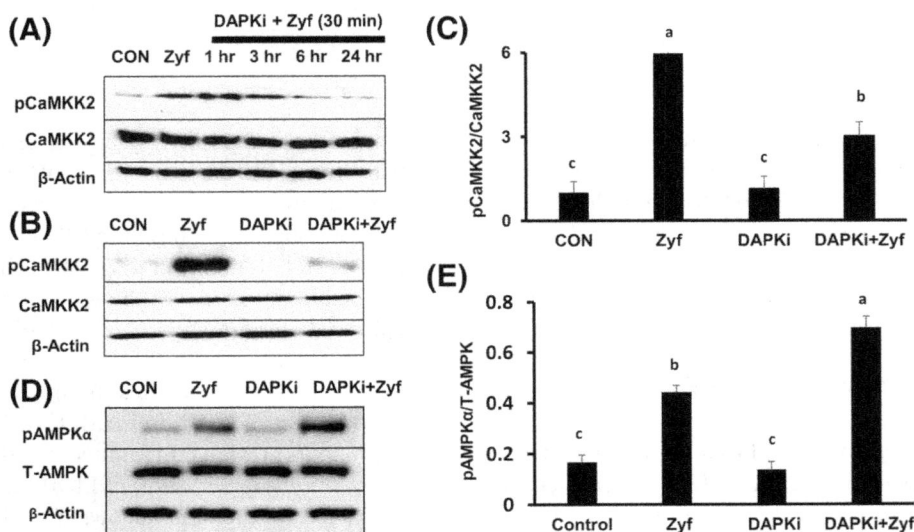

Fig. 4 The effects of Zyflamend and an inhibitor of DAPK on the phosphorylation of CaMKK2 (at Ser511), in CWR22Rv1 cells. **A** Western blot of pCaMKK2 ± Zyflamend (200 µg/mL, 30 min) and following treatment of DAPKi (20 µM, 1 h – 24 h) followed by the treatment of Zyflamend (200 µg/mL, 30 min). **B, C** Western blot and graph comparison of pCaMKK2 following treatment of DAPKi (20 µM, 24 h) ± Zyflamend (200 µg/mL, 30 min). (**D, E**) Western blot and graph comparison of pAMPK following treatment of Zyflamend (200 µg/mL, 30 min) and DAPKi (20 µM, 24 h) ± Zyflamend (200 µg/mL, 30 min). Data are presented as mean ± SEM, $n = 3$. Bars with different letters are statistically different at $p < 0.05$. Abbreviations: CON, Control; DAPKi, DAPK inhibitor; Zyf, Zyflamend

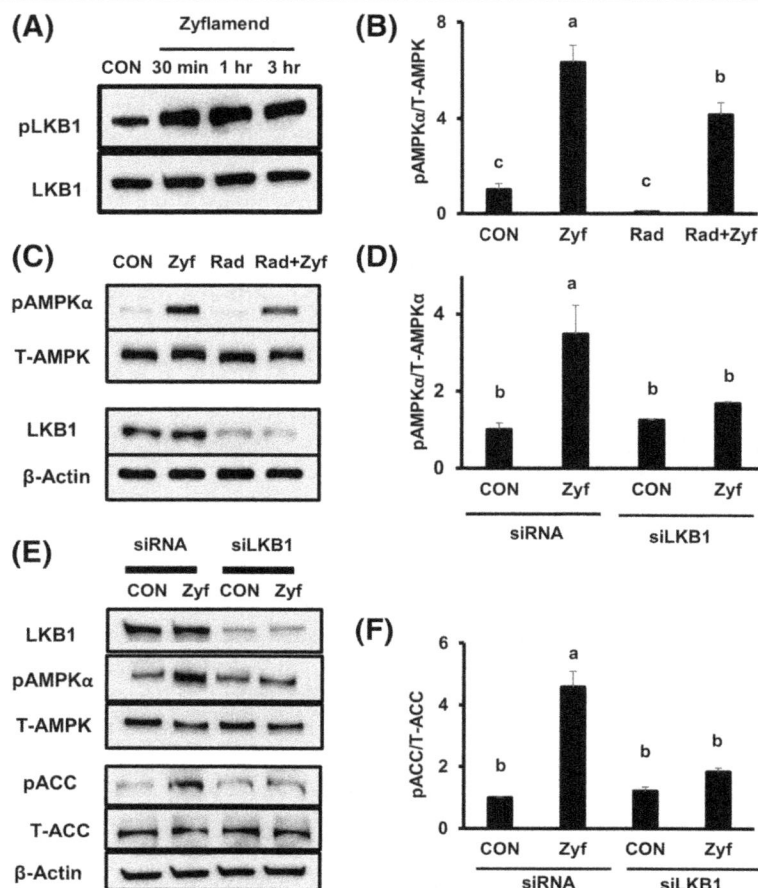

Fig. 5 The effects of Zyflamend on phosphorylation of LKB1 (at Ser428) and AMPKα (at Thr172) following inhibition with radicicol and knockdown of LKB1 in CWR22Rv1 cells. **A** Western blot of pLKB1 ± Zyflamend (200 μg/mL, 30 min – 3 h). **B, C** Western blot of pAMPKα following treatment with radicicol (5 μM, 24 h) ± Zyflamend (200 μg/mL, 30 min). **D-F** Western blot of pAMPKα and pACC (at Ser79) following knockdown of LKB1 ± Zyflamend (200 μg/mL, 30 min). Data are presented as mean ± SEM, $n = 3$. Bars with different letters are statistically different at $p < 0.05$. Abbreviations: CON, Control; Rad, Radicicol; Zyf, Zyflamend

non-specific inhibitor of LKB1 that results in reduction of total LKB1 protein levels (Fig. 5C, row 3, column 3), phosphorylation of AMPK failed to be fully restored upon Zyflamend treatment (Fig. 5B and C). Likewise, knockdown of LKB1 by siRNA (Fig. 5d-f) inhibited Zyflamend-induced phosphorylation of AMPK (Fig. 5D and E) and its downstream target ACC (Fig. 5E and F).

Zyflamend-induced AMPK phosphorylation is LKB1 dependent

To confirm that Zyflamend-induced phosphorylation of AMPK is LKB1 dependent and CaMKK2 independent, we treated LKB1-null HeLa cells, that constitutively express CaMKK2, with AICAR (an activator of AMPK that is commonly used as a positive control), ionomycin (activator of CaMKK2) and Zyflamend (Fig. 6a). The same experiment was conducted on HeLa cells that were stably transfected with the wild-type (WT) or the catalytically dead (KD) mutants of the human LKB1. Two different constructs of the

KD mutants were used, Flag-tagged or green fluorescent protein (KD-LKB1 Flag or KD-LKB1 GFP, respectively) (Fig. 6b). In both mutants, lysine 78 was mutated to isoleucine, abolishing auto-phosphorylation and activation of LKB1 [41, 42]. Ionomycin (Fig. 6b, column 3), but not AICAR (column 2) or Zyflamend (column 4), induced phosphorylation of AMPK in LKB1-null HeLa cells (control) (Fig. 6b, columns 1–5). Following transfection with WT-LKB1 (Fig. 6b, columns 6–8), Zyflamend induced phosphorylation of LKB1 and AMPK (column 7), an effect more pronounced with co-treatment of AICAR (column 8). However, no phosphorylation of LKB1 and AMPK was observed in the KD mutants following treatment with Zyflamend and Zyflamend+AICAR (Fig. 6b, columns 9–14).

Zyflamend-mediated LKB1 phosphorylation is linked to PKCzeta

In an effort to determine how Zyflamend may be mediating the phosphorylation of LKB1, PKCζ was investigated

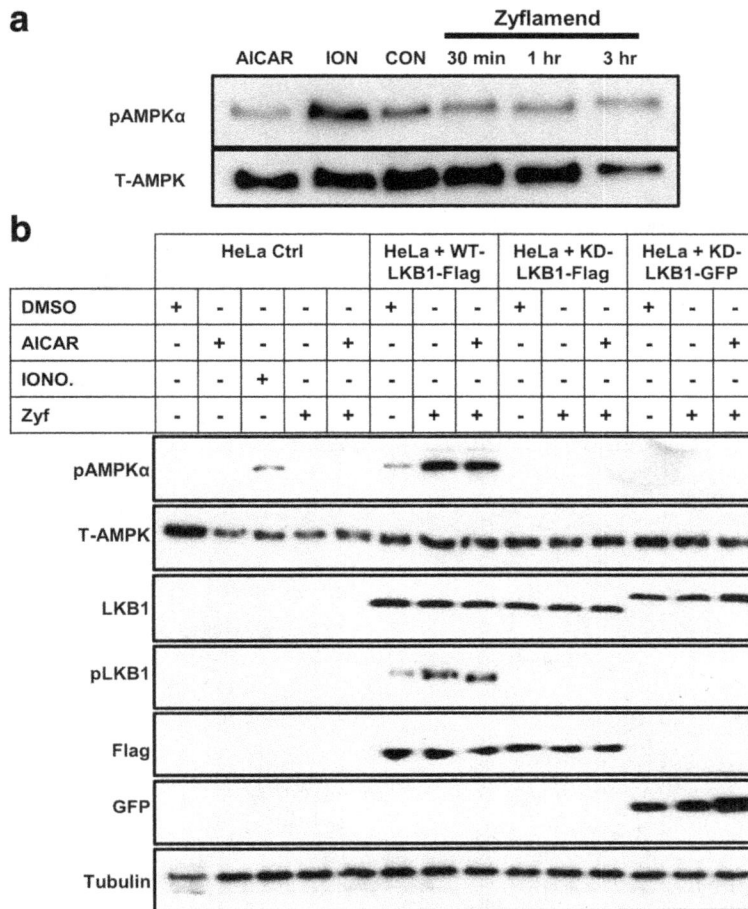

Fig. 6 Effects of Zyflamend on pAMPK (at Thr172) and pLKB1 (at Ser428) in HeLa cells null for LKB1, transfected with wild type (WT) LKB1 or with two catalytically dead (KD) mutants of LKB1. **a** Western blot of pAMPK in HeLa cells ± AICAR, (1 mM, 1 h), ionomycin (1 μM, 1 h) or Zyflamend (200 μg/mL, 30 min – 3 h). (**b**) Western blot of pAMPK in HeLa cells, WT-LKB1 HeLa cells, and KD-LKB1 HeLa cells ± AICAR (1 mM, 1 h), ionomycin (1 μM, 1 h), and/or Zyflamend (200 μg/mL, 1 h). Representative immunoblots from 3 independent experiments are shown. Abbreviations: Con, Control; DMSO, dimethyl sulfoxide; Ion, ionomycin; Zyf, Zyflamend

as a possible upstream target (Fig. 7). Phosphorylation of PKCζ and LKB1 increased when CWR22Rv1 cells were treated with Zyflamend (Fig. 7A). However, in the presence of a highly selective PKCζ pseudo-substrate inhibitor, phosphorylation of LKB1 could not be restored to control levels following Zyflamend treatment (Fig. 7B and C). Using our informative HeLa cell constructs, null for LKB1 and transfected with WT-LKB1 or KD-LKB1, we further investigated the relationship between PKCζ and LKB1 (Fig. 7D). In HeLa cells devoid of LKB1 (control cells), PKCζ is located in the cytosol (Fig. 7D, row 1, column 3), but appears to translocate to the nucleus upon treatment with Zyflamend (Fig. 7D, row 1, column 2). In cells transfected with WT-LKB1, PKCζ is located in the cytosol (Fig. 7D, row 1, column 7) and LKB1 is located in the nucleus (Fig. 7D, row 2, column 5). Following Zyflamend treatment, their locations switch, where PKCζ translocates to the nucleus (Fig. 7D, row 1, column

6) and LKB1 is found in the cytosol (Fig. 7D, row 2, column 8). This translocation following Zyflamend treatment appears to be independent of a catalytically active protein, as the same results were observed with the KD-LKB1 mutant (Fig. 7D, columns 9–12).

Discussion

Zyflamend is a unique blend of ten herbal extracts with tumor suppressor properties whose biochemical and physiological effects have been replicated in different laboratories, at different times, using different lots, with similar doses/concentrations [6–8, 10, 11, 13–17, 19, 21, 43]. The quality control of this preparation has been summarized elsewhere [7] and is most likely responsible for the reproducibility of results. Importantly, the effects of Zyflamend have been reported in a variety of cell lines, not just prostate cancer cells (CWR22, CWR22R, CWR22Rv1, PC3, LNCaP, RWPE-1, RAW 264.7, H1299, KBM-5, U266, MeW0, A365,

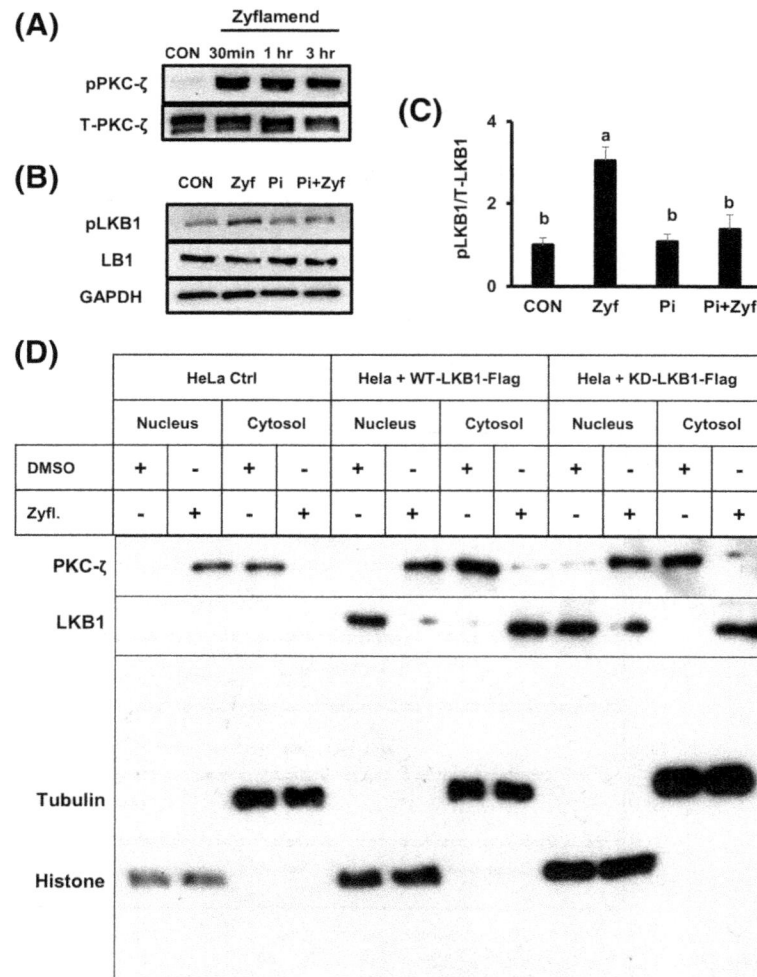

Fig. 7 The effects of Zyflamend on phosphorylation of PKCζ (at Thr410) and cellular location of PKCζ and LKB1 in HeLa cells null for LKB1, transfected with wild type (WT) LKB1 or with a catalytically dead (KD) mutant of LKB1. **A** Western blot of phosphorylation of PKCζ ± Zyflamend (200 μg/mL, 30 min – 3 h). **B, C** Western blot of pLKB1 (at Ser428) following treatment with Zyflamend, PKCζ inhibitor (5 μM, 30 min) or pretreatment with the PKCζ inhibitor plus Zyflamend (200 μg/mL, 30 min). **D** Western blot for PKCζ and LKB1 following subcellular fractionation (cytosol and nucleus) in HeLa cells null for LKB1, transfected with WT LKB1 or with a KD mutant of LKB1 treated with or without Zyflamend (200 μg/mL, 1 h). Representative immunoblots from 3 independent experiments are shown. Abbreviations: CON, Control; Pi, PKCζ inhibitor; Zyf, Zyflamend

MSK-Leuk1, HaCaT, HCT116, THP-1, HEK293) [6–8, 10–19, 21, 43]. While there is clinical evidence for the beneficial effects of Zyflamend on prostate cancer [9, 18, 20, 44], it is not possible to tease out the contributions and/or interactions of each constituent due to the high number of possible combinations (as many as 1024). However, recent studies have demonstrated that combining components from this blend enhances their cellular and molecular effects by orders of magnitude as compared to isolated components, indicating highly synergistic interactions when combined [22]. The ability of this mixture to function at human equivalent doses and in clinical trials is most likely due to this synergy. This combination has been shown to be clinically effective in prostate cancer patients by reducing levels of prostate

specific antigen (PSA), a biomarker used to monitor prostate cancer progression. Case studies from M.D. Anderson Cancer Center report dramatic reductions in PSA levels following treatment with Zyflamend and/or metformin (an activator of AMPK) in patients whose prostate cancer no longer responds to a variety of standard therapies [9], an effect also observed in our recent clinical trial with prostate cancer patients undergoing radical prostatectomy [44].

Castrate-resistant prostate cancer is the focus of this research and the research in our laboratory. To study mechanisms of action, we use human prostate cancer cells derived from the CWR22 lineage [6–8, 10, 45, 46]. Similar to the progression of human prostate cancer, these cells are originally androgen dependent and can transform to a castrate-resistant line in vivo (i.e., CRW22R) following hormone ablation [46–48]. Unlike some other prostate cancer cell lines (i.e., PC3 cells), the CWR22Rv1 cells express a constitutively active androgen receptor and PSA, characteristics shared by castrate-resistant prostate cancer in humans.

The effectiveness of Zyflamend on prostate cancer rests, in part, with its ability to upregulate AMPK, an effect observed in other cell types and tissues (i.e., HCT116, PC3, adipose) suggesting a general effect [10, 44]. However, the mechanism as to how Zyflamend upregulates AMPK is unknown, although many of its constituents have been shown to independently activate AMPK by modifying mitochondrial ATP production (as reviewed in [49]). This is the first paper to delineate the coordination of potential upstream pathways involved in the activation of AMPK, viz., LKB1 and CaMKK2, and to do so using natural products.

The role of AMPK in prostate cancer is controversial in the sense that upstream kinases responsible for its activation appear to have contradictory effects on cancer [29]. CaMKK2 is a known tumor promotor whose expression is linked to the upregulation of the androgen receptor, a key step in castrate-resistant prostate cancer [4, 31]. Interestingly, Zyflamend down regulates the androgen receptor and its nuclear localization [6]. DAPK is a differentially methylated gene where most of its effects on cancer have focused on its epigenetic regulation [33–36]. Uniquely, a catalytic downstream target of DAPK is CaMKK2 where it phosphorylates CaMKK2 at Ser511 [37], a site adjacent to the Ca^{+2}-calmodulin regulatory domain, preventing autophosphorylation and inhibiting catalytic activity [37].

In contrast, LKB1 exhibits tumor suppressor properties, where loss of LKB1 is involved in a variety of cancers [24, 30]. LKB1-mediated activation of AMPK is dependent upon increases in the AMP(ADP):ATP ratios. Zyflamend significantly decreases ATP in the cells. LKB1 contains a nuclear localization domain and is typically (but not always exclusively) found in the nucleus. Following activation, LKB1 co-localizes with STE20-related adaptor (known as STRAD) protein and scaffolding mouse 25 (known as MO25) protein and translocates to the cytosol where it exerts its kinase activity on a number of downstream targets, including AMPK [50]. Nuclear export, in part, appears to involve phosphorylation at Ser428 by PKCζ [51].

A key finding from this research is that Zyflamend antithetically regulates two parallel pathways important in the phosphorylation of AMPK that is potentially important in castrate-resistant prostate cancer. These effects are summarized in Fig. 8. Zyflamend-mediated activation of AMPK appears to be LKB1 dependent, while coordinately and negatively regulating CaMKK2 activity. This was observed using LKB1-null and KD-LKB1 transfected HeLa cells that constitutively express CaMKK2. The addition of ionomycin (activator of CaMKK2) robustly increased phosphorylation of AMPK, but Zyflamend (with and without AICAR, an AMP analog) had no effect. Our results suggest that Zyflamend inhibits CaMKK2 following DAPK-mediated phosphorylation at Ser511, as this effect is prevented by the presence of a DAPK inhibitor.

On the other hand, Zyflamend robustly increased the phosphorylation of AMPK only in HeLa cells transfected with WT LKB1. Using the various constructs of the HeLa cells, we confirmed nuclear localization of LKB1, with translocation to the cytosol following Zyflamend treatment (Fig. 7). Zyflamend increased phosphorylation

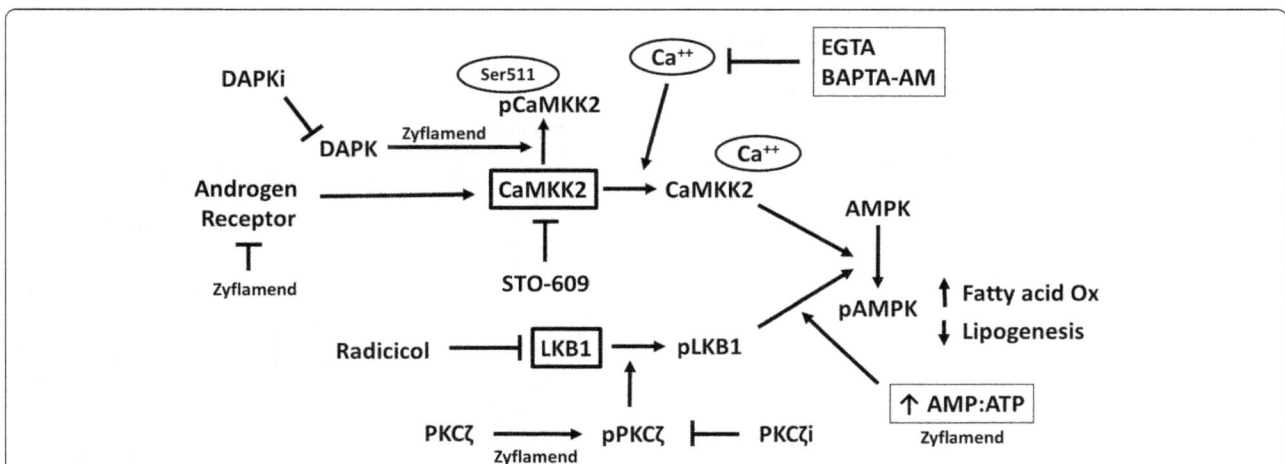

Fig. 8 Summary of the effects of Zyflamend on AMPK regulation by signaling pathways of LKB1 and CaMKK2. Zyflamend has been shown to inhibit castrate-resistant prostate cancer, in part, through the activation of AMPK. This activation is mediated by the increase in AMP:ATP ratio and the activation of the tumor suppressor protein LKB1 following phosphorylation by PKCζ. Simultaneously, Zyflamend inhibits the tumor promotor CaMKK2 via phosphorylation at Ser511 by DAPK

of PKCζ, a known activator of LKB1, and inhibition of PKCζ reduced LKB1 phosphorylation in the presence of Zyflamend. Importantly, translocation of PKCζ from the cytosol to the nucleus occurred concomitantly.

These results help explain why inhibitors of CaMKK2 (STO-609, BAPTA-AM, EGTA, DAPKi) failed to prevent the activation of AMPK in the presence of Zyflamend in CWR22Rv1 cells. This was due to the simultaneous activation of LKB1, and this was confirmed when activation of AMPK (in the presence of Zyflamend) was not completely rescued following inhibition (radicicol) and knockdown (siRNA) of LKB1.

Conclusions

In summary, Zyflamend has been shown to inhibit castrate-resistant prostate cancer, in part, through the activation of AMPK, results confirmed using chemical and molecular interventions [10]. In conjunction with reducing ATP levels, this activation is mediated by the tumor suppressor protein LKB1, via activation of PKCζ. Simultaneously, Zyflamend inhibits CaMKK2, a tumor promotor that is over-expressed in many cancers, including castrate-resistant prostate cancer. This inhibition appears to be uniquely mediated by DAPK. More studies are warranted to interrogate the relationship of Zyflamend with DAPK signaling. In conclusion, this is the first evidence that multiple upstream pathways involved in the activation of AMPK, an important signaling molecule in cancer, can be simultaneously regulated using a well-defined natural product.

Abbreviations

ACC: Acetyl CoA carboxylase; AICAR: 5-aminoimidazole-4-carboxamide ribonucleotide; AMPK: 5'-adenosine monophosphate-activated protein kinase; ANOVA: Analysis of variance; BAPTA-AM: 1,2-bis(o-aminophenoxy)ethane-N,N,N',N'-tetraacetic acid acetoxymethyl ester; CaMKK,2: Calcium-calmodulin kinase kinase-2; CR-PCa: Castrate-resistant prostate cancer; DAPK: Death-associated protein kinase Inhibitor; DTT: Dithiothreitol; EGTA: Ethylene glycol-bis(β-aminoethyl ether)-N,N,N',N'-tetraacetic acid; GAPDH: Glyceraldehyde 3-phosphate dehydrogenase; GFP: Green fluorescent protein; LKB1: Liver kinases B1; MLK3: Mixed lineage kinase 3; MO25: Scaffolding mouse 25 protein; MOPS: 3-(N-morpholino)propanesulfonic acid; PKCζ: Protein kinase C-zeta; PMSF: Phenylmethylsulfonyl fluoride; RIPA: Radioimmunoprecipitation assay; STRAD: STE20-related adaptor protein; TAK1: Transforming growth factor-β activated protein kinase-1

Acknowledgements

GFP-LKB1 was a gift from Junying Yuan (Addgene plasmid # 21147), while pcDNA3-FLAG-LKB1 was a gift from Lewis Cantley (Addgene plasmid # 8590).

Funding

This work was supported, in part, by a USDA HATCH grant (#TEN00441) through the Tennessee Agricultural Experiment Station, (JW), University of Tennessee, Knoxville, TN 37996, and by a grant from the National Institutes for Health (R00DK100736) (AB). The University of Tennessee Institute of Agriculture, the University of Tennessee Agricultural Experiment Station, the National Institutes for Health, the manufacturer of Zyflamend (New Chapter, Brattleboro, VT) or anyone affiliated with them, have not been consulted or associated with the research in this paper, or involved in the study design; in the collection, analysis, or interpretation of data; in the writing or review of the manuscript; or in the decision to submit the paper for publication.

Authors' contributions

All of the authors have read and approved the manuscript. AFM conducted the research, analyzed the data, help write the paper, read and approved the final manuscript. AB helped in the design of the experiments, provided essential technical expertise/supplies/materials, conducted research, read, commented on, approved the final manuscript and provide some financial support through his NIH grant. DRD helped in the design of the experiments, provided essential technical expertise, supplies/materials, conducted research, read, commented on and approved the final manuscript. DSA provided essential technical expertise to the research, read, and approved the final manuscript. AH provided essential technical expertise to the research, read, commented on and approved the final manuscript. YZ provided essential technical expertise to the research, generated preliminary data for this research, read, commented on and approved the final manuscript. JW was primarily responsible for the design of the research, oversite and supervision of the research, writing of the manuscript, had final responsibility for the content and funded the project through his USDA Hatch grant.

Author's information

The impact of food and food components (including natural products) on delaying or inhibiting the promotion and progression of cancer and modifying the ability of relapse following the use standard therapies is the focus and line of research of the primary author (JW). If you are unfortunate enough to get an advanced form of prostate cancer (castrate-resistant prostate cancer), what can be done to enhance the effectiveness of standard therapies? This research focuses on castrate-resistant prostate cancer, a potentially deadly form of the disease, using an experimental design consistent with this condition to explore underlying mechanisms.

Competing interests

The authors have no conflicts of interest. They have not received any reimbursement fees or funding from the manufacturers or distributors of Zyflamend as outlined by the publisher. None of the authors hold stock or shares that can result in financial gain in anyway, nor have applied for patents or reimbursements or fees that would constitute a conflict of interest. The University of Tennessee Agricultural Experiment Station, the National Institutes for Health, the manufacturer of Zyflamend (New Chapter, Brattleboro, VT) or anyone affiliated with them, have not been consulted or associated with this study, or involved in the study design; in the collection, analysis, or interpretation of data; in the writing or review of the manuscript; or in the decision to submit the paper for publication. No financial support or product has been provided by New Chapter (Brattleboro, VT), manufacturer of Zyflamend, for this study. This research has been reviewed and accepted by all authors. It has not been published or submitted for publication elsewhere.

Author details
[1]Department of Nutrition, University of Tennessee, 1215 West Cumberland Avenue, 229 Jessie Harris Building, Knoxville, TN 37996, USA. [2]Tennessee Agricultural Experiment Station, University of Tennessee, Knoxville, TN 37996, USA. [3]Department of Nutrition, Laboratory for Cancer Research, University of Tennessee, 1215 West Cumberland Avenue, Room 229 Jessie Harris Building, Knoxville, TN 37996-1920, USA. [4]Present addresses: Kellogg Eye Center, University of Michigan, 1000 Wall St, Ann Arbor, MI 48105, USA. [5]Present addresses: Department of Cancer Biology, Thomas Jefferson University, 233 S.10th Street, Philadelphia, PA 19107, USA.

References

1. Siegel RL, Miller KD, Jemal A. Cancer statistics, 2017. CA-Cancer J Clin. 2017; 67(1):7–30.

2. Miller KD, Siegel RL, Lin CC, Mariotto AB, Kramer JL, Rowland JH, Stein KD, Alteri R, Jemal A. Cancer treatment and survivorship statistics, 2016. CA-Cancer J Clin. 2016;66(4):271–89.

3. Whelan J, Zhao Y, Huang EC, MacDonald A, Donohoe D. In: Hardman R, Harikumar KB, editors. Zyflamend and prostate cancer therapy In Complementary and Alternative Medicines in Prostate Cancer: A Comprehensive Approach. Boca, Raton, FL: CRC Press; 2017. p. 197–220.

4. Conteduca V, Wetterskog D, Sharabiani MTA, Grande E, Fernandez-Perez MP, Jayaram A, Salvi S, Castellano D, Romanel A, Lolli C, et al. Androgen receptor gene status in plasma DNA associates with worse outcome on enzalutamide or abiraterone for castration-resistant prostate cancer: a multi-institution correlative biomarker study. Ann Oncol. 2017;28:1508–16.

5. Taplin ME, Balk SP. Androgen receptor: a key molecule in the progression of prostate cancer to hormone independence. J Cell Biochem. 2004;91(3):483–90.

6. Huang EC, Chen G, Baek SJ, McEntee MF, Collier JJ, Minkin S, Biggerstaff JP, Whelan J. Zyflamend reduces the expression of androgen receptor in a model of castrate-resistant prostate cancer. Nutr Cancer. 2011;63(8):1287–96.

7. Huang EC, McEntee MF, Whelan J. Zyflamend, a combination of herbal extracts, attenuates tumor growth in murine xenograph models of prostate cancer. Nutr Cancer. 2012;64(5):749–60.

8. Huang EC, Zhao YCG, Baek SJ, McEntee MF, Minkin S, Biggerstaff JP, Whelan J. Zyflamend, a polyherbal mixture, down regulates class I and class II histone deacetylases and increases p21 levels in castrate-resistant prostate cancer cells. BMC Complement Altern Med. 2014;14:68.

9. Bilen MA, Lin SH, Tang DG, Parikh K, Lee MH, Yeung SC, Tu SM. Maintenance therapy containing metformin and/or Zyflamend for advanced prostate Cancer: a case series. Case Rep Oncol Med. 2015;2015:471861.

10. Zhao Y, Donohoe D, Huang EC, Whelan J. Zyflamend, a polyherbal mixture, inhibits lipogenesis and mTORC1 signalling via activation of AMPK. J Funct Foods. 2015;18:147–58.

11. Mohebati A, Guttenplan JB, Kochhar A, Zhao ZL, Kosinska W, Subbaramaiah K, Dannenberg AJ. Carnosol, a constituent of Zyflamend, inhibits aryl hydrocarbon receptor-mediated activation of CYP1A1 and CYP1B1 transcription and mutagenesis. Cancer Prev Res. 2012;5(4):593–602.

12. Subbaramaiah K, Sue E, Bhardwaj P, Du B, Hudis CA, Giri D, Kopelovich L, Zhou XK, Dannenberg AJ. Dietary polyphenols suppress elevated levels of proinflammatory mediators and aromatase in the mammary gland of obese mice. Cancer Prev Res. 2013;6(9):886–97.

13. Sandur SK, Ahn KS, Ichikawa H, Sethi G, Shishodia S, Newman RA, Aggarwal BB. Zyflamend, a polyherbal preparation, inhibits invasion, suppresses osteoclastogenesis, and potentiates apoptosis through down-regulation of NF-kappa B activation and NF-kappa B-regulated gene products. Nutr Cancer. 2007;57(1):78–87.

14. Kunnumakkara AB, Sung B, Ravindran J, Diagaradjane P, Deorukhkar A, Dey S, Koca C, Tong Z, Gelovani JG, Guha S, et al. Zyflamend suppresses growth and sensitizes human pancreatic tumors to gemcitabine in an orthotopic mouse model through modulation of multiple targets. Int J Cancer. 2012; 131(3):E292–303.

15. Kim JH, Park B, Gupta SC, Kannappan R, Sung B, Aggarwal BB. Zyflamend sensitizes tumor cells to TRAIL-induced apoptosis through up-regulation of death receptors and down-regulation of survival proteins: role of ROS-dependent CCAAT/enhancer-binding protein-homologous protein pathway. Antioxid Redox Signal. 2012;16(5):413–27.

16. Ekmekcioglu S, Chattopadhyay C, Akar U, Gabisi A Jr, Newman RA, Grimm EA. Zyflamend mediates therapeutic induction of autophagy to apoptosis in melanoma cells. Nutr Cancer. 2011;63(6):940–9.

17. Bemis DL, Capodice JL, Anastasiadis AG, Katz AE, Buttyan R. Zyflamend, a unique herbal preparation with nonselective COX inhibitory activity, induces apoptosis of prostate cancer cells that lack COX-2 expression. Nutr Cancer. 2005;52(2):202–12.

18. Rafailov S, Cammack S, Stone BA, Katz AE. The role of Zyflamend, an herbal anti-inflammatory, as a potential chemopreventive agent against prostate cancer: a case report. Integr Cancer Ther. 2007;6(1):74–6.

19. Yang P, Cartwright C, Chan D, Vijjeswarapu M, Ding J, Newman RA. Zyflamend-mediated inhibition of human prostate cancer PC3 cell proliferation: effects on 12-LOX and Rb protein phosphorylation. Cancer Biol Ther. 2007;6(2):228–36.

20. Capodice JL, Gorroochurn P, Cammack AS, Eric G, McKiernan JM, Benson MC, Stone BA, Katz AE. Zyflamend in men with high-grade prostatic intraepithelial neoplasia: results of a phase I clinical trial. J Soc Integr Oncol. 2009;7(2):43–51.

21. Yan J, Xie B, Capodice JL, Katz AE. Zyflamend inhibits the expression and function of androgen receptor and acts synergistically with bicalutamide to inhibit prostate cancer cell growth. Prostate. 2012;72(3):244–52.

22. Zhao Y, Collier JJ, Huang EC, Whelan J. Turmeric and Chinese goldthread synergistically inhibit prostate cancer cell proliferation and NF-kB signaling. Funct Foods Health Dis. 2014;4(7):312–39.

23. Jeon SM. Regulation and function of AMPK in physiology and diseases. Exp Mol Med. 2016;48(7):e245.

24. Cheng J, Zhang T, Ji H, Tao K, Guo J, Wei W. Functional characterization of AMP-activated protein kinase signaling in tumorigenesis. Biochim Biophys Acta. 2016;1866(2):232–51.

25. Hawley SA, Davison M, Woods A, Davies SP, Beri RK, Carling D, Hardie DG. Characterization of the AMP-activated protein kinase kinase from rat liver and identification of threonine 172 as the major site at which it phosphorylates AMP-activated protein kinase. J Biol Chem. 1996;271(44):27879–87.

26. Hawley SA, Pan DA, Mustard KJ, Ross L, Bain J, Edelman AM, Frenguelli BG, Hardie DG. Calmodulin-dependent protein kinase kinase-beta is an alternative upstream kinase for AMP-activated protein kinase. Cell Metab. 2005;2(1):9–19.

27. Herrero-Martin G, Hoyer-Hansen M, Garcia-Garcia C, Fumarola C, Farkas T, Lopez-Rivas A, Jaattela M. TAK1 activates AMPK-dependent cytoprotective autophagy in TRAIL-treated epithelial cells. EMBO J. 2009;28(6):677–85.

28. Luo L, Jiang S, Huang D, Lu N, Luo Z. MLK3 phosphorylates AMPK independently of LKB1. PLoS One. 2015;10(4):e0123927.

29. Khan AS, Frigo DE. A spatiotemporal hypothesis for the regulation, role, and targeting of AMPK in prostate cancer. Nat Rev Urol. 2017;14(3):164–80.

30. Gan RY, Li HB. Recent progress on liver kinase B1 (LKB1): expression, regulation, downstream signaling and cancer suppressive function. Int J Mol Sci. 2014;15(9):16698–718.

31. Karacosta LG, Foster BA, Azabdaftari G, Feliciano DM, Edelman AM. A regulatory feedback loop between Ca2+/calmodulin-dependent protein kinase kinase 2 (CaMKK2) and the androgen receptor in prostate cancer progression. J Biol Chem. 2012;287(29):24832–43.

32. Lin F, Marcelo KL, Rajapakshe K, Coarfa C, Dean A, Wilganowski N, Robinson H, Sevick E, Bissig KD, Goldie LC, et al. The camKK2/camKIV relay is an essential regulator of hepatic cancer. Hepatology. 2015;62(2):505–20.

33. Yuan W, Chen J, Shu Y, Liu S, Wu L, Ji J, Liu Z, Tang Q, Zhou Z, Cheng Y, et al. Correlation of DAPK1 methylation and the risk of gastrointestinal cancer: a systematic review and meta-analysis. PLoS One. 2017;12(9):e0184959.

34. Li L, Guo L, Wang Q, Liu X, Zeng Y, Wen Q, Zhang S, Kwok HF, Lin Y, Liu J. DAPK1 as an independent prognostic marker in liver cancer. PeerJ. 2017;5:e3568.

35. Xie JY, Chen PC, Zhang JL, Gao ZS, Neves H, Zhang SD, Wen Q, Chen WD, Kwok HF, Lin Y. The prognostic significance of DAPK1 in bladder cancer. PLoS One. 2017;12(4):e0175290.

36. Cai F, Xiao X, Niu X, Zhong Y. Association between promoter methylation of DAPK gene and HNSCC: a meta-analysis. PLoS One. 2017;12(3):e0173194.

37. Schumacher AM, Schavocky JP, Velentza AV, Mirzoeva S, Watterson DM. A calmodulin-regulated protein kinase linked to neuron survival is a substrate for the calmodulin-regulated death-associated protein kinase. Biochemistry. 2004;43(25):8116–24.

38. Laemmli UK. Cleavage of structural proteins during the assembly of the head of bacteriophage T4. Nature. 1970;227(5259):680–5.

39. Bettaieb A, Averill-Bates DA. Thermotolerance induced at a mild

temperature of 40 degrees C protects cells against heat shock-induced apoptosis. J Cell Physiol. 2005;205(1):47–57.

40. Samali A, Cai J, Zhivotovsky B, Jones DP, Orrenius S. Presence of a pre-apoptotic complex of pro-caspase-3, Hsp60 and Hsp10 in the mitochondrial fraction of jurkat cells. EMBO J. 1999;18(8):2040–8.

41. Shaw RJ, Kosmatka M, Bardeesy N, Hurley RL, Witters LA, DePinho RA, Cantley LC. The tumor suppressor LKB1 kinase directly activates AMP-activated kinase and regulates apoptosis in response to energy stress. Proc Natl Acad Sci U S A. 2004;101(10):3329–35.

42. Karuman P, Gozani O, Odze RD, Zhou XC, Zhu H, Shaw R, Brien TP, Bozzuto CD, Ooi D, Cantley LC, et al. The Peutz-Jegher gene product LKB1 is a mediator of p53-dependent cell death. Mol Cell. 2001;7(6):1307–19.

43. Yang P, Sun Z, Chan D, Cartwright CA, Vijjeswarapu M, Ding J, Chen X, Newman RA. Zyflamend reduces LTB4 formation and prevents oral carcinogenesis in a 7,12-dimethylbenz[alpha]anthracene (DMBA)-induced hamster cheek pouch model. Carcinogenesis. 2008;29(11):2182–9.

44. Tague ED, Bourdon AK, MacDonald A, Lookadoo MS, Kim ED, White WM, Terry PD, Campagna SR, Voy BH, Whelan J. Metabolomics approach in the study of the well-defined Polyherbal preparation Zyflamend. J Med Food; 2018;21:306–316.

45. Pretlow TG, Wolman SR, Micale MA, Pelley RJ, Kursh ED, Resnick MI, Bodner DR, Jacobberger JW, Delmoro CM, Giaconia JM, et al. Xenografts of primary human prostatic carcinoma. J Natl Cancer Inst. 1993;85:394–8.

46. Nagabhushan M, Miller CM, Pretlow TP, Giaconia JM, Edgehouse NL, Schwartz S, Kung HJ, de Vere White RW, Gumerlock PH, Resnick MI, et al. CWR22: the first human prostate cancer xenograft with strongly androgen-dependent and relapsed strains both in vivo and in soft agar. Cancer Res. 1996;56(13):3042–6.

47. Tepper CG, Boucher DL, Ryan PE, Ma AH, Xia L, Lee LF, Pretlow TG, Kung HJ. Characterization of a novel androgen receptor mutation in a relapsed CWR22 prostate cancer xenograft and cell line. Cancer Res. 2002;62(22):6606–14.

48. Sramkoski RM, Pretlow TG, Giaconia JM, Pretlow TP, Schwartz S, Sy MS, Marengo SR, Rhim JS, Zhang D, Jacobberger JW. A new human prostate carcinoma cell line, 22Rv1. In Vitro Cell Dev Biol Anim. 1999;35(7):403–9.

49. Hardie DG. AMPK: a target for drugs and natural products with effects on both diabetes and cancer. Diabetes. 2013;62(7):2164–72.

50. Korsse SE, Peppelenbosch MP, van VW. Targeting LKB1 signaling in cancer. Biochim Biophys Acta. 2013;1835(2):194–210.

51. Song P, Xie Z, Wu Y, Xu J, Dong Y, Zou MH. Prot10, lines 222 and 224. Ein kinase Czeta-dependent LKB1 serine 428 phosphorylation increases LKB1 nucleus export and apoptosis in endothelial cells. J Biol Chem. 2008;283(18): 12446–55.

7

Identification of antitumoral agents against human pancreatic cancer cells from Asteraceae and Lamiaceae plant extracts

Lamia Mouhid[1], Marta Gómez de Cedrón[1*], Teodoro Vargas[1], Elena García-Carrascosa[1], Nieves Herranz[2], Mónica García-Risco[2], Guillermo Reglero[1,2], Tiziana Fornari[2] and Ana Ramírez de Molina[1*]

Abstract

Background: Pancreatic cancer is one of the most aggressive and mortal cancers. Although several drugs have been proposed for its treatment, it remains resistant and new alternatives are needed. In this context, plants and their derivatives constitute a relevant source of bioactive components which might efficiently inhibit tumor cell progression.

Methods: In this study, we have analyzed the potential anti-carcinogenic effect of different Asteraceae (*Achillea millefolium* and *Calendula officinalis*) and Lamiaceae (*Melissa officinalis* and *Origanum majorana*) plant extracts obtained by different green technologies (Supercritical CO_2 Extraction –SFE- and Ultrasonic Assisted Extraction –UAE-) to identify efficient plant extracts against human pancreatic cancer cells that could constitute the basis of novel treatment approaches.

Results: Asteraceae extracts showed better results as antitumoral agents than Lamiaceae by inducing cytotoxicity and inhibiting cell transformation, and SFE extracts were most efficient than UAE extracts. In addition, SFE derived plant extracts from *Achillea millefolium* and *Calendula officinalis* displayed synergism with the chemotherapeutic 5-Fluororacil.

Conclusion: These results show how Yarrow and Marigold SFE-derived extracts can inhibit pancreatic cancer cell growth, and could be proposed for a comprehensive study to determine the molecular mechanisms involved in their bioactivity with the final aim to propose them as potential adjuvants in pancreatic cancer therapy.

Keywords: Pancreatic cancer, Asteraceae, Lamiaceae, Chemotherapeutic agents, 5-Fluororacil

Background

As reported by the European Society for Medical Oncology (ESMO), pancreatic cancer is the seventh most common cancer in Europe, accounting for 2.8% of cancer in men and 3.2% in women. It is the fifth leading cause cancer-related death with 70,000 estimated deaths each year [1]. Depending on the tumor stage and if surgery is possible, current treatments are based on the use of the antimetabolite 5-fluorouracil (5-FU), but also gemcitabine, nab-paclitaxel, or in combination with acid folic, such as Folfirinox (folic acid+ 5-FU or irinotecan or oxaliplatin) [2]. A reduced percentage of patients respond to these antitumor agents due to the advanced stage of the

tumor when it is diagnosticated and due to the appearance of resistances. In this scenario, plants are an important source to obtain new compounds that could be used as chemotherapeutic drugs.

In the last decades, plant-derived compounds have been clinically used as anti-cancer agents [3, 4], as they demonstrate the ability to modulate several molecular pathways involved in tumor development and progression. In this sense, the expected intervention for a plant-derived extract as antitumoral agent should exert a cytotoxic effect in tumor cells, without affecting cell viability of normal cells.

In a recent work, we produced and chemically characterized several extracts obtained from Lamiaceae (*Melissa officinalis* or Balm and *Origanum majorana* or Marjoram) and Asteraceae (*Achillea millefolium* or Yarrow, and *Calendula officinalis* or Marigold) plant families. For this purpose, we produced two different extracts from each

* Correspondence: marta.gomezdecedron@imdea.org; ana.ramirez@imdea.org
[1]Molecular Oncology and Nutritional Genomics of Cancer, Madrid Institute for Advanced Studies on Food (IMDEA-Food), Ctra de Cantoblanco, 8, 28049 Madrid, Spain
Full list of author information is available at the end of the article

plant by applying two sequential extraction steps: first Supercritical Fluid Extraction (SFE) and then, the remained vegetal raw material was re-extracted by Ultrasonic Assisted Extraction (UAE) [5].

Herein, in the present work, we investigated the antitumoral activity of those extracts obtained from Balm, Marjoram, Yarrow and Marigold SFE and UAE extracts in pancreatic cancer cell lines models (MIA PaCa-2 and PANC-1), and we have compared their biological activity and efficiency between the two extraction approaches (Fig. 1). Furthermore, additional UAE extracts were produced using the original vegetal matrix (OVM) for comparison with those produced previously [4] using the SFE residual vegetal matrix (RVM).

Although previous works have been described the antitumoral properties exerted by Marjoram [6, 7], Balm [8, 9], Yarrow [10, 11], and Marigold [12, 13], to our knowledge, the novelty of the present work lies in the analysis of extracts produced by environmentally friendly extraction techniques together with advanced biological methods in order to obtain, test and characterize natural extracts that could be potentially used for cancer therapies. After identifying the most efficient extracts inducing pancreatic cells toxicity, we further studied the

mechanisms through which they induce cell death (apoptosis or necrosis) and their potentiality to inhibit cell malignancy and invasion. We also have evaluated the putative synergism with 5-FU to propose an efficient antitumoral product as a potential adjuvant in pancreatic cancer treatment. Our findings indicate that the SFE extracts obtained from Yarrow and Marigold meet the requirements to be proposed as a promising antitumoral approach.

Methods
Reagents
DMEM (Dulbecco's Modified Eagle Medium), PBS (Phosphate-buffered saline), glutamine and trypsin were purchased from Lonza Spain; and FBS from Thermo Fisher Scientific. DMSO (Dimethyl Sulfoxide) and Ethanol were purchased from Scharlab S.L. MTT (3-(4,5-dimethylthiazol-2-yl)-2,5-diphenyltetrazolium bromide) and Staurosporine were purchased from Sigma Aldrich. Plants leaves for producing the extracts were purchased from Herboristería Murciana (Murcia, Spain), and commercial extracts were purchased from Soria Natural, S.A.

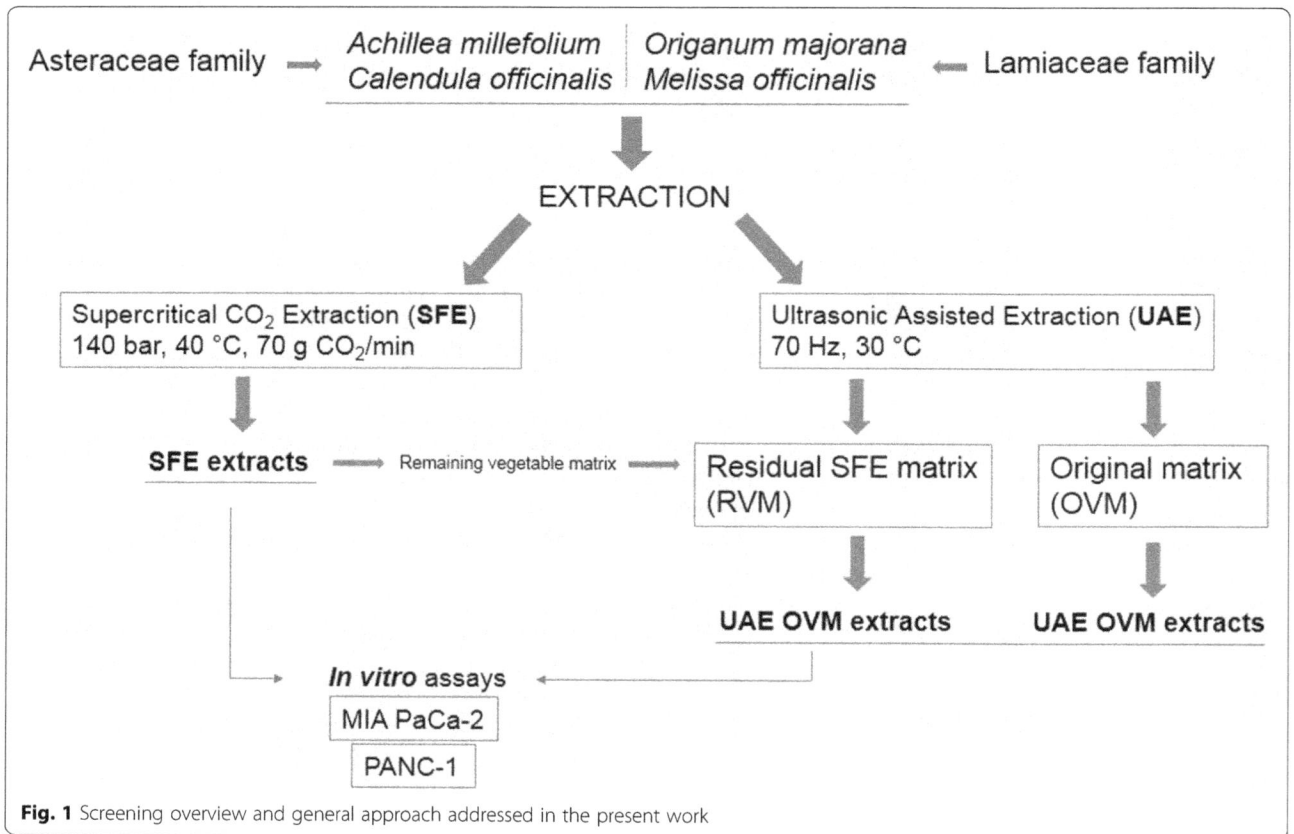

Fig. 1 Screening overview and general approach addressed in the present work

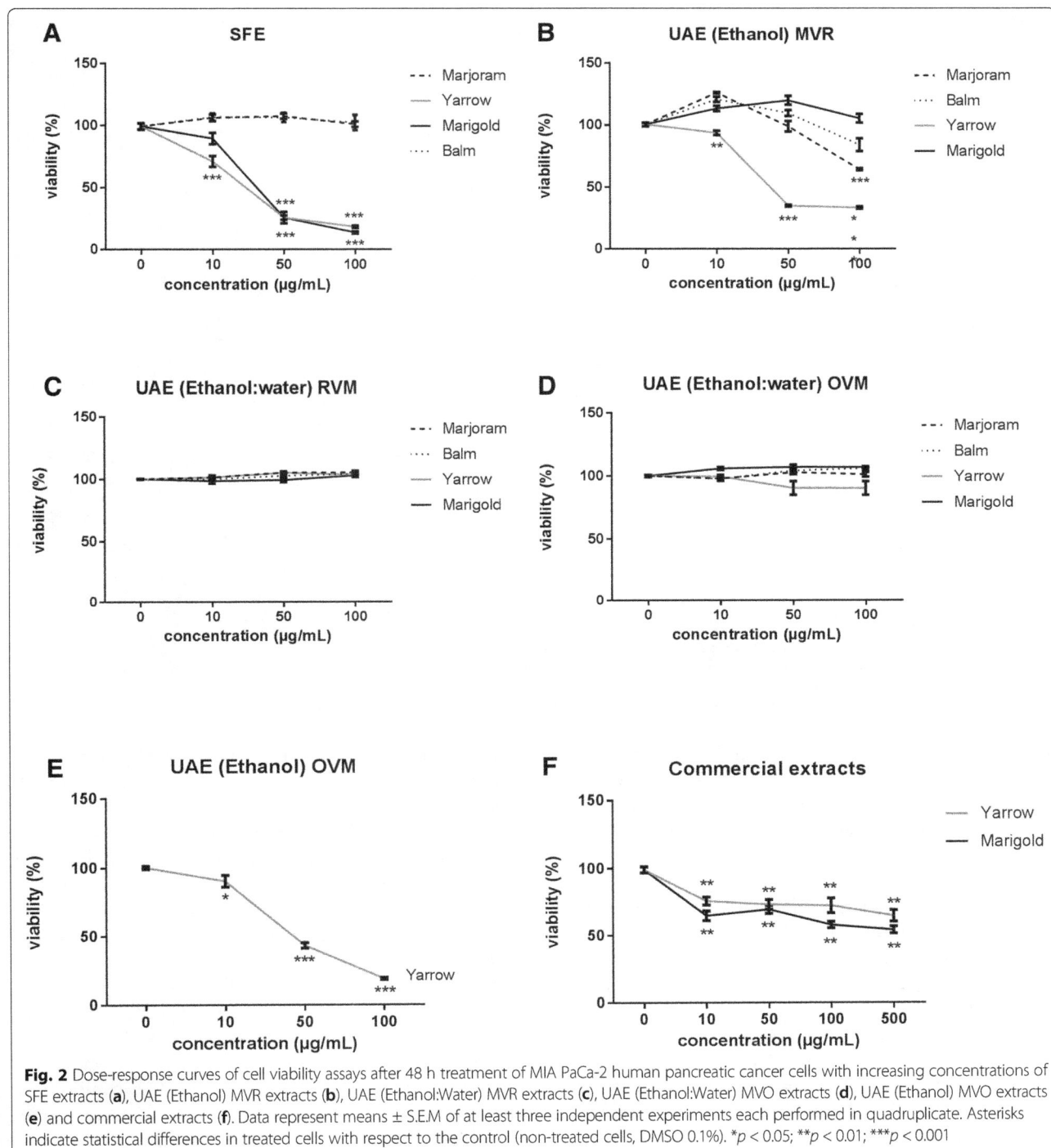

Fig. 2 Dose-response curves of cell viability assays after 48 h treatment of MIA PaCa-2 human pancreatic cancer cells with increasing concentrations of SFE extracts (**a**), UAE (Ethanol) MVR extracts (**b**), UAE (Ethanol:Water) MVR extracts (**c**), UAE (Ethanol:Water) MVO extracts (**d**), UAE (Ethanol) MVO extracts (**e**) and commercial extracts (**f**). Data represent means ± S.E.M of at least three independent experiments each performed in quadruplicate. Asterisks indicate statistical differences in treated cells with respect to the control (non-treated cells, DMSO 0.1%). *$p < 0.05$; **$p < 0.01$; ***$p < 0.001$

Extraction procedures

Extracts were obtained by mean of two different green technologies as described previously [[5]]. Briefly, SFE was carried out using supercritical CO_2 (140 bar, 40 °C, 70 g CO_2/min), and UAE derived extracts using ethanol or ethanol: water – 50:50- (70 Hz, 30 °C). In addition, and regarding UAE, two different extracts were

compared in the present work: the extracts produced from the Original Vegetable Matrix (OVM) and the those produced from the Residual Vegetable Matrix (RVM) after the SFE extraction. Fig. 1 shows a schematic overview of all the extracts evaluated in this study.

Chemical composition of the extracts is described in a previous work [4]. The extracts obtained by ultrasonic

Table 1 Concentration parameters of the selected plant extracts on MIA PaCa-2 cell line sensitivity depending on the extraction method

Plant extract	Concentration Parameter	SFE	UAE RVM Ethanol	RVM Ethanol:Water	OVM Ethanol	OVM Ethanol:Water	Commercial
Marjoram	IC50	> 100[a]	> 100[a]	> 100[a]	–	> 100	–
	GI50	> 100	75,89 ± 2,05	> 100	–	> 100	–
	TGI	> 100	> 100	> 100	–	> 100	–
	LC50	> 100	> 100	> 100	–	> 100	–
Balm	IC50	> 100[a]	> 100[a]	> 100[a]	–	> 100	–
	GI50	> 100	> 100	> 100	–	> 100	–
	TGI	> 100	> 100	> 100	–	> 100	–
	LC50	> 100	> 100	> 100	–	> 100	–
Yarrow	IC50	31,4 ± 8,5[a]	48,5 ± 2,5[a]	> 100	28,8 ± 15,8	> 100	> 500
	GI50	37,4 ± 7,3	> 100	> 100	49,4 ± 25,7	> 100	> 500
	TGI	56 ± 1,4	65,1 ± 6,1	> 100	86,6 ± 3,4	> 100	> 500
	LC50	70,6 ± 7,1	> 100	> 100	> 100	> 100	> 500
Marigold	IC50	39,8 ± 4,6[a]	> 100[a]	> 100[a]	–	> 100	> 500
	GI50	–	> 100	> 100	–	> 100	> 500
	TGI	54, ± 3,1	> 100	> 100	–	> 100	> 500
	LC50	78,5 ± 1,4	> 100	> 100	–	> 100	> 500

Data (> 100): not significant activity found at 100 µg/mL concentration; (–): not determined; *SFE* Supercritical Fluid Extraction, *UAE* Ultrasound Assisted Extraction, *RVM* Residual Vegetable Matrix, *OVM* Original Vegetable Matrix. [a]Data acquired from a previous work [4]
Data are presented as IC50 (µg/mL) (concentration needed to induce 50% cell viability inhibition [4, 5] [5], GI50 (µg/mL) (concentration needed for 50% growth inhibition), TGI (µg/mL) (concentration needed for total growth inhibition) and LC50 (µg/mL) (concentration needed for 50% cell death) after 48 h treatment as mean ± SEM of at least three independent experiments each performed in quadruplicate

probe are rich in flavonoids and phenols, whereas those obtained by supercritical CO_2 are rich in sesquiterpenes and monoterpenes, which were detailed by a gas-chromatography analysis [4].

Cell culture

Human pancreatic cancer cells MIA PaCa-2 and PANC-1, obtained from American Type Culture Collection (ATCC), were cultured in DMEM supplemented with 10% FBS. Cells were kept under standard conditions of temperature (37 °C), humidity (95%) and carbon dioxide (5%).

For tridimensional culture, MIA PaCa-2 cells were grown in Matrigel Growth Factor Reduced (Corning® Life Sciences) 80%, and media was renewed every two days, until the 3D-spheres were formed. Treatments with extracts were then applied for 72 h.

Cell viability assay

The cytotoxic and antiproliferative activities of the different extracts in human pancreatic tumor cell lines were determined by MTT assay. Briefly, cells in the exponential growth phase were plated in 96-multiwell plates. After 24 h, media was replaced with 200 µL media containing serial concentrations of each extract (dissolved in DMSO) for 48 h. The number of viable

cells was determined at time zero (control growth wells) and after treatments. To determine the number of viable cells, tetrazolium MTT salt solution (Sigma) (5 mg/mL in phosphate- buffered saline) was added for 3 h. Then, the formazan produced in each well was solubilized by adding 200 µL DMSO and measured using a spectrophotometer reader ($\lambda = 560$ nm) (Biochrom Asys UVM 340 Microplate Reader; ISOGEN). Parameters for 50% of cell viability inhibition (IC50), 50% of cell growth inhibition (GI50), total cell growth inhibition (TGI), and 50% of cell death (LC50) were calculated accordingly to NIH definitions using a logistic regression [14].

The synergism between 5-FU and Yarrow and Marigold SFE extracts was analyzed by the combination index (CI) obtained using the Calcusyn software (Biosoft), based on the Chou-Talalay method [15].

Flow cytometry

After 24 h' culture in DMEM, pancreatic cancer MIA PaCa-2 cells were treated with increasing concentrations of Yarrow and Marigold SFE extracts for 24 h. Marjoram SFE extract was used as a negative control and staurosporine 1.5 µM as a positive control for apoptosis. The Annexin V and Propidium iodide (PI) staining was carried out by using Annexin V-FITC Apoptosis Detection

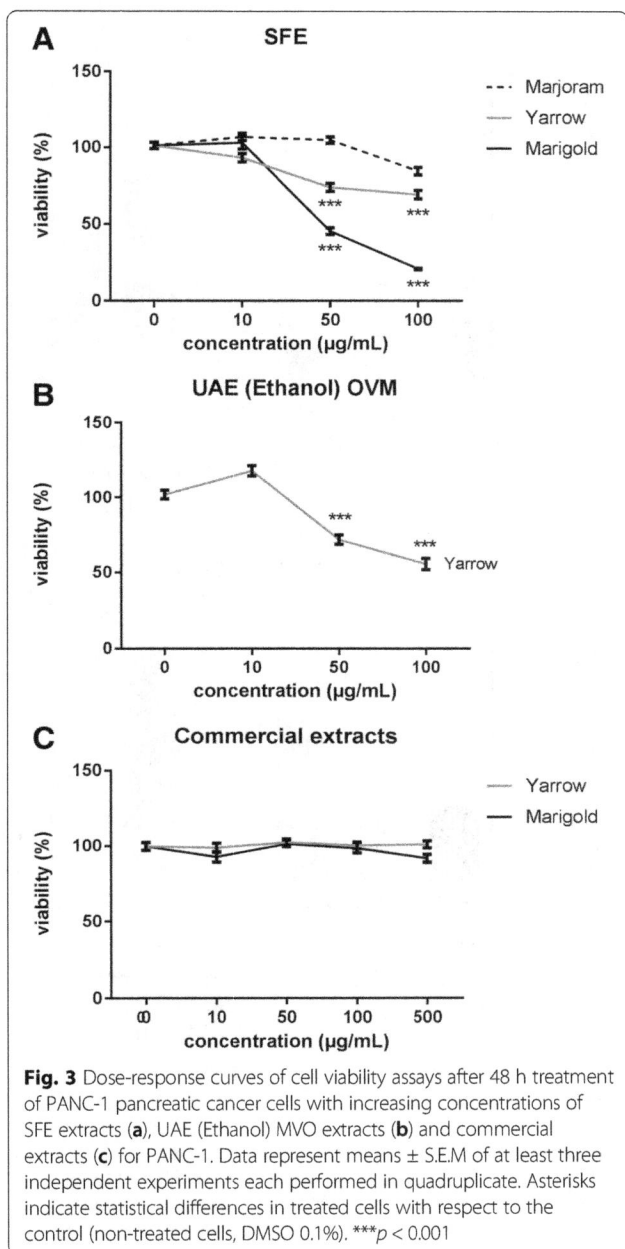

Fig. 3 Dose-response curves of cell viability assays after 48 h treatment of PANC-1 pancreatic cancer cells with increasing concentrations of SFE extracts (**a**), UAE (Ethanol) MVO extracts (**b**) and commercial extracts (**c**) for PANC-1. Data represent means ± S.E.M of at least three independent experiments each performed in quadruplicate. Asterisks indicate statistical differences in treated cells with respect to the control (non-treated cells, DMSO 0.1%). ***$p < 0.001$

Table 2 Concentration parameters of the selected plant extracts on PANC-1 cell line sensitivity depending on the extraction method

Plant extract	Concentration Parameter	Extraction Method		
		SFE	UAE OVM Ethanol	Commercial
Marjoram	IC50	> 100	–	–
	GI50	> 100	–	–
	TGI	> 100	–	–
	LC50	> 100	–	–
Yarrow	IC50	> 100	> 100	> 500
	GI50	24,5 ± 0,26	> 100	> 500
	TGI	96,4 ± 6,2	69,2 ± 1,1	> 500
	LC50	> 100	> 100	> 500
Marigold	IC50	43,2 ± 7,9	–	> 500
	GI50	> 100	–	> 500
	TGI	45,9 ± 1,8	–	> 500
	LC50	74,2 ± 6,6	–	> 500

Data (> 100): not significant activity found at 100 µg/mL concentration; (–): not determined; *SFE* Supercritical Fluid Extraction, *UAE* Ultrasound Assisted Extraction, *OVM* Original Vegetable Matrix
Data are presented as IC50 (µg/mL) (concentration needed for 50% inhibition of cell proliferation), GI50 (µg/mL) (concentration needed for 50% growth inhibition), TGI (µg/mL) (concentration needed for total growth inhibition) and LC50 (µg/mL) (concentration needed for 50% cell death) after 48 h' treatment as mean ± SEM of at least three independent experiments each performed in quadruplicate

determined using the Caspase-Glo 3/7 assay kit (Promega), following manufacturer's instructions.

Statistical analysis
Results were analyzed by ANOVA non-parametric with Bonferroni post hoc tests. Data were represented as mean ± S.E.M of at least three independent experiments. Statistical differences were defined as $p < 0,05$. Statistical analysis was performed with Graph Pad Prim 6 statistical software.

Results
Effect of Asteraceae and Lamiaceae families plant derived extracts on MiaPaca-2 cell viability
We first determined the effect of all extracts on MIA PaCa-2 cell viability by MTT assay. In this assay, viable cells with active metabolism can convert MTT into a colored product by reducing the MTT into formazan [16]. MIA PaCa-2 cells were treated for 48 h with all extracts in a range of concentrations between 0 and 100 µg/ml. As observed in Fig. 2a, Yarrow and Marigold SFE extracts decreased cell viability in a dose-dependent manner (IC50 = 31,5 ± 8,6 µg/mL and 39,8 ± 4,6 µg/mL respectively [5]), while Balm and Marjoram SFE extracts did not affected cell viability at any of the doses tested.

Regarding UAE (Ethanol), Yarrow extracts, both obtained from RVM and from OVM, inhibited cell proliferation in a

kit (Immunostep, Spain) accordingly to manufacturer's instructions. Stained cells were conducted on a Cytomics FC500 (Beckam Coulter) cytometer. Early apoptosis was defined as Ann+/PI- cells, whereas Ann+/PI+ cells was defined as late apoptosis and Ann-/PI+ cells were considered as necrotic cells.

Caspase activation assay
MIA Paca-2 cells were plated in 96-multiwell and treated for 48 h with increasing concentrations of the extracts. The activation of caspase 3 and caspase 7 was

higher manner than the rest of the UAE plant extracts (Marigold, Marjoram and Balm) (Fig. 2b, e). We also checked UAE extracts obtained with a mix of ethanol: water (50:50) as solvent from both vegetal matrices (OVM, RVM), but none of them affected cell viability in any of the tested doses (Fig. 2c, d). Table 1 summarizes concentrations corresponding to 50% cell viability inhibition (IC50), 50% cell growth inhibition (GI50), total cell growth inhibition (TGI), and 50% of cell death (LC50) for all the extracts tested.

With these preliminary results, SFE extracts from Asteraceae family (Marigold and Yarrow) seems to compromise cell viability by inducing lethal toxicity (Yarrow: LC50 = 70,6 ± 8,6 μg/mL and Marigold: LC50 = 78,5 ± 1,4 μg/mL) suggesting that these two extracts might act as promising antitumor agents against pancreatic cancer.

Effect of yarrow and Marigold extracts on PANC-1 metastatic pancreatic cancer cell line

We next studied the effect of the most effective extracts from Asteraceae plants (Yarrow SFE and Marigold SFE) on PANC-1 pancreatic cancer cell line, described to be more resistant to treatments [14, 15]. As shown in Fig. 3a and Table 2, Marigold displayed the strongest cell growth inhibition (IC50 = 43,2 ± 7,9 μg/mL) and lethal effect (LC50 = 74,2 ± 6,6), while Yarrow did not exert any effect at the doses tested (IC50 > 100 μg/mL).

Regardless UAE derived extracts, we only tested Yarrow UAE (Ethanol) from the OVM, as it has been shown to be the most effective UAE extracts tested in MIA PaCa-2. As shows Fig. 3b, IC50 value was much higher in PANC-1 compared to MIA PaCa-2 value (Fig. 2b).

In the other hand, we compared the effect on cell viability of commercial extracts obtained industrially by glycerin tincture, with Yarrow and Marigold SFE extracts and Yarrow UAE (ethanol) OVM extract. As shown in Tables 1 and 2, commercial extracts from Yarrow or Marigold did not exerted any effect on cell viability of MIA PaCa-2 and PANC-1 in the range of the doses tested (Fig. 2f and Fig. 3c, respectively) (GI50, TGI and LC50 values were higher than 500 μg/mL).

Finally, we have determined the effect on cell viability in a non-tumoral cell line (Additional file 1: Table S1, Additional file 1: Figure S1) to ensure the nontoxic response. The IC50 in the non-tumoral cells is 81,6 ± 14,1 μg/mL for Yarrow and 84,3 ± 21,2 for Marigold SFE extract.

Yarrow and Marigold SFE extracts induce pancreatic cancer cell death through apoptosis

To assess the mechanism by which Yarrow and Marigold SFE extracts induce cell growth inhibition, we have analyzed caspase 3/7 activation and the apoptotic populations.

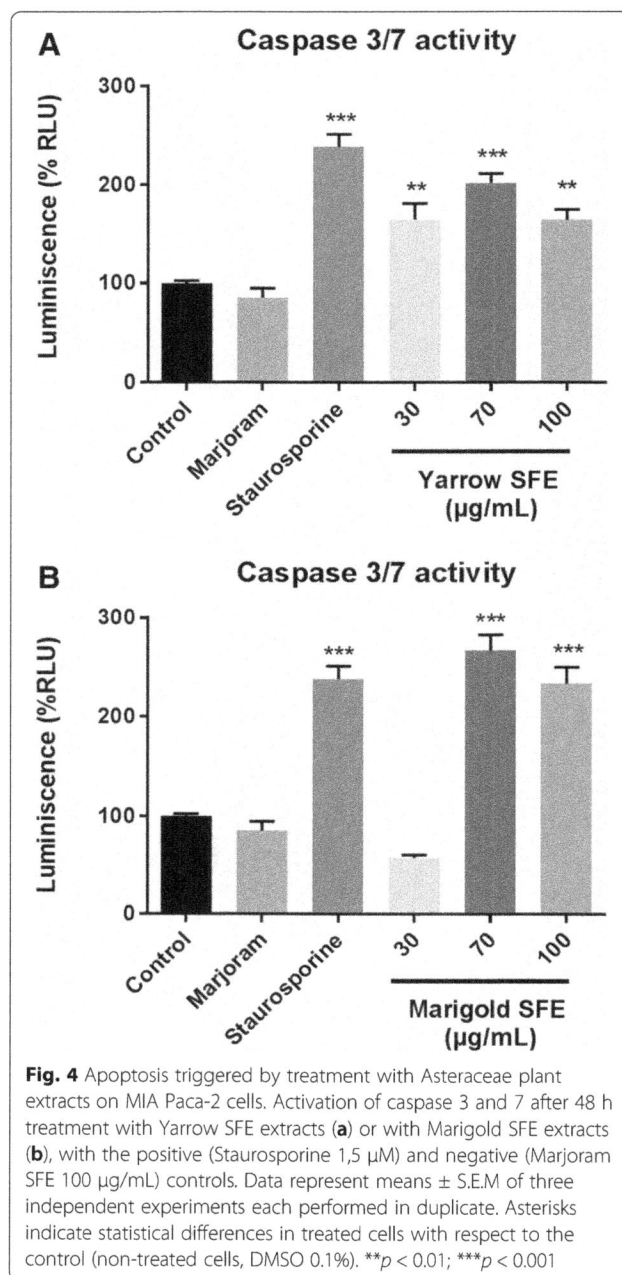

Fig. 4 Apoptosis triggered by treatment with Asteraceae plant extracts on MIA Paca-2 cells. Activation of caspase 3 and 7 after 48 h treatment with Yarrow SFE extracts (a) or with Marigold SFE extracts (b), with the positive (Staurosporine 1,5 μM) and negative (Marjoram SFE 100 μg/mL) controls. Data represent means ± S.E.M of three independent experiments each performed in duplicate. Asterisks indicate statistical differences in treated cells with respect to the control (non-treated cells, DMSO 0.1%). **$p < 0.01$; ***$p < 0.001$

Firstly, and as shown in Fig. 4, after 48 h of treatment, both Yarrow and Marigold SFE increased the levels of active (cleaved) caspases 3/7.

In addition, we have also determined, by flow cytometry with Annexin-V and PI staining, the distribution of apoptotic and necrotic cell subpopulations. Fig. 5a shows percentages of early apoptotic cells (PI–/Annexin V+), late apoptotic cells (PI+/Annexin V+) and necrotic cells (PI+/Annexin V-). Both extracts induced late apoptosis at 100 μg/mL (Fig. 5a). Interestingly Marigold gave rise to a higher percentage of necrotic cells (Fig. 5b). Fig. 5c

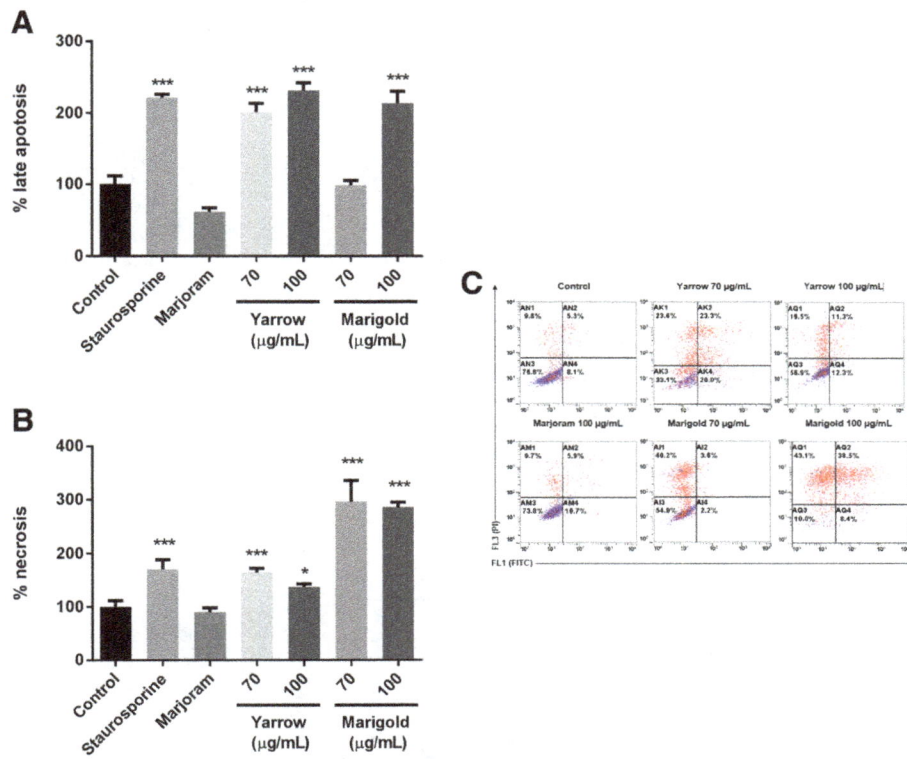

Fig. 5 Different phases of cell death after 24 h treatment with Asteraceae plants on MIA Paca-2. The % of apoptotic cells depending on Yarrow and Marigold SFE extracts (**a**) and the % of necrotic populations after those treatments (**b**). A representative flow cytometry diagram (**c**). Annexin V-FITC/PI double staining discriminates the live cells (Annexin V−/PI−; bottom left quadrant), early apoptotic cells (Annexin V+/PI−; bottom right quadrant), late apoptotic (Annexin V+/PI+; upper right quadrant), and necrotic or dead cells (Annexin V−/PI+; upper left quadrant). Data represent means ± S.E.M of at least four independent experiments each performed in triplicate. Asterisks indicate statistical differences in treated cells with respect to the control (non-treated cells, DMSO 0.1%). *$p < 0.05$; ***$p < 0.001$

shows a representative flow cytometry plot indicating the gates for the different subpopulations.

Yarrow and Marigold SFE extracts inhibit colony growth in 3D

We were interested in determining if Yarrow and Marigold SFE extracts affect the ability of MIA PaCa-2 epithelial cancer cells to form colonies when grown in 3D culture.

We first plated MIA PaCa-2 in Matrigel and 72 h later, when the colonies were formed, we treated the cells with 30, 50 and 70 μg/mL of the extracts, and the control with DMSO (0.1% v/v) (Fig. 6a). Yarrow reduced the size and number of the spheres maintaining their integrity (Fig. 6b), while Marigold affected significantly both parameters when cells were treated with 70 μg/mL (Fig. 6c), promoting the disruption of colonies (Fig. 6a). Both extracts diminished colony integrity suggesting that stem or progenitor cells are not able to sustain the tumor in vivo when treated with Yarrow or Marigold.

Yarrow and Marigold SFE extracts exhibit synergizes with 5-FU treatment

Finally, we analyzed the effect of Yarrow SFE and Marigold SFE in combination with the antitumoral drug 5-fluororacil (5-FU) on MIA PaCa-2, which is usually proposed in clinic to treat pancreatic cancer. Cells were treated with different concentrations of 5-FU for 72 h. We have observed that both Yarrow and Marigold markedly potentiate the antiproliferative effect of 5-FU when cells were pre-treated with these extracts, showing a higher cytotoxic effect when combining a plant extract with the antimetabolite 5-FU (Fig. 7), with a significant decrease in cell viability. Thus, according to the Chou–Talalay method [16], the combination of Yarrow with 5-FU and the combination of Marigold with 5-FU resulted in a synergistic effect displaying a (combinatory index) CI value < 1 in every combination assayed (Fig. 7).

Discussion

In this work, we have evaluated the antitumoral properties of four plants (Yarrow, Marigold, Balm and Marjoram) derived extracts in pancreatic cancer cell lines.

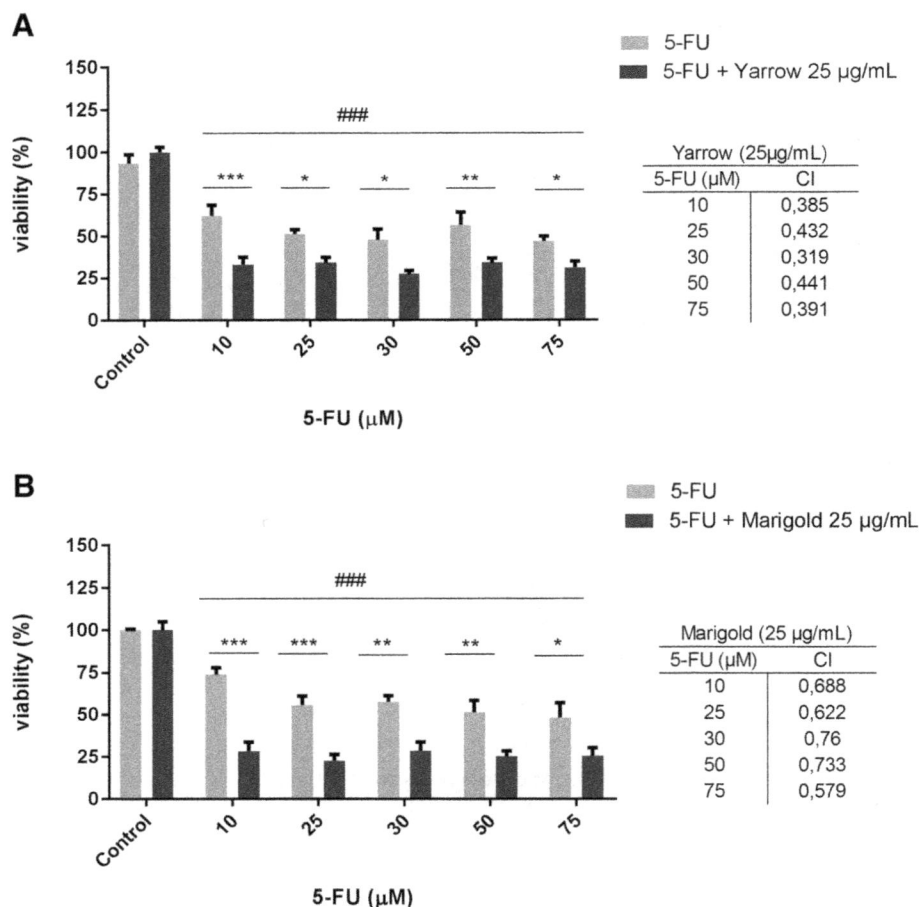

Fig. 6 MIA PaCa-2 response and Combination Index (CI) when cells were pre-treated 8 h with A) Yarrow or B) Marigold, followed by an exposure of increased doses of 5-FU for 72 h. Data represent means ± S.E.M of at three independent experiments each performed in quadruplicate. Asterisks (*) indicate statistical differences between 5-FU and Yarrow/Marigold+ 5-FU treatments *$p < 0.05$; **$p < 0.01$ ***$p < 0.001$. # indicates statistical differences in treated cells with respect to the control (DMSO 0.1%). ### $p < 0.001$

Importantly, two different green technologies have been used to obtain the bioactive components from these plants: Supercritical Fluid Extraction (SFE) and Ultrasonic Assisted Extraction (UAE). For UAE extractions, two different raw materials were compared -the Residual Vegetable Material obtained after the SFE step (RVM), and the Original Vegetable Material (OVM)-.

Yarrow and Marigold extracts obtained by SFE were the most effective ones on inhibiting cell proliferation, exhibiting similar values of IC50, TGI and LC50 in MIA PaCa-2 cells (Table 1). These results are within the range of those previously reported for Marigold extract obtained by Laser extraction in pancreatic cancer, leukemia and fibrosarcoma (IC50 = 60 µg/mL) [12]; or by those obtained by ethyl alcohol maceration in melanoma (IC50 = 50 µg/mL) [17].

Yarrow extracts obtained by UAE (Ethanol) from OVM and RVM were also effective on inhibiting cell viability. The concentration needed to achieve 50% of growth inhibition (GI50 = 49,4 ± 25,7 µg/mL) is within the interval of that obtained in other works by methanolic stirring extraction in hepatocellular (39.02 ± 2.9 µg/mL) and cervical carcinomas (47.1 ± 1.8 µg/mL) models [18].

Conversely and related to Lamiaceae family plants (Balm and Marjoram), none of the extracts (nor SFE, nor UAE) had any effect on the range of concentration tested (Table 1, Fig. 2). Although it has been described ethanolic Marjoram extract to promote lymphoblastic leukemia cell death [19], and Balm extract in hepatocellular and gastric carcinomas [20], in both cases the range of concentrations were around one thousand times higher than the ones tested in this work (IC50 = 8 mg/mL for Marjoram and around 70 mg/mL for Balm).

Thus, Marigold and Yarrow SFE extracts displayed better dose-dependence activity compared to the UAE and other extraction methodologies, both in MIA PaCa-2 and in the more resistant model, PANC-1.

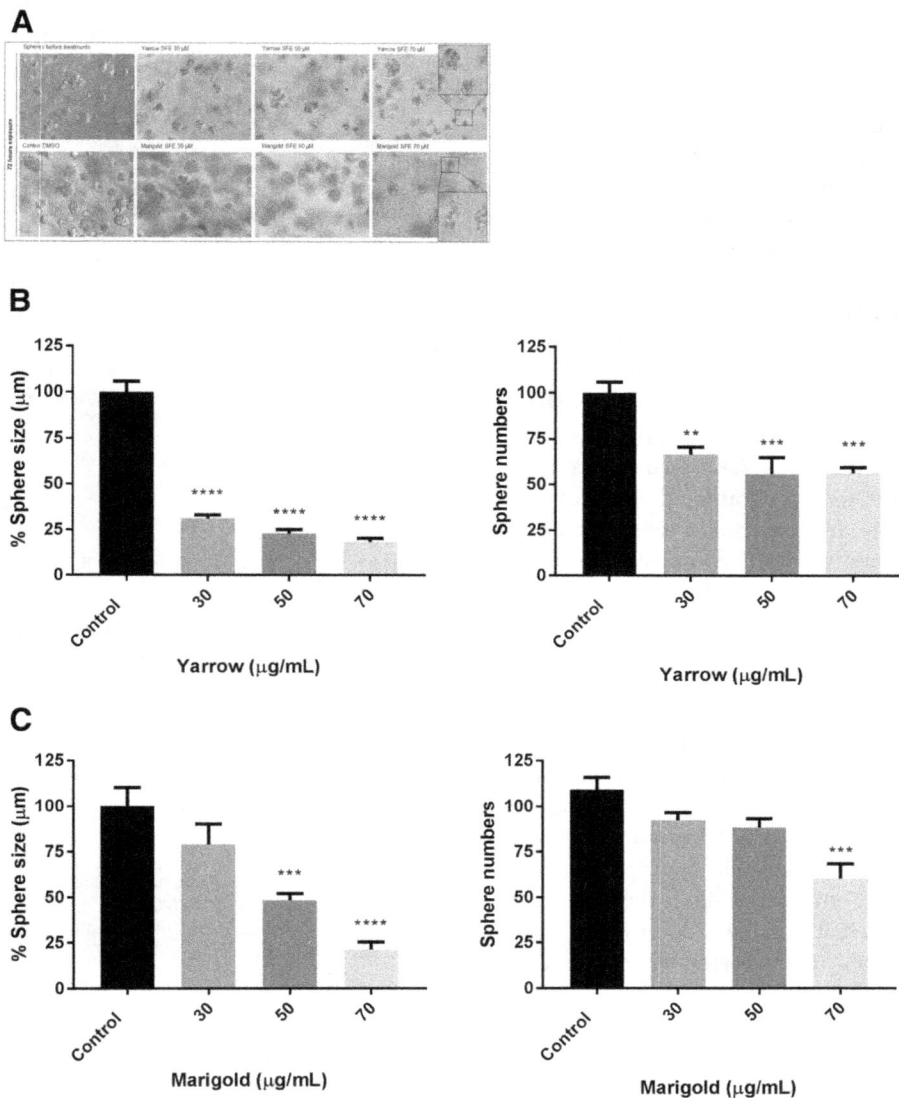

Fig. 7 Tridimensional MIA PaCa-2 cells when exposed to Asteraceae Extracts. **a**) Representative images of spheres after Yarrow (up) and Marigold (down) treatments for 72 h. Sphere number, size and morphology after Yarrow (**b**) and Marigold (**c**) exposures. Data represent means ± S.E.M of three independent experiments each performed in duplicate. Asterisks indicate statistical differences in treated cells with respect to the control (DMSO, 0.1%) ***$p < 0.001$; ****$p < 0.0001$

Indeed, here, Yarrow and Marigold SFE extracts have a IC50 dose much higher in a colon non-cancer cell line (CCD18), comparing the IC50 in a colon cancer cell line (SW-620) (Additional file 1: Figure S1, Additional file 1: Table S1), which supports a therapeutic window for the use of the extracts in combination with current therapy.

In the other hand, current treatment in clinic is mostly based on 5-fluorouracil (5-FU) and gemcitabine, even combined with other drugs. In this sense, we wanted to determine a possible synergism of Yarrow and Marigold SFE extracts with 5-FU. Thus, when pre-conditioning MIA PaCa-2 cells with Yarrow or Marigold, the cytotoxic

effect mediated by the subsequent 5-FU exposure has been increasing (Fig. 7). This enhancement in 5-FU effect has been previously described for other SFE extracts, such as Rosemary in colon cancer model [21], but Yarrow and Marigold are here described for the first time. In this sense, this synergism could be considered a promise as a co-adjuvant treatment, improving patient survival, given that both extracts potentiate the effect of a first-line chemotherapeutic agent. Until date, plants extracts, as a grouped set of molecules, have been tested and used to reduce chemotherapy side effects and for improve patient's quality of life [22], with few approaches proposing their use as a second-line therapy [23]. Thus, there is a need to promote clinical trials with plant extracts, as an ensemble of phytochemicals, after validating the antiproliferative hypothesis in murine models.

Further describing the effect of Yarrow and Marigold SFE extracts, and regarding their mechanism of action, we have found that both extracts induce apoptosis through caspase 3/7 cleavage (Fig. 4), although Marigold has also shown to promote the accumulation of high levels of a necrotic cell population. These results suggest that different signaling pathways may be implicated in the induction of cell death for each extract. In this context, restoring apoptotic signaling pathways has been proposed as a strategy for cancer treatment. In fact, most of the antitumoral agents exert their effect through induction of apoptosis [24, 25]. Particularly, these results are in accordance with those described previously for Marigold [12] related with programmed cell death. Concerning Yarrow, there are few studies which describe its involvement in the induction of apoptosis, contributing this study to the first evidences of them.

Finally, we also have demonstrated that Yarrow and Marigold SFE inhibit transforming activity (Fig. 7). Growing and giving rise to 3D colonies is a way to monitor cell malignancy and the ability of stem and progenitor cells to sustain the tumor. If the proposed extracts affect the colony formation, cells are not able to evade signals that restraint their growth. In this sense, herein, we have seen that Yarrow induces a dose-dependent decrease in cell transformation and brakes the 3D sphere growth, while, Marigold induces disruption of the integrity of 3D colonies that may be due to the loose of their mesenchymal phenotype associated with an increased motility.

These results also suggest differences in the specific antitumoral mechanism of both extracts. They demonstrate that even both plants are from the same family (Asteraceae), there are differences in the way they exert their bioactive effect against pancreatic tumor cells. These differences encourage further studies to better understand the molecular action of the extracts, conducting individual approaches for each plant type. Once we a deeper understanding of their anticancer profile reached, the extracts could be registered for this purpose, beyond their current use as herbal preparation in most of the European Union countries.

Conclusion

This work has demonstrated that Yarrow and Marigold supercritical fluid extracts (SFE), besides avoiding chemical agents for their obtaining, allow to get effective amounts of antitumor phytochemical agents with effects not only in cell viability and 3D grown, but also in sensitizing tumor cells to chemotherapeutic agents such as 5-FU.

Related to Marjoram and Balm, their derived extracts have shown no cytotoxic effect in the pancreatic cell lines tested.

Abbreviations
DMSO: Dimethyl Sulphoxide; GI50: concentration to induce 50% growth inhibition; IC50: concentration to induce 50% cell viability inhibition; LC50: lethal concentration; OVM: Original Vegetable Matrix; RVM: Residual Vegetable Matrix; SFE: Supercritical Fluid Extraction; TGI: concentration to induce total growth inhibition; UAE: Ultrasound Assisted Extraction

Funding
This work has been supported by Ministerio de Economía y Competitividad del Gobierno de España (MINECO, Plan Nacional I + D + i) AGL2016–76736-C3/FEDER, and Gobierno Regional de la Comunidad de Madrid (P2013/ABI-2728, ALIBIRD-CM).

Authors' contributions
Conception and design of in vitro experiments: ARdM, LM, MGdC. Conducted in vitro experiments: LM. Conception and design of the extractions: TF, MRGR, GR. Conducted extractions LM, NHM. Data analysis and interpretation: LM, MGdC, TV, EGC. Manuscript drafting: LM, MGdC. Final approval and critical revision: ARdM. All authors read and approved the final manuscript.

Competing interests
The authors declare that they have no competing interests.

Author details
[1]Molecular Oncology and Nutritional Genomics of Cancer, Madrid Institute for Advanced Studies on Food (IMDEA-Food), Ctra de Cantoblanco, 8, 28049 Madrid, Spain. [2]Production and Characterization of Novel Foods Department, Institute of Food Science Research (CIAL) CEI UAM + CSIC, Madrid, Spain.

References
1. Jemal A, Bray F, Center MM, Ferlay J, Ward E, Forman D. Global cancer statistics. CA Cancer J Clin. 2011;61(2):69–90.
2. Ducreux M, Caramella C, Hollebecque A, Burtin P, Goéré D, Seufferlein T, Haustermans K, Van Laethem J, Conroy T, Arnold D. Cancer of the pancreas: ESMO clinical practice guidelines for diagnosis, treatment and follow-up. Ann Oncol. 2015;26(suppl_5):v56–68.
3. Mouhid L, Corzo-Martínez M, Torres C, Vázquez L, Reglero G, Fornari T. Ramírez de Molina a: improving in vivo efficacy of bioactive molecules: an overview of potentially antitumor phytochemicals and currently available lipid-based delivery systems. Journal of Oncology. 2017;2017.
4. Gonzalez-Vallinas M, Gonzalez-Castejon M, Rodriguez-Casado A. Ramirez de Molina a: dietary phytochemicals in cancer prevention and therapy: a complementary approach with promising perspectives. Nutr Rev. 2013;71(9):585–99.
5. García-Risco MR, Mouhid L, Salas-Pérez L, López-Padilla A, Santoyo S, Jaime L, de Molina AR, Reglero G, Fornari T: Biological activities of Asteraceae (Achillea millefolium and Calendula officinalis) and Lamiaceae (Melissa officinalis and Origanum majorana) plant extracts. Plant Foods Hum Nutr 2017, 72(1):96–102.
6. Savini I, Arnone R, Catani MV and Avigliano L. Origanum vulgare induces apoptosis in human colon cancer caco2 cells. Nutr Cancer. 2009;61(3):381–9.
7. Erenler R, Sen O, Aksit H, Demirtas I, Yaglioglu AS, Elmastas M, Telci İ. Isolation and identification of chemical constituents from Origanum

majorana and investigation of antiproliferative and antioxidant activities. J Sci Food Agric. 2015.

8. Weidner C, Rousseau M, Plauth A, Wowro S, Fischer C, Abdel-Aziz H, Sauer S. Melissa officinalis extract induces apoptosis and inhibits proliferation in colon cancer cells through formation of reactive oxygen species. Phytomedicine. 2014.

9. Saraydin SU, Tuncer E, Tepe B, Karadayi S, Ozer H, Sen M, Karadayi K, Inan D, Elagoz S, Polat Z. Antitumoral effects of Melissa officinalis on breast cancer in vitro and in vivo. Asian Pac J Cancer Prev. 2012;13(6):2765–70.

10. Csupor-Löffler B, Hajdú Z, Zupkó I, Réthy B, Falkay G, Forgo P, Hohmann J. Antiproliferative effect of flavonoids and sesquiterpenoids from Achillea millefolium sl on cultured human tumour cell lines. Phytother Res. 2009; 23(5):672–6.

11. Ghavami G, Sardari S, Shokrgozar MA. Anticancerous potentials of Achillea species against selected cell lines. J Medicinal Plants Research. 2010;4(22): 2411–7.

12. Ukiya M, Akihisa T, Yasukawa K, Tokuda H, Suzuki T, Kimura Y. Anti-inflammatory, anti-tumor-promoting, and cytotoxic activities of constituents of marigold (Calendula officinalis) flowers. J Nat Prod. 2006;69(12):1692–6.

13. Jimenez-Medina E, Garcia-Lora A, Paco L, Algarra I, Collado A, Garrido F. A new extract of the plant Calendula officinalis produces a dual in vitro effect: cytotoxic anti-tumor activity and lymphocyte activation. BMC Cancer. 2006;6:119.

14. Monks A, Scudiero D, Skehan P, Shoemaker R, Paull K, Vistica D, Hose C, Langley J, Cronise P, Vaigro-Wolff A. Feasibility of a high-flux anticancer drug screen using a diverse panel of cultured human tumor cell lines. J Natl Cancer Inst. 1991;83(11):757–66.

15. Chou T, Talalay P. Quantitative analysis of dose-effect relationships: the combined effects of multiple drugs or enzyme inhibitors. Adv Enzym Regul. 1984;22:27–55.

16. Riss TL, Moravec RA, Niles AL, Duellman S, Benink HA, Worzella TJ, Minor L. Cell Viability Assays. In: Sittampalam GS, Coussens NP, Brimacombe K, et al., editors. Assay Guidance Manual: Bethesda (MD); 2004.

17. Fryer RA, Barlett B, Galustian C, Dalgleish AG. Mechanisms underlying gemcitabine resistance in pancreatic cancer and sensitisation by the iMiD lenalidomide. Anticancer Res. 2011;31(11):3747–56.

18. Huanwen W, Zhiyong L, Xiaohua S, Xinyu R, Kai W, Tonghua L. Intrinsic chemoresistance to gemcitabine is associated with constitutive and laminin-induced phosphorylation of FAK in pancreatic cancer cell lines. Mol Cancer. 2009;8(125):21.

19. Preethi KC, Siveen KS, Kuttan R, Kuttan G. Inhibition of metastasis of B16F-10 melanoma cells in C57BL/6 mice by an extract of Calendula officinalis L flowers. Asian Pac J Cancer Prev. 2010;11(6):1773–9.

20. Dias MI, Barros L, Dueñas M, Pereira E, Carvalho AM, Alves RC, Oliveira MBP, Santos-Buelga C, Ferreira IC. Chemical composition of wild and commercial Achillea millefolium L. and bioactivity of the methanolic extract, infusion and decoction. Food Chem. 2013;141(4):4152–60.

21. Abdel-Massih RM, Fares R, Bazzi S, El-Chami N, Baydoun E. The apoptotic and anti-proliferative activity of Origanum majorana extracts on human leukemic cell line. Leuk Res. 2010;34(8):1052–6.

22. Lin J, Chen Y, Lee Y, Hou CR, Chen F, Yang D. Antioxidant, anti-proliferative and cyclooxygenase-2 inhibitory activities of ethanolic extracts from lemon balm (Melissa officinalis L.) leaves. LWT-Food Science and Technology. 2012; 49(1):1–7.

23. González-Vallinas M, Molina S, Vicente G, de la Cueva A, Vargas T, Santoyo S, García-Risco MR, Fornari T, Reglero G, de Molina AR. Antitumor effect of 5-fluorouracil is enhanced by rosemary extract in both drug sensitive and resistant colon cancer cells. Pharmacol Res. 2013;72:61–8.

24. Kienle GS, Kiene H. Review article: influence of Viscum album L (European mistletoe) extracts on quality of life in cancer patients: a systematic review of controlled clinical studies. Integrative cancer therapies. 2010;9(2):142–57.

25. Tröger W, Galun D, Reif M, Schumann A, Stanković N, Milićević M. Viscum album [L.] extract therapy in patients with locally advanced or metastatic pancreatic cancer: a randomised clinical trial on overall survival. Eur J Cancer. 2013;49(18):3788–97.

8

Isolation of anticancer constituents from *Cucumis prophetarum* var. prophetarum through bioassay-guided fractionation

Abdulrhman Alsayari[1], Lucas Kopel[2], Mahmoud Salama Ahmed[3], Hesham S. M. Soliman[4], Sivakumar Annadurai[1] and Fathi T. Halaweish[5*]

Abstract

Background: *Cucumis prophetarum* var. prophetarum is used in Saudi folk medicine for treating liver disorders and grows widely between Abha and Khamis Mushait City, Saudi Arabia.

Methods: Bioassay-guided fractionation and purification were used to isolate the main active constituents of *Cucumis prophetarum* var. prophetarum fruits. These compounds were structurally elucidated using NMR spectroscopy, mass spectral analyses and x-ray crystallography. All fractions, sub-fractions and pure compounds were screened for their anticancer activity against six cancer cell lines.

Results: The greatest cytotoxic activity was found to be in the ethyl acetate fraction, resulting in the isolation of five cucurbitacin compounds [E, B, D, F-25 acetate and Hexanorcucurbitacin D]. Among the cucurbitacins that were isolated and tested cucurbitacin B and E showed potent cytotoxicity activities against all six human cancer cell lines.

Conclusion: Human breast cancer cell lines were found to be the most sensitive to cucurbitacins. Preliminary structure activity relationship (SAR) for cytotoxic activity of Cucurbitacins against human breast cancer cell line MDA-MB-231 has been reported.

Keywords: Bioassay-guided fractionation, Cucurbitacins, *Cucumis prophetarum* var. prophetarum, Anticancer, Breast cancer, Preliminary SAR

Background

The advances in natural product screening coupled with the growing appreciation for functional assays and phenotypic screens have contributed to the re-emergence of natural products for drug discovery in the genomics era [1]. Natural products have played a significant role in human disease therapy and compounds derived from natural products have always been noted as a valuable source for drug discovery [2]. Saudi flora contains 2250 species arranged in 142 families; among these, more than 1200 species are expected to be medicinal [3]. Several plant families in Saudi flora have been reported to have medicinal properties, such as the Cucurbitaceae family which is commonly used in Saudi folk medicine, a number of plant species from the Cucurbitaceae family, such as *Citrullus colocynthis*, have been utilized for the treatment of various health disorders [4–6].

Cucurbitacins are a group of highly oxygenated tetracyclic triterpenoids existing widely in the plant kingdom, especially in the Cucurbitaceae family [7]. A total of 12 classes of cucurbitacins have been recognized based on their structural characteristics and designated alphabetically from A to T with over 200 derivatives. Eight most active cucurbitacin components against cancer are cucurbitacin B, D, E, I, IIa, L glucoside, Q and R [8]. A number of cucurbitacins have been reported to be isolated from the genus Cucumis. Cucurbitacin (B, E, I, O, P and Q1); dihydrocucurbitacin (D and E), isocucurbitacin (B, D and E) and dihydroisocucurbitacin (D and E) have been reported to be isolated from *Cucumis prophetarum* L. Cucurbitacin B and Dihydrocucurbitacin B isolated from *Cucumis prophetarum* L., were studied for their cytotoxic

* Correspondence: fathi.halaweish@sddtate.edu
[5]Department of Chemistry and Biochemistry, South Dakota State University, Brookings, SD 57007, USA
Full list of author information is available at the end of the article

activity towards human cancer cell lines, mouse embryonic fibroblast (NIH3T3) and virally transformed form (KA3IT) cells [9]. Recently the antidiabetic and antioxidant activity of the different fractions of fruits of *Cucumis prophetarum* L. has been reported [10].

Cucumis prophetarum var. prophetarum (Cucurbitaceae), which is locally called as Shari-al-deeb, is used in Saudi folk medicine for the treatment of liver disorders and grows widely between Abha and Khamis Mushait City, Saudi Arabia. To the best of our knowledge there are no studies reported on this variety.

The aim of the present study was the extraction, isolation, and structural elucidation of the active constituents with potential anti-cancer activity from *Cucumis prophetarum* var. prophetarum using bioassay-guided fractionation. The anticancer activities of the extracts, fractions, and pure isolated compounds obtained from the bioassay-guided fractionation were evaluated in vitro using six human cancer cell lines: breast (MCF7, MDA-MB-231), colon (HCT-116), ovarian (A2780/ A2780CP), and liver (HepG2). The chemical structures of the pure isolated compounds were elucidated using NMR spectroscopy, mass spectral analyses, and x-ray crystallography.

Methods

^{1}H-NMR, ^{13}C-NMR, and 2D-NMR were conducted using Bruker AVANCE-400 MHz and 600 MHz NMR spectrometers at 22 °C, in deuterated chloroform (CDCl$_3$) using tetramethylsilane (TMS) as the internal standard; chemical shifts are given in ä (ppm) values. High-resolution ESI mass spectra were measured on a ThermoFinnigan MAT 95 XL mass spectrometer at the mass spectroscopy facility located at the University of Buffalo (Buffalo, NY, USA). X-ray crystal structure was obtained with a Bruker-AXS Photon-100 diffractometer at the X-Ray Crystallographic Laboratory, University of Minnesota (Minneapolis, MN, USA). Column chromatography was carried out using silica gel (230–400 mesh) purchased from Sorbent Technologies (Norcross, GA, USA). TLC was performed using pre-coated silica gel PE Sheets purchased from Sorbent Technologies (Norcross, GA, USA), visualized under ultraviolet at 254 nm, and stained with Ceric Ammonium Molybdate (CAM) followed by heating. All solvents were obtained from commercial suppliers and used as received.

Dimethyl sulfoxide (DMSO), 3-(4,5-Dimethyl-2-thiazolyl)-2,5-diphenyl-2H-tetrazolium bromide (MTT), sodium dodecyl sulfate (SDS), and RPMI 1640 medium were purchased from Sigma-Aldrich (St. Louis, MO, USA). Dulbecco's modified Eagle medium (DMEM), antibiotics, phosphate buffered saline (PBS) 1X solution, and trypsin were purchased from Gibco (Grand Island, NY, USA). Fetal bovine serum (FBS) was purchased from HyClone (Logan, UT, USA).

Plant materials

Fresh fruits of *Cucumis prophetarum* var. prophetarum were collected in June 2010 from the wild near Abha-Khamis Road, Abha, Saudi Arabia. The plant was botanically authenticated and a voucher specimen was deposited in the Pharmacognosy Department Herbarium, College of Pharmacy, King Khalid University, Abha, Saudi Arabia.

Preparation of plant extracts and fractions

The fruits of *Cucumis prophetarum* var. prophetarum (6.5 kg) were cut into pieces and homogenized in methanol (a blender was filled to 1/3 volume with fruits, 1.5 L of methanol was added, then the mixture was homogenized for 5 min). The mixture was then macerated in methanol for a further 72 h. The methanol extract was filtered, concentrated under reduced pressure at 40 °C using a rotary evaporator, and lyophilized to afford a residue (200 g, 3.07%). The dried methanol extract (160 g) was divided into several portions of 20 g and each of them was dispersed in de-ionized water (500 ml) and partitioned sequentially with n-hexane (500 ml × 3), ethyl acetate (500 ml × 3), and n-butanol (500 ml × 3). The combined solvent of each partitioned extract was concentrated under reduced pressure at 40 °C using the rotary evaporator and freeze dried for 72 h to yield an n-hexane fraction (2.5 g, 0.03%), an ethyl acetate fraction (4.5 g, 0.07%), n-butanol (4.5 g, 0.07%), and the remainder of the water fraction (91 g, 1.40%). All fractions were dissolved in DMSO, with the exception of the water fraction which was dissolved in media, and they were tested for their anti-cancer activities using six human cancer cell lines [11].

Isolation

According to the bioassay-guided fractionation, the ethyl acetate fraction showed the greatest anti-cancer activity, and thus was selected for the present study (Table 4). The EtOAc fraction was subjected to column chromatography on silica gel (300 g) and eluted with stepwise gradients of n-hexane/EtOAc (100:0, 90:10, 80:20, 70:30, 60:40, 50:50, 45:55, 40:60, 30:70, 20:80, 10:90, 0:100 *v/v*) and finally with 2 L methanol. A total of 475 fractions (25 mL each) were collected and combined on the basis of their TLC profiles into three main fractions as follows: fraction I (1–186) (766.8 mg, 0.011%), Fraction II (187–226) (655 mg, 0.010%), and Fraction III (227–475) (1.206 g, 0.018%).

Fraction I (306 mg) was subjected to preparative TLC using (n-hexane/EtOAc, 7:3) to yield band 1 (a mixture of compound 1 and 2) (15.8 mg, 0.00024%) and band 2 (pure compound 2) (35.3 mg, 0.00054%). Fraction II crystallized (on standing) yielding compound 2 (655 mg, 0.010%). Fraction III (933.7 mg) was chromatographed again on a silica gel (80 g) and eluted with dichloromethane/ methanol (100:0, 98:2). A total number of 154 subfractions (10 mL each) were collected and combined on the basis of their TLC profiles into three main subfractions, as follows: subfraction A (1–72) (222.25 mg, 0.0034%), subfraction B (73–97) (423.8 mg, 0.0065%), and subfraction C (98–15) (79.9 mg, 0.0012%).

Subfraction A yielded compound 3 (106.6 mg, 0.0016%), subfraction B yielded compound 4 (99.8 mg, 0.0015%), and subfraction C yielded compound 5 (51.6 mg, 0.00079%).

Cell cultures

Human cancer breast cell lines (MCF7, MDA-MB-231), human cancer colon cell lines (HCT-116), human ovarian carcinoma cell lines (A2780/ A2780CP), and human liver carcinoma cell lines (HepG2) were obtained from American Type Cell Culture (ATCC, Rockville, MD, USA). The MDA-MB-231, A2780, and A2780CP cell lines were maintained at 37 °C in a humidified atmosphere of 5% CO_2 in RPMI-1640 medium containing 10% fetal bovine serum and antibiotics (100 IU/mL penicillin and 100 μg/mL streptomycin). The HepG2, HCT-116, and MCF7 cell lines were maintained at 37°C in a humidified atmosphere of 5% CO_2 in a DMEM medium containing 10% fetal bovine serum and antibiotics (100 IU/mL penicillin and 100 μg/mL streptomycin).

MTT assay

The effects of all fractions and pure compounds were tested on six human cancer cell lines (MCF7, MDA-MB-231, HCT-116, A2780, A2780CP and HepG2) using a 3-(4,5-dimethylthiazol-2-yl)-2,5-diphenyltetrazolium bromide (MTT) assay, which measures the ability of metabolically active cells to convert tetrazolium salt into a blue formazan product. Cells (1×10^4 cells/well) were seeded into a 96-well plate and allowed to attach to the well over night. All plant fractions or pure compounds were dissolved in DMSO at 10 mM and then diluted in culture medium (The final DMSO concentration did not exceed 1%). Plant fractions or pure compounds were added at different concentrations (0, 1.6, 8, 40, 200, 1000 μg/ml for each fraction and 0, 0.16, 0.8, 4, 20, 100 μM for pure compounds) and cells were incubated for a further 48 h. After incubation, 10 μL of 5 mg/mL of MTT dye were added to the cells for 4 h at 37 °C, followed by the addition of 100 μL of 10% SDS in 0.01 N HCl as a solubilizing agent. The absorbance at 570 nm was recorded using an ELISA microplate reader. The results of viability were expressed as a percentage of the control and IC_{50} concentrations with 50% growth inhibitory effects were calculated from a dose–response curve.

Results

Isolation and structural elucidation

The methanolic extract of the fruits of *Cucumis prophetarum* var. *prophetarum* was dispersed in deionized water and partitioned sequentially with n-hexane, ethyl acetate, and n-butanol. Based on the bioassay-guided fractionation, the ethyl acetate fraction showed higher anticancer activity and thus it was subjected to a series of chromatography techniques to yield five Cucurbitacin compounds (Fig. 1).

Compound 2 was isolated as a white powder. It showed a molecular ion peak at m/z 581.30697 $[M + Na]^+$ (calcd. 581.30849) in the HR-ESIMS spectrum, which corresponded to the molecular formula $C_{32}H_{46}O_8$. The ^{1}H-NMR spectral data of 2 (Table 1) exhibited nine tertiary methyl group signals at δ_H 0.99 (3H, s, H-18); 1.08(3H, s, H-19); 1.29 (3H, s, H-28); 1.35(3H, s, H-29); 1.36 (3H, s, H-30); 1.43 (3H, s, H-21); 1.55 (3H, s, H-26); 1.57 (3H, s, H-27); 2.02 (3H, s, OAc), an olefinic proton at δ_H 5.80 (1H, d, J = 5.60 Hz, H-6), two *trans*-coupled olefinic protons on a side chain at δ_H 6.48 (1H, d, J = 15.6 Hz, H-23) and 7.07 (1H, d, J = 15.6 Hz, H-24), two hydroxymethine protons at δ_H 4.43 (1H, dd, J = 4.4, 12.9 Hz, H-2) and 4.36 (1H, m, H-16), and a pair of doublets at δ_H 2.69 (1H, d, J = 14.7 Hz, H-12β) and 3.25 (1H, d, J = 14.4 Hz, H-12α). The ^{13}C-NMR spectral data of compound 2 revealed the presence of 30 carbon signals for a triterpene skeleton, in addition to two carbon signals for an acetate moiety. The ^{13}C-NMR data (Table 2) showed nine methyl signals at δ_C 18.8, 19.8, 20.0, 21.2, 23.9, 25.9, 26.3, 29.3, 21.9 were assigned for C -30, C-18, C-19, C-29, C-21,C-27, C-26, C-28 and CH_3CO, respectively, three carbonyls at δ_C 202.5, 212.3 213.6 were assigned for C-22, C-11, C-2, respectively, four olefinic signals at δ_C 120.3, 120.4, 140.2, 151.9 were assigned for C-23, C-6, C-5, C-24, respectively, and four oxygenated functions at δ_C 71.2, 71.6, 78.2, 79.3 were assigned for C-16, C-2, C-20 and C-25. The presence of a singlet methyl signal at δ_H 2.02 in ^{1}H NMR spectra and two carbon signals at 21.9 and 170.3 in ^{13}C NMR spectra indicated the presence of an acetate moiety at C-25. The above data indicated the presence of a cucurbitacin tetracyclic triterpene skeleton; a comparison of the data with those published [10, 12–14] indicated that structure 2 was characterized as cucurbitacin B. Further confirmation of compound 2 was achieved by comparison with an authentic sample of cucurbitacin B from our lab.

Band 1 was obtained as a white amorphous powder and displayed two molecular ion peaks at m/z 579.29530 $[M + Na]^+$ (calcd. 579.29284) and m/z 581.30967 $[M + Na]^+$ (calcd. 581.30849) in its HR-ESIMS, corresponding to the molecular formulas $C_{32}H_{44}O_8$ and $C_{32}H_{46}O_8$, respectively. A comparison of the ^{1}H-NMR spectrum of 1 with published data [15–17] led us to characterize

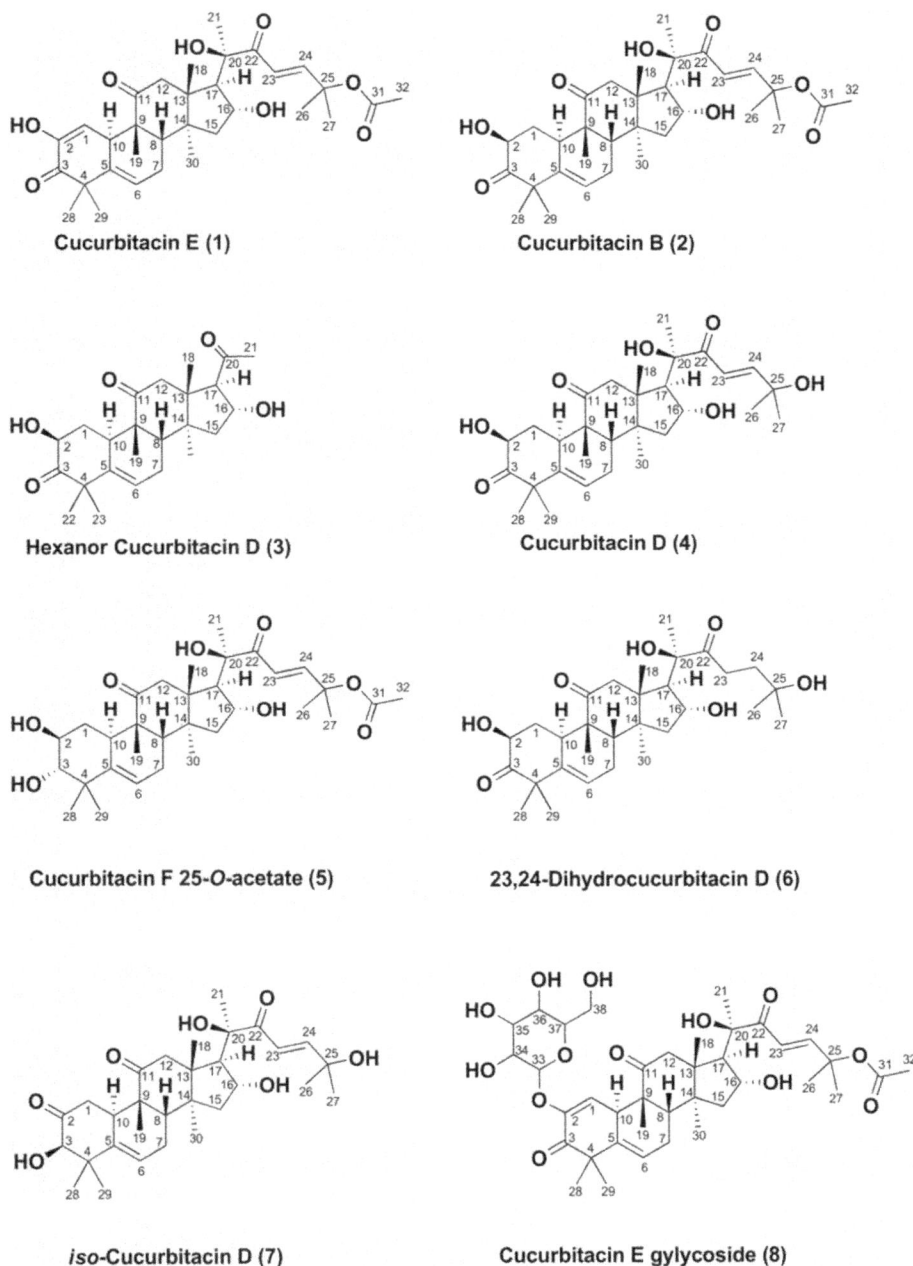

Fig. 1 Chemical Structures of Isolated Cucurbitacins

band **1** as a mixture of cucurbitacin E (**1**) and cucurbitacin B (**2**).

Compound **4** was isolated as a yellow amorphous powder. It showed a molecular ion peak at m/z 539.29854 [M + Na]$^+$ (calcd. 539.29792) in the HR-ESI-MS spectrum, which corresponded to the molecular formula $C_{30}H_{44}O_7$. The ^1H NMR spectral data of **4** (Table 1) exhibited eight tertiary methyl group signals at δ_H 0.98 (3H, s, H-18); 1.30 (3H, s, H-28); 1.33 (3H, s, H-29); 1.34 (3H, s, H-30); 1.35 (3H, s, H-26); 1.35 (3H, s, H-27); 1.39 (3H, s, H-21); 1.8

(3H, s, H-19), an olefinic proton at δ_H 5.79 (1H, m, J = 5.60 Hz, H-6), two *trans*-coupled olefinic protons on a side chain at δ_H 6.60 (1H, d, J = 15.16 Hz, H-23) and 7.14 (1H, d, J = 15.17 Hz, H-24), two hydroxymethine protons at δ_H 4.46 (1H, dd, J = 6.5, 12.8 Hz, H-2) and 4.33 (1H, m, H-16), and a pair of doublets at δ_H 2.7 (1H, d, J = 14.6 Hz, H-12β) and 3.32 (1H, d, J = 14.3 Hz, H-12α). The ^{13}C-NMR spectral data of compound **4** revealed the presence of 30 carbon signals for a triterpene skeleton. The ^{13}C-NMR data (Table 2) showed eight methyl signals at

Table 1 ^{1}H-NMR spectral data for compounds 2, 3, 4 and 5 in CDCl$_3$[a] (400 MHz)

H	(2)	(3)	(4)	(5)
1 α	2.32 ddd (3.3/ 5.8 /12.5)	2.24 m	2.33 ddd (3.3/ 5.8 /12.5)	s.o.
1β	1.21 d (13.0)	1.21 d (12.8)	1.21 m	1.15 d (6.30)
2	4.43 dd (4.44/12.9)	4.43 dd (6.0/12.8)	4.46 dd (6.5/12.8)	3.59 m
3	–	–	–	2.98 d (9.0)
4	–	–	–	–
5	–	–	–	–
6	5.80 d(5.6)	5.78 d br (5.6)	5.79 br m	5.73 d (5.4)
7α	s.o.	s.o.	1.94 m	s.o
7β	2.41 dm	2.41 dd (7.5/19.1)	2.40 dd (8.2/19.8)	2.39 m
8	1.98 br d (7.8)	2.01 d (6.8)	1.97 d br (7.9)	1.93 br d (7.6)
9	–	–	–	–
10	2.75 br d (13.1)	2.50 d (14.3)	2.78 d (13.7)	2.62 br d (14.4)
11	–	–	–	–
12α	3.25 d (14.4)	3.32 d (14.5)	3.32 d (14.3)	3.18 d (14.4)
12β	2.69 d (14.7)	2.76 d (12.7)	2.7 d (14.6)	2.52 d (6.81)
13	–	–	–	–
14	–	–	–	–
15α	1.88 dd(9.4/13.5)	s.o	s.o.	s.o.
15β	1.45 d (5.8)	1.93 dd (11.7/19.8)	1.84 dd (8.2/13.1)	1.85 m
16	4.36 m	4.92 m	4.33 m br	4.33 m
17	2.51 d (7.3)	3.17 d (6.45)	2.55 d (6.88)	2.48 d (7.03)
18	0.99 s	0.66 s	0.98 s	0.96 s
19	1.08 s	1.05 s	1.8 s	1.27 s
20	–	–	–	–
21	1.43 s	2.16 s	1.39 s	1.55 s
22	–	–	–	–
23	6.48 d (15.6)	–	6.60 d (15.1)	6.46 d (15.6)
24	7.07 d (15.6)	–	7.14 d (15.1)	7.07 d (15.6)
25	–	–	–	–
26	1.55 s	–	1.35 s	1.57 s
27	1.57 s	–	1.35 s	1.55
28	1.29 s	1.27 s	1.30 s	1.27 s
29	1.35 s	1.33 s	1.33 s	1.20 s
30	1.36 s	1.37 s	1.34 s	1.10 s
O$_2$CMe	2.02 s	–	–	2.02 s

[a] j values in Hz are given in parentheses, (so) signal obscured, (s) singlet, (d) doublet, (dd) doublet of doublets, (m) multiplet, (br) broad

δ_C 19.2, 19.9, 20.1, 21.2, 23.9, 28.9, 26.3, 29.3, 29.5 which were assigned for C-30, C-18, C-19, C-29, C-21, C-28, C-27 and C-26, respectively; three carbonyls at δ_C 202.6, 212.3213.1 which were assigned for C-22, C-11 and C-3, respectively: four olefinic signals at δ_C 118.9, 120.2, 140.3, 155.7 which were assigned for C-23, C-6, C-5 and C-24, respectively, and four oxygenated functions at δ_C 71.3, 71.6, 78.1, and 71.1 which were assigned for C-16, C-2, C-20 and C-25, respectively.

The above ^{1}H- and ^{13}C-NMR data of Compound **4** were similar to that of Compound **2**, except for the absence of a singlet methyl signal at δ_H 2.02 in the ^{1}H-NMR spectrum and two carbon signals at 21.9 and 170.3 in the ^{13}C-NMR spectra, indicating that the acetate group at C-25 of **2** was replaced by a proton in compound **4**. Thus, on the basis of spectral data and published data [18] compound **4** was defined as cucurbitacin D. Further confirmation of compound **4** was

Table 2 ^{13}C-NMR spectral data for compounds 2, 3, 4 and 5 in CDCl$_3$

C	(2)[a]	(3)[a]	(4)[a]	(5)[b]
1	36.0	35.9	35.9	34.0
2	71.6	71.5	71.6	71.4
3	213.6	212.9	213.1	81.1
4	50.2	50.2	50.2	50.8
5	140.2	140.3	140.3	140.7
6	120.4	120.1	120.2	120.5
7	23.8	23.9	23.8	24.1
8	42.3	42.7	42.3	42.7
9	48.4	48.6	48.3	48.4
10	33.7	33.6	33.7	33.4
11	212.3	211.1	212.3	213.1
12	48.6	49.8	48.6	48.7
13	50.6	48.9	50.7	51.7
14	48.1	44.9	48.2	48.1
15	45.3		45.4	45.4
16	71.2	71.4	71.3	71.1
17	58.1	67.5	57.3	58.2
18	19.8	19.7	19.9	19.9
19	20.0	19.9	20.1	20.4
20	78.2	208.2	78.1	78.4
21	23.9	31.5	23.9	24.7
22	202.5	–	202.6	202.6
23	120.3	–	118.9	119.4
24	151.9	–	155.7	152.0
25	79.3	–	71.1	79.4
26	26.3	–	29.5	26.5
27	25.9	–	29.3	26.1
28	29.3	21.2	28.9	21.7
29	21.2	29.3	21.2	23.8
30	18.8	19.9	19.2	19.1
CH$_3$COO	170.3, 21.9			170.4, 21.6

[a] Measured at 100 MHz. [b] Measured at 150 MHz

achieved by comparison with an authentic sample of cucurbitacin D in our lab.

Compound **3** was isolated as a yellow amorphous powder. It showed a molecular ion peak at m/z 425.23082 [M + Na]$^+$ (calcd. 525.22985) in the HR-ESI-MS spectrum, which corresponded to the molecular formula C$_{24}$H$_{34}$O$_5$. The ^{1}H NMR spectral data of **3** (Table 1) suggested that the chemical shift of rings of A, B, and C were in agreement with those of compound **4**. However, the shifts of the two trans-coupled olefinic protons of the side chain were not detected and only five tertiary methyl group signals were found at δ$_H$ 0.66 (3H, s, H-18), 1.05 (3H, s, H-19), 1.27 (3H, s, H-28), 1.33 (3H,

s, H-29), and 1.37 (3H, s, H-30), in addition to a new tertiary methyl group signal at δ$_H$ 2.16 (3H, methyl ketone). This is somewhat different than the eight tertiary methyl signals in compound **4**. The ^{13}C-NMR data (Table 2) revealed the presence of 24 carbon signals, including six methyl signals at δ$_C$ 19.7, 19.9, 19.9, 21.2, 29.3, 31.5 which were assigned for C-18, C-19, C-30, C-28, C-29, and C-21, respectively; two carbonyls at δ$_C$ 211.1, 212.9 which were assigned for C-11 and C-3, respectively; two olefinic signals at δ$_C$ 120.1, 140.3 which were assigned for C-6 and C-5, respectively, and two oxygenated functions at δ$_C$ 71.4 and 71.5 which were assigned for C-16 and C-2, respectively. This suggests a hexanorcucurbitacin skeleton [19]. As evident from the mass spectra, 114 amu differences were observed between the molecular ion peak of compound **3** (m/z 425) and that of compound **4** (m/z 539), indicating the loss of a side chain by the cleavage between C-20 and C-22 and the formation of a methyl ketone at C-21. On the basis of the above spectral data, along with reported ^{13}C-NMR data in the literature [20] compound **3** was identified as hexanorcucurbitacin D.

Compound **5** was obtained as a white amorphous powder and displayed a molecular ion peak at m/z 583.32388 [M + Na]$^+$ (calcd. 583.32414) in its HR-ESI-MS, corresponding to the formula C$_{32}$H$_{48}$O$_8$. The ^{1}H-NMR spectral data of compound **5** (Table 1) showed nine tertiary methyl group signals at δ$_H$ 0.96 (3H, s, H-18), 1.10 (3H, s, H-30), 1.20 (3H, s, H-29), 1.27 (3H, s, H-28), 1.27 (3H, s, H-19), 1.55 (3H, s, H-21), 1.57 (3H, s, H-26), 1.55 (3H, s, H-27), and 2.02(3H, s, OAc), while resonances at δ$_H$ 2.98 (1H, d, J = 9.0 Hz, H-3), 3.59 (1H, m, H-2), and 4.33 (1H, m, H-16) were assigned to proton signals attached to three oxygenated methine carbons. An olefinic proton at δ$_H$ 5.73 (1H, d, J = 5.49 Hz, H-6) and two trans-coupled olefinic protons on the side chain at δ$_H$ 6.46 (1H, d, J = 15.6 Hz, H-23) and 7.07 (1H, d, J = 15.6 Hz, H-24) were observed in the ^{1}H NMR spectrum. In addition, a pair of coupled doublet protons was recognized at δ$_H$ 2.52 (1H, d, J = 6.81 Hz, H-12β) and 3.18 (1H, d, J = 14.4 Hz, H-12α). The ^{13}C-NMR spectrum of **5** displayed 32 carbon signals, of which 30 carbon signals were attributed to the triterpene skeleton and two carbon signals for an acetate moiety. As evident from the DEPT experiment, the ^{13}C-NMR data (Table 2) showed nine tertiary methyl signals at δ$_C$ 19.1, 19.9, 20.4, 21.7, 23.8, 24.7, 26.1, 26.5, and 21.6 which were assigned for C -30, C-18, C-19, C-28, C-29, C-21, C-27, C-26, and CH$_3$CO, respectively; two carbonyls at δ$_C$ 202.6 and 213.1 which were assigned for C-22 and C-11, respectively; four olefinic signals at δ$_C$ 119.4, 120.5, 140.7 and 152.0 which were assigned for C-23, C-6, C-5, and C-24, respectively; and five oxygenated functions at δ$_C$ 71.1, 71.4, 78.4, 79.3, and 81.1 which were assigned for C-16,C-2,C-20,C-25 and C-3, respectively. The presence of a singlet methyl signal at δ_H 2.02 in the ^{1}H-NMR spectra and two carbon signals at 21.6 and 170.4 in the ^{13}C-NMR spectra indicated the presence of an acetate moiety at C-25. A comparison of the ^{1}H- and ^{13}C-NMR spectroscopic data between 5 and 2 showed similarities, although compound 5 exhibits the absence of a carbonyl signal and the presence of a new oxygenated carbon signal, suggesting the carbonyl in 2 was replaced by a hydroxyl group in 5. This assumption was also supported by the analyses of the two-dimensional NMR spectrum (Table 3).

In the ^{1}H-^{1}H COSY spectrum, the methine proton at δ_H 2.98 (1H, d, J = 9.0 Hz, H-3) correlated with a methine proton at δ_H 3.59 (1H, m, H-2) while the HMQC spectrum showed a correlation between a methine proton at δ_H 2.98 (1H, d, J = 9.0 Hz, H-3) and an oxygenated carbon at δ_C 81.1 (C-3), as well as between a methine proton at δ_H 3.59 (1H, m, H-2) and an oxygenated carbon at δ_C 71.1, (C-2). Further confirmation for the proposed structure was obtained by X-ray single crystal (Fig. 2). Therefore, on the basis of above spectral evidence, the structure of 5 was identified as Cucurbitacin F 25 O-acetate.

Biological evaluation

The potential effects of the n-hexane, ethyl acetate, n-butanol and aqueous extracts and fractions (I and III) from the fruits of *Cucumis prophetarum* var. prophetarum on the proliferation of MCF7, MDA-MB-231,

Table 3 NMR spectroscopic data of compound 5

NO	^{13}C/ppm[a]	1H/ppm[b] multiplicities (J/Hz)	HMBC
1	34.0	s.o., 1.15 d (6.30)	C-2, C-19, C-10, C-3,C-5,C-8,C-9
2	71.4	3.59 m	C-1, C-3,C-4,C-10
3	81.1	2.98 d (9.08)	C-28,C-29,C-1
4	50.8	–	C-28,C-29,C-6
5	140.7	–	C-7,C-1,C-10
6	120.5	5.73 d (5.49)	C-4,C-5,C-7,C-10,C-8
7	24.1	s.o., 2.39 m	C-6,C-8
8	42.7	1.93 br d (7.66)	C-30,C-19,C-7,C-15,C-6,C-10
9	48.4	–	C-19,C-12,C-10,C-8
10	33.4	2.62 br d (14.43)	C-6,C-8,C-19,C-1
11	213.1	–	C-12,C-19
12	48.7	3.18 d (14.49), 2.52 d (6.81)	C-18, C-17, C-11, C-13
13	51.7	–	C-12, C-15, C-17, C-18, C-30
14	48.1	–	C-30, C-18, C-12, C-7, C-16,C-8, C-15
15	45.4	s.o., 1.85 m	C-30, C-8
16	71.1	4.33 m	C-17, C-15
17	58.2	2.48 d (7.03)	C-18, C-21, C-12, C-16
18	19.9	0.96 s	C-12, C-13, C-14, C-17
19	20.4	1.27 s	C-10, C-8
20	78.4	–	C-21, C-16, C-17
21	24.7	1.55 s	–
22	202.6	–	C-24, C-23
23	119.4	6.46 d (15.6)	C-24
24	152.0	7.07 d (15.6)	C-27, C-26, C-23
25	79.4	–	C27, C26, C23
26	26.5	1.57 s	C-27, C-24
27	26.1	1.55 s	C-26
28	21.7	1.27 s	C-29
29	23.8	1.20 s	C-28
30	19.1	1.10 s	C-15, C-21, C-8

[a]Measured at 150 MHz, [b] Measured at 400 MHz

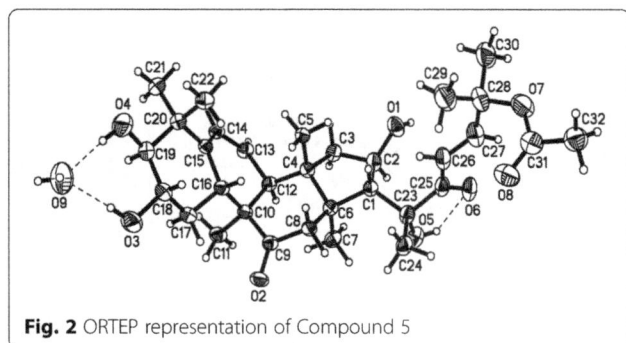

Fig. 2 ORTEP representation of Compound 5

HCT-116, A2780, A2780CP, and HepG2 were investigated using the MTT assay for 48 h. Cell viability was measured in the concentration range of 0 µg/mL to 1000 µg/mL for each fraction (Fig. 3) and 0 µM to 100 µM for each pure compound (Fig. 4). As shown in (Table 4) the ethyl acetate fraction exhibits potential cytotoxic effects on the MCF-7, MDA MB-231, A2780, A2780 CP, and HCT-116 cell lines with IC_{50} 17.5, 0.35, 2.82, 19.2, and 14.2 µg/mL, respectively, while the

n-hexane fraction was found to be active against the MCF-7, MDA MB-231, and A2780 cell lines with IC_{50} 19.7, 0.76, and 7.15 µg/mL, respectively. The n-butanol fractions demonstrated very weak cytotoxic activity against all cell lines, with IC_{50} values ranging from 43 to 358 µg /mL, whereas the water fraction showed no cytotoxic activity against any of the tested cell lines (> 1000 µg /mL). In addition, the ethyl acetate fraction showed a concentration-dependent inhibitory effect in the MCF-7, MDA MB-231, A2780, A2780 CP, and HCT-116 cell lines at ≥ 8 µg /mL, as did the n-hexane fraction suggesting that the ethyl acetate fraction possesses the highest cytotoxicity and led us to carry out a study to determine the active constituents that may be potential anticancer compounds.

Discussion

Bioassay guided fractionation of the methanolic extract of fruits of *Cucumis prophetarum* var. prophetarum led to the identification of ethyl acetate fraction as the most active fraction. The subsequent chromatographic

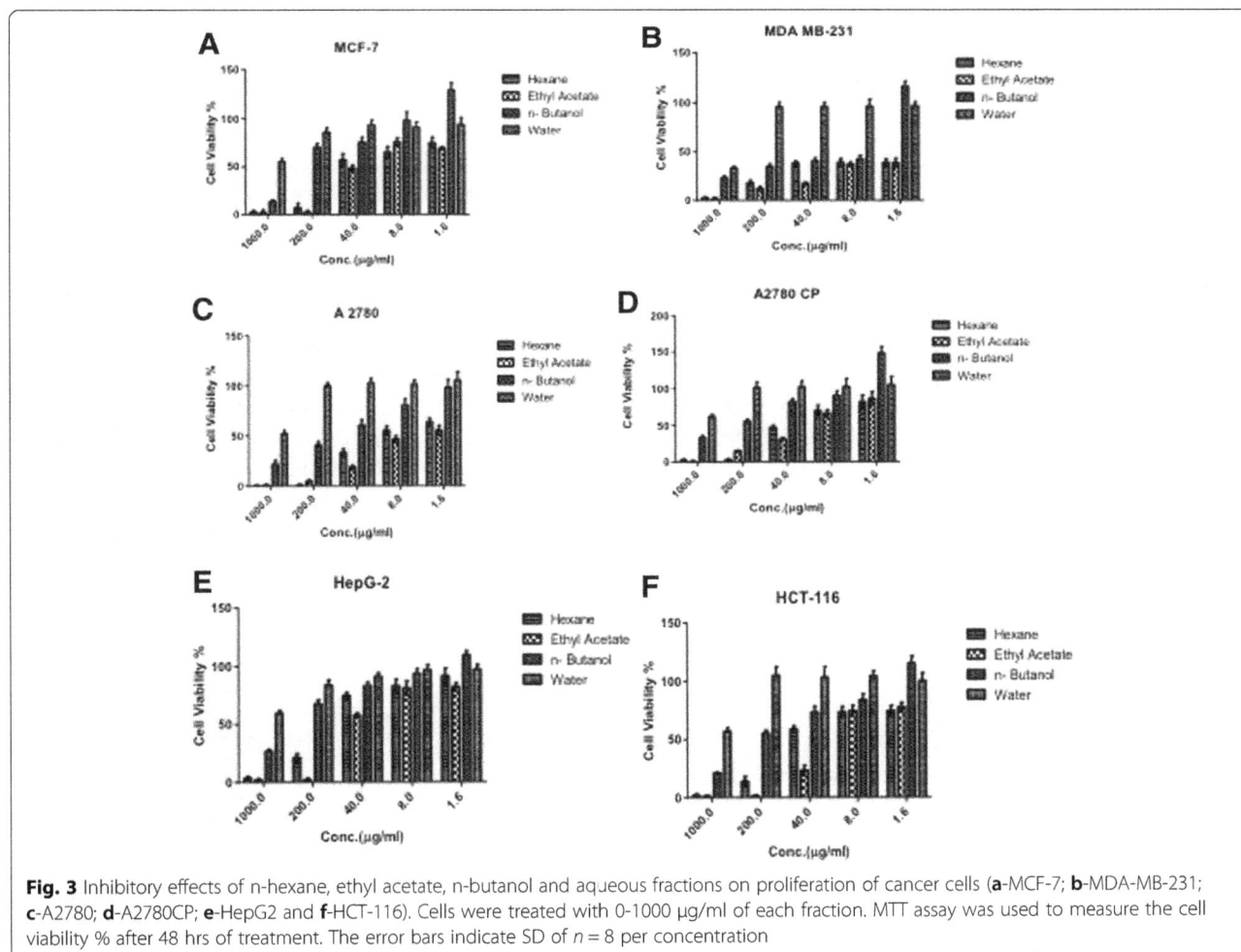

Fig. 3 Inhibitory effects of n-hexane, ethyl acetate, n-butanol and aqueous fractions on proliferation of cancer cells (**a**-MCF-7; **b**-MDA-MB-231; **c**-A2780; **d**-A2780CP; **e**-HepG2 and **f**-HCT-116). Cells were treated with 0-1000 µg/ml of each fraction. MTT assay was used to measure the cell viability % after 48 hrs of treatment. The error bars indicate SD of *n* = 8 per concentration

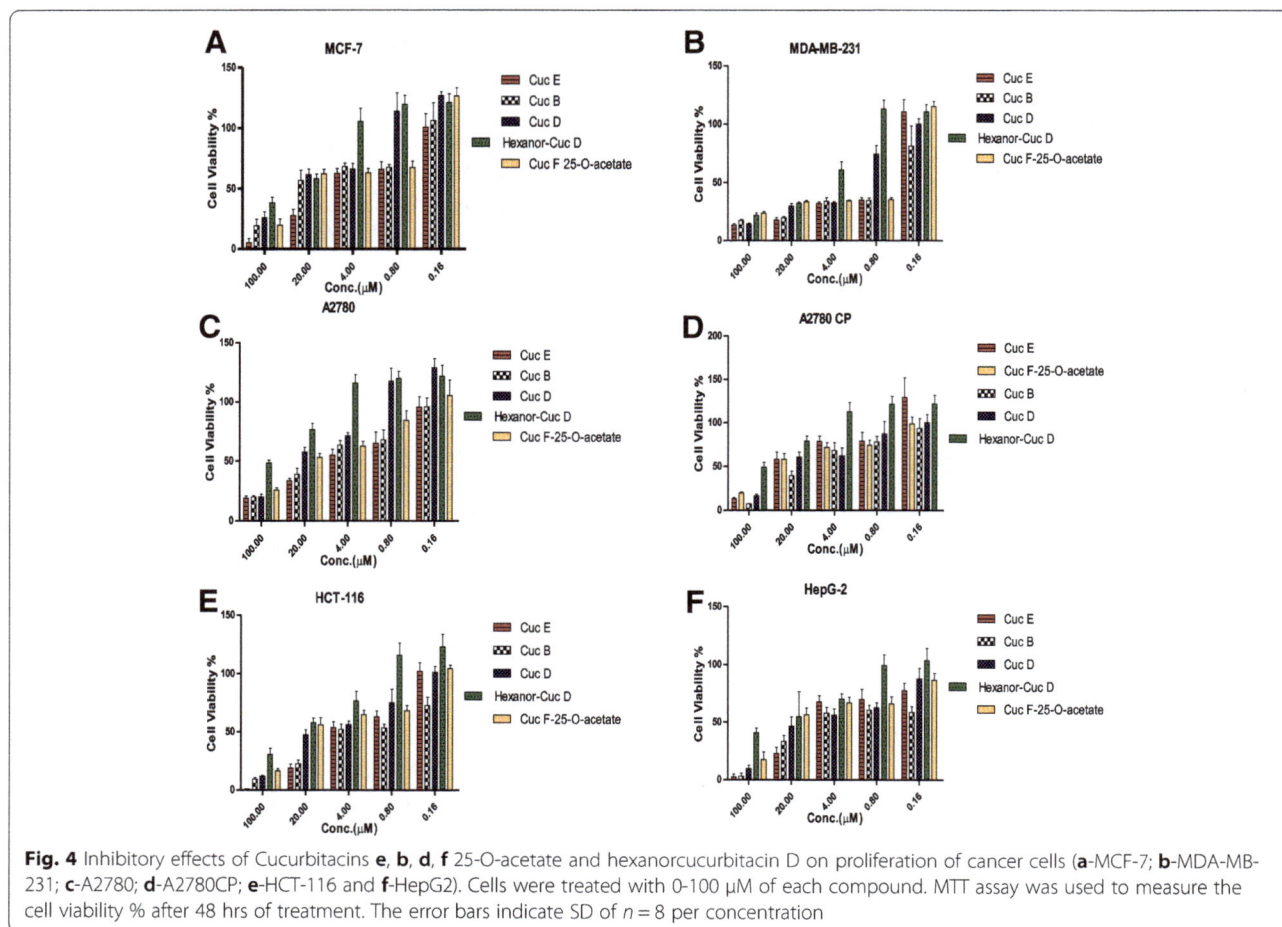

Fig. 4 Inhibitory effects of Cucurbitacins e, b, d, f 25-O-acetate and hexanorcucurbitacin D on proliferation of cancer cells (**a**-MCF-7; **b**-MDA-MB-231; **c**-A2780; **d**-A2780CP; **e**-HCT-116 and **f**-HepG2). Cells were treated with 0-100 μM of each compound. MTT assay was used to measure the cell viability % after 48 hrs of treatment. The error bars indicate SD of $n = 8$ per concentration

purification of the ethyl acetate fraction resulted in the isolation of five Cucurbitacin compounds. The compounds were characterized based on NMR and mass spectral data.

The ethyl acetate fraction was subjected to column chromatography on silica gel to give three main fractions (I, II, and III). Fraction II afforded pure cucurbitacin B (2) (Fig. 1). Both fractions I and III demonstrated very active cytotoxicity profiles against all cell lines in a concentration-dependent manner, with the IC_{50} value range from 0.15 to 5.9 μg/mL for fraction I and 0.12 to 20.5 μg/mL for fraction III (Table 3). The bioassay guided purification of fractions I and III resulted in the isolation and identification of four cucurbitane-type triterpenes, cucurbitacin E (1), hexanorcucurbitacin D (3), cucurbitacin D (4), and cucurbitacin F 25-O-acetate (5) (Fig. 1). Previously, several cucurbitacin compounds were reported to inhibit the growth of several types of cancers in time-dependent and dose-dependent manners [21]. Cucurbitacin B exhibited inhibitory effects on the

Table 4 Cytotoxic effects of the tested fractions

Fractions	IC_{50} [a] (μg/mL)					
	MCF-7	MDA MB 231	A2780	A2780 CP	HepG2	HCT-116
Hexane fraction	19.7	0.76	7.15	20.27	55.4	25
Ethyl acetate fraction	17.5	0.35	2.82	19.2	28.5	14.2
n-Butanol fraction	218.4	43	94.01	273	358.5	169.5
Water fraction	>1000	>1000	>1000	>1000	>1000	>1000
Fraction I	3.5	0.15	4.9	5.9	0.27	0.15
Fraction III	6.80	0.12	20.5	17.5	0.52	0.65

Inhibitory effects of the fractions from the extract of *Cucumis prophetarum* var. prophetarum fruits on the proliferation of MCF7, MDA-MB-231, HCT-116, A2780, A2780CP, and HepG2. Cell were treated with 0–1000 μg/ml. [a] IC_{50}: is the concentration that inhibited cell proliferation by 50%. $n = 8$

proliferation of breast cancer cell lines MDA-MB-231, ZR-75-1, BT474 [22], MDA-MB-453, T47D [22, 23] and MCF-7 [23]; the hepatic carcinoma cell lines BEL-7402 [24] and HepG2 [25]; and the colon cancer cell lines SW480 [26] and HCT-116 [27]. In the same manner, cucurbitacin D and E have shown significant cytotoxicity on the colon cancer cell line HCT-116 [27] and the breast cancer cell line MCF-7 [27, 28]. To the best of our knowledge, cucurbitacin compounds have not been investigated against the human ovarian cancer cell lines A2780 and A2780CP. In addition, this is the first report of screening hexanorcucurbitacin D and cucurbitacin F 25-O-acetate against the six human cancer cell lines used in this study.

Here, we report the inhibitory effects of five cucurbitacin compounds (cucurbitacin E, B, D, F 25-O-acetate, and hexanorcucurbitacin D) obtained from the ethyl acetate fraction on the proliferation of six human cancer cell lines for 48 h. Compounds were re-evaluated against the same cell lines in order to establish a structure activity relationship (SAR) as we describe in the manuscript. Another reason was to ensure that the cytotoxicity activity was consistent with the literature data.

Cell viability was measured in the concentration range of 0 µM to 100 µM for each pure compound. All compounds exhibited antiproliferative activities to the cells in a concentration-dependent manner (Table 5, Fig. 4). Among the cucurbitacins that we tested, cucurbitacin B and E showed potent cytotoxicity activities against all six human cancer cell lines at different concentrations, with the IC_{50} value ranging from 0.96 to 16 µM for cucurbitacin B and from 2.1 to 15.9 µM for cucurbitacin E. Meanwhile, cucurbitacin D and Q demonstrated less cytotoxic activity on all six human tumor cell lines than cucurbitacin B and E, with the IC_{50} ranging from 3.4 to 18.4 µM for cucurbitacin F 25-O-acetate and 4 to 26.7 µM for cucurbitacin D. Hexanorcucurbtacin D was the least active of the five cucurbitacins examined, with an IC_{50} ranging from 12.0 to > 100 µM. Interestingly, all cucurbitacin compounds exhibited significant cytotoxic

activity against the estrogen-receptor negative human breast cancer cell line (MDA MB-231) compared to the estrogen-receptor. Positive human breast cancer cell line (MCF-7). This significant difference in the biological activities may be related to the status of the estrogen receptor in both cell lines [14]. This was confirmed by using an estrogen- receptor (ER) competitive-binding assay to determine the affinity of cucurbitacin compounds to an estrogen-receptor (alpha and beta). The results confirmed that cucurbitacin compounds possessed very weak affinity toward estrogen receptors and this may explain the significant growth inhibitory effect associated with treatment MDA MB-231.

Furthermore, the inhibitory effects of the five cucurbitacin compounds were quite consistent with the trend observed for the activity of fractions I and III, where fraction I demonstrated a more potent cytotoxic activity (IC_{50} value range from 0.15 to 5.9 µg/mL) than fraction III (IC_{50} value range from 0.12 to 20.5 µg/mL). The strong activity of fraction I is probably related to the presence of cucurbitacins B and E, the most active compounds in this study, suggesting that the activity of the two cucurbitacins are synergistic.

In order to establish structure-activity relationships for cytotoxicity against the human breast cancer cell line MDA MB-231, additional cucurbitacin compounds [dihydrocucurbitacin D (6), isocucurbitacin D (7), cucurbitacin E glucoside (8)] were isolated in our laboratory [11] and screened against MDA MB-231 [29].

Our results indicate that the most important structural features for cytotoxicity which are listed below:

(i) The presence of a side chain attached to the four-ringed core structure in the cucurbitacin skeleton. Cucurbitacins B and D, which contain the side chain, exhibited significantly more potent cytotoxic activity (2, 4 IC_{50} = 0.96, 4 µM, respectively) than hexanorcucurbitacin D, without the side chain (3, IC_{50} = 12). This clearly indicated the importance of

Table 5 Cytotoxic effects of tested compounds

Isolated compounds	IC$_{50}$ (µM)					
	MCF-7	MDA MB 231	A2780	A2780 CP	HepG2	HCT-116
Cucurbitacin E (1)	7.2	2.1	5.4	15.9	3.4	3.4
Cucurbitacin B (2)	16.0	0.96	7.6	14.2	1.7	1.7
Hexanor-Cucurbitacin D (3)	47.9	12.0	> 100	> 100	37.8	30.7
Cucurbitacin D (4)	26.7	4.0	21.6	6.9	5.0	7.6
Cucurbitacin F 25-O-acetate (5)	18.4	3.4	15.8	15.2	10.2	11.2
Dihydrocucurbitacin D (6)	–	> 100	–	–	–	–
Isocucurbitacin D (7)	–	1.0	–	–	–	–
Cucurbitacin E glucoside (8)	–	27.3	–	–	–	–

Inhibitory effects of compounds from the ethyl acetate extract fraction of *Cucumis prophetarum* var. prophetarum fruits on the proliferation of MCF7, MDA-MB-231, HCT-116, A2780, A2780CP, and HepG2. Cell were treated with 0–100 µM. [a] IC_{50} is the concentration that inhibited cell proliferation by 50%. $n = 8$

the side chain since the hydroxyl group at C-16 forms a hydrogen bond with carbonyl group at C-22 on the side chain, leading to the activation of α, β unsaturated ketone [13].

(ii) The presence of an α, β unsaturated ketone in the side chain. Thus, cucurbitacin D, in particular, showed potent cytotoxic activity (4, IC_{50} = 4 μM), while dihydrocucurbitacin D (without an α, β unsaturated ketone in its side chain) showed no activity (6, IC_{50} > 100). This is understandable because α, β unsaturated ketone play important role in nucleophlic attack and consequently alkylation of thiol groups [13].

(iii) The presence of an acetoxyl group at C-25 in the side chain. Cucurbitacin B, which contains this feature, displayed very strong cytotoxic activity (2, IC_{50} = 0.96 μM) compared with cucurbitacin D, which has no an acetoxyl group at C-25 in the side chain (4, IC_{50} = 4 μM). Lipophilicity plays a significant role in transport, absorption and distribution of chemicals in biological systems. Since the presence of acetate group increases lipophilicity, acetylation of C-25 hydroxyl may explain the increase in the cytotoxicity of cucurbitacin B [30].

(iv) The presence of a keto and hydroxyl group on ring A. Thus, cucurbitacin B displayed high activity (2 IC_{50} = 0.96 μM) compared to cucurbitacin F 25-O-acetate, with two hydroxyl groups on ring A (5, IC_{50} = 3.4 μM).

(v) The position of a keto and hydroxyl group on ring A. Isocucurbitacin D, with the keto group at C-2 and the hydroxyl at C-3, demonstrates better activity (7, IC_{50} = 1 μM) than cucurbitacin D, with the keto group at C-3 and the hydroxyl at C-2, (4, IC_{50} = 4 μM).

(vi) The presence of a 2-glucosyl substituent. The cucurbitacin E glycoside (8) has a C-2 glucoside moiety and showed lower activity (4, IC_{50} = 27.3 μM) than cucurbitacin E (1, IC_{50} = 2.1 μM). This is understandable, since the presence of the glucose moiety increased the polarity and the volume of structure, consequently reduces the lipophilicity and transportation through the lipid bilayer of the cell membrane [30, 31]

Conclusion

Cucumis prophetarum var. prophetarum (Cucurbitaceae), called Shari-al-deeb in Arabic, is used in Saudi folk medicine for the treatment of liver disorders. The chemical constituents were defined to determine potential toxicity, mutagenicity, and carcinogenicity. In the present study, bioassay-guided fractionation and purification were used to isolate the cytotoxic compounds of an extract of *Cucumis prophetarum* var. prophetarum

frutis. All fractions, sub-fractions, and pure compounds were screened for their cytotoxic activity against six human cancer cell lines. The greatest cytotoxic activity was found to be in the ethyl acetate fraction, resulting in the isolation of five cucurbitacin compounds identified as cucurbitacin E (1), cucurbitacin B (2), hexanorcucurbitacin D (3), cucurbitacin D (4), and cucurbitacin F 25-O-acetate (5). Among the cucurbitacins that were isolated and tested, cucurbitacin B and E showed potent cytotoxicity activities against all six human cancer cell lines at different concentrations. Interestingly, the estrogen-receptor negative human breast cancer cell line (MDA MB-231) was the most sensitive to cucurbitacins B, D, and E, compared to other cell lines. This finding may help us to identify new anticancer compounds against estrogen receptor negative breast cancer.

Abbreviations

^{13}C-NMR: Carbon- Nuclear Magnetic Resonance; ^{1}H-NMR: Proton-Nuclear magnetic resonance; 2D-NMR: Two dimensional- Nuclear Magnetic Resonance; CAM: Ceric Ammonium Molybdate; $CDCl_3$: Dueterated chloroform; COSY: Homonuclear correlation spectroscopy; DMEM: Dulbecco's modified eagle medium; DMSO: Dimethyl sulfoxide; ELISA: Enzyme linked immunosorbent assay; EtOAC: Ethyl acetate; FBS: Fetal bovine serum; HCl: Hydrochloric acid; HMQC: Heteronuclear Multiple-Quantum Correlation; HR-ESIMS: High resolution electron spray ionization mass spectrometry; IC_{50}: Half maximal inhibitory concentration; mM: Milli molar; MTT: 3-(4,5-Dimethyl-2-thiazolyl)-2,5-diphenyl-2H-tetrazolium bromide; PBS: Phosphate buffered saline; RPMI: Rosewell Park Memorial Institute; SDS: Sodium dodecyl sulfate; TLC: Thin layer chromatography; TMS: Tetramethyl silane; var.: Variety; μg: Microgram; μL: Microliter; μM: Micromolar

Acknowledgments

The authors would like to express their gratitude to King Khalid University, Saudi Arabia for providing administrative and technical support.

Authors' contributions

AA, MSA and FTH were involved in the extraction, isolation of compounds, performed the assays and analyzed the data. LK was involved in the spectroscopic characterization. HSMS authenticated the plant material. SA formatted and edited the manuscript. All authors have read and approved the manuscript.

Competing interests

The authors declare that they have no competing interests.

Author details

[1]Department of Pharmacognosy, College of Pharmacy, King Khalid University, Abha, Saudi Arabia. [2]Kalexsyn, 4502 Campus Drive, Kalamazoo, MI 49008, USA. [3]Department of Pharmaceutical Chemistry, Faculty of Pharmacy, The British University in Egypt, Al-Sherouk City, Cairo, Egypt. [4]Department of Pharmacognosy, Helwan University, Cairo, Egypt. [5]Department of Chemistry and Biochemistry, South Dakota State University, Brookings, SD 57007, USA.

References

1. Harvey AL, Edrada-Ebel R, Quinn RJ. The re-emergence of natural products for drug discovery in the genomics era. Nat Rev Drug Disccv. 2015;14:111–29.

2. Veeresham C. Natural products derived from plants as a source of drugs. J Adv Pharm Technol Res. 2012;3(4):200–1.

3. Rahman MA, et al. Medicinal plant diversity in the flora of Saudi Arabia 1: a report on seven plant families. Fitoterapia. 2004;75(2):149–61.

4. Khan SA, et al. Colocynth toxicity. A possible cause of bloody diarrhea. Saudi Med J. 2003;24(8):904–6.

5. Khalil M, et al. The Effect of *Citrullus colocynthis* Pulp Extract on the Liver of Diabetic Rats a Light and Scanning Electron Microscopic Study. Am J. Biochem Biotechnol. 2010;6(3):155.

6. Youssef S. Medicinal and non-medicinal uses of some plants found in the middle region of Saudi Arabia. J Med Plants Res. 2013;7(34):2501–17.

7. Chung SO, Kim YJ, Park SU. An updated review of cucurbitacins and their biological and Pharmacological activities. EXCLI J. 2015;14:562–6.

8. Cai Y, Fang X, He C, Li P, Xiao F, Wang Y, Chen M. Cucurbitacins: A systematic review of the phytochemistry and anticancer activity. Am J Chin Med. 2015;43:1331.

9. Ayyad SN, Abdel-lateff A, Basaif SA, Shier T. Cucurbitacins-type triterpene with potent activity on mouse embryonic fibroblast from *Cucumis prophetarum*, cucurbitaceae. Pharmacognosy Res. 2011;3(3):189–93.

10. Gawli K, Lakshmidevi N. Antidiabetic and antioxidant potency evaluation of different fractions obtained from *Cucumis prophetarum* fruit. Pharm Biol. 2015;53(5):689–94.

11. Abdulrhman Saleh Alsayari Doctoral thesis, Anticancer and Antiviral activities of Cucurbotacins isolated from *Cucumis prophetarum* var. prophetarum growing in the southwestern region of Saudi Arabia (2014)

12. Alghasham AA. Cucurbitacins-a promising target for cancer therapy. Int J Health Sci. 2013;7(1):77–89.

13. Zhang M, et al. Targeted constitutive activation of signal transducer and activator of transcription 3 in human hepatocellular carcinoma cells by cucurbitacin B. Cancer Chemother Pharmacol. 2009;63(4):635–42.

14. Alongkornsopit J, et al. Anticancer activity of ethyl acetate and n-butanol extracts from rhizomes of Agapetes megacarpa WW Smith. Afr J Biotechnol. 2013;10(17):3455–62.

15. Wiart C. Lead compounds from medicinal plants for the treatment of cancer: Academic Press; 2013; p 97-265.

16. Afifi MS, Ross SA, Elsohly MA, Naeem ZE, Halaweish FT. Cucurbitacins of Cucumis prophetarum and *Cucumis prophetarum*. J Chem Ecol. 1999; 25(40):847–59.

17. Velde VV, Lavie D. 13C NMR spectroscopy of cucurbitacins. Tetrahedron. 1983;39(2):317–21.

18. Fang X, et al. Plant anticancer agents, XXXIV. Cucurbitacins from Elaeocarpus dolichostylus. J Nat Prod. 1984;47(6):988–93.

19. Seger C, et al. 1H and 13C NMR signal assignment of cucurbitacin derivatives from *Citrullus colocynthis* (L.) Schrader and *Ecballium elaterium* L. (Cucurbitaceae). Magn Reson Chem. 2005;43(6):489–91.

20. Seger C, et al. NMR Signal assignment of 22-Deoxocucurbitacin D and Cucurbitacin D from *Ecballium elaterium* L.(Cucurbitaceae). Monatsh.Chem. 2005;136(9):1645–9.

21. Fujita S, et al. Dammarane glycosides from aerial parts of Neoalsomitra integrifoliola. Phytochemistry. 1995;38(2):465–72.

22. Suffness M, Pezzuto JM. Assays related to cancer drug discovery. Methods in Plant Biochemistry: Assays for bioactivity. 1990;6:71–133.

23. Chen X, et al. Biological activities and potential molecular targets of cucurbitacins: a focus on cancer. Anti-Cancer Drugs. 2012;23(8):777–87.

24. Wakimoto N, et al. Cucurbitacin B has a potent antiproliferative effect on breast cancer cells in vitro and in vivo. Cancer Sci. 2008;99(9): 1793–7.

25. Kongtun S, Jiratchariyakul W, Kummalue T, Tan-ariya P, Kunnachak S, Frahm AW. Cytotoxic properties of root extract and fruit juice of *Trichosanthes cucumerina*. Planta Med. 2009;75(8):839–42.

26. Chan KT, et al. Cucurbitacin B induces apoptosis and S phase cell cycle arrest in BEL-7402 human hepatocellular carcinoma cells and is effective via oral administration. Cancer Lett. 2010;294(1):118–24.

27. Yasuda S, et al. Cucurbitacin B induces G2 arrest and apoptosis via a reactive oxygen species-dependent mechanism in human colon adenocarcinoma SW480 cells. Mol Nutr Food Res. 2010;54(4):559–65.

28. Jayaprakasam B, Seeram NP, Nair MG. Anticancer and antiinflammatory activities of cucurbitacins from *Cucurbita andreana*. Cancer Lett. 2003; 189(1):11–6.

29. Bartalis J, Halaweish FT. In vitro and QSAR studies of cucurbitacins on HepG2 and HSC-T6 liver cell lines. Bioorg Med Chem. 2011;19(8):2757–66.

30. Bartalis J, Halaweish FT. Relationship between cucurbitacins reversed-phase high-performance liquid chromatography hydrophobicity index and basal cytotoxicity on HepG2 cells. J Chromatogr B. 2005;818(2):159–66.

31. Sahranavard S, Naghibi F, Ghaffari S. Cytotoxic activity of extracts and pure compounds of Bryonia aspera. Int J Pharm Pharm Sci. 2012;4(3):541–3.

9

Regulatory effect of Phikud Navakot extract on *HMG-CoA reductase* and *LDL-R*: potential and alternate agents for lowering blood cholesterol

Napatara Tirawanchai[1], Sudarat Supapornhemin[1], Anchaleekorn Somkasetrin[1], Bhoom Suktitipat[1] and Sumate Ampawong[2]* (iD)

Abstract

Background: For decades, various cardiovascular symptoms have been relieved by the use of Ya-Hom Navakot, which is a formulation comprising 54 herbal medicines. The Thailand Ministry of Public Health listed Ya-Hom Navakot's nine active principle and nomenclative herbal ingredients and termed them 'Phikud Navakot' (PN). Several reports have confirmed that PN has cardiovascular benefits similar to Ya-Hom Navakot. However, whether PN facilitates lipid-lowering activity remains unclear.

Methods: The present study investigated an in vitro model for examining the gene expression levels of 3-hydroxyl-3-methylglutaryl-CoA reductase (*HMGCR*) and low-density lipoprotein receptor (*LDL-R*) in HepG2 cells using qRT-PCR. The ethanol and water extractions of Ya-Hom Navakot, PN and Ya-Hom Navakot without PN were compared.

Results: One mg/ml of both NYEF and NYWF were found to significantly lower cholesterol by either the up-regulation of *LDL-R* or down-regulation of *HMGCR* compared with negative controls and 1 mg/ml simvastatin ($p < 0.05$). PNEF also up-regulated *LDL-R* gene expression, even more than NYEF ($p < 0.05$). In addition, the ethanol and water extracts of PN significantly down-regulated *HMGCR* gene expression compared with those of Ya-Hom Navakot without PN ($p < 0.05$).

Conclusion: The use of Ya-Hom Navakot or PN may provide an alternative treatment to lower cholesterol through *HMGCR* gene inhibition and *LDL-R* gene enhancement.

Keywords: Cholesterol, HMG-CoA reductase, Low-density lipoprotein receptor, Phikud Navakot, Ya-Hom Navakot

Background

In Thailand, traditional medicines are used in primary healthcare for treating illnesses and diseases because of their effectiveness and minimal side effects. Thai traditional medicines and Thai herbal formulae are promoted by the Thailand Ministry of Public Health for use as alternative medicine in the treatment of health problems. Thai herbal medicines are recorded in the List of Herbal Medicinal Products (LHMP) A.D. 2012, which contains numerous polyherbal formulations. All polyherbal formulations are considered to provide maximal therapeutic efficacy with less toxicity [1].

Ya-Hom Navakot is a well-known Thai polyherbal formulation that originated as a product of Thai wisdom. It comprises 54 herbal medicines and is frequently used in primary healthcare and Thai traditional household. Ya-Hom Navakot improves blood circulation and reduces dizziness, nausea and vomiting [2]. However, when the Ministry of Public Health included Ya-Hom Navakot in LHMP A.D. 2012, the 54 herbal medicines were reduced to nine principle herbal ingredients and termed as 'Phikud Navakot' (PN), while the rest were excluded. All the nine herbs are mixed in equal proportions and include the following: Kot Soa (*Angelica dahurica*), Kot Chiang (*A. sinensis*), Kot Kradook (*Saussurea costus*), Kot Khamao

* Correspondence: am_sumate@hotmail.com
[2]Department of Tropical Pathology, Faculty of Tropical Medicine, Mahidol University, 420/6 Ratchawithi Road, Ratchathewi, Bangkok 10400, Thailand
Full list of author information is available at the end of the article

(*Atractylodes lancea*), Kot Huabua (*Ligusticum chuanxiong*), Kot Kanprao (*Picrorhiza kurrooa*), Kot Jatamansi (*Nardostachys jatamansi*), Kot Chulalumpa (*Artemisia pallens*) and Kot Pungpla (*Terminalia chebula*).

Even without the 45 excluded herbal plants of Ya-Hom Navakot, it is still claimed that PN improves the functioning of the cardiovascular system. Moreover, PN is reported to be effective in improving blood circulation [3]. The hydro-ethanolic extract of PN significantly attenuates carbachol-induced vasorelaxation in endothelium-intact rat aorta, partly through its antagonistic effect on the muscarinic receptor [2]. Moreover, the hydro-ethanolic extract of PN possesses antioxidant properties; it finds reactive oxygen species (ROS) and reactive nitrogen species (RNS) in human endothelial ECV304 cells more effectively than the water-extract of PN [4]. The antioxidant properties of PN also preserve the integrity and osmotic ability of red blood cells throughout the induced oxidative stress [5]. Furthermore, it is considered safe because no treatment-related mortality events have been observed among acute and sub-chronic toxicity studies in PN-fed rats [6].

Based on the documented effects of PN, it is also possible that Ya-Hom Navakot has a lipid-lowering activity. In the present study, the expression of the genes encoding 3-hydroxyl-3-methylglutaryl-CoA reductase (*HMGCR*) and low-density lipoprotein receptor (*LDL-R*), both of which are crucial enhancing factors for cholesterol biosynthesis, were examined in HepG2 cell lines for demonstrating the hypocholesterolaemic activities of PN and Ya-Hom Navakot. In vitro cultures and quantitative reverse transcription-polymerase chain reaction (qRT-PCR) were used. The results provide a better understanding of the effect of PN on blood lipid homeostasis and propose it as a candidate for anti-lipidaemic therapy or adjunct treatment for patients with hypercholesterolaemia.

Methods
Reagents
Dulbecco's modified Eagle's medium (DMEM), minimal essential medium (MEM), foetal bovine serum (FBS), penicillin–streptomycin, glutamine, non-essential amino acids and sodium pyruvate were purchased from GIBCO Laboratories (Grand Island, NY, USA). Dimethyl sulfoxide (DMSO) was obtained from Prolabo (Paris, France). Simvastatin (Zocor®) was obtained from Berlin Pharmaceutical Co. Ltd. (Bangkok, Thailand). GENEzol™ reagents, which were used for RNA extraction, were obtained from Geneaid (New Taipei, Taiwan). Reagents for first-strand cDNA synthesis were available at Thermo Fischer Scientific (Waltham, MA, USA). FastStart Essential DNA Green Master Kit, which was used in qRT-PCR, was obtained from Roche (Mannheim, Germany). MTT [3-(4, 5 di-methylthiazol-2-yl)-2, 5-diphenyltetrazolium bromide] was purchased from

Sigma-Aldrich (St. Louis, MO, USA). All other chemical reagents were of analytical grade and highest quality.

Plant materials and preparation of PN extracts
The roots of *A. dahurica* (Fisch.) Benth, et Hook. f. (Apiaceae), *A. sinensis* (Oliv.) Diels (Apiaceae) and *S. costus* (Falc.) Lipsch. (Asteraceae), rhizomes of *A. lancea* (Thunb.) DC. (Asteraceae), *L. chuanxiong* Hort. (Apiaceae) and *P. kurrooa* Royle ex Benth. (Scrophulariaceae), roots and rhizomes of *N. jatamansi* (D. Don) DC. (Valerianaceae), aerial parts of *A. pallens* Walls ex DC. (Asteraceae) and galls of *T. chebula* Retz. (Combretaceae) were purchased in October 2009 from traditional drugstores in Bangkok, Thailand. Dr. Sanya Hokputsa, who is affiliated with the Research and Development Institute, Government Pharmaceutical Organisation, examined all the specimens. Voucher specimens (NVK10–52) have been deposited at the Phytochemical Research Group, Research and Development Institute, Government Pharmaceutical Organisation, Thailand. All herbal materials were examined according to the quality control parameters of Thai Herbal Pharmacopoeia and compared with authentic specimens, which were generously provided by Associate Professor Dr. Noppamas Soonthornchareonnon, Faculty of Pharmacy, Mahidol University, Thailand.

PN extracts were prepared as previously described by Nalintara [4] using ethanol reflux as demonstrated in the previous report [7]. Briefly, each dried plant material was powdered and equally mixed before sieving through a No. 40 mesh. The powdered herbs (1 kg each) were extracted with 2×5 L of either 50% ethanol or water (PNEF and PNWF, respectively) under reflux for 3 h. Extracts were then spray-dried or freeze-dried. Stock solutions of the extracted PN were prepared by dissolving 1 g of the extract in 5 ml of 100% DMSO to a final concentration of 200 mg/ml. Aliquots of the stock solutions were prepared and stored at $-20\ °C$ until use.

Ethanolic and water extracts of Ya-Hom Navakot polyherbal formulation
In October 2009, all the 54 herbs included in the Ya-Hom Navakot polyherbal formulation were purchased from traditional drugstores in Bangkok, Thailand, examined by Dr. Sanya Hokputsa, dried and mixed. The herbal mixtures were extracted using 50% ethanol or water (NYEF and NYWF, respectively) as previously described. For control, plant materials excluding PN were prepared and extracted using 50% ethanol (NBEF) or water (NBWF).

In vitro culture of HepG2 cells
HepG2 cell lines purchased from American Type Culture Collection (ATCC, HB 8065) were cultured in DMEM containing MEM supplemented with 10% FBS,

penicillin (100 units/ml), streptomycin (100 µg/ml), 2.0 mM glutamine, 0.1 mM non-essential amino acids and 1.0 mM sodium pyruvate. The cells were cultured at 37 °C under 5% CO_2 and 98% relative humidity until they reached 80% confluence.

MTT assay

The viability of HepG2 cells was assessed using the MTT assay [8, 9]. Briefly, HepG2 cells were plated at a density of 1×10^4 cells/well in 100-µl DMEM complete medium in a 96-multiwell plate and cultured at 37 °C under 5% CO_2 and 98% relative humidity for 24 h. DMEM complete medium was aspirated before treatment with a test medium containing the DMEM complete medium and standard concentrations (0.01, 0.05, 0.1, 0.5 and 1 mg/ml) of PNEF, PNWF, NYEF, NYWF, NBEF, or NBWF for 24 h. The experimental medium was aspirated, and MTT solution was added to each well at a concentration of 0.25 mg/ml before incubation for another 2 h at 37 °C. After the addition of 100-µl DMSO/well, the absorbance of purple formazan at 570 nm was determined. Simvastatin was used as the positive control. Cytotoxicity for all herbal extracts and their respective concentrations was calculated using the percentage of living cells in relation to the percentage of cells treated with only 0.5% DMSO (negative control).- Cytotoxicity of all herbal extracts was calculated as the percentage of cell viability using the following equation:

$$\%\text{cell viability} = \frac{(OD_{570}\text{of the test condition} - OD_{570} \text{ of the blank}) \times 100}{(OD_{570} \text{ of the standard control} - OD_{570} \text{ of the blank})}$$

RNA preparation and qRT-PCR

For assessing the effect of PNEF, PNWF, NYEF, NYWF, NBEF and NBWF on the expressions of *HMGCR* and *LDL-R*, HepG2 cells were seeded at 1×10^6 cells/ml and cultured in DMEM complete medium for 24 h before treatment with 1 mg/ml of herbal extracts. The cells were also treated with 0.5% DMSO and 1 mg/ml of simvastatin as negative and positive controls, respectively. After 24 h of treatment, total RNA was extracted using GENEzol™ reagents following the manufacturer's protocol. The concentration of the extracted RNA was measured using a spectrophotometer (NanoPhotometer™, Implen GmBH, Munich, Germany). One microgram of total RNA was subjected to reverse transcription to obtain cDNA using the RevertAid First-Strand cDNA Synthesis Kit (Thermo Fischer Scientific) according to the manufacturer's instructions. qRT-PCR was performed using the FastStart Essential DNA Green Master Kit (Roche, Mannheim, Germany) according to the manufacturer's instructions. qRT-PCR included a heat

inactivation step at 95 °C for 10 min, followed by 40 cycles of denaturation at 95 °C for 30 s, annealing at 60 °C for 45 s and extension at 72 °C for 1 min using a Stratagene quantitative PCR Mx3005 (Stratagen, USA). Oligonucleotide primers designed using OLIGO 7 primer analysis software were ordered from Sigma-Aldrich (Singapore). For the amplification of *HMGCR*, forward and reverse primers used were 5′-TACCATGTCAGGG GTACGTC-3′ and 5′-CAAGCCTAGAGACATAAT-3′, respectively (amplicon size = 247 bp). In addition, forward and reverse primers for amplifying *LDL-R* were 5′-TGCAGTGGGCGACAGATGCG-3′ and 5′-GGTT GACACGGCCCCCACAG-3′, respectively (amplicon size = 179 bp). The expression of each specific gene was normalised to that of the housekeeping gene GAPDH using the forward and reverse primers 5′-CAGCCTCAAGATCA TCAGCA-3′ and 5′-CATGAGTCCTTCCACGATAC-3′ (amplicon size = 100 bp).

Statistical analysis

All the results were expressed as the mean ± standard deviation (SD) from at least three independent experiments. Prism software package version 6.01 and GraphPad Software Inc. (CA, USA) were used for both statistical analysis and graph plotting. Unpaired Student's *t-tests* or one-way analysis of variance with Tukey's post-hoc test were used for determining statistical significance. A *p*-value of < 0.05 with 95% confidence interval was considered statistically significant.

Results
Cytotoxicity of all herbal extracts in HepG2 cells

The cytotoxicity of PNEF, PNWF, NYEF, NYWF, NBEF, NBWF and simvastatin in HepG2 cells was assessed using the MTT assay. Results were generated from independent experiments performed in triplicate (Figs. 1, 2, 3 and 4). Inhibitory concentration at 50% (IC_{50}) for each assay was calculated using the MTT assay. No cytotoxicity was noted for any herbal extract examined in HepG2 cells ($IC_{50} \geq 1$ mg/ml).

Effect of all herbal extracts on *LDL-R* and *HMGCR* gene expression

The effect of PNEF, PNWF, NYEF, NYWF, NBEF and NBWF on *LDL-R* transcripts was assessed using qRT-PCR (Fig. 5). Furthermore, qRT-PCR-amplified DNA was detected using agarose gel electrophoresis (Fig. 6). We found that 1 mg/ml of PNEF, PNWF, NYEF and NYWF were effective and significantly enhanced the synthesis of *LDL-R* compared with the negative control DMSO and simvastatin (PNEF = 9.31 ± 0.77, NYEF = 5.68 ± 0.11, PNWF = 3.98 ± 0.08, NYWF = 5.41 ± 0.09 and simvastatin = 1.40 ± 0.21). *LDL-R* expression was up-regulated the most when using PNEF. The effects of NBEF and NBWF on *LDL-R*

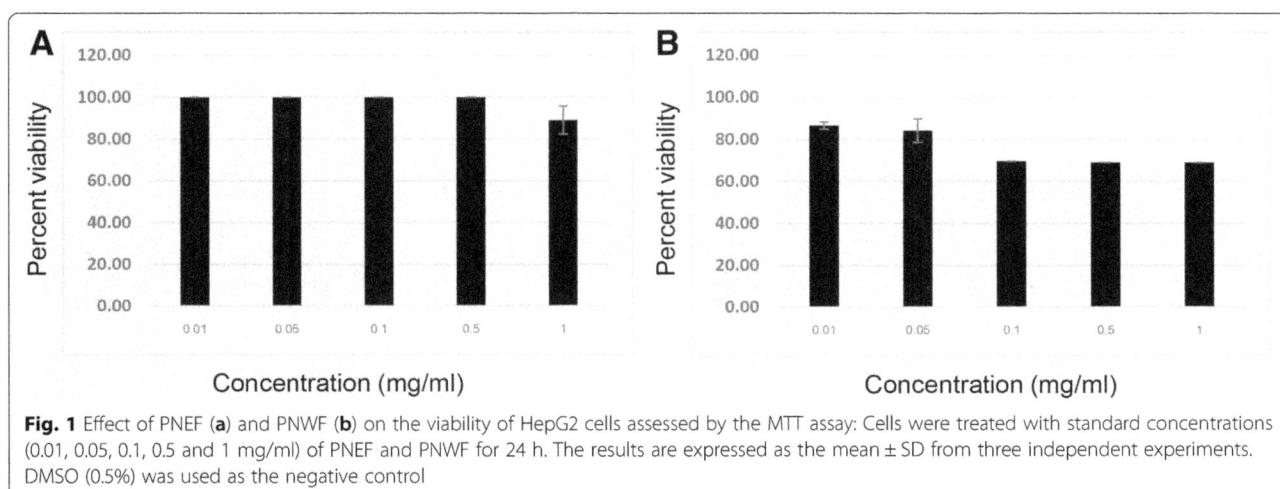

Fig. 1 Effect of PNEF (**a**) and PNWF (**b**) on the viability of HepG2 cells assessed by the MTT assay: Cells were treated with standard concentrations (0.01, 0.05, 0.1, 0.5 and 1 mg/ml) of PNEF and PNWF for 24 h. The results are expressed as the mean ± SD from three independent experiments. DMSO (0.5%) was used as the negative control

were intermittent, indicating that PN plays a major role in either regulating or modulating cholesterol-lowering effects and the associated gene expression.

Similar to *LDL-R*, the effects of 1 mg/ml of PN (PNEF and PNWF), Ya-Hom Navakot (NYEF and NYWF) and Ya-Hom Navakot without PN (NBEF and NBWF) on *HMGCR* transcripts were determined using qRT-PCR (Fig. 7). The qRT-PCR-amplified DNA was also detected using agarose gel electrophoresis (Fig. 6). PNEF, PNWF, NYEF and NYWF significantly inhibited the expression of *HMGCR* compared with the negative control (PNEF = − 2.91 ± 0.53, PNWF = − 5.8 ± 0.57, NYEF = − 2.3 ± 0.1 and NYWF = − 1.74 ± 0.24) and down-regulated the synthesis of *HMGCR* compared with simvastatin (2.41 ± 0.03).

On the contrary, 1 mg/ml extracts of NBEF and NBWF significantly up-regulated the expression of *HMGCR* compared with the DMSO negative control (NBEF = 1.54 ± 0.25 and NBWF = 0.51 ± 0.38). However, the *HMGCR* gene expression level was lower than that observed using simvastatin (2.41 ± 0.03). Unlike *LDL-R*, PNWF exhibited

a higher potential for reducing *HMGCR* gene expression than its ethanolic extract and other groups. Therefore, PN may play an important role in the inhibition of *HMGCR* gene expression.

Discussion

The incidence of cardiovascular diseases (CVDs) has been increasing worldwide. In 2015, it was estimated that there were 422.7 million cases of CVD and 17.92 million CVD-related deaths [10]. Hypercholesterolaemia is a major risk factor for CVD progression and is rapidly becoming more prevalent in developing countries. Interestingly, in 2016, ischaemic heart disease, which is a CVD, was the primary cause of mortality in Thailand. The incidence of hypercholesterolaemia is increasing in Thailand owing to changes in the lifestyle and behaviour to adapt to the Western culture [11]. Approximately 14% and 17% of Thai men and women have hypercholesterolaemia, respectively [12]. Cholesterol biosynthesis primarily occurs in the liver as a result of the HMGCR

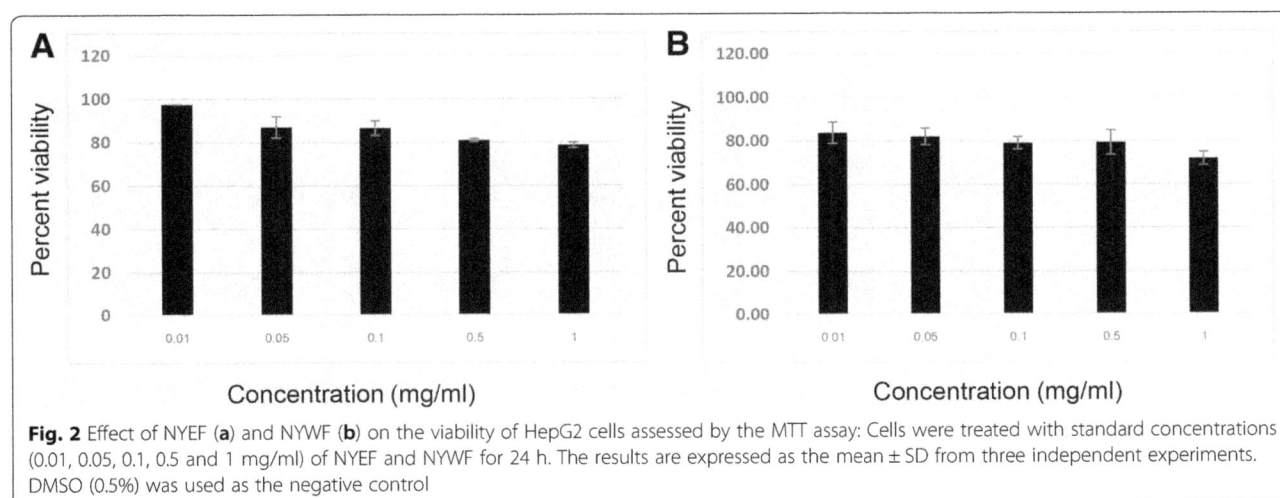

Fig. 2 Effect of NYEF (**a**) and NYWF (**b**) on the viability of HepG2 cells assessed by the MTT assay: Cells were treated with standard concentrations (0.01, 0.05, 0.1, 0.5 and 1 mg/ml) of NYEF and NYWF for 24 h. The results are expressed as the mean ± SD from three independent experiments. DMSO (0.5%) was used as the negative control

A

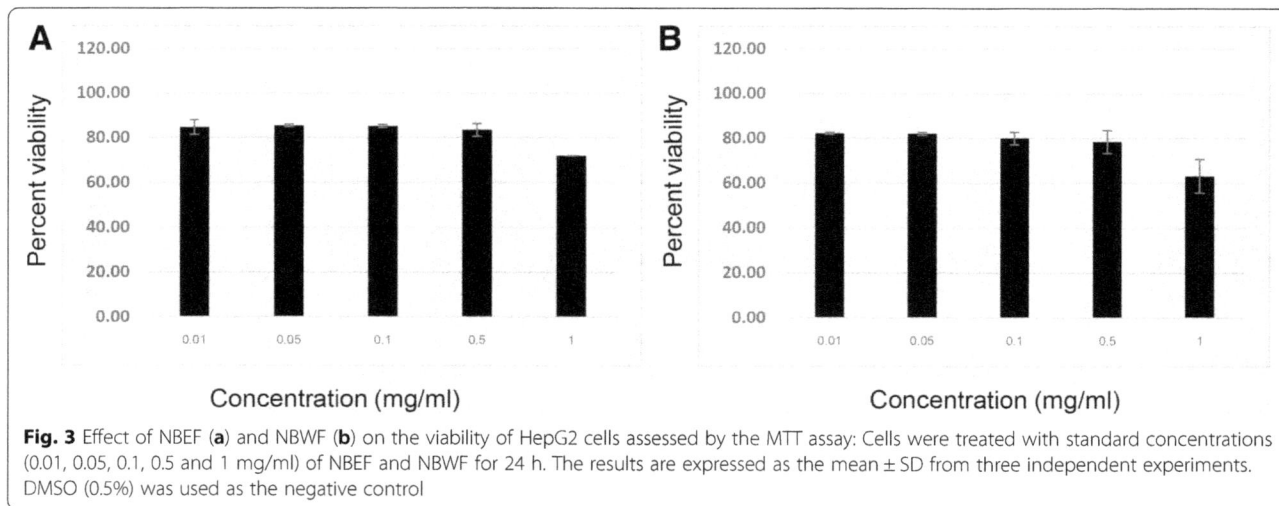

B

Fig. 3 Effect of NBEF (**a**) and NBWF (**b**) on the viability of HepG2 cells assessed by the MTT assay: Cells were treated with standard concentrations (0.01, 0.05, 0.1, 0.5 and 1 mg/ml) of NBEF and NBWF for 24 h. The results are expressed as the mean ± SD from three independent experiments. DMSO (0.5%) was used as the negative control

enzyme, which is a regulatory enzyme in the mevalonate pathway [13]. This enzyme is considered a therapeutic target for lowering blood cholesterol.

Low-density lipoprotein-cholesterol (LDL-C), which is an important atherogenic lipoprotein, is metabolised in the liver by LDL-R. High levels of LDL-C in the blood can increase the risk of atherosclerosis and CVD [14, 15]. High levels of LDL-C are present in 29.6% of Thai adults [16]. As such, LDL-C has largely replaced total cholesterol as a risk marker and primary treatment target for hyperlipidaemia [17]. A reduction in LDL-C levels can lead to a reduced risk of CVD development [18].

Simvastatin, which is a widely used lipid-lowering drug, increases the mRNA synthesis of *HMGCR* and *LDL-R* [19]. It is a synthetic derivative of the fermentation product of *Aspergillus terreus* [20] and blocks cholesterol synthesis by the competitive inhibition of the HMGCR enzyme, the

rate-limiting step of cholesterol biosynthesis in the human body. Simvastatin is a powerful lipid-lowering drug, primarily used for treating dyslipidaemia and preventing atherosclerosis-related complications in high-risk individuals. However, statin therapies are associated with numerous adverse effects [21–28]. Hence, alternative treatments to alleviate hyperlipidaemic conditions and substitute statins are warranted.

Several herbal extracts have been shown to affect the synthesis of HMGCR and LDL-R genes. A phenol-enriched extract of *Moringa oleifera* leaf significantly increased the expression of both *HMGCR* and *LDL-R* in HepG2 cells [29]. GINST, a hydrolysed ginseng extract, also decreased the expression of *HMGCR* via AMPKα activation in HepG2 cells [30]. In addition, hydrolic extract of lemongrass [*Cymbopogon citratus* (DC) Stapf.] suppressed the expression of sterol regulatory element binding protein-1c and *HMGCR*

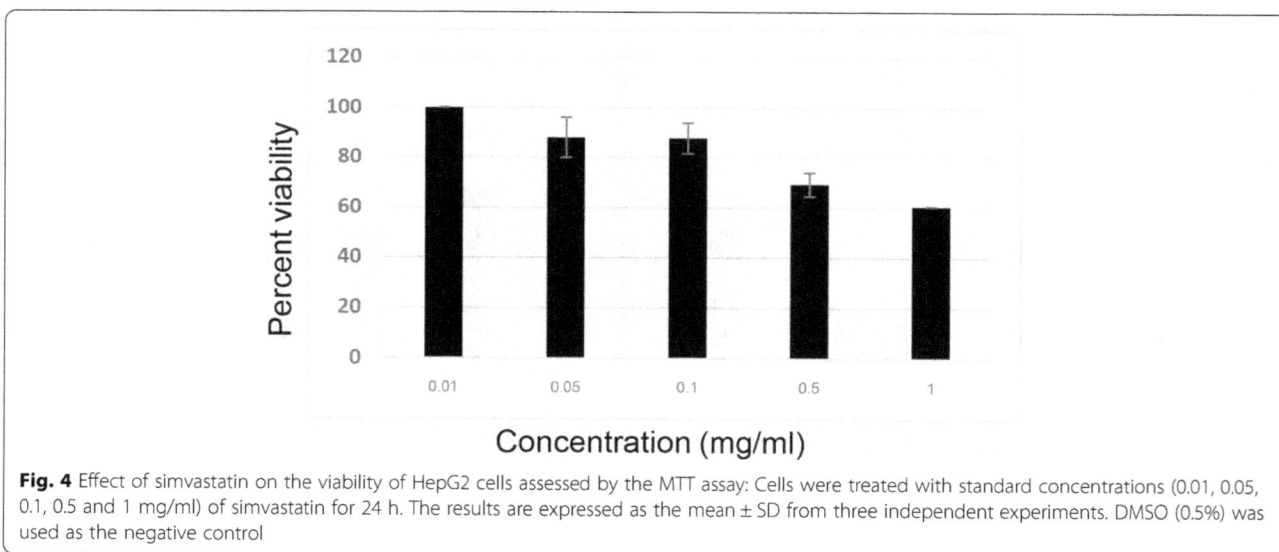

Fig. 4 Effect of simvastatin on the viability of HepG2 cells assessed by the MTT assay: Cells were treated with standard concentrations (0.01, 0.05, 0.1, 0.5 and 1 mg/ml) of simvastatin for 24 h. The results are expressed as the mean ± SD from three independent experiments. DMSO (0.5%) was used as the negative control

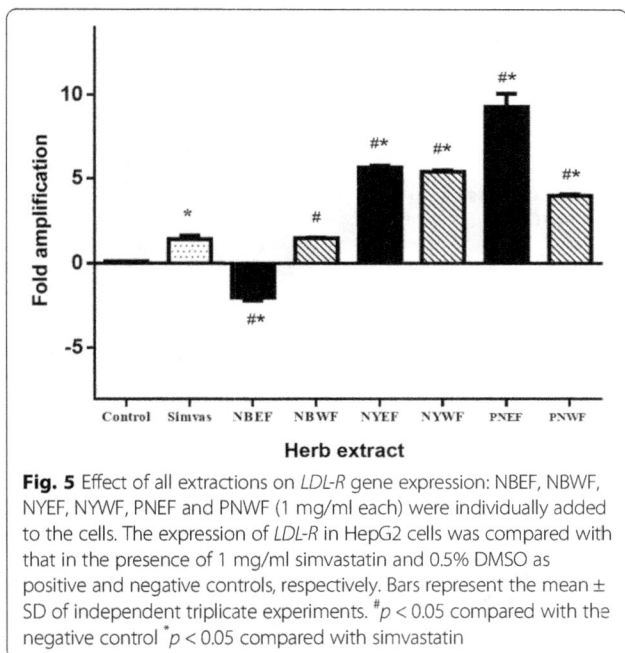

Fig. 5 Effect of all extractions on *LDL-R* gene expression: NBEF, NBWF, NYEF, NYWF, PNEF and PNWF (1 mg/ml each) were individually added to the cells. The expression of *LDL-R* in HepG2 cells was compared with that in the presence of 1 mg/ml simvastatin and 0.5% DMSO as positive and negative controls, respectively. Bars represent the mean ± SD of independent triplicate experiments. $^{#}p < 0.05$ compared with the negative control $^{*}p < 0.05$ compared with simvastatin

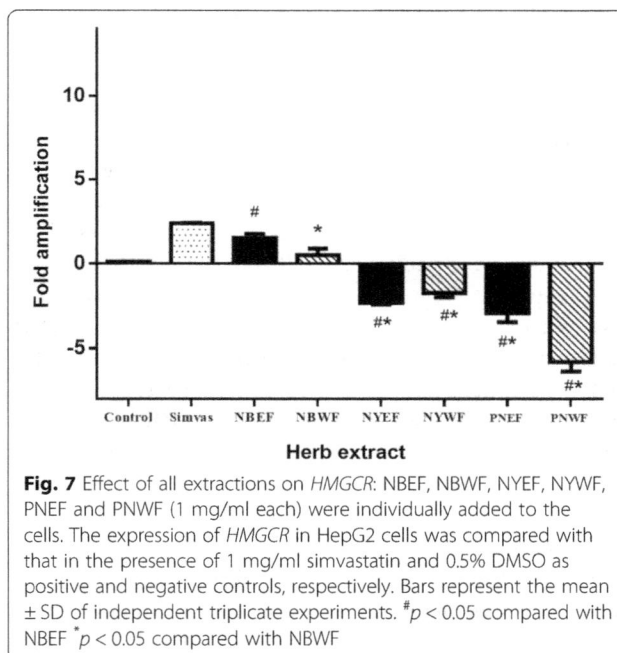

Fig. 7 Effect of all extractions on *HMGCR*: NBEF, NBWF, NYEF, NYWF, PNEF and PNWF (1 mg/ml each) were individually added to the cells. The expression of *HMGCR* in HepG2 cells was compared with that in the presence of 1 mg/ml simvastatin and 0.5% DMSO as positive and negative controls, respectively. Bars represent the mean ± SD of independent triplicate experiments. $^{#}p < 0.05$ compared with NBEF $^{*}p < 0.05$ compared with NBWF

in rats [31]. Furthermore, low concentrations of anthocyanin (200 mg/L) extracted from Thai black sticky rice significantly enhanced the expression of *LDL-R* in HepG2 cells [32]. In this study, both PNEF and NYEF demonstrated a significant down-regulation of *HMGCR* mRNA and

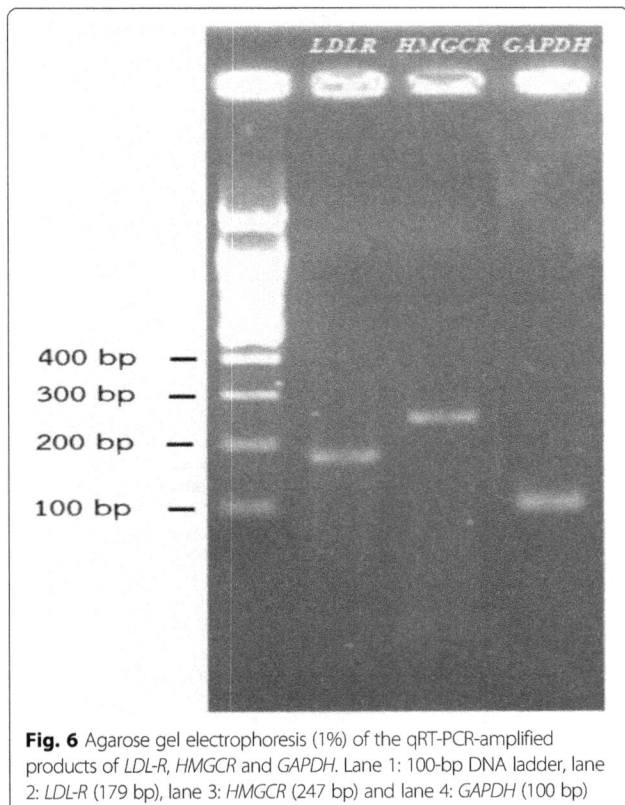

Fig. 6 Agarose gel electrophoresis (1%) of the qRT-PCR-amplified products of *LDL-R*, *HMGCR* and *GAPDH*. Lane 1: 100-bp DNA ladder, lane 2: *LDL-R* (179 bp), lane 3: *HMGCR* (247 bp) and lane 4: *GAPDH* (100 bp)

up-regulation of *LDL-R* mRNA compared with simvastatin. However, NBEF and NBWF effects did not differ from those of simvastatin.

In this study, different methods of extraction led to a variety of effects on target genes, depending on the composition and proportion of the extracted ingredients. In agreement with other studies, active ingredients extracted using different solvents resulted in different effects. For example, many phenolic compounds are extracted using chloroform, n-butanol and ethyl acetate rather than ethanol, ethanol/water or water [33, 34]. In this study, PNEF up-regulated *LDL-R* gene expression the most, whereas PNWF down-regulated *HMGCR* gene expression (Figs. 5 and 7). This demonstrated the board spectrum of activity when using different extraction methods. In addition, PNEF scavenged ROS and RNS better than PNWF [4].

Thus, it is suggested that PN contains herbs with the following two mechanisms involving cholesterol metabolism: (i) up-regulation of *LDL-R* resulting in the increased uptake of LDL-C and (ii) down-regulation of *HMGCR* resulting in the suppression of cholesterol biosynthesis. Although PNWF had the highest ability to decrease *HMGCR* gene expression compared with other groups, NYEF and PNEF still exhibited better effects on cholesterol metabolism than NBEF, NBWF, simvastatin and DMSO negative control. Indeed, ethanol extraction should be considered as the appropriate method for herbal extraction because it is safe, quick, consumes little energy and preserves heat-labile components. However, the mechanisms underlying the increased expression of *LDL-R* or decreased expression of *HMGCR* remain unknown.

Recently, traditional Thai medicines and herbal formulae have been promoted by the Ministry of Public Health for use as alternative medicines in the treatment of health problems [3]. Ya-Hom Navakot is one of the Thai herbal formulae listed in the Herbal Medicinal Products A.D. 2006 announced by the Ministry of Public Health. Based on traditional knowledge, it has a therapeutic effectiveness against circulatory disorders. It effectively improves blood circulation in the body through its cholesterol-lowering effect. However, the mechanisms involved in this hypocholesterolaemic effect of Ya-Hom Navakot or PN are yet to be clarified. To the best of our knowledge, this study is the first report describing the cholesterol-lowering effect of both Ya-Hom Navakot and its PN formulation and their association with *HMGCR* down-regulation and *LDL-R* up-regulation.

Conclusion

Ya-Hom Navakot and its PN formulation create a cholesterol-lowering effect, primarily by inhibiting *HMGCR* and enhancing *LDL-R* gene expressions. The effect of these herbal extracts is greater than that of the standard cholesterol treatment using statins. Ethanol-extracted PN up-regulated *LDL-R* gene expression best, while Ya-Hom Navakot without PN down-regulated both *HMGCR* and *LDL-R* gene expressions.

Abbreviations
DMEM: Dulbecco's modified Eagle's medium; LDL-C: Low-density lipoprotein-cholesterol; *A. dahurica*: Angelica dahurica; *A. lancea*: Atractylodes lancea; *A. pallens*: Artemisia pallens; *A. sinensis*: Angelica sinensis; CA: California; CVDs: Cardiovascular diseases; DMSO: Dimethyl sulfoxide; FBS: Foetal bovine serum; HMGCR: 3-hydroxyl-3-methylglutaryl-CoA reductase; IC$_{50}$: Inhibitory concentration at 50%; *L. chuanxiong*: Ligusticum chuanxiong; LDL-R: Low-density lipoprotein receptor; LHMP: List of Herbal Medicinal Products; MA: Massachusetts; MEM: Minimal Essential Medium; MO: Missouri; MTT: 3-(4, 5 di-methylthiazol-2-yl)-2, 5-diphenyltetrazolium bromide; *N. jatamansi*: Nardostachys jatamansi; NBEF: Ya-Hom Navakot without PN ethanolic extraction; NBWF: Ya-Hom Navakot without PN water extraction; NY: New York; NYEF: Ya-Hom Navakot ethanolic extraction; NYWF: Ya-Hom Navakot water extraction; *P. kurrooa*: Picrorhiza kurrooa; PN: Phikud Navakot; PNEF: Phikud Navakot ethanolic extraction; PNWF: Phikud Navakot water extraction; qRT-PCR: Quantitative reverse transcription-polymerase chain reaction; RNS: Reactive nitrogen species; ROS: Reactive oxygen species; *S. costus*: Saussurea costus; *T. chebula*: Terminalia chebula; USA: United States of America

Acknowledgements
This research was supported by National Research Council of Thailand (NRCT) under the project 'Development of Standardized Extracts from Herbs in Phikud Navakot'. The Faculty of Medicine Siriraj Hospital and Faculty of Tropical Medicine at Mahidol University kindly provided additional support for the publication.

Funding
National Research Council of Thailand (NRCT) under the project 'Development of Standardized Extracts from Herbs in Phikud Navakot'.

Authors' contributions
NT and SA designed the experimental study. SS, AS and NT conducted the experiments. BS assisted in statistical analyses. NT and SA interpreted the data and drafted the manuscript. All authors have read and approved the final manuscript.

Competing interests
The authors declare that they have no competing interest.

Author details
[1]Department of Biochemistry, Faculty of Medicine Siriraj Hospital, Mahidol University, 2 Bangkok Noi Road, Bangkok Noi, Bangkok 10700, Thailand. [2]Department of Tropical Pathology, Faculty of Tropical Medicine, Mahidol University, 420/6 Ratchawithi Road, Ratchathewi, Bangkok 10400, Thailand.

References
1. Disayavanish C, Disayavanish P. Introduction of the treatment method of Thai traditional medicine: its validity and future perspectives. Psychiatry Clin Neurosci. 1998;52(Suppl):S334–7.
2. Nusuetrong P, Sotanaphun U, Tep-Areenan P: Effects of Phikud Navakot extract on vascular reactivity in the isolated rat aorta. J Med Assoc Thai 2012, 95 Suppl 12:S1–S7.
3. Nusuetrong P, Gerdprasert O, Wetchasit P, Nakchat O, Sotanaphun U: Effect of short-term oral administration of Phikud Navakot in rats. J Med Assoc Thai 2015, 98 Suppl 10:S52–S60.
4. Nalinratana N, Kaewprem W, Tongumpai S, Luechapudiporn R, Sotanaphun U, Meksuriyen D. Synergistic antioxidant action of Phikud Navakot ameliorates hydrogen peroxide-induced stress in human endothelial cells. Integrative medicine research. 2014;3(2):74–82.
5. Kengkoom K, Ampawong S. In vitro protective effect of Phikud Navakot extraction on erythrocyte. Evidence-based complementary and alternative medicine : eCAM. 2016;2016:1961327.
6. Kengkoom K, Chaimongkolnukul K, Cherdyu S, Inpunkaew R, Ampawong S. Acute and sub-chronic oral toxicity study of the extracts from herbs in Phikud Navakot. Afr J Biotechnol. 2012;11(48):10903–11.
7. Gong X, Zhang Y, Pan J, Qu H. Optimization of the ethanol recycling reflux extraction process for saponins using a design space approach. PLoS One. 2014;9(12):e114300.
8. Mosmann T. Rapid colorimetric assay for cellular growth and survival: application to proliferation and cytotoxicity assays. J Immunol Methods. 1983;65(1–2):55–63.
9. Sangkitikomol W, Rocejanasaroj A, Tencomnao T. Effect of Moringa oleifera on advanced glycation end-product formation and lipid metabolism gene expression in HepG2 cells. Genet Mol Res. 2014;13(1):723–35.
10. Roth GA, Johnson C, Abajobir A, Abd-Allah F, Abera SF, Abyu G, Ahmed M, Aksut B, Alam T, Alam K, et al. Global, regional, and national burden of cardiovascular diseases for 10 causes, 1990 to 2015. J Am Coll Cardiol. 2017; 70(1):1–25.
11. Le D, Garcia A, Lohsoonthorn V, Williams MA. Prevalence and risk factors of hypercholesterolemia among Thai men and women receiving health examinations. The Southeast Asian journal of tropical medicine and public health. 2006;37(5):1005–14.
12. Khonputsa P, Veerman JL, Vos T, Aekplakorn W, Bertram M, Abbott-Klafter J, Hogan MC, Lim SS. Joint prevalence and control of hypercholesterolemia and hypertension in Thailand: third national health examination survey. Asia Pac J Public Health. 2012;24(1):185–94.
13. Ness GC. Physiological feedback regulation of cholesterol biosynthesis: role of translational control of hepatic HMG-CoA reductase and possible involvement of oxylanosterols. Biochim Biophys Acta. 2015;1851(5):667–73.
14. Ference BA, Ginsberg HN, Graham I, Ray KK, Packard CJ, Bruckert E, Hegele RA, Krauss RM, Raal FJ, Schunkert H, et al. Low-density lipoproteins cause atherosclerotic cardiovascular disease. 1. Evidence from genetic, epidemiologic, and clinical studies. A consensus statement from the European atherosclerosis society consensus panel. Eur Heart J. 2017;38(32):2459–72.

15. Pirillo A, Bonacina F, Norata GD, Catapano AL. The interplay of lipids, lipoproteins, and immunity in atherosclerosis. Curr Atheroscler Rep. 2018;20(3):12.

16. Aekplakorn W, Taneepanichskul S, Kessomboon P, Chongsuvivatwong V, Putwatana P, Sritara P, Sangwatanaroj S, Chariyalertsak S. Prevalence of dyslipidemia and management in the Thai population. National Health Examination Survey IV, 2009. Journal of lipids. 2014;249584:2014.

17. Wadhera RK, Steen DL, Khan I, Giugliano RP, Foody JM. A review of low-density lipoprotein cholesterol, treatment strategies, and its impact on cardiovascular disease morbidity and mortality. Journal of clinical lipidology. 2016;10(3):472–89.

18. Soran H, Dent R, Durrington P. Evidence-based goals in LDL-C reduction. Clin Res Cardiol. 2017;106(4):237–48.

19. Morikawa S, Umetani M, Nakagawa S, Yamazaki H, Suganami H, Inoue K, Kitahara M, Hamakubo T, Kodama T, Saito Y. Relative induction of mRNA for HMG CoA reductase and LDL receptor by five different HMG-CoA reductase inhibitors in cultured human cells. J Atheroscler Thromb. 2000;7(3):138–44.

20. Endo A. The origin of the statins. Atherosclerosis Supplements. 2004;5(3):125–30.

21. Bruckert E, Hayem G, Dejager S, Yau C, Begaud B. Mild to moderate muscular symptoms with high-dosage statin therapy in hyperlipidemic patients--the PRIMO study. Cardiovasc Drugs Ther. 2005;19(6):403–14.

22. Fallouh N, Chopra V. Statin withdrawal after major noncardiac surgery: risks, consequences, and preventative strategies. J Hosp Med. 2012;7(7):573–9.

23. Golomb BA, Evans MA, Dimsdale JE, White HL. Effects of statins on energy and fatigue with exertion: results from a randomized controlled trial. Arch Intern Med. 2012;172(15):1180–2.

24. Hoffman KB, Kraus C, Dimbil M, Golomb BA. A survey of the FDA's AERS database regarding muscle and tendon adverse events linked to the statin drug class. PLoS One. 2012;7(8):e42866.

25. Puccetti L, Pasqui AL, Scarpini F, Cappellone R, Ghezzi A, Ceccatelli L, Auteri A. Statins discontinuation in compliant chronic users induces atherothrombotic profile despite baseline clinical setting and treatments. Int J Cardiol. 2011;153(3):328–9.

26. Xue Y, Tao L, Wu S, Wang G, Qian L, Li J, Liao L, Tang J, Ji K. Red yeast rice induces less muscle fatigue symptom than simvastatin in dyslipidemic patients: a single center randomized pilot trial. BMC Cardiovasc Disord. 2017;17(1):127.

27. Peng D, Fong A, Pelt AV. Original research: the effects of red yeast Rice supplementation on cholesterol levels in adults. Am J Nurs. 2017;117(8):46–54.

28. Tshongo Muhindo C, Ahn SA, Rousseau MF, Dierckxsens Y, Hermans MP. Efficacy and safety of a combination of red yeast rice and olive extract in hypercholesterolemic patients with and without statin-associated myalgia. Complementary therapies in medicine. 2017;35:140–4.

29. Tabboon P, Sripanidkulchai B, Sripanidkulchai K. Hypocholesterolemic mechanism of phenolics-enriched extract from *Moringa oleifera* leaves in HepG2 cell lines. Songklanakarin Journal of Science and Technology. 2016;38(2):155–61.

30. Han JS, Sung JH, Lee SK. Inhibition of cholesterol synthesis in HepG2 cells by GINST-decreasing HMG-CoA reductase expression via AMP-activated protein kinase. J Food Sci. 2017;82(11):2700–5.

31. Somparn N, Saenthaweeuk S, Naowaboot J, Thaeomor A, Kukongviriyapan V. Effect of lemongrass water extract supplementation on atherogenic index and antioxidant status in rats. Acta Pharma. 2018;68(2):185–97.

32. Sangkitikomol W, Tencomnao T, Rocejanasaroj A. Effects of Thai black sticky rice extract on oxidative stress and lipid metabolism gene expression in HepG2 cells. Genet Mol Res. 2010;9(4):2086–95.

33. Kamiya T, Nishihara H, Hara H, Adachi T. Ethanol extract of Brazilian red propolis induces apoptosis in human breast cancer MCF-7 cells through endoplasmic reticulum stress. J Agric Food Chem. 2012;60(44):11065–70.

34. Sun C, Wu Z, Wang Z, Zhang H. Effect of ethanol/water solvents on phenolic profiles and antioxidant properties of Beijing propolis extracts. Evid Based Complement Alternat Med. 2015;2015:595393.

10

Protective effects of Liuweiwuling tablets on carbon tetrachloride-induced hepatic fibrosis in rats

Huimin Liu[1], Zhenfang Zhang[1], Huangwanyin Hu[1], Congen Zhang[1], Ming Niu[1], Ruishen Li[2], Jiabo Wang[1], Zhaofang Bai[1*] and Xiaohe Xiao[3*]

Abstract

Background: Liuweiwuling tablets (LWWL) are an herbal product that exerts remarkable effects on liver protection and aminotransferase levels, and they have been approved by the Chinese State Food and Drug Administration (CFDA). Clinical studies have found that LWWL can inhibit collagen production and reduce the levels of liver fibrosis markers in the serum. Thus, LWWL is expected to have beneficial effects in the treatment of liver fibrosis. The purpose of this study was to evaluate the pharmacological effects of LWWL.

Methods: Hepatic fibrosis was induced in rats via carbon tetrachloride (CCl_4) treatment. The rats were treated twice weekly for 8 weeks with either 2 $mL \cdot kg^{-1}$ body weight of a 50% solution of CCl_4 in olive oil or olive oil alone by oral gavage. A subset of rats received daily intraperitoneal injections of either colchicine (0.2 mg/kg per day), LWWL (0.4, 1.6, or 6.4 g/kg per day), or vehicle ($N = 12$ for all groups) during weeks 9–12. The rats were sacrificed after 12 weeks. Pathological changes in hepatic tissue were examined using hematoxylin and eosin (H&E) and Sirius Red staining. Immunohistochemistry was performed to observe α-smooth muscle actin (α-SMA) and collagen type I (collagen I) protein expression. Western blotting was also used to detect α-SMA protein expression. Real-time quantitative reverse-transcription polymerase chain reaction (RT-qPCR) was used to detect transforming growth factor-1 (TGF-β1), platelet-derived growth factor (PDGF), tissue inhibitor of metalloproteinase-1 (TIMP1), and tissue inhibitor of metalloproteinase-2 (TIMP2) mRNA expression.

Results: LWWL significantly reversed histological fibrosis and liver injury, reduced the hydroxyproline content in liver tissue, and decreased α-SMA and collagen I expression. LWWL also suppressed hepatic stellate cell (HSC) activation by reducing the expression of the profibrogenic factors TGF-β1 and PDGF. The expression levels of TIMP1 and TIMP2, which regulate extracellular matrix (ECM) degradation, were decreased after CCl_4 injury in LWWL-treated rats.

Conclusions: These data suggest that LWWL may serve as a promising therapeutic agent to reduce fibrogenesis.

Keywords: Traditional Chinese medicine, Liuweiwuling tablets, Hepatic fibrosis, Hepatic stellate cell, TGF-β1, TIMPs

Background

Liver fibrosis is a wound-healing process that occurs in response to chronic liver injury from a variety of etiologies and eventually progresses to liver cirrhosis following persistent inflammation and fibrogenesis [1, 2]. Characteristic features of liver fibrosis include agglutination in the extracellular matrix (ECM) of the liver, increased collagen fiber content, and decreased ECM degradation. Hepatic parenchymal cell injury is the initiating factor in liver fibrosis. Hepatic stellate cell (HSC) activation, proliferation, and transdifferentiation into myofibroblasts are considered pivotal mechanisms of hepatic fibrosis and of the activation of HSC secretion of ECM, including α-smooth muscle actin (α-SMA) and collagen I [3]. The activated HSCs secrete matrix metalloproteinases (MMPs) and matrix metalloproteinase tissue inhibiting factors (TIMPs) and affect the deposition and degradation of the

* Correspondence: Baizf2008@126.com; pharmacy302xxh@126.com
[1]Department of Pharmacy, 302 Hospital of People's Liberation Army, Beijing, People's Republic of China
[3]China Military Institute of Chinese Medicine, 302 Hospital of People's Liberation Army, Beijing, People's Republic of China
Full list of author information is available at the end of the article

ECM in the liver. Among the MMPs is the main ECM-degrading enzyme, while TIMPs are specific inhibitors of MMPs. Thus, TIMPs inhibit the expression of TIMP1 and weaken the inhibition of MMP1, which promotes ECM degradation and exerts an anti-liver fibrosis effect [4, 5]. Transforming growth factor-1 (TGF-β1), a highly potent fibrogenic cytokine, simulates both small mothers against decapentaplegic homolog (Smad) and mitogen-activated protein kinase (MAPK) signaling in HSCs, thus stimulating collagen I gene expression [6, 7]. TGF-β signaling also plays an important role in the reduction of MMPs and the increase in TIMPs during liver fibrosis [8]. Platelet-derived growth factor (PDGF), a potent proliferative cytokine in HSCs, stimulates mitogen-activated protein kinase/extracellular signal-regulated kinase (MAPK/ERK) and PI3K/Akt/P70S6K signaling in HSCs. These signaling pathways lead to the activation, migration, proliferation, survival, and contraction of HSCs as well as the promotion of ECM secretion and deposition, thus potentially causing hepatic fibrogenesis [9, 10].

Recent studies of the pathophysiological mechanisms and diagnosis of hepatic fibrosis have made considerable progress. Moreover, possible drug targets against hepatic fibrosis have been identified [11]; however, biological or chemical drugs that target hepatic fibrosis have not yet been approved by the FDA (food and Drug Administration) for clinical applications. Traditional Chinese medicine (TCM) has proven to be effective in the treatment of liver fibrosis due to its unique advantages, which have been demonstrated over many years of clinical validation [12]. LWWL is classified under a new category of TCM drugs approved by the CFDA. LWWL is composed of six herbs: *Schisandrae chinensis fructus, Fructus Ligustri Lucidi, Forsythiae fructus, Curcumae rhizoma, Perennial sow thistle*, and *Ganoderma spore*. Clinically, LWWL effectively improves collagenase activity, thus increasing collagen degradation in liver tissue and the serum protein content, reduces the liver tissue collagen content, and effectively reduces liver fibrosis markers in the serum. Chronic liver injury is significantly improved and reversed, which promotes ECM degradation and reabsorption to prevent and delay the occurrence of progressive liver fibrosis [12, 13]. Moreover, long-term colchicine treatment in patients with liver fibrosis showed anti-inflammatory, anti-fibrotic, and immunomodulatory effects as well as the relief of portal hypertension [14, 15]. Therefore, colchicine was used as a positive control. In this study, we evaluated the therapeutic effect of LWWL in the treatment of hepatic fibrosis and investigated the mechanism of its antifibrotic effects.

Methods
Experimental animals
Sprague-Dawley rats (male, Grade III, 180 ± 20 g, 8 weeks old) were purchased from the Laboratory Animal Center of the Academy of Military Medical Sciences. All the animals were kept in an environmentally controlled breeding room (20–22 °C, 45–50% humidity). This study protocol strictly adhered to the recommendations of the Guidelines for the Care and Use of Laboratory Animals of 302 Military Hospital (No. IACUC-2015-008).

Experimental drugs
LWWL was purchased from the Shandong Shibojindu Pharmaceutical Company (batch Nos. 150,709, 150,805, 150,804, and 150,812). Colchicine was purchased from Sigma-Aldrich (USA). Olive oil was purchased from Sinopharm (China). Carbon tetrachloride (CCl_4) was purchased from Beihua.

Reagents
Hydroxyproline, alanine transaminase (ALT) and aspartate aminotransferase (AST) testing kits were purchased from Nanjing Jiancheng Co., Ltd., China. PCR primers were purchased from Invitrogen. Maxima SYBR Green qPCR Master Mix (2×) and the First Strand cDNA Synthesis Kit were purchased from Thermo Fisher Scientific, Inc. The bicinchoninic acid (BCA) Protein Quantification Kit was purchased from CWBIO (China). Primary antibodies against α-SMA and collagen I were purchased from Abcam (UK), and that against DAPDH was purchased from Cell Signaling Technology (USA).

Animal model and protocol
Hepatic fibrosis was induced by CCl_4 as previously described. Male Sprague-Dawley rats were treated twice weekly for 8 weeks with either 2 $mL \cdot kg^{-1}$ body weight of a 50% solution of CCl_4 in olive oil or olive oil alone by oral gavage. A subset of rats received daily intraperitoneal injections of either colchicine (0.2 mg/kg per day), LWWL (0.4, 1.6, or 6.4 g/kg per day), or vehicle ($N = 12$ for all groups) during weeks 9–12. The rats were sacrificed after 12 weeks. After sample collection, the rats were euthanized by cervical dislocation. The rat was placed on the lid of the feeding box, and then, the research grabbed the rat's tail with their right hand, pulled the tail back slightly, quickly pressed the thumb and forefinger of their left hand down on the head, and dislocated the rat's neck with both hands. All the animals received humane care in compliance with the Chinese Animal Protection Act and according to National Research Council criteria. The protocol was approved by the Committee on the Ethics of Animal Experiments of the 302 Military Hospital.

Histological analysis and immunohistochemistry
Tissues were fixed in 4% paraformaldehyde and embedded in paraffin. Sections (5-μm thickness) were prepared for H&E and Sirius Red staining as well as α-SMA (1:500)

and collagen I (1:200) immunohistochemistry. All the procedures were performed as previously described.

Measurement of the hydroxyproline content and serum ALT/AST levels

Hydroxyproline, ALT, and AST kits were utilized in accordance with the manufacturers' protocols. Briefly, serum samples were obtained by separating the supernatant from the blood. After centrifugation (3000 rpm for 10 min), serum ALT and AST levels and the hydroxyproline content were measured using an Olympus AU5400 Automatic Biochemistry Analyzer (Olympus Optical, Tokyo, Japan).

RNA isolation and quantitative reverse-transcription polymerase chain reaction (RT-PCR) analysis

The total RNA was isolated from liver tissue using TRIzol reagent (Invitrogen). RNA (1 μg) was reverse-transcribed to complementary DNA (cDNA) using a First Strand cDNA Synthesis Kit (Thermo Fisher Scientific, Inc.). Quantitative RT-PCR was performed to measure Acta2 (encoding α-SMA), collagen I, TGF-β1, PDGF, TIMP1, and TIMP2 mRNA expression using Power SYBR Green PCR Master Mix (Life Technologies, Thermo Fisher Scientific, Inc.) on an ABI Prism 7500 Sequence Detection System. Data analysis was performed using the $2^{-\Delta\Delta CT}$ method for relative quantification. All the gene expression levels were calculated relative to GADPH. Primer sequences are shown in Table 1.

Western blot analysis

Liver tissues were homogenized in lysis buffer (150 mM of NaCl, 1% Nonidet P-40, 0.1% SDS, 50 mM of Tris-HCl, pH = 7.4, 1 mM of EDTA, 1 mM of PMSF, and 1× Roche Complete Mini Protease Inhibitor Cocktail), and protein concentrations were determined using the BCA Protein Assay Kit according to the manufacturer's protocol. The proteins were separated by gel electrophoresis and transferred to membranes, followed by blocking with 5% w/v skim milk in 1× TBST for 1 h at room temperature and overnight incubation with primary antibodies against α-SMA (1:200) and GAPDH (1:1000) at 4 °C with gentle shaking. After incubation with the secondary antibody (anti-rabbit IgG) for 1 h, the blot was processed according to the recommended procedure. The gray densities of the protein bands were normalized by using the GAPDH density as an internal control, and the results were further normalized to the control.

Statistical analysis

All the data are presented as the means ± standard deviation (x ± s) and were analyzed using SPSS 23.0. Differences between experimental groups were analyzed by analysis of variance (ANOVA) followed by post-hoc tests. $P < 0.01$ was regarded as highly statistically significant, and $P < 0.05$ was regarded as statistically significant.

Results

LWWL inhibited CCl₄-induced liver fibrosis in rats

The effects of LWWL on fibrogenesis were tested using the well-characterized CCl_4 rat model. The rats that were injured with CCl_4 by oral gavage reliably developed liver fibrosis after 8 weeks. The experimental design is shown in Fig. 1a. Liver pathological observation is the gold standard for the clinical diagnosis of liver fibrosis. Compared with the control group, the liver tissues of the model group showed severe adhesion of liver tissue, and the texture was significantly stiffened, the surface roughened, and the luster was lost, forming a lumpy mass. After treatment with LWWL (0.4, 1.6, or 6.4 g/kg) dramatically inhibited CCl_4-induced hepatic fibrogenesis, the adhesion of liver tissues decreased, and the texture became soft and lustrous, as indicated by the striking morphological alteration (Fig. 1b). H&E and Sirius Red staining results showed that compared with the control group, the livers of the model group had a remarkable ECM area. Furthermore, the groups treated with LWWL showed markedly reduced collagen levels in H&E and Sirius Red staining sections (Fig. 1c, d).

LWWL attenuated liver function and the hydroxyproline content in rats

Liver function tests were used to assess injury. Hydroxyproline, an indicator of collagen deposition. CCl_4 significantly increased the levels of the serum ALT and hydroxyproline in liver tissue compared with those of the control group, and the effects of LWWL revealed decreased ALT levels but no changes in serum AST levels. Meanwhile, LWWL also reduced the level of hydroxyproline, which directly reflects the amount of liver fibrosis (Fig. 2a, b, c).

Table 1 Primer Sequences Used in This Study

Target gene	Forward primer (5'- 3')	Reverse primer (5'- 3')
Acta2	GAACACGGCATCATCACCAA	CAAGGTCGGATGCTCCTCTG
Collagen I	CTCCTGGCAAGAACGGAGA	CCAGCTGTTCCAGGCAATC
TGF-β1	CCGCAACAACGCAATCTATG	AGTTCTACGTGTTGCTCCACAGT
PDGF	TCTGCTGCTACCTGCGTCTG	AGGCGCTGAAGGTCATCAA
TIMP1	GCCTCTGGCATCCTCTTGTT	CCAGGTCCGAGTTGCAGAA
TIMP2	TATTGTGCCCTGGGACACG	GTCCATCCAGAGGCACTCATC
GAPDH	GCATCCTGCACCACCAACT	GCAGTGATGGCATGGACTGT

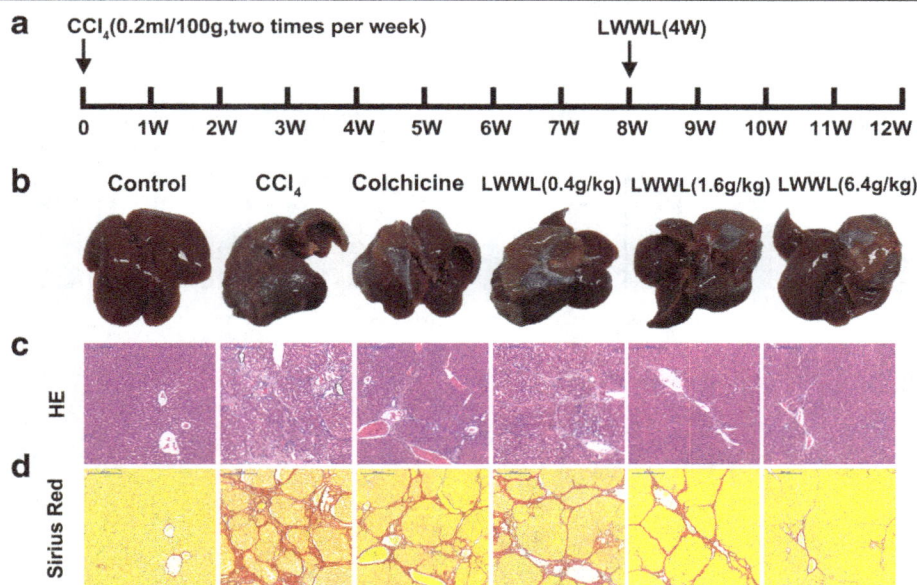

Fig. 1 LWWL inhibited CCl₄-induced rat liver fibrosis. **a** Schematic representation of the CCl₄-induced hepatic fibrosis in rats; **b** Representative rat livers at the time of sacrifice; **c** Representative rat livers stained with HE at the time of sacrifice; **d** Representative rat livers stained with Sirius Red (× 100) at the time of sacrifice

LWWL inhibited HSC activation in CCl₄-induced hepatic fibrosis in rats

HSCs have been recognized as the main matrix-producing cells during the process of liver fibrosis. α-SMA is a commonly used marker for the activated HSCs [16]. Collagen I is the prototype constituent of the fibril-forming matrix in fibrotic liver, and its expression is regulated by transcriptionally as described in several reviews [17, 18]. In this animal model, LWWL reduced liver injury, which is one potential mechanism by which fibrosis progression was inhibited. CCl₄ injury markedly increased the α-SMA and collagen I mRNA and protein levels. In contrast, LWWL treatment dramatically suppressed the messenger RNA (mRNA) expression of markers for HSC activation, such as α-SMA and collagen I, in a dose-dependent manner in CCl₄-injured fibrotic livers (Fig. 3a, c, d). In line with the former, the protein expression of α-SMA was significantly inhibited in the LWWL-treated rat livers (Fig. 3b).

LWWL inhibited the progression of profibrogenic factors and collagen deposition in CCl₄-induced hepatic fibrosis in rats

Several profibrogenic factors (e.g., TGF-β1 and PDGF) that bind to their cognate receptors on the HSC surface activate the corresponding signaling pathway, as well as the proliferation of HSCs, excessive ECM deposition, and hepatic fibrogenesis [19, 20]. The proliferation and activation of HSCs is critical during the process of liver fibrosis, and TGF-β1 and PDGF are the most effective factors that promote HSC proliferation and liver fibrosis. We observed that TGF-β1 expression normally increases over time in CCl₄-injured rats. We also observed a consistent increase in the expression of PDGF but a decrease in LWWL-treated livers (Fig. 4a, b). TIMPs are an important family of enzymes that regulate the activity of MMPs. TIMPs can inhibit the activity of MMPs and reduce ECM degradation, leading to liver fibrosis. TIMP-1 and TIMP-2 are mainly produced by HSCs and are upregulated in various human liver diseases [21]. TIMP-1 production can be attributed to activated HSCs [22]. Thus, TIMP-1 is a central molecule in liver fibrosis. In cultured liver cells, TIMP-2 mRNA expression has not been detected in native hepatocytes, but it has been detected in activated HSCs, Kupffer cells, and rat liver myofibroblasts [23]. In fibrogenesis, TIMP-2 mRNA expression is restricted to the early stages, during which a transient increase in TIMP-2 activates MMP-2, followed by the pericellular degradation of the normal liver matrix [24]. In this study, we assessed the TIMP1 and TIMP2 mRNA expression in CCl₄-injured livers, which was increased compared with that in the control. However, treatment with LWWL decreased TIMP mRNA levels in a dose-dependent manner in CCl₄-injured rats (Fig. 4c, d).

Discussion

Hepatic fibrosis results in severe hepatic injury following ECM accumulation. This phenomenon causes many chronic liver diseases, including chronic HCV and HBV infections, chronic alcoholic liver disease,

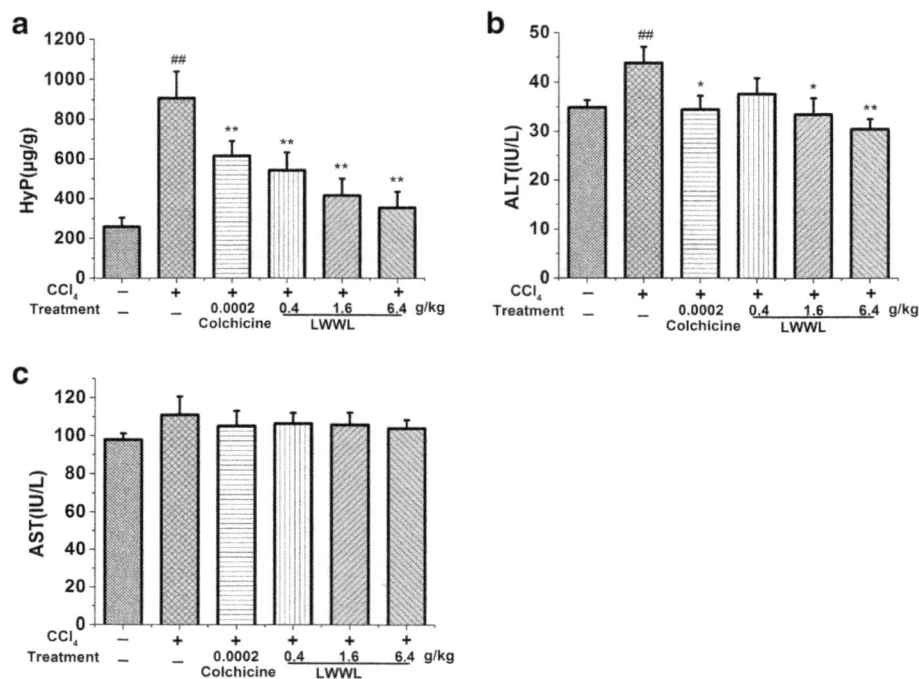

Fig. 2 LWWL attenuated liver function and the hydroxyproline content in rats. **a** Effect of LWWL on hydroxyproline levels in liver tissue; **b** Effect of LWWL on serum ALT levels; **c** Effect of LWWL on serum AST levels. ##$P < 0.01$ vs. normal group; *$P < 0.05$, **$P < 0.01$ vs. model group

and nonalcoholic steatohepatitis. These occurrences can lead to cirrhosis or hepatocellular carcinoma (HCC). Thus, preventing hepatic fibrosis represents an important strategy for the treatment of chronic liver disease. A variety of small molecules and biological agents are being developed to treat hepatic fibrosis [20]. However, several pathogenic mechanisms mediate hepatic fibrosis, and these agents have not yet been successfully employed in anti-hepatic fibrosis treatment regimens in a clinical setting. Many clinical and experimental studies have shown that TCMs are advantageous because they exert pharmacological effects by acting on multiple targets during the treatment of complex diseases [25, 26], which can delay or curb liver fibrosis and even cirrhosis. Their mechanism of action includes liver injury prevention, inhibition of ECM synthesis, activation of HSCs, and ECM degradation. Thus, TCMs with anti-liver fibrosis properties are becoming the focus of studies on the prevention and treatment of this disease [27–30].

LWWL, a Chinese medicinal formula, has historically been used to reduce ALT levels in patients with chronic hepatitis. Moreover, LWWL-specific adverse drug reactions have not yet been observed in a clinical setting. The present study investigated the herbal prescription LWWL, which exerts protective effects on the liver by reducing serum ALT levels. In the pharmacodynamic evaluation section of this study, LWWL did not significantly interfere with the level of AST in the serum of rats with CCl_4-induced hepatic fibrosis. The above results were repeated at least two times, and the error of detection could be eliminated as a cause. Some studies on anti-hepatic fibrosis exist, but only ALT data were available, and AST data did not appear [31, 32]. A possible reason for the above results is that the model is a classic model of hepatic fibrosis, but the modeling time is as long as 8 weeks. Therefore, it may be that long-term stimulation by CCl_4 is not sensitive to changes in AST. LWWL inhibited HSC activation associated with a reduction in the mRNA and protein levels of α-SMA. LWWL administration also markedly suppressed fibrotic pathological changes and elevated the hydroxyproline content in parallel with a reduction in the mRNA levels of collagen I in the liver treated with CCl_4. In fact, we gathered the protein expression of collagen I several times before; during the experiment, we changed to different antibodies, and the experimental conditions were constantly improved, but the band was blurred. Thus, the result was very difficult to determine, and the final data are not displayed. Because there is currently no reliable anti-hepatic fibrosis drug, it is difficult to determine which drug concentrations should be utilized for antifibrotic experiments. Upon designing this experiment, we decided to use colchicine as the positive control drug, but taking into account that the mechanism may be different from that of LWWL, it did not appear in the later data.

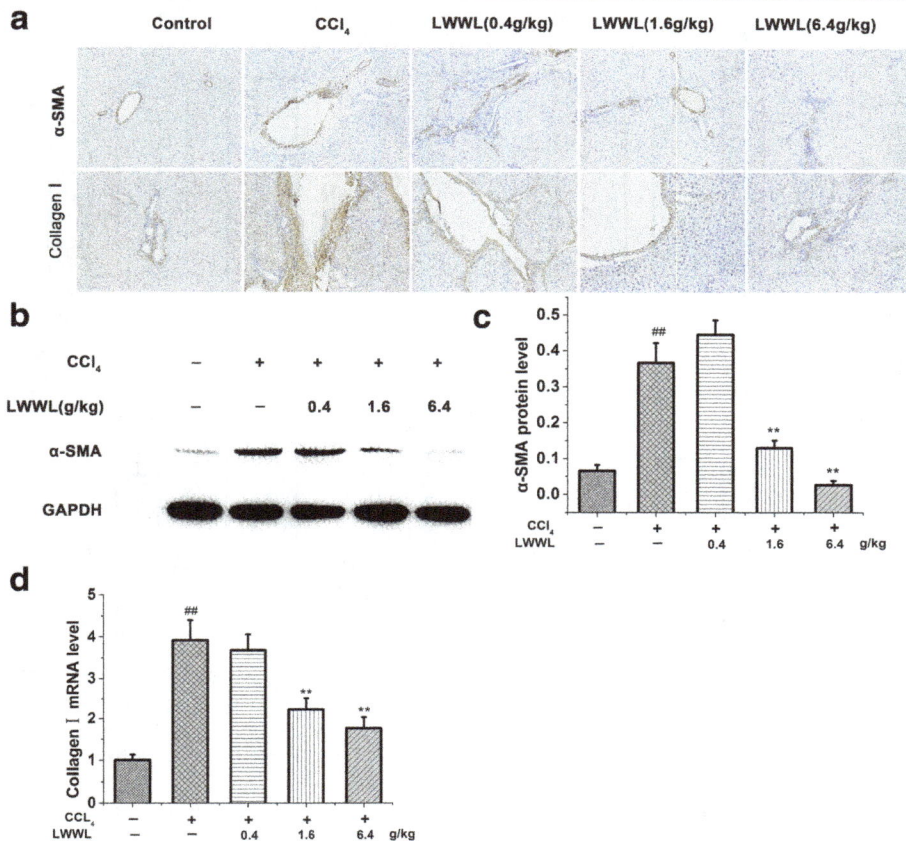

Fig. 3 LWWL inhibited HSCs activation in CCl4-induced hepatic fibrosis rats. **a** Immunohistochemical analysis of α-SMA and collagen I (× 200); **b** Western blot analysis of α-SMA; **c** Densitometry of α-SMA expression levels; **d** RT-PCR for collagen I. ##$P < 0.01$ vs. normal group; **$P < 0.01$ vs. model group

Activated HSCs proliferate and migrate to injured sites, secreting large amounts of ECM, which alters the normal architecture of the liver and initiates several positive feedback pathways that lead to liver fibrosis [33, 34]. Therefore, strategies to eliminate or normalize activated HSCs are critical for liver fibrosis therapy. Fibrotic pathologies are associated with increased levels of TGF-β1 that initially recruit inflammatory cells and fibroblasts into an area of injury and then stimulate these cells to produce cytokines and ECM [35]. TGF-β directly increases the synthesis of ECM components such as Collagen I. In addition, a significant increase in the TGF-β expression is observed in the activated HSCs and MFBs, thus indicating that TGF-β acts as an autocrine positive regulator for ECM production [36]. In the present study, LWWL markedly decreased the expression of TGF-β1 and PDGF in the livers of experimental rats after treatment with CCl4. TGF-β inhibits the expression of tissue collagenase, which is a specific enzyme for degradation of mammalian intestinal collagens, and enhances the production of inhibitors of such ECM-degrading enzymes as TIMPs [37]. In this respect, TIMPs are the main targets of

the TGF-β signaling pathway [38, 39]. LWWL caused significant reductions in TIMP-1 and TIMP-2 mRNA levels in CCl4-treated rats. Thus, decreasing TIMP-1 or TIMP-2 levels may lead to an increase in ECM degradation. In the present study, TGF-β1 mRNA expression was significantly inhibited by LWWL, which may be one mechanism by which TIMP expression is regulated. Because of their importance in fibrosis, TIMPs may represent an attractive therapeutic target. These results suggest that LWWL prevents hepatic fibrosis, at least in part, by negatively regulation of TGF-β signaling pathway to inhibit the activation and proliferation of HSCs. Salidroside is a phenolic glycoside and possesses various pharmacological properties which can isolated from *Fructus Ligustri Lucidi* in the herbal prescription LWWL. It's reported that treatment with salidroside can protects against bleomycin-induced pulmonary fibrosis via inhibition of NF-κB and TGF-β1/Smad-2/– 3 pathways [40]. Therefore, understanding the regulatory mechanisms of the TGF-β signal between physiologic and pathologic situations will be essential in the design of new therapeutic approaches for various diseases caused by a deregulation of the TGF-β signal. Thus,

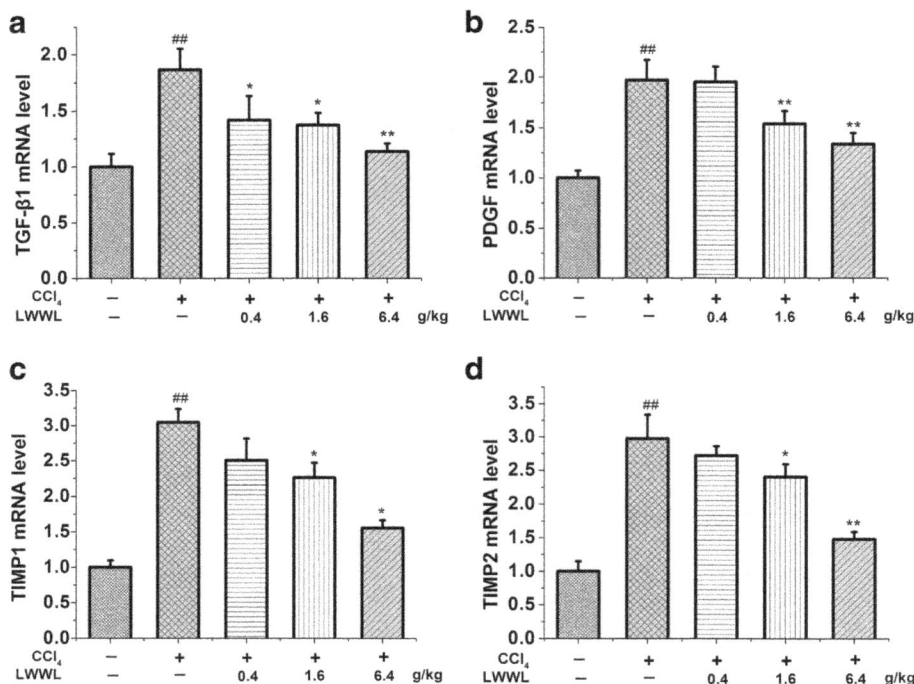

Fig. 4 LWWL inhibited the progression of profibrogenic factors and deposition of collagen in rats with CCl_4-induced hepatic fibrosis. **a** RT-PCR for TGF-β1; **b** RT-PCR for PDGF; **c** RT-PCR for TIMP1; **d** RT-PCR for TIMP2. ##$P < 0.01$ vs. normal group; *$P < 0.05$, **$P < 0.01$ vs. model group

antagonists of the TGF-β signal could be applied in liver fibrosis. If the active compounds are available to the public, our present knowledge base of the physiologic regulation in activated HSCs and pathologic deregulation in MFBs of autocrine TGF-β signal will help elucidate the clinical application of such drugs for liver fibrosis in the future.

Conclusions

In summary, we used the well-characterized CCl_4 rat model to examine the antifibrotic effects of LWWL. In the present study, LWWL attenuated CCl_4-induced liver fibrosis and improved liver function. The antifibrotic effects of LWWL were associated with its reduction of collagen synthesis, suppression of HSC activation, and promotion of ECM degradation. Taken together, the results of this study provide new opportunities for the use of LWWL in the treatment of liver fibrosis. However, the specific mechanism involved still needs to be determined.

Abbreviations

ALT: alanine transaminase; ANOVA: analysis of variance; AST: aspartate aminotransferase; BCA: bicinchoninic acid; CCl_4: carbon tetrachloride; cDNA: complementary DNA; CFDA: Chinese State Food and Drug Administration; collagen I: collagen type I; ECM: extracellular matrix; ELISA: enzyme-linked immunosorbent assay; FDA: food and Drug Administration; HE: hematoxylin and eosin; LWWL: Liuweiwuling tablets; MAPK/ERK: mitogen-activated protein kinase/extracellular signal-regulated kinase; MFB: myofibroblasts; MMPs: matrix metalloproteinases; PDGF: platelet-derived growth factor; RT-qPCR: real-time quantitative reverse-transcription polymerase chain reaction; TCM: traditional Chinese medicine; TGF-β1: transforming growth factor β1; TIMPs: tissue inhibitor of metalloproteinases; VEGF: vascular endothelial growth factor; α-SMA: α-smooth muscle actin

Acknowledgments
The authors thank the China Military Institute of Chinese Materia & Integrative Medical Center, 302 Military Hospital, for technical support.

Funding
This work was supported by the National Key Technology R&D Program (no. 2017ZX09301022) and the Key Research and Development Project of Shandong Province (2016ZDJQ0108).

Authors' contributions
XX, ZB, JW and HL participated in the research design; HL and ZB conducted the experiments; HL and CZ contributed new reagents or analytical tools and revised the manuscript; HL, RL and MN performed the data analysis; and HL, ZB and WH wrote or contributed to the writing of the manuscript. All authors read and approved the final manuscript.

Competing interests
The authors declare that they have no competing interests.

Author details

[1]Department of Pharmacy, 302 Hospital of People's Liberation Army, Beijing, People's Republic of China. [2]Animal Laboratory Center, 302 Hospital of People's Liberation Army, Beijing, People's Republic of China. [3]China Military Institute of Chinese Medicine, 302 Hospital of People's Liberation Army, Beijing, People's Republic of China.

References

1. Wree A, Eguchi A, Mcgeough MD, Pena CA, Johnson CD, Canbay A, et al. NLRP3 inflammasome activation results in hepatocyte pyroptosis, liver inflammation, and fibrosis in mice. Hepatology. 2014;59:898.
2. Lee UE, Friedman SL. Mechanisms of hepatic fibrogenesis. Best Pract Res Clin Gastroenterol. 2011;25:195–206.
3. Yang C, Zeisberg M, Mosterman B, Sudhakar A, Yerramalla U, Holthaus K, et al. Liver fibrosis: insights into migration of hepatic stellate cells in response to extracellular matrix and growth factors. Gastroenterology. 2003;124:147–59.
4. Hemmann S, Graf J, Roderfeld M, Roeb E. Expression of MMPs and TIMPs in liver fibrosis-a systematic review with special emphasis on anti-fibrotic strategies. J Hepatol. 2007;46:955–75.
5. Schuppan D, Ruehl M, Somasundaram R, Hahn EG. Matrix as a modulator of hepatic Fibrogenesis. Semin Liver Dis. 2001;21:351–72.
6. Heldin CH, Miyazono K, Ten DP. TGF-beta signalling from cell membrane to nucleus through SMAD proteins. Nature. 1997;390:465–71.
7. Liu B, Xuan Z, Zhang FC, Zong JB, Zhang W, Zhao Y. Aberrant TGF-β1 signaling contributes to the development of primary biliary cirrhosis in murine model. World J Gastroenterol. 2013;19:5828–36.
8. Han YP, Zhou L, Wang J, Xiong S, Garner WL, French SW, et al. Essential role of matrix metalloproteinases in interleukin-1-induced myofibroblastic activation of hepatic stellate cell in collagen. J Biol Chem. 2004;279:4820–8.
9. Mann DA, Marra F. Fibrogenic signalling in hepatic stellate cells. J Hepatol. 2010;52:949–50.
10. Adachi T, Togashi H, Suzuki A, Kasai S, Ito J, Sugahara K, et al. NAD (P) H oxidase plays a crucial role in PDGF-induced proliferation of hepatic stellate cells. Hepatology. 2005;41:1272–81.
11. Zhang DY, Friedman SL. Fibrosis-dependent mechanisms of Hepatocarcinogenesis. Hepatology. 2012;56:769–75.
12. Wu JL. Therapeutic effect of Liuweiwuling tablets on hepatic fibrosis. Chinese J Liver Dis. 2011;3:8–10.
13. Zhao SF, Kan QC. Protective effects of Liuweiwulingpian on hepatic fibrosis induced by carbon tetrachloride in rats. Chin Pharmacol Bull. 2011;27:872–5.
14. Poo JL, Feldmann G, Moreau A, Gaudin C, Lebrec D. Early colchicine administration reduces hepatic fibrosis and portal hypertension in rats with bile duct ligation. J Hepatol. 1993;19:90–4.
15. Nikolaidis N, Kountouras J, Giouleme O, Tzarou V, Chatzizisi O, et al. Colchicine treatment of liver fibrosis. Hepato-Gastroenterology. 2006;53:281–5.
16. Gressner AM, Weiskirchen R. Modern pathogenetic concepts of liver fibrosis suggest stellate cells and TGF-beta as major players and therapeutic targets. J Cell Mol Med. 2006;10:76–99.
17. Stefanovic B, Stefanovic L, Schnabl B. TRAM2 protein interacts with endoplasmic reticulum Ca2+ pump Serca2b and is necessary for collagen type I synthesis. Mol Cell Biol. 2004;24:1758–68.
18. Inagaki Y, Okazaki I. Emerging insights into transforming growth factor beta Smad signal in hepatic fibrogenesis. Gut. 2007;56:284–92.
19. Tahashi Y, Matsuzaki K, Date M, Yoshida K, Furukawa F, Sugano Y, et al. Differential regulation of TGF-beta signal in hepatic stellate cells between acute and chronic rat liver injury. Hepatology. 2002;35:49–61.
20. Fallowfield JA. Therapeutic targets in liver fibrosis. Am J Physiol Gastrointest Liver Physiol. 2011;300:G709–15.
21. Benyon RC, Iredale JP, Goddard S, Winwood PJ, Arthur MJ. Expression of tissue inhibitor of metalloproteinases 1 and 2 is increased in fibrotic human liver. Gastroenterology. 1996;110:821–31.
22. Iredale JP, Benyon RC, Arthur MJ, Ferris WF, Alcolado R, Winwood PJ, et al. Tissue inhibitor of metalloproteinase-1 messenger RNA expression is enhanced relative to interstitial collagenase messenger RNA in experimental liver injury and fibrosis. Hepatology. 1996;24:176–84.
23. Knittel T, Mehde M, Kobold D, Saile B, Dinter C, Ramadori G. Expression patterns of matrix metalloproteinases and their inhibitors in parenchymal and non-parenchymal cells of rat liver: regulation by TNF-alpha and TGF-beta1. J Hepatol. 1999;30:48–60.
24. Wang Z, Juttermann R, Soloway PD. TIMP-2 is required for efficient activation of proMMP-2 in vivo. J Biol Chem. 2000;275:26411–5.
25. Qian Q, Liu X, He W, An Y, Chen Q, Wu J, et al. TG accumulation inhibitory effects of Jinqi formula by AMPK signaling pathway. J Ethnopharmacol. 2012;143:41–8.
26. Du CY, Choi RC, Zheng KY, Dong TT, Lau DT, Tsim KW. Yu ping Feng san, an ancient Chinese herbal decoction containing Astragali Radix, Atractylodis Macrocephalae Rhizoma and Saposhnikoviae Radix, regulates the release of cytokines in murine macrophages. PLoS One. 2013;8:e78622.
27. Guo SG, Zhang W, Jiang T, Dai M, Zhang LF, Meng YC, et al. Influence of serum collected from rat perfused with compound Biejiaruangan drug on hepatic stellate cells. World J Gastroenterol. 2004;10:1487–94.
28. Wang QL, Yuan JL, Tao YY, Yue Z, Ping L, Liu CH. Fuzheng Huayu recipe and vitamin E reverse renal interstitial fibrosis through counteracting TGF-β1-induced epithelial-to-mesenchymal transition. J Ethnopharmacol. 2010; 127:631–40.
29. Yang MD, Chiang YM, Higashiyama R, Asahina K, Mann DA, Mann J, et al. Rosmarinic acid and baicalin epigenetically de-repress Pparγ in hepatic stellate cells for their anti-fibrotic effect. Hepatology. 2012;55:1271–81.
30. Zhang L, Schuppan D. Traditional Chinese medicine (TCM) for fibrotic liver disease: hope and hype. J Hepatol. 2014;61:166–8.
31. Tan Y, Lv ZP, Bai XC, Liu XY, Zhang XF. Traditional Chinese medicine Bao Gan Ning increase phosphorylation of CREB in liver fibrosis in vivo and in vitro. J Ethnopharmacol. 2006;105(1–2):69–75.
32. Hsieh CC, Fang HL, Lina WC. Inhibitory effect of Solanum nigrum on thioacetamide-induced liver fibrosis in mice. J Ethnopharmacol. 2008;119(1):117–21.
33. Thompson AI, Conroy KP, Henderson NC. Hepatic stellate cells: central modulators of hepatic carcinogenesis. BMC Gastroenterol. 2015;15:63.
34. Yang C, et al. Liver fibrosis: insights into migration of hepatic stellate cells in response to extracellular matrix and growth factors. Gastroenterology. 2003; 124:147–59.
35. Ogawa K, Chen F, Kuang C, Chen Y. Suppression of matrix metalloproteinase-9 transcription by transforming growth factor-b is mediated by a nuclear factor-kB site. Biochem J. 2004;381:413–22.
36. Bissell DM, Wang S-S, Jarnagin WR, Roll FJ. Cell-specific expression of transforming growth factor-b in rat liver. Evidence for autocrine regulation of hepatocyte proliferation. J Clin Invest. 1995;96:447–55.
37. Massague J. The transforming growth factor-b family. Annu Rev Cell Biol. 1990;6:597–641.
38. Yan C, Boyd DD. Regulation of matrix metalloproteinase gene expression. J Cell Physiol. 2007;211:299–356.
39. Krstic J, Santibanez JF. Transforming growth factor-beta and matrix metalloproteinases: functional interactions in tumor stroma-infiltrating myeloid cells. ScientificWorldJournal. 2014;2014:521754.
40. Tang H, Gao L, Mao J, He H, Liu J, Cai X, Lin H, Wu T. Salidroside protects against bleomycin-induced pulmonary fibrosis: activation of Nrf2-antioxidant signaling, and inhibition of NF-κB and TGF-β1/Smad-2/−3 pathways. Cell Stress Chaperones. 2016;21:239–49.

11

Cytotoxic properties of the anthraquinone derivatives isolated from the roots of *Rubia philippinensis*

Vivek K. Bajpai[1]📷, Md Badrul Alam[2,3], Khong Trong Quan[4], Hee-Jeong Choi[2], Hongyan An[2], Mi-Kyoung Ju[2], Sang-Han Lee[2,3*], Yun Suk Huh[5], Young-Kyu Han[1*] and MinKyun Na[4*]

Abstract

Background: Cancer is one of the most frequently occurring diseases and is the second leading cause of death worldwide. In this study, anthraquinone derivatives (Compounds 1–5) were evaluated for their anti-cancer potential against various skin and breast cancer cell lines to assess whether these anthraquinone derivatives may serve as a lead for the augmentation of anti-cancer drug.

Methods: Anthraquinone derivatives, 2-methyl-1,3,6-trihydroxy-9,10-anthraquinone-3-O-(6′-O-acetyl)-α-rhamnosyl(1 → 2)-β-glucoside (Comp 1), 2-methyl-1,3,6-trihydroxy-9,10-anthraquinone (Comp 2), and alizarin (Comp 3) were isolated from the dichloromethane fraction of the roots of *Rubia philippinensis*., whereas ethyl acetate fraction yielded xanthopurpurin (Comp 4) and lucidin-ω-methyl ether (Comp 5). Structures of all the isolated compounds were determined by spectral data analysis. All isolated compounds (Comp 1–5) were assessed for cytotoxicity by the 3-(4,5-dimethylthiazol-2-yl)-2,5-diphenyltetrazolium bromide (MTT) assay against four different cancer cell lines, i.e. human melanoma (SK-MEL-5), murine melanoma (B16F10), and human breast adenocarcinoma (MCF7 and MDA-MB-231).

Results: Significant activity of the compounds 4 and 5 was observed against the breast cancer cell line MDA-MB-231 with IC_{50} values of 14.65 ± 1.45 and 13.03 ± 0.33 μM, respectively. Encouragingly, IC_{50} values of 67.89 ± 1.02 and 79.01 ± 0.03 μM against normal kidney epithelial cells (MDCK) were also obtained for compounds 4 and 5, respectively, which indicated very low toxicity and favorable selectivity indices for compounds 4 and 5 in the range of 1.85 to 3.95 and 2. 11 to 6.06 against skin cancer cell lines (SK-MEL-5, and B16F10), and breast cancer cell lines (MCF7 and MDA-MB-231), respectively.

Conclusion: Our results suggested that the compounds 4 (xanthopurpurin) and 5 (lucidin-ω-methyl ether) showed high selective toxicity towards breast cancer cells at lower concentrations without showing toxicity towards normal cells, thus could be of potential as new lead molecules in cancer treatment.

Keywords: *Rubia philippinensis*, Anthraquinone, Cytotoxicity, Breast cancer, Skin cancer

Background

Cancer is one of the most frequently occurring diseases and is the second leading cause of death worldwide, while chemotherapy is most extensively used among a wide range of anti-cancer therapies, and its high toxicity, being expensive as well as activating alternative cell signaling pathways are limiting its applications [1]. For centuries to date, being safe, low cost and easily accessible, medicinal herbs are viewed as the main sources of new drugs to treat cancer worldwide while various pharmacological studies continue to validate their uses [1]. Moreover, herbal medicines are widely assumed in complementary and alternative medicine especially in cancer patients with poor socioeconomic condition. Mounting evidences suggest that plants possessing anticancer properties, such as *Soymida fembrifuga*

---

* Correspondence: sang@knu.ac.kr; ykenergy@dongguk.edu; mkna@cnu.ac.kr
[2]Department of Food Science and Biotechnology, Graduate School, Kyungpook National University, Daegu 41566, Republic of Korea
[1]Department of Energy and Materials Engineering, Dongguk University-Seoul, Seoul 04620, Republic of Korea
[4]College of Pharmacy, Chungnam National University, Daejeon 34134, Republic of Korea
Full list of author information is available at the end of the article

(Miliaceae), *Tinospora cordifolia* (Menispermaceae), *Lavandula bipinnata* (Lamiaceae), *Helicteres isora* (Sterculiaceae), *Urtica membranacea* (Urticaceae), *Artemesia monosperma* (Asteraceae), and *Origanum dayi post* (Labiatae) etc., are the source of alternative medicine for cancer therapy in various regions of the globe [2–4]. However, a large number of plant species remain to be screened for their therapeutic potential; consequently, they can be used as a continual source of new medicines for present and future health problems of humans, including cancer.

Rubia philippinensis is a rambling and low climbing perennial herb that grows in the Southern part of Vietnam. Local communities have long utilized this medicinal plant to treat ordinary ailments such as wounds, inflammation, and skin infections. Previous investigations of the species have resulted in the purification of arborinane triterpenoids, which show promising effects on the prevention and treatment of atherosclerosis [5]. Additionally, rubiarbonone C, a popular chemical entity isolated from *R. philippinensis*, has been shown to inhibit abnormal proliferation and migration of vascular smooth muscle cells, which plays an important role in the pathophysiology of atherosclerosis. The mechanism by which rubiarbonone C regulates vascular remodeling was further clarified through focal adhesion kinase (FAK), MAPK, and STAT3 Tyr705 [6]. In searching for bioactive components from *R. philippinensis*, in this study, derivatives of anthraquinone were isolated as the major compounds.

Anthraquinones possessing three benzene rings represent a class of compounds belonging to quinone family. The divergence of the anthraquinone molecules relies on the nature and the setting of the substituents. Anthraquinones display a number of biological functions, including laxative [7], diuretic [8], phytoestrogen [9], anti-platelet [10], anti-fungal [11], anti-viral [12], and anti-cancer properties [13]. Moreover, they have a significant industrial potential of being used as textile dyes, food colorants and bugs repellents.

As a part of continuous attempts to probe the potential nature-derived drug templates for the treatment of cancer [5, 14], the current study delineates the isolation and characterization of five anthraquinone derivatives (compound 1–5) from *R. philippinensis*. These compounds were evaluated for their anti-cancer potential against various skin cancer cells (SK-MEL-5 and B16F10) and breast cancer cells (MCF7 and MDA-MB-231) to assess whether these anthraquinone derivatives may serve as a lead for the development of anti-cancer drugs.

Methods

Plant materials

Root samples of *Rubia philippinensis* were procured from Bidoup-Nui Ba National Park, Lamdong province, Vietnam and identified by the expert Dr. Phuong Thien Thuong at the Department of Pharmaceutical Analysis and Herbal Standardization, NIMM, Hanoi, Vietnam. An authenticated root voucher sample was deposited at the laboratory of the NIMM (VDL20140801) and at the Pharmacognosy Laboratory, College of Pharmacy, Chungnam National University (CNU1409), Daejeon, Korea.

Extraction, isolation, and characterization of anthraquinone derivatives

Anthraquinones were isolated from the root samples of *R. philippinensis* by chromatographic techniques. In brief, the ethanol extract of *R. philippinensis* (150 g) was suspended in H_2O (1.5 L) and sequentially partitioned with CH_2Cl_2 (2 L × 3) and EtOAc (2 L × 3) to yield the CH_2Cl_2 and EtOAc extracts. The CH_2Cl_2-soluble fraction (50 g) was loaded into silica gel VLC and eluted with *n*-hexane-EtOAc (20:1, 10:1, 5:1, 3:1, 2:1) and $CHCl_3$-MeOH (8:1) to afford six fractions (D-1 → D-6). Fraction D-4 (6.1 g) was divided into 10 sub-fractions (D-4-1 → D-4-10) using MPLC with a step-wise gradient of Acetone-H_2O (60:40, 72:28, 75:25, 95:5, 100:0, each 1.5 L). Xanthopurpurin (4) (t_R 33.5 min, 28 mg) and lucidin-ω-methyl ether (5) (t_R 36.0 min, 31 mg) were obtained from D-4-4 (320 mg) by HPLC eluting with MeCN-H_2O (54.5:45.5, 4 mL/min, UV 360 nm). The EtOAc fraction (14.0 g) was subjected to silica gel VLC and eluted with *n*-hexane/ EtOAc/MeOH (2:1:0.2) and $CHCl_3$-MeOH (8:1, 5:1, 3:1, 0:1) to yield five fractions (EA-1 → EA-5). Eight sub-fractions (EA-1-1 → EA-1-8) were collected from fraction EA-1 (1.8 g) by utilizing MPLC, eluting with MeOH-H_2O (10:90, 50:50, 67:33, 80:20, 100:0, each 500 mL). Alizarin (3) (t_R 44.0 min, 2 mg) was isolated from EA-1-5 (100 mg) by HPLC eluting with MeCN-H_2O (44.5:55.5, 4 mL/min, UV 360 nm). Two sub-fractions EA-1-6 and EA-1-7 were combined (EA-1-6,7; 500 mg), then purified one more time by MPLC, eluted with Acetone-H_2O (40:60, 60:40, 100:0, each 500 mL) to afford 2-methyl-1,3,6-trihydroxy-9,10-anthraquinone (2) as orange crystals (200 mg). Fraction EA-4 (2.6 g) was separated by MPLC applying mixtures of solvent MeOH-H_2O (23:77, 37:63, 47:53, 52:48, 60:40, 67:33, 100:0, each 400 mL) to yield 11 sub-fractions (EA-4-1 → EA-4-11). 2-methyl-1,3,6-trihydroxy-9,10-anthraquinone-3-*O*-(6'-*O*-acetyl)-α-rhamnosyl(1 → 2)-β-glucoside (1) (t_R 40 min, 800 mg) was purified from sub-fractions EA-4-8 (706 mg) and EA-4-9 (410 mg) by HPLC utilizing MeOH-H_2O (65:35, 6 mL/min, UV 254 nm).

2-methyl-1,3,6-trihydroxy-9,10-anthraquinone-3-*O*-(6'-*O*-acetyl)-α-rhamnosyl(1 → 2)-β-glucoside (1): yellow powder, ^1H NMR (300 MHz, DMSO-d_6): δ_H 13.28 (1H, s, OH-1), 8.08 (1H, d, *J* = 8.4 Hz, H-8), 7.45 (1H, d, *J* = 2.4 Hz, H-5), 7.40 (1H, s, H-4), 7.20 (1H, dd, *J* = 8.4, 2.4 Hz, H-7), 5.45 (1H, d, *J* = 6.9 Hz, Glu-H-1'), 5.28 (1H, d, *J* = 0.9 Hz, Rha-H-1''), 2.15 (3H, s, CH_3–2), 1.93 (3H, s, OAc-6'), 1.09

(3H, d, $J = 6.3$ Hz, Rha-CH$_3$–6″). ^{13}C NMR (150 MHz, DMSO-d_6) δ_C *Aglycone*: 164.2 (C-1), 120.5 (C-2), 160.0 (C-3), 105.2 (C-4), 135.4 (C-4a), 112.8 (C-5), 161.3 (C-6), 121.6 (C-7), 129.7 (C-8), 124.1 (C-8a), 186.3 (C-9), 110.7 (C-9a), 181.8 (C-10), 131.9 (C-10a), 8.7 (CH$_3$–2). *Glucose*: 97.3 (C-1′), 76.3 (C-2′), 77.0 (C-3′), 70.0 (C-4′), 74.0 (C-5′), 63.3 (C-6′), 170.3 (OAc-6′), 20.4 (OAc-6″). *Rhamnose*: 100.2 (C-1″), 70.3 (C-2″), 70.5 (C-3″), 72.0 (C-4″), 68.5 (C-5″), 18.1 (C-6″).

2-methyl-1,3,6-trihydroxy-9,10-anthraquinone (**2**): orange crystal, ^{1}H NMR (300 MHz, DMSO-d_6): δ_H 13.31 (1H, s, OH-1), 8.05 (1H, d, $J = 8.4$ Hz, H-8), 7.43 (1H, d, $J = 2.4$ Hz, H-5), 7.20 (1H, s, H-4), 7.20 (1H, dd, $J = 8.4, 2.4$ Hz, H-7), 2.05 (3H, s, CH$_3$–2). ^{13}C NMR (75 MHz, DMSO-d_6) δ_C 162.3 (C-1), 117.4 (C-2), 163.1 (C-3), 107.1 (C-4), 135.2 (C-4a), 112.5 (C-5), 162.1 (C-6), 121.3 (C-7), 129.4 (C-8), 124.7 (C-8a), 185.8 (C-9), 108.6 (C-9a), 182.0 (C-10), 131.8 (C-10a), 8.1 (CH$_3$–2).

Alizarin (**3**): brownish red powder, ^{1}H NMR (300 MHz, DMSO-d_6) δ_H 7.51 (1H, d, $J = 8.1$, H-4), 7.18 (1H, d, $J = 8.1$, H-3). ^{13}C NMR (150 MHz, DMSO-d_6) δ_C 151.0 (C-1), 153.3 (C-2), 120.8 (C-3), 121.3 (C-4), 126.5 (C-5), 134.0 (C-6), 135.1 (C-7), 126.7 (C-8), 188.8 (C-9), 180.5 (C-10), 123.5 (C-4a), 132.9 (C-10a), 133.7 (C-8a), 116.2 (C-9a).

Xanthopurpurin (**4**): orange powder, ^{1}H NMR (300 MHz, DMSO-d_6) δ_H 7.79 (1H, d, $J = 2.1$, H-4), 7.27 (1H, d, $J = 2.1$, H-3). ^{13}C NMR (75 MHz, DMSO-d_6) δ_C 164.7 (C-1), 107.6 (C-2), 165.5 (C-3), 108.4 (C-4), 126.7 (C-5), 134.5 (C-6), 134.3 (C-7), 126.2 (C-8), 185.6 (C-9), 181.6 (C-10), 134.7 (C-4a), 132.7 (C-10a), 132.8 (C-8a), 109.1 (C-9a).

Lucidin-ω-methyl ether (**5**): orange powder, ^{1}H NMR (300 MHz, CDCl$_3$) δ_H 13.24 (1H, s, OH-1), 4.89 (2H, s, CH$_2$OCH$_3$–2), 3.55 (3H, s, CH$_2$OCH$_3$–2). ^{13}C NMR (75 MHz, CDCl$_3$) δ_C 162.0 (C-1), 114.5 (C-2), 164.2 (C-3), 109.7 (C-4), 127.5 (C-5), 134.3 (C-6), 134.2 (C-7), 126.8 (C-8), 187.0 (C-9), 182.3 (C-10), 133.6 (C-4a), 134.2 (C-10a), 133.6 (C-8a), 109.9 (C-9a), 69.0 (CH$_2$OCH$_3$–2), 59.5 (CH$_2$OCH$_3$–2).

Cell culture and cell viability assay

The potential cytotoxicity of the isolated anthraquinone derivatives was studied against various cancer cell lines, including SK-MEL-5 (human melanoma), B16F10 (murine melanoma) MCF7 (human breast adenocarcinoma), and MDA-MB-231 (human breast adenocarcinoma) and the normal cell line MDCK (normal kidney epithelial) using the MTT assay [15]. All cell lines were cultured in DMEM medium supplemented with 10% foetal bovine serum (FBS) and streptomycin–penicillin (100 µg/ml each; Hyclone) in a 5% CO_2 humidified incubator. An MTT assay was employed to determine the percentage of the viability of various cancer cells as well as MDCK cells. All cells were first cultured in 96-well plates (1×10^5 cells/mL for all cancerous cells and 5×10^5 cells/mL for MDCK cells) for 24 h,

and treated with indicated concentration of isolated compounds (6.25–100 µM for cancerous cells and 6.25–400 µM for MDCK cells). Various dilutions of stock culture were made in the culture medium to get the final concentration of the sample with a 0.1% of DMSO concentration, including the control. After 24 h incubation, MTT reagent was added to each well and the plate was incubated at 37 °C for 1 h. After removing the medium, the plate was washed twice with PBS (pH 7.4). The intracellular insoluble formazan was dissolved in 100% DMSO. A microplate reader was used to measure the absorbance of each cell line at 570 nm, and the percentage of cell viability was calculated. The absorbance value for the average of wells of cells treated with each test sample concentration was expressed as a percentage of this control and the IC$_{50}$ values for each sample on each cell line were calculated. The anti-cancer drug oxaloplatin was used as a positive control.

Statistical analysis

All the results were presented as the mean ± SD following the analysis of one-way ANOVA. A value of $p < 0.05$ was recognized as significant for the differences. An SPSS version of Windows' (Chicago, Illinois, USA) was performed for all the analyses.

Results

Identification and characterization of anthraquinone derivatives (Fig. 1)

The ^{1}H NMR data of compound 1 displayed signals of the anthraquinone aglycone, including one aromatic singlet proton δ_H 7.40 (1H, s, H-4), one ABX ring system δ_H 8.08 (1H, d, $J = 8.4$ Hz, H-8), 7.45 (1H, d, $J = 2.4$ Hz, H-5), 7.20 (1H, dd, $J = 8.4, 2.4$ Hz, H-7), and one singlet methyl δ_H 2.15. The glycosidic linkage, meanwhile, contained resonances of two anomeric protons of the sugar moiety at δ_H 5.45 (glucose), δ_H 5.28 (rhamnose), one secondary methyl (δ_H 1.09, rhamnose), and one acetyl group (δ_H 1.93). The ^{13}C NMR data showed 14 signals of a typical anthraquinone, including two ketones (δ_C 186.3, 181.8), and resonances for glucose (δ_C 97.3, 76.3, 77.0, 70.0, 74.0, 63.3), acetoxy (δ_C 170.3, 20.4), and rhamnose (δ_C 100.2, 70.3, 70.5, 72.0, 68.5, 18.1) moieties. On the basis of NMR spectroscopic data analyses, the compound was identified as 2-methyl-1,3,6-trihydroxy-9,10-anthraquinone-3-O-(6′-O-acetyl)-α-rhamnosyl(1 → 2)-β-glucoside.

Similar to compound 1, compound 2 also showed resonances of one aromatic singlet proton, one ABX ring system, and one singlet methyl at δ_H 7.20 (1H, s, H-4); [δ_H 8.05 (1H, d, $J = 8.4$ Hz, H-8; 7.43 (1H, d, $J = 2.4$ Hz, H-5; 7.20 (1H, dd, $J = 8.4, 2.4$ Hz, H-7)]; and δ_H 2.05 (3H, s, CH$_3$–2), respectively in ^{1}H NMR spectrum. On the other hand, the skeleton of 14 carbon signals along with two ketonic carbonyls (δ_C 185.8, 182.0) and one methyl functionality (δ_C 8.1) was representative of ^{13}C NMR data of an

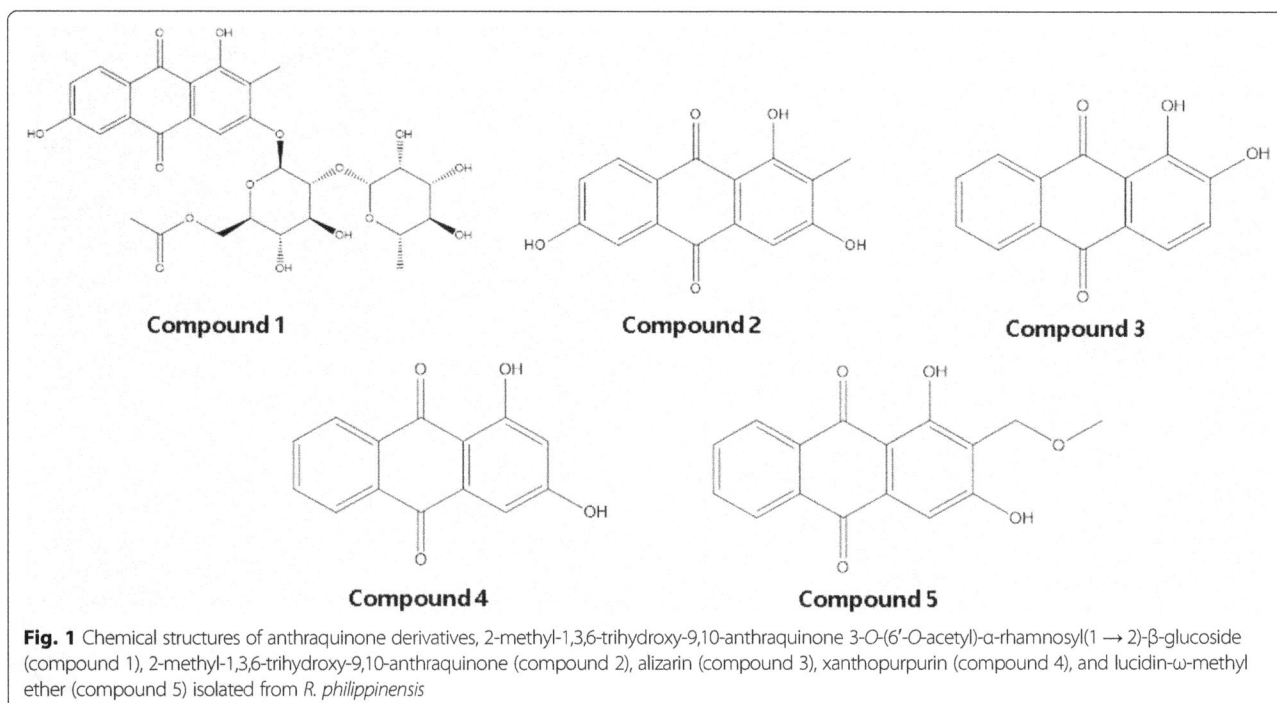

Fig. 1 Chemical structures of anthraquinone derivatives, 2-methyl-1,3,6-trihydroxy-9,10-anthraquinone 3-O-(6'-O-acetyl)-α-rhamnosyl(1 → 2)-β-glucoside (compound 1), 2-methyl-1,3,6-trihydroxy-9,10-anthraquinone (compound 2), alizarin (compound 3), xanthopurpurin (compound 4), and lucidin-ω-methyl ether (compound 5) isolated from *R. philippinensis*

anthraquinone. The 1D NMR of compound 2 resemble closely to those of compound 1, except for the absence of signals belonging to sugar units. In comparison with reference values, compound 2 was determined as 2-methyl-1,3,6-trihydroxy-9,10-anthraquinone. Compound 3, 4, and 5 are also anthraquinone derivatives and their structures were elucidated as alizarin, xanthopurpurin, and lucidin-ω-methyl ether, respectively, based on the NMR data analysis. NMR data of all anthraquinone has been provided in Additional file 1: Figures S1-S5).

Cytotoxicity of anthraquinone derivatives

All compounds were tested for cytotoxicity by MTT assay on cell lines SK-MEL-5, B16F10, MCF7, MDA-MB-231, and MDCK cells as a normal cell line, which showed significant cytotoxicity (Table 1, Additional file 1: Figures S6-S10). Our results showed that the IC_{50} values for cancer cell lines treated ranged from 48.68 ± 0.10 to 91.04 ± 1.88 μM for compound 1; 46.75 ± 1.39 to 79.96 ± 1.14 μM for compound 2; 48.64 ± 0.33 to 98.79 ± 2.10 μM for compound 3, 14.65 ± 1.45 to 23.71 ± 1.71 μM for compound 4, and 13.03 ± 0.33 to 42.79 ± 1.32 μM for compound 5. Regarding the normal cell line MDCK cells, the IC_{50} values were 192.34 ± 0.49, 168.76 ± 0.61, 199.32 ± 1.88, 67.89 ± 1.02 and 79.01 ± 0.03 μM for compounds 1, 2, 3, 4, and 5, respectively. Interestingly, among all the compounds, compounds 4 and 5 showed strong cytotoxicity towards breast cancer cells (MCF7 and MDA-MB-231) than skin cancer cells (SK-MEL-5 and B16F10) with IC_{50} value of 15.75 ± 1.00 and 24.10 ± 1.06 for MCF7 as well as 14.65 ± 1.45 and 13.03 ± 0.33 for MDA-MB-231, respectively.

Table 1 IC_{50} values of anthraquinone derivatives (compound 1–5) on various skin cancer cells (SK-MEL5 and B16F10) and breast cancer cells (MCF7 and MBA-MD-231)

Compounds	IC_{50} (μM)[a]				
	SK-MEL-5	B16F10	MCF7	MDA-MB-231	MDCK
1	91.04 ± 1.88	48.68 ± 0.10	65.48 ± 1.10	49.44 ± 0.78	192.34 ± 0.49
2	46.75 ± 1.39	77.88 ± 0.34	79.96 ± 1.14	59.22 ± 0.40	168.76 ± 0.61
3	53.08 ± 0.30	98.79 ± 2.10	49.17 ± 0.85	48.64 ± 0.33	199.32 ± 1.88
4	21.35 ± 0.99	23.71 ± 1.71	15.75 ± 1.00	14.65 ± 1.45	67.89 ± 1.02
5	42.79 ± 1.32	29.48 ± 2.61	24.10 ± 1.06	13.03 ± 0.33	79.01 ± 0.03
Oxaloplatin	14.25 ± 1.02	10.51 ± 0.92	8.59 ± 1.22	7.95 ± 1.92	24.02 ± 1.04

[a]The values are mean ± standard deviation. IC_{50} (concentration inhibiting 50% growth). SK-MEL-5 (human melanoma); B16F10 (murine melanoma); MCF-7 (human breast adenocarcinoma); MDA-MB-231 (human breast adenocarcinoma), MDCK (normal kidney epithelial cells)

In addition, compound 4 and 5 were more cytotoxic to MDA-MB-231 cancer cell line (IC_{50} = 14.65 ± 1.45 and 13.03 ± 0.33 μM, respectively) than to normal cells (IC_{50} = 67.89 ± 1.02 and 79.01 ± 0.03 μM (Table 1), respectively with their respective selectivity indices of 4.63 and 6.06 (Table 2).

Table 2 shows the selectivity indices of the isolated compounds tested against the various cancer cell lines and the non-tumor cell line (MDCK). In the current study, treatments with compound 4 and 5 afforded the highest selectivity indices in breast cancer cell than skin cancer cells. Compound 4 showed the selectivity indices as 4.31 and 4.63 whereas compound 5 showed 3.28 and 6.06 in MCF7 and MDA-MB-231 cells, respectively (Table 2).

Discussion

A number of natural compounds have been isolated from different plant sources which have shown enormous biological potential [16–19]. In this study, five anthraquinone derivatives, such as 2-methyl-1,3,6-trihydroxy-9,10-anthraquinone 3-O-(6'-O-acetyl)-α-rhamnosyl(1 → 2)-β-glucoside (compound 1), 2-methyl-1,3,6-trihydroxy-9,10-anthraquinone (compound 2), alizarin (compound 3), xanthopurpurin (compound 4), and lucidin-ω-methyl ether (compound 5) were isolated from the root of *R. philippinensis.*, and were characterized based on the spectral data analysis [16–19].

These anthraquinone derivatives showed significant anticancer potential as confirmed by their cytotoxicity effects against various cancer cell lines, such as cell lines SK-MEL-5, B16F10, MCF7, MDA-MB-231, including normal MDCK cell line. However, according to American National Center Institute, extract/compounds with IC_{50} values lower than 30 μM against experimental cancer cell lines constitute promising anticancer agents for drug development [20]. Therefore, compound 4 and 5 showed IC_{50} values greater than 30 μM against all cell lines tested, and were more cytotoxic to normal line to which the cancer cell lines. Moreover, among the testest compounds,

anthraquinone derivatives xanthopurpurin (compound 4), and lucidin-ω-methyl ether (compound 5) showed highest selectivity indices in breast cancer cell than skin cancer cells.

Mounting evidences have considered that a value greater than or equals to 2.0 is an interesting selectivity index [21]. This value means that the compound is more than twice more cytotoxic to the cancer cell line as compared with the normal cell line [21]. These findings demonstrated that compound 4 and 5 can be considered promising lead molecules for the development of anticancer drugs, especially for breast cancer, because they provided indices value greater than 2.

Conclusions

It is very important to consider natural compounds as a chemotherapeutic agent for cancer which have minimum or no side effects on normal body cells of patients. To achieve this goal among various ways, one of the way is by employing lower doses of drug at which drug shows highly potent activity as well as exhibits high degree of selectivity. In this study, we presented the cytotoxicity potential of five anthraquinone derivatives isolated from the roots of *Rubia philippinensis*. The results of in vitro studies demonstrate the ability of the compounds 4 (xanthopurpurin) and 5 (lucidin-ω-methyl ether) for high selective toxicity at lower concentrations (Table 1) without showing toxicity towards normal cells, confirming that compounds 4 and 5 may have the potentiality to be developed as anticancer drugs, especially for breast cancer. Further research strategies should investigate cytotoxic potential of compound 4 and 5 against multifactorial drug-resistant cancers for their pharmaceutical formulations.

Abbreviations
ANOVA: Analysis of variance; DMEM: Dulbecco"s Modified Eagle"s Medium; DMSO: Dimethyl sulfoxide; FAK: Focal adhesion kinase; FBS: Foetal bovine serum; HPLC: High-performance liquid chromatography; MAPK: Mitogen-activated protein kinase; MPLC: Medium pressure liquid chromatography; MTT: 3-(4,5-dimethylthiazol-2-yl)-2,5-diphenyltetrazolium bromide; NMR: Nuclear magnetic resonance; SD: Standard deviation; UV: Ultraviolet; VLC: Vacuum liquid chromatography

Acknowledgements
This study was supported by the research fund of Chungnam National University.

Authors' contributions
Designed the experiments: VKB, MBA, KTQ, HJC. Performed the experiments: MBA, KTQ, HA, MKJ. Analyzed the data: VKB, MBA, SHL, YKH, MN. Conception and design, analysis and interpretation of data, and contribution of reagents/materials/analysis tools: MKN, SHL. Manuscript preparation and revision: VKB, MBA, YKH, MN. All authors have approved the final draft of the manuscript.

Table 2 Selectivity of the cytotoxicity of anthraquinone derivatives (compound 1–5) to various cancer cells as compared with MDCK cells

Compounds	IC_{50} (μM)[a]			
	SK-MEL-5	B16F10	MCF7	MDA-MB-231
1	2.11	3.95	2.94	3.89
2	3.61	2.17	2.11	2.85
3	3.76	2.02	4.05	4.10
4	3.18	2.86	4.31	4.63
5	1.85	2.68	3.28	6.06

[a]The selectivity index is the ratio of the IC_{50} values of the treatments on MDCK cells to those in the cancer cell lines. SK-MEL-5 (human melanoma); B16F10 (murine melanoma); MCF-7 (human breast adenocarcinoma); MDA-MB-231 (human breast adenocarcinoma)

Competing interests
The authors declare that they have no competing interests.

Author details
[1]Department of Energy and Materials Engineering, Dongguk University-Seoul, Seoul 04620, Republic of Korea. [2]Department of Food Science and Biotechnology, Graduate School, Kyungpook National University, Daegu 41566, Republic of Korea. [3]Food and Bio-Industry Research Institute, Kyungpook National University, Daegu 41566, Republic of Korea. [4]College of Pharmacy, Chungnam National University, Daejeon 34134, Republic of Korea. [5]Department of Biological Engineering, Biohybrid Systems Research Center (BSRC), Inha University, 100 Inha-ro, Nam-gu, Incheon 22212, Republic of Korea.

References
1. El-Kashak WA, Osman SM, Gaara AH, El-Toumy SA, Mohamed TK, Brouard I, et al. Phenolic metabolites, biological activities, and isolated compounds of Terminalia muelleri extract. Pharm Biol. 2017;55:2277–84.
2. Graham JG, Quinn ML, Fabricant DS, Farnsworth NR. Plants used against cancer - an extension of the work of Jonathan Hartwell. J Ethnopharmacol. 2000;73:347–77.
3. Solowey E, Lichtenstein M, Sallon S, Paavilainen H, Solowey E, Lorberboum-Galaski H, et al. Evaluating medicinal plants for anticancer activity. Sci World J. 2014;2014:e721402.
4. Shaikh R, Pund M, Dawane A, Iliyas S. Evolution of anticancer, antioxidant, and possible anti-inflammatory properties of selected medicinal plants used in Indian traditional medication. J Tradit Complement Med. 2014;4:253–7.
5. Quan KT, Park HS, Oh J, Park HB, Ferreira D, Myung CS, Na M, et al. Arborinane triterpenoids from Rubia philippinensis inhibit proliferation and migration of vascular smooth muscle cells induced by the platelet-derived growth factor. J Nat Prod. 2016;79:2559–69.
6. Park HS, Quan KT, Han JH, Jung SH, Lee DH, Jo E, et al. Rubiarbonone C inhibits platelet-derived growth factor-induced proliferation and migration of vascular smooth muscle cells through the focal adhesion kinase, MAPK and STAT3 Tyr705 signaling pathways. Br J Pharmacol. 2017;174:4140–54.
7. Sakulpanich A, Gritsanapan W. Determination of anthraquinone glycoside content in Cassia fistula leaf extracts for alternative source of laxative drug. Int J Biomed Pharm Sci. 2009;3:42–5.
8. Zhou XM, Chen QH. Biochemical study of Chinese rhubarb. XXII. Inhibitory effect of anthraquinone derivatives on Na+-K+-ATPase of the rabbit renal medulla and their diuretic action. Acta Pharm Sin. 1988;23:17–20.
9. Matsuda H, Shimoda H, Morikawa T, Yoshikawa M. Phytoestrogens from the roots of Polygonum cuspidatum (Polygonaceae): structure-requirement of hydroxyanthraquinones for estrogenic activity. Bioorg Med Lett. 2001;11:1839–42.
10. Aburjai TA. Anti-platelet stilbenes from aerial parts of Rheum palaestinum. Phytochemistry. 2000;55(5):407–10.
11. Agarwal SK, Singh SS, Verma S, Kumar S. Antifungal activity of anthraquinone derivatives from Rheum emodi. J Ethnopharmacol. 2000;72:43–6.
12. Semple SJ, Pyke SM, Reynolds GD, Flower RL. In vitro antiviral activity of the anthraquinone chrysophanic acid against poliovirus. Antivir Res. 2001;49:169–78.
13. Nemeikaite-Ceniene A, Sergediene E, Nivinskas H, Cenas N. Cytotoxicity of natural hydroxyanthraquinones: role of oxidative stress. J Biosci. 2002;57:822–7.
14. Alam MB, Bajpai VK, Lee J, Zhao P, Byeon JH, Ra JS, et al. Inhibition of melanogenesis by jineol from Scolopendra subspinipes mutilans via MAP-kinase mediated MITF downregulation and the proteasomal degradation of tyrosinase. Sci Rep. 2017;7:e45858.
15. Bajpai VK, Alam MB, Quan KT, Kwon KR, Ju MK, Choi HJ, et al. Antioxidant efficacy and the upregulation of Nrf2-mediated HO-1 expression by (+)-lariciresinol, a lignan isolated from Rubia philippinensis, through the activation of p38. Sci Rep. 2017;7:e46035.
16. Itokawa H, Mihara K, Takeya K. Studies on a novel anthraquinone and its glycosides isolated from Rubia cordifolia and R. akane. Chem Pharm Bull. 1983;31:2353–8.
17. Berger Y, Castonguay A, Brassard P. Carbon-13 nuclear magnetic resonance studies of anthraquinones. Org Mag Reson. 1980;14:103–8.
18. Chung MI, Jou SJ, Cheng TH, Lin CN. Antiplatelet constituents of Formosan Rubia akane. J Nat Prod. 1994;57:313–6.
19. Banthorpe DV, White JJ. Novel anthraquinones from undifferentiated cell cultures of Galium verum. Phytochemistry. 1995;38:107–11.
20. Badisa RB, Darling-Reed SF, Joseph P, Cooperwood JS, Latinwo LM, Goodman CB, et al. Selective cytotoxic activities of two novel synthetic drugs on human breast carcinoma MCF-7 cells. Anticancer Res. 2009;29(8):2993–6.
21. de Oliveira PF, Alves JM, Damasceno JL, Machado Oliveira RA, Dias HJ, Miller Crotti AE, Tavares DC. Cytotoxicity screening of essential oils in cancer cell lines. Rev Bras Farmacogn. 2015;25(2):183–88.

12

The leaves of *Crataeva nurvala* Buch-Ham. modulate locomotor and anxiety behaviors possibly through GABAergic system

Md Moniruzzaman[1,3]* ⓘ, Md Abdul Mannan[1], Md Farhad Hossen Khan[1], Ariful Basher Abir[1] and Mirola Afroze[2]

Abstract

Background: *Crataeva nurvala* Buch-Hum is an indigenous herb, extensively used in traditional medicines of the South Asian countries to treat inflammation, rheumatic fever, gastric irritation, and constipation. Despite this wide range of uses, very little information is known regarding its effects on the central nervous system (CNS). Therefore, this study evaluated the neuropharmacological properties of methanolic extract of *Crataeva nurvala* leaves (MECN) using a number of behavioral models in animals. This study also identified potentially active phytochemicals in MECN.

Methods: Following MECN administration (at 50, 100 and 200 mg/kg; b.w.) the animals (male Swiss albino mice) were employed in hole-cross test (HCT), open field test (OFT), and rota-rod test (RRT) to evaluate sedative properties, where anxiolytic activities were investigated using elevated plus maze (EPM), light dark box (LDB), and marble burying test (MBT). The involvement of GABAergic system was evaluated using thiopental sodium (TS)-induced sleeping time determination test. Moreover, colorimetric phytochemical tests as well as GC/MS-MS were also conducted to define the phytochemical constituents of MECN.

Results: MECN possesses sedative properties indicated through the dose-dependent inhibition of locomotor activities of the animals in HCT and OFT and motor coordination in RRT. MECN also exhibited prominent anxiolytic properties through decreased burying behavior in MBT, increased time spent and transitions in open arm of EPM, and increased time spent in light compartment of LDB. In addition, the treatments potentiated TS-mediated hypnosis indicating a possible participation of GABAergic system in the observed sedative and anxiolytic activities. Phytochemical screening of MECN revealed 48 different compounds in it. We reviewed and conceive that the sedative and anxiolytic effects could be due to the presence of neuroactive compounds such as phytol, D-allose, and α-Tocopherol in MECN.

Conclusion: The present study showed that MECN possesses sedative and anxiolytic potential which could be beneficial in treatment of anxiety and insomnia associated with different psychological disorders.

Keywords: Capparidaceae, *Crataeva nurvala*, Sedative, Anxiolytic, Medicinal plant, GC/MS-MS

Background

Sleep disturbance and anxiety are the very common mental health problems world-wide, which have been regarded as underpinning factors to exacerbate different psychiatric diseases. Now-a-days the treatments for insomnia and anxiety consist of several synthetic and semisynthetic chemical compounds such as benzodiazepines, barbituric acids, and buspirone. However, these drugs have a number of undesirable side effects including amnesia, muscle relaxation, dependence, and tolerance [1, 2]. Therefore, searching for novel pharmacotherapy particularly from natural sources for neurological and psychiatric diseases has progressed significantly, owing to their better tolerability and fewer side effects. It is also evident that phytotherapies play a beneficial role for the patients who poorly respond to the conventional therapies [3, 4]. Therefore, the present study aimed to investigate *Crataeva nurvala* Buch. -Ham., a well-known

* Correspondence: moniruzzaman.babu@yahoo.com
[1]Department of Pharmacy, Stamford University Bangladesh, 51 Siddeswari road, Dhaka 1217, Bangladesh
[3]Mater Research Institute – UQ at Translational Research Institute, Faculty of Medicine, The University of Queensland, Brisbane QLD 4102, Australia
Full list of author information is available at the end of the article

member of Capparidaceae family, for its sedative and anxiolytic properties.

C. nurvala is a very common, medium-sized branched deciduous tree found in all over South Asian countries including Bangladesh, where the plant is known as Borun or Bonna [5]. Borun is extensively used in the traditional medicines due to its beneficial properties as memory enhancer, promoter of wound healing [6], laxative, lithotrophic, anti-inflammatory, contraceptive, febrifuge, and tonic. The traditional medicine practitioners also use this plant in treatment of kidney and bladder stone, vomiting, rheumatic fever, and gastric irritation [7]. Due to these diverse pharmacological properties, researchers have tried to validate the scientific basis of use of this plant. Their findings provided scientific evidence regarding the analgesic, antidiarrheal, and antinociceptive properties of the ethanol and methanol extracts of the leaves in mice, respectively [8]. On the other hand, Capparidaceae family particularly the genus *Crataeva* is almost unknown in their effects on the central nervous system. *Crataeva religiosa* is the only member reviewed to have stimulatory effects of autonomic nervous system [9]. Previously, we have shown that MECN has the potential to alleviate pain responses through controlling CNS, particularly the opioid system [8]. Therefore, we hypothesized that the chemical constituents of MECN might cross blood brain barrier and have capability to modulate brain functions directly. In 2014, Ali et al. and his colleagues reported the sedative effects of MECN using HCT, OFT, and EPM models with a single high dose (400 mg/kg) of the extract [10]. In our opinion, research outcomes from a single higher dose and a limited number of experimental models are unable to claim a specific pharmacological property, dose dependency, as well as mechanism of action of an agent. Moreover, the phytochemical constituents of MECN is still unknown.

Therefore, these limited study of the family Capparidaceae especially *C. nurvala* on the central nervous system (CNS) influenced us to design present study to investigate the sedative and anxiolytic properties of the extract using different behavioral models in mice.

Methods
Plant material and extraction
The leaves of *C. nurvala* were collected from Comilla, Bangladesh, in October 2012. The samples were then authenticated by Bushra Khan, Principal Scientific Officer of Bangladesh National Herbarium, Dhaka, Bangladesh. A voucher specimen (DACB: 37942) has been deposited in the Herbarium for further reference. 250 g of shed dried powdered leaves were macerated with 500 ml of methanol with occasional stirring for 72 h at 25 ± 2 °C temperature. The filtrate was then collected and made it dry using rotary evaporator and normal air flow resulting in 10.31 g extract (Yield 4.12%). This crude extract was further used for the acute toxicity, sedative, anxiolytic activity studies, and phytochemical analysis.

Reagents
Diazepam and thiopental sodium were purchased from Square Pharmaceuticals Ltd. (Dhaka, Bangladesh). Methanol and tween 20 were procured from Merck (Darmstadt, Germany).

Animals
Male *Swiss albino* mice of 20–25 g body weight were collected from icddr,b. Animals were housed in a standard environment maintaining 12 h light/dark cycle (7.00 am to 7.00 pm), 25 ± 2 °C room temperature, and 55–65% relative humidity. Flake wood shavings were used as bedding materials and icddr,b formulated standard diet and clean water ad libitum were provided in their regular meal. Prior to the experiments, 14 days of acclimatization period was maintained. All experimental animals were treated following the Health guide for the care and use of Laboratory animals (1978) formulated by the National Institute of Health. All protocols conducted in this study comply with the ARRIVE guidelines and were approved by the Institutional Animal Ethics Committee of Stamford University Bangladesh (SUB/IAEC/14.09). Moreover, pentobarbital was used to euthanize the animals following AVMA guidelines for the Euthanasia of Animals (2013).

Drugs and treatments
Mice were divided into 5 different groups containing 5 animals in each. In all experiments, diazepam at 1 mg/kg was used as a reference standard and administered through intraperitoneal (i.p.) route 15 min before the experiments. On the other hand, MECN was dissolved in 0.2% tween 20 and orally administered to the animals at the doses of 50, 100 and 200 mg/kg body weight (adjusted volume 0.1 ml/mouse). Animals from the control group only received 0.2% tween 20 (vehicle; p.o.) 30 min prior to the experiments. Moreover, thiopental sodium (20 mg/kg; i.p.) in sleeping time measurement test was injected 15 min after MECN or diazepam treatments.

Acute toxicity test
The animals were divided into five consecutive groups containing five animals in each. Animals were kept in close observation for 72 h and in a total of seven days following the oral treatments with vehicle or MECN at 500, 1000, 2000, and 3000 mg/kg doses (adjusted volume 0.1 ml/mouse) to check any allergic reaction, swelling, vomiting, diarrhea, and mortality induced by MECN. In the meantime they were allowed to have access to food and water ad libitum [11].

Sedative activity analysis

Hole cross test

The hole cross box is a cage of $(30 \times 20 \times 14)$ cm^3 in size with a partition in the middle having a hole of 3 cm in diameter. Mice were treated with vehicle, MECN or diazepam and placed in one chamber of the cage. Then the total number of passages of a mouse through the hole from one compartment to another was counted for a period of 3 min before and after 30, 60, 90 and 120 min of the treatments [12]. The percentage of inhibition was calculated for each time point according to the following formula:

$$\%\text{Inhibition} = [(\text{Control}-\text{Treatment})/\text{Control}] \times 100$$

Open field test

This test is one of the most frequently used methods to evaluate locomotor activity and emotionality of the rodents. The apparatus is a square box consisting of a 50 cm high wall and a wooden floor with a series of squares alternatively painted in black and white. Animals were administered with vehicle, MECN, or diazepam and placed in the middle of the open field allowing free exploration. The animals were then scored with the number of squares they visited for 3 min before and at 30, 60, 90 and 120 min post treatments [13]. The percentage of inhibition was calculated for each time point as described in hole cross test.

Test for motor co-ordination (Rota-rod test)

The apparatus consists of a non-slippery plastic rod of 3 cm in diameter (Ugo Basile, Varese, Italy) which rotates at the speed of 20 rpm. The animals which were able to stay in the rotating rod for more than 180 s were selected for the study. Animals were then treated with vehicle or MECN or diazepam and placed on the rotating rod to register their falling latency from the rod within 180 s [14, 15]. The percentage of inhibitions were calculated as described in hole cross test.

Anxiolytic activity analysis

Elevated plus-maze test (EPM)

The plus-maze apparatus is consisting of two open arms $(15 \times 5$ cm$^2)$ and two closed arms $(15 \times 5 \times 5$ cm$^3)$ extending from a central platform $(5 \times 5$ cm$^2)$, and raised 50 cm above the floor level. Animals were randomly selected for each group and treated with vehicle, MECN, or drug. Then each animal was placed at the center of the plus-maze and allowed them to freely access the maze for 3 min. The number of entries and total time spent in open arms were then recorded within the indicated time [16].

Light-dark box exploration test (LDB)

The apparatus is an open-topped rectangular box $(46 \times 27 \times 30$ cm$^3)$, divided into a small $(18 \times 27$ cm$^2)$ and a large $(27 \times 27$ cm$^2)$ compartments with a fixed partition containing a small hole (3 cm in diameter) in the middle. The small compartment was closed with a lid, painted black and illuminated with a dim light. On the other hand, the large compartment was painted in white and a 60 W electric bulb was hanged on at the top (120 cm above) to brightly illuminate it. Mice were treated with vehicle, MECN, or diazepam and placed in the middle of the open compartment. Then the time spent by the animals in open compartment and total number of transitions between the compartments were recorded for 3 min [17, 18].

Marble burying test (MBT)

A normal glass cage with bedding materials was used in this experiment. Before testing, individual animal was acclimatized in one cage for 30 min. After removal of the animal, 25 glass marbles were uniformly distributed on top of the 4 cm layer of bedding materials. Following MECN, vehicle, or diazepam treatment, each animal was replaced in the cage for 30 min. The number of buried marbles were then counted as a score of anxiety [19]. The percentage of inhibitions were calculated as described in hole cross test.

Table 1 Effect of MECN on hole cross test

Treatment	Dose (mg/kg)	Number of hole crossed (% of Inhibition)				
		Pretreatment	30 min	60 min	90 min	120 min
Control	0.1 ml/mouse	23.40 ± 1.21	18.60 ± 1.44	18.20 ± 1.36	17.00 ± 1.22	15.60 ± 1.08
Diazepam	1	21.40 ± 2.32	6.20 ± 1.07*** (66.67)	3.80 ± 0.58*** (79.12)	2.60 ± 0.51*** (84.71)	1.40 ± 0.24*** (91.03)
MECN	50	22.80 ± 1.28	15.40 ± 0.93 (17.20)	11.80 ± 0.73*** (35.16)	7.80 ± 0.86*** (54.12)	6.00 ± 0.71*** (61.54)
MECN	100	20.60 ± 1.86	10.60 ± 0.75*** (43.01)	9.00 ± 0.71*** (50.55)	4.60 ± 0.93*** (72.94)	3.80 ± 0.86*** (75.64)
MECN	200	21.20 ± 1.85	8.00 ± 0.71*** (56.99)	5.20 ± 0.73*** (71.43)	2.40 ± 0.51*** (85.88)	1.60 ± 0.24*** (89.74)

Effect of MECN on hole cross test. Values are presented as the Mean ± SEM ($n = 5$). MECN = Methanolic extract of *Crataeva nurvala*; ***$p < 0.001$ compared with the control group (two-way ANOVA followed by Bonferroni's test)

Table 2 Effect of MECN on open field test

Treatment	Dose (mg/kg)	Number of square crossed (% of Inhibition)				
		Pretreatment	30 min	60 min	90 min	120 min
Control	0.1 ml/mouse	103.80 ± 3.51	94.40 ± 4.31	83.20 ± 3.09	74.60 ± 3.20	66.80 ± 2.58
Diazepam	1	101.60 ± 3.89	49.20 ± 2.13*** (47.88)	33.20 ± 1.88*** (60.10)	14.80 ± 1.28*** (80.16)	5.40 ± 1.12*** (91.92)
MECN	50	98.00 ± 2.83	67.40 ± 3.79*** (28.60)	42.00 ± 2.49*** (49.52)	31.60 ± 2.87*** (57.64)	16.20 ± 2.40*** (75.75)
MECN	100	100.80 ± 2.62	46.40 ± 2.75*** (50.85)	35.80 ± 2.48*** (56.97)	16.20 ± 4.53*** (78.28)	5.60 ± 0.75*** (91.62)
MECN	200	102.20 ± 3.44	34.40 ± 3.23*** (63.56)	22.20 ± 3.88*** (73.32)	10.80 ± 2.89*** (85.52)	4.20 ± 0.58*** (93.71)

Effect of MECN on open field test. Values are presented as the Mean ± SEM ($n = 5$). MECN = Methanolic extract of *Crataeva nurvala*; ***$p < 0.001$ compared with the control group (two-way ANOVA followed by Bonferroni's test)

Thiopental sodium-induced sleeping time test

The animals were randomly divided into desired groups and administered with vehicle, MECN, or diazepam. Thirty min after vehicle or MECN and 15 min after standard drug, thiopental sodium (TS) was administered to each animal i.p. at a dose of 20 mg/kg. Then animals were observed for the latent period (time between TS administration and loss of their righting reflex) and the duration of sleep (time between the loss and recovery of righting reflex)-induced by TS [14].

Phytochemical analysis

MECN was qualitatively evaluated to detect the presence of alkaloids, carbohydrates, glycosides, flavonoids, tannins, and reducing sugars according to the protocols described by Ghani et al. [20].

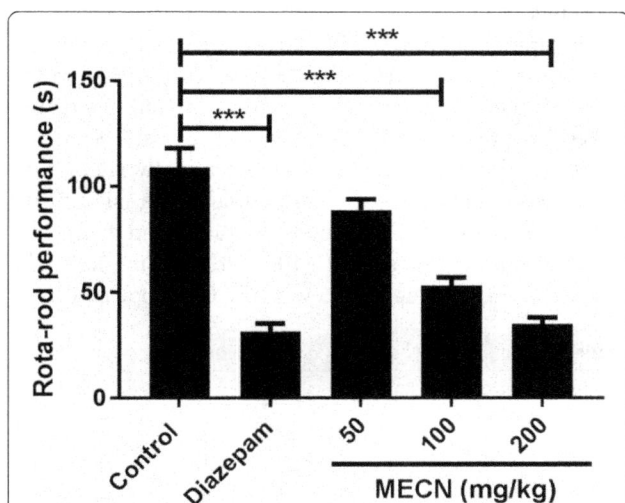

Fig. 1 Rota-rod performance of mice. Animals were administered with MECN and exposed to the rota-rod to record their falling latency as described in the methods. Data are presented as Mean ± SEM ($n = 5$). pED$_{50}$ value is 2.05 with the Hill slope of 1.55. MECN = Methanolic extract of *Crataeva nurvala*; *$p < 0.05$; **$p < 0.01$; ***$p < 0.001$ compared with the control group (one-way ANOVA followed by Dunnett's test)

GC/MS-MS analysis

GC/MS-MS analysis of the methanolic extract of the leaves of *C. nurvala* was carried out using GCMS-TQ8040 gas chromatograph mass spectrometer (Shimadzu Corp., Kyoto, Kyoto Prefecture, Japan) with a Rxi-5 ms fused silica capillary column (30 m × 0.25 mm × 0.25 μm film thickness). For GC, the injection temperature was set at 250 °C. The oven temperature was programmed at 50 °C for 1 min, 25 °C/min to 125 °C for 0 min, and 10 °C/min to 300 °C for 10 min. Total analysis time was 31.50 min where the column flow rate was 1.69 ml/min Helium gas. The MS was electron ionization (EI) type and set in Q3 scan mode. The ion source temperature was maintained at 200 °C and the interface at 250 °C. The detector voltage was set at 0.2 kV and the mass range was 50–1000 m/z. The individual compound was searched and identified using "NIST-MS Library 2009". Total Ionic Chromatogram (TIC) was used to determine the peak area as well as the percentage amounts of each compound.

Statistical analyses

The results are presented as Mean ± SEM. The statistical analysis was performed using one-way analysis of variance (ANOVA) followed by Dunnett's post hoc test, except for the HCT and OFT. For these tests, two-way ANOVA followed by Bonferroni's post hoc tests was adopted. In all the cases $P < 0.05$ was considered as significant. All statistical analysis was performed using SPSS software. Moreover, the pED$_{50}$ and Hill Slope values were calculated using Graphpad Prism software.

Results

Hole cross and open field tests

Our results demonstrated that MECN significantly decreased the spontaneous locomotor activity in mice which is evident in both HCT ($F_{4,100} = 90.67$, $p < 0.001$) and OFT ($F_{4,100} = 232.9$, $p < 0.001$) models. The suppressive effect was observed at 30 min after oral administration with all MECN doses (50, 100 and 200 mg/kg) and continued up to 120 min of the observation period. However, the major drawbacks of these models are the

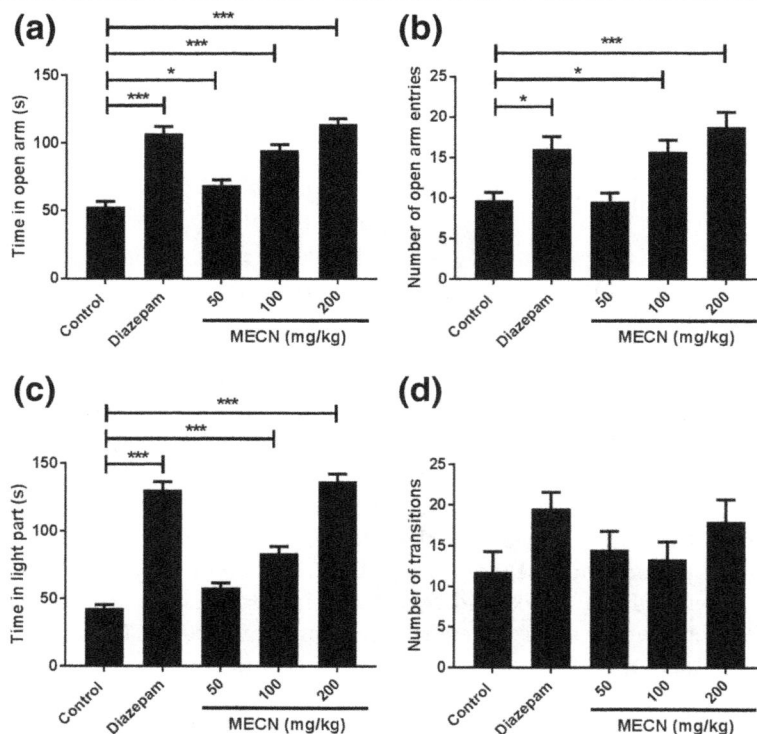

Fig. 2 Effects of MECN on elevated plus maze (EPM) and light-dark box (LDB) tests. Following 30 min of drugs administration, animals were placed in the EPM to record the time they spent (pED$_{50}$: 1.81; Hill slope: 3.55) (**a**) as well as number of transitions (pED$_{50}$: 1.97; Hill slope: 6.71) (**b**) in the open arm. In LDB, mice were observed for the time spent (pED$_{50}$: 1.74; Hill slope: 6.65) (**c**) and total number of transitions (pED$_{50}$: 2.33; Hill slope: 1.35) (**d**) in the open lighted compartment. Data are presented as Mean ± SEM (n = 5). MECN = Methanolic extract of *Crataeva nurvala*; *$p < 0.05$; **$p < 0.01$; ***$p < 0.001$ compared with the control group (one-way ANOVA followed by Dunnett's test)

animals get habituated and lost their curiosity due to repeated exposure in the same environment, which result in a decrease in their ambulatory activities. As expected, we observed the same results with animals from the control group. However, the decrements with MECN doses are higher and dose-dependent. As the locomotor activity of the animals has been decreased with time and doses, we performed two-way ANOVA analysis followed by Bonferroni's post hoc test and found the effects of MECN are significantly ($P < 0.05$) different from the control group (Tables 1 and 2).

Test for motor co-ordination

As depicted in Fig. 1, the results showed that acute oral administration with MECN (50, 100 and 200 mg/kg doses) decreased the time that the mice were able to stay on the rota-rod. The highest performance inhibitions were observed with diazepam (71.01%) and MECN at 200 mg/kg (67.76%). Although, MECN dose-dependently suppressed motor co-ordination of the animals, the significant ($F_{4,20} = 39.13$, $p < 0.001$) inhibition was found with only higher doses of the extract (100 and 200 mg/kg). The estimated pED$_{50}$ value is 2.05 with the Hill slope of 1.55.

Table 3 Effect of MECN on marble burying test

Treatment	Dose (mg/kg)	Responses	
		Numbers of marbles buried	% Inhibition
Control	0.1 ml/mouse	11.80 ± 2.52	0
Diazepam	1	1.20 ± 0.20**	89.83
MECN	50	9.40 ± 2.23	20.34
MECN	100	5.00 ± 2.10*	57.63
MECN	200	2.20 ± 0.58**	81.36

Effect of MECN on marble burying test. Values are presented as the Mean ± SEM (n = 5). MECN = Methanolic extract of *Crataeva nurvala*; *$p < 0.05$; **$p < 0.01$; compared with the control group (one-way ANOVA followed by Dunnett's test)

Table 4 Effect of MECN on thiopental sodium induced hypnosis

Treatment	Dose (mg/kg)	Responses	
		Onset of sleeping	Sleeping duration
Control	0.1 ml/mouse	9.24 ± 0.25	50.20 ± 1.86
Diazepam	1	6.97 ± 0.19***	98.40 ± 3.83***
MECN	50	8.87 ± 0.60	49.00 ± 4.85
MECN	100	7.92 ± 0.27*	69.60 ± 3.12*
MECN	200	7.18 ± 0.28**	92.20 ± 2.44***

Effect of MECN on thiopental sodium induced hypnosis. Values are presented as the Mean ± SEM (n = 5). MECN = Methanolic extract of *Crataeva nurvala*; *$p < 0.05$; **$p < 0.01$; ***$p < 0.001$ compared with the control group (one-way ANOVA followed by Dunnett's test)

The leaves of Crataeva nurvala Buch-Ham. modulate locomotor and anxiety behaviors possibly through...

117

Table 5 Groups of phytochemicals identified in MECN

Phytochemicals	Names of the tests	Expected changes	Results
Alkaloids	Mayer's test	Yellowish buff color precipitate	+
	Hager's test	Yellow crystalline precipitate	–
	Wagner's test	Brown or deep brown precipitate	+
	Dragendorff's test	Orange or orange-brown precipitate	+
	Tannic acid test	Buff color precipitate	+
Tannins	Ferric chloride test	Blue green color	+
	Alkaline reagent test	Yellow to red precipitate	+
Glycosides	General test	Yellow color	+
	Test for glucoside	Production of brick-red precipitation	+
Carbohydrates	Molisch's test	A red or reddish violet ring is formed at the junction of two layers, and on shaking a dark purple solution is formed	+
	Barfoed's test (general test for monosaccharides)	Red precipitate	+
	Fehling's test	A red or brick-red precipitate	+
	Test for reducing sugar	A brick-red precipitate	+
Flavonoids	Hydrochloric acid reduction test	Red color	+

Elevated plus-maze test

In EPM test, as expected for a positive control, diazepam at 1 mg/kg produced a selective anxiolytic effect in mice characterized by a significant ($F_{4,20} = 36.28$, $p < 0.001$) increase in the time spent as well as the number of entries in the open arm of EPM. Besides, treatments with the methanolic extract of *C. nurvala* at 100 and 200 mg/kg doses significantly ($F_{4,20} = 36.28$, $p < 0.001$) increased the spending time (pED$_{50}$: 1.81; Hill slope: 3.55) and total number of entries ($F_{4,20} = 8.50$, $p < 0.001$; pED$_{50}$: 1.97; Hill slope: 6.71) in the open arm (Fig. 2a, b).

Light-dark box exploration test

The results obtained in this test demonstrated a significant ($F_{4,20} = 78.56$, $p < 0.001$) increase in time spent in LDB light chamber by MECN (pED$_{50}$: 1.74; Hill slope: 6.65). It also increased the number of transitions between compartments in a dose-dependent manner (pED$_{50}$: 2.33; Hill slope: 1.35) (Fig. 2c, d).

Marble burying test

In this study, the oral administration of MECN at 50, 100 and 200 mg/kg doses showed dose-dependent and

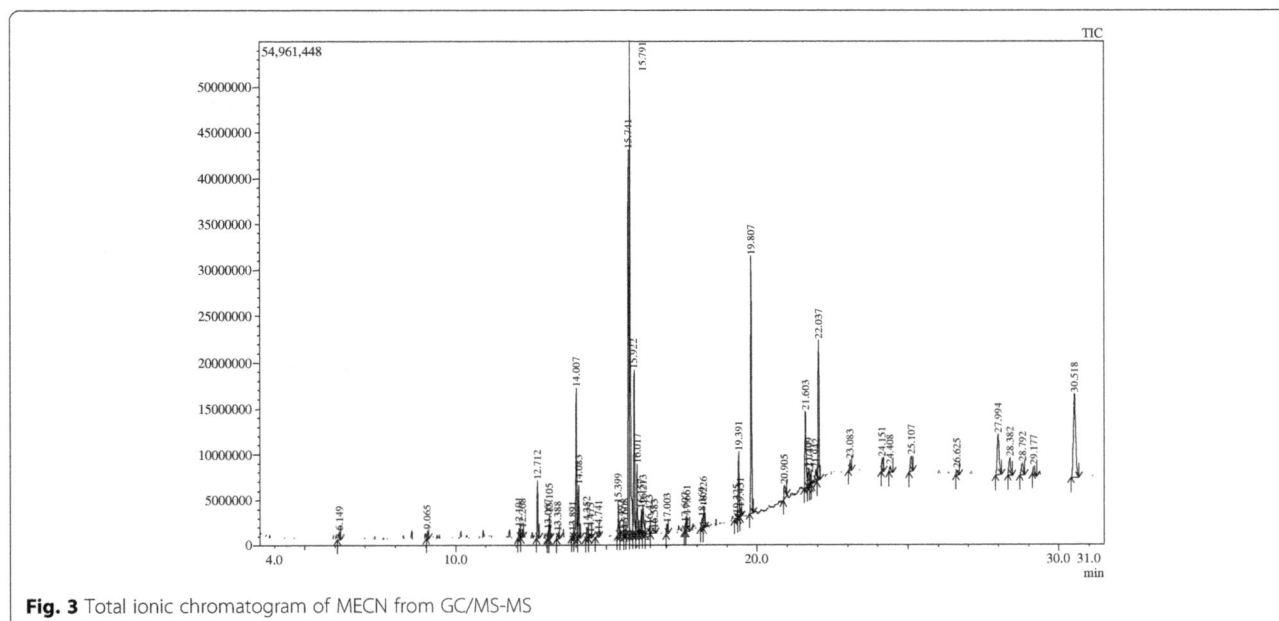

Fig. 3 Total ionic chromatogram of MECN from GC/MS-MS

Table 6 Phytochemicals detected in MECN using GC/MS-MS

SN	RT (min)	% PA	Compound name	Biological activity	References
1	6.04	0.55	Catechol	Antioxidant	[39]
2	6.15	0.64	Butanenitrile, 3-chloro-3-methyl-	Not found	–
3	8.98	0.44	n-Tridecan-1-ol	Anti-alcoholic	[40]
4	9.07	0.84	D-Allose	Hepatoprotective, immunosuppressant, antioxidant, and anticancer.	[41–44]
5	10.92	0.96	Megastigmatrienone	Not found	–
6	11.1	0.70	2-Cyclohexen-1-one, 4-(3-hydroxy-1-butenyl)-3,5,5-trimethyl-	Not found	–
7	11.78	0.90	Ethanol, 2-(dodecyloxy)-	Antithyroid, supress varicose veins formation.	[45, 46]
8	11.96	0.44	Cedrol	Prevent chemotherapy-induced alopecia, promote hair growth, anticancer.	[47–49]
9	12.1	1.28	(E)-4-(3-Hydroxyprop-1-en-1-yl)-2-methoxyphenol	Not found	–
10	12.21	1.05	6-Hydroxy-4,4,7a-trimethyl-5,6,7,7a-tetrahydrobenzofuran-2(4H)-one	Not found	–
11	12.4	0.35	5,5,8a-Trimethyl-3,5,6,7,8,8a-hexahydro-2H-chromene	Not found	–
12	12.71	5.24	(S,E)-4-Hydroxy-3,5,5-trimethyl-4-(3-oxobut-1-en-1-yl)cyclohex-2-enone	Anticholinesterase and antioxidant	[50]
13	12.94	0.44	1(2H)-Naphthalenone, 3,4,5,6,7,8-hexahydro-	Not found	–
14	13.07	0.93	N,N-Diethylhexylamine	Not found	–
15	13.11	1.98	Neophytadiene	Not found	–
16	13.18	0.58	Z-28-Heptatriaconten-2-one	Not found	–
17	13.39	1.02	Bicyclo[4.1.0]heptan-3-one, 4,7,7-trimethyl-, [1R-(1.alpha.,4.beta.,6.alpha.)]-	Not found	–
18	13.392	1.02	2,3a-Dimethylhexahydrobenzofuran-7a-ol	Not found	–
19	13.89	0.73	1-(3-Hydroxymethyl-phenyl)-heptan-1-ol	Not found	–
20	14.09	4.36	7,9-Di-tert-butyl-1-oxaspiro(4,5)deca-6,9-diene-2,8-dione	Not found	–
21	14.47	0.81	9-(3,3-Dimethyloxiran-2-yl)-2,7-dimethylnona-2,6-dien-1-ol	Not found	–
22	14.48	0.84	1,4-Dimethyladamantane	Not found	–
23	14.74	0.49	Diethylene glycol monododecyl ether	Not found	–
24	14.79	0.61	trans-Sinapyl alcohol	Not found	–
25	15.92	14.84	Phytol	Anxiolytic, antitubercular and anticancer	[36, 51, 52]
26	16.21	4.07	Ethanol, 2,2'-(dodecylimino)bis-	Not found	–
27	16.69	0.52	Hexadecane	Not found	–
28	18.37	0.55	(2,2,6-Trimethyl-bicyclo[4.1.0]hept-1-yl)-methanol	Not found	–
29	18.79	0.61	7-Hexadecenal, (Z)-	Pheromone	[53]
30	19.32	1.02	2-Methylhexacosane	Not found	–
31	19.92	0.73	Ethyl 13-docosenoate(ethyl erucate)	Not found	–
32	20.13	0.58	Hexacontane	Not found	–
33	20.39	0.47	7-Methyl-6-oxo-1,2,3,4-tetrahydro-6H-pyrimido[1,2-a]pyrimidine	Not found	–
34	21.43	1.16	Cyclopentane, (4-octyldodecyl)-	Not found	–
35	21.6	8.73	13-Docosenamide, (Z)-	Not found	–
36	22.29	0.52	α-Tocospiro A	Not found	–
37	22.49	1.28	α-Tocospiro B	Not found	–
38	24.15	1.86	.gamma.-Tocopherol	Anti-inflammatory	[54, 55]

Table 6 Phytochemicals detected in MECN using GC/MS-MS *(Continued)*

SN	RT (min)	% PA	Compound name	Biological activity	References
39	25.11	3.23	Vitamin E	Antioxidant	[56]
40	26.63	0.93	Ergost-5-en-3-ol, (3.beta.)-	Not found	–
41	27.08	0.49	Stigmasterol	Anti-asthmatic, anti-inflammatory, anti-proliferative, anti-bacterial, acetylcholinesterase inhibitor	[57–60]
42	28.38	3.40	β-Amyrone	Not found	–
43	28.79	3.49	4-Campestene-3-one	Not found	–
44	28.96	0.55	Cholestan-3-one, (5.alpha.)-	Not found	–
45	29.18	2.30	Lup-20(29)-en-3-one	Melanogenesis, hypolipidemic, anti-inflammatory, antidiabetic	[61–64]
46	29.35	1.08	4,22-Cholestadien-3-one	Not found	–
47	30.52	19.44	γ-Sitostenone	Not found	–
48	31.14	0.93	Cholesta-4,6-dien-3-one	Not found	–

SN serial number, *RT* retention time, *PA* peak area

significant ($F_{4,20} = 6.60$, $p < 0.01$) inhibition of burying behavior of the animals (Table 3). The calculated pED_{50} value for MBT is 1.96 with the Hill slope of 2.09. Therefore, keeping with the results obtained in EPM and LDB tests, these findings support the anxiolytic potential of MECN.

Thiopental sodium-induced sleeping time test

Our results demonstrated that the acute oral administration of MECN at 50, 100 and 200 mg/kg reduced the TS-mediated induction of sleep in the animals. However, the significant ($F_{4,20} = 8.31$, $p < 0.01$) effects were observed with the higher doses of MECN (100 and 200 mg/kg) for sleeping onset. These result in prolonged duration of sleep ($F_{4,20} = 46.14$, $p < 0.001$; pED_{50}: 2.07; Hill slope: 3.50) as summarized in Table 4.

Acute toxicity test

The acute toxicity test revealed that the oral administration of MECN at the doses of 500, 1000 2000, and 3000 mg/kg did not show any mortality or allergic manifestations during 7 days of the observation period. Therefore, it can be assumed that MECN possesses low toxicity profile and safe within our experimental doses up to the 3000 mg/kg.

Phytochemical analysis

The preliminary phytochemical analysis revealed the presence of alkaloids, glycosides, carbohydrates, flavonoids, and tannins in MECN (Table 5).

GC/MS-MS analysis

The GC/MS-MS analysis of MECN confirmed the presence of 48 different compounds (Fig. 3, Table 6). The major 25 compounds identified with % peak area are γ-Sitostenone (19.44%), Phytol (14.84%), 13-Docosenamide, (Z)- (8.73%), (S,E)-4-Hydroxy-3,5,5-trimethyl-4-(3-oxobut-1-en-1-yl)cyclohex-2-enone (5.24%), 7,9-Di-tert-butyl-1-oxaspiro(4,5)deca-6,9-diene-2,8-dione (4.36%), Ethanol, 2,2′-(dodecylimino)bis- (4.07%), 4-Campestene-3-one (3.49%), β-Amyrone (3.40%) Vitamin E (3.23%), Lup-20(29)-en-3-one (2.30%), Neophytadiene (1.98%), γ-Tocopherol (1.86%), (E)-4-(3-Hydroxyprop-1-en-1-yl)-2-methoxyphenol (1.28%), α-Tocospiro B (1.28%), Cyclopentane, (4-octyldodecyl)- (1.16%), 4,22-Cholestadien-3-one (1.08%), 6-Hydroxy-4,4,7a-trimethyl-5,6,7,7a-tetrahydrobenzofuran-2(4H)-one (1.05%), Bicyclo[4.1.0]heptan-3-one, 4,7,7-trimethyl-, [1R-(1.alpha., 4.beta.,6.alpha.)]- (1.02%), 2,3a-Dimethylhexahydrobenzofuran-7a-ol (1.02%), 2-Methylhexacosane (1.02%), Megastigmatrienone (0.96%), N,N-Diethylhexylamine (0.93%), Ergost-5-en-3-ol, (3.beta.)- (0.93%), Cholesta-4,6-dien-3-one (0.93%), and D-Allose (0.84%).

Discussion

The present study was carried out to investigate the effects of MECN on the central nervous system (Fig. 4), which is the first extensive study reporting the psychoactive potential of a member of the genus *Crataeva*. In hole cross and open field tests, the oral administration of MECN significantly suppressed spontaneous locomotor behavior of the animals indicating that MECN possesses at least some sedative properties. These observations were supported by a previously reported work, where the locomotor activity of

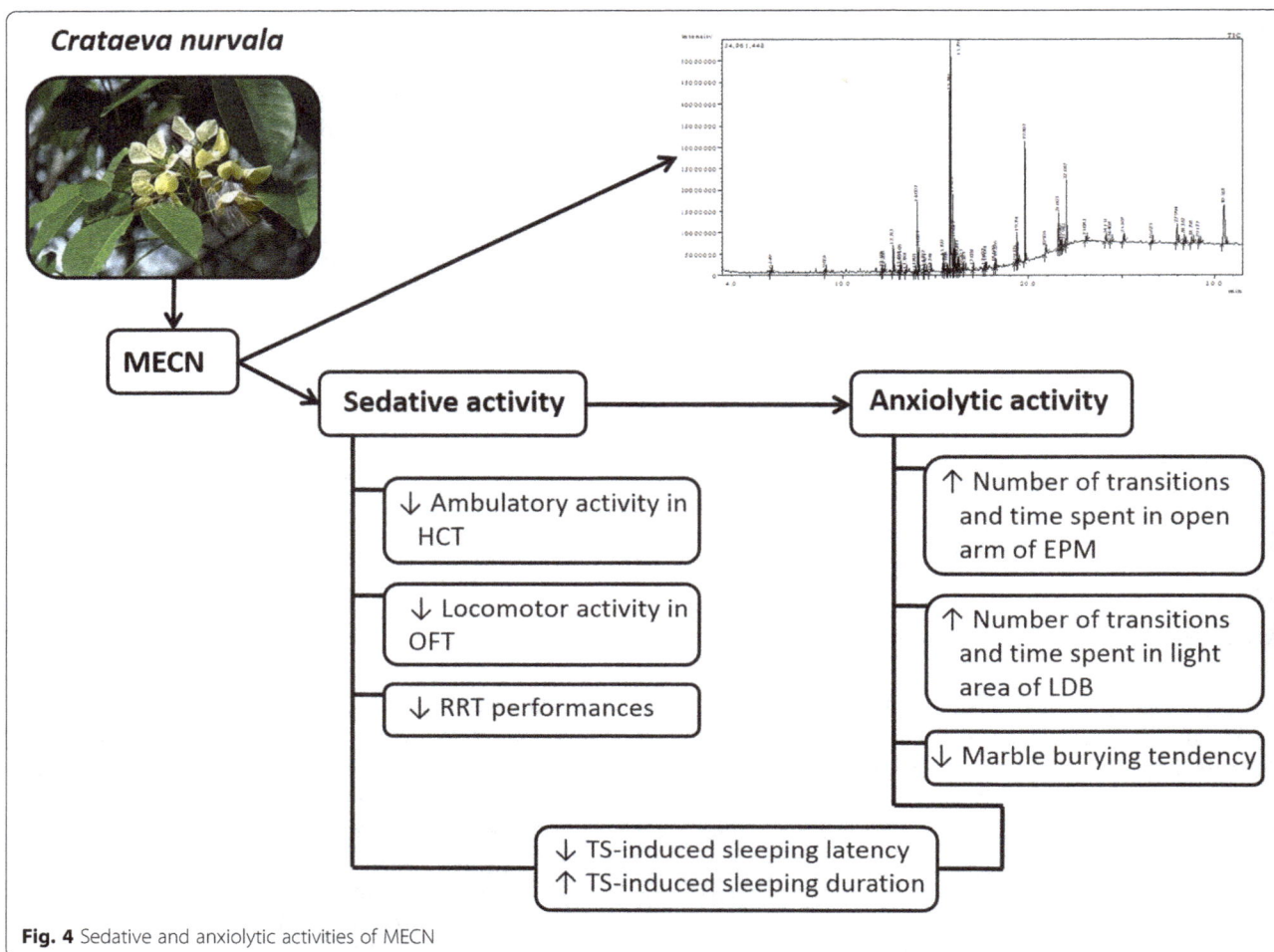

Fig. 4 Sedative and anxiolytic activities of MECN

the animals was suppressed by MECN at 400 mg/kg dose [10]. Moreover, our earlier study revealed that MECN involves opioid system to show its antinociceptive effect in mice which was confirmed by using a non-specific opioid receptors antagonist, naloxone [8]. It has been reported that the opioid system inhibits GABAergic interneurons and directly affect the dopaminergic system to control locomotor behaviors [21]. Therefore, in agreement with these reports, it is conceivable that MECN may also involve opioid pathway to exhibit its sedative activity.

Motor coordination is a complex behavioral domain that reflects muscle strength, balance, and patterned gait [22]. It has been reported that barbiturates, benzodiazepines, and similar compounds can cause muscle weakness [23], sedation, and decrease ambulatory activity resulting in an impaired performance in rota-rod [24]. In our study, the administration of MECN and standard drug diazepam parallelly impaired motor co-ordination in rota-rod test, indicating that MECN has the capability to produce sedation that affects general activity and motor coordination of the mice.

To investigate the anxiolytic effect of MECN, we used EPM, a widely used animal model to scrutinize anxiolytic drugs. This experimental model acts based on the innate aversion of mice/rats to open place. In this test, the number of entries and total time spent in the open arms have generally been used as the indication of anxiolytic effect [25]. Like EPM, LDB is also a classical model of screening anxiolytic or anxiogenic drugs. LDB works based on the inherent unwillingness of rodents to enter into the brightly illuminated areas and on their spontaneous exploratory behaviors in response to mild stressors like light and novel environment. It has been reported that not the number of transitions but the time spent in the light area is the most consistent and useful parameter in investigation of anxiolytic action [26]. We found that MECN treatments influenced the animals to come in open and lighted areas of EPM and LDB, disclosing the anxiolytic potential of MECN. Moreover, the glass marbles in marble burying test provide an effective unconditioned stimulus which incites burying. This aversive stimulus has been reported sensitive to diazepam or chlordiazepoxide and suggested that the decrease in burying behavior will indicate the anxiolytic action of a drug candidate [19, 27]. Therefore, our findings in MBT suggest the prominent anxiolytic action of MECN which is consistent with the results obtained from EPM and LDB tests.

To confirm the possible involvement of GABAergic system in MECN-mediated sedative and anxiolytic activity, we co-administered thiopental sodium (TS) with MECN or diazepam. It is well established that the sedative and anxiolytic effect of benzodiazepines are due to their binding to $GABA_A$ receptor at a site distinct from the GABA binding site [28]. However, when barbiturates like TS binds with the barbituric acid binding sites of $GABA_A$ receptor complex, it potentiates GABA-mediated hyperpolarization of postsynaptic neurons [29]. Therefore, it has been suggested that the agents including natural products and chemical compounds which potentiate thiopental-induced sleeping, will potentially affect GABAergic neurotransmission [30, 31]. In corroboration with our results it is therefore conceivable that GABAergic system might have the contribution at least in a part in MECN-induced modulation of the sleeping behavior of animals produced by TS.

The qualitative phytochemical analysis identified the presence of alkaloids, glycosides, carbohydrates, flavonoids, and tannins in MECN. Although GC is mainly effective for identification of volatile compounds, we further analyzed MECN using GC/MS-MS due to the instrument availability and accessibility. Among others, D-Allose is the most active compound in MECN, reported to inhibit mitochondrial reactive oxygen species in Neuro2A cells [32] as well as protect the brain from transient ischemic neural death [33]. During cerebral ischemia, this compound also inhibited the production of inflammatory cytokines and translocation of NF-κB components to protect blood-brain barrier [34, 35]. Phytol was found to produce significant anxiolytic activity in mice which is mediated through its interaction with GABAergic system [36]. Moreover, it has also been reported that α-Tocopherol (vitamin E) and other alkaloids, flavonoids, tannins, and terpenoids containing plant extracts possess strong sedative and anxiolytic and anticonvulsant effects on Swiss albino mice [37, 38]. Although the direct involvements of individual components are yet to be revealed, accumulated evidence raise the possibility of these reported neuro-active components to participate at least in a part in the mechanism of sedative and anxiolytic actions of MECN.

Conclusion

Taken together, we conclude that MECN possesses strong sedative-and anxiolytic-like properties which may be mediated through the interactions with GABAergic system that affect the general activity, motor coordination and muscle strength of the animals. We also hypothesize that the observed effects are due to the presence of several psychoactive phytochemicals including phytol, D-allose, and α-tocopherol in MECN. Therefore, further in-depth studies are required to isolate the bioactive phytochemical(s) and understand the precise molecular mechanisms underlying the observed pharmacological activities. In addition, we also believe that this work will act as an eye-opener regarding the central nervous system effect of the genus Crataeva and will serve as a basis for future research of MECN.

Abbreviations

CNS: Central nervous system; EPM: Elevated plus maze; GC/MS-MS: Gas chromatography-mass spectroscopy-mass spectroscopy; HCT: Hole cross test; icddr,b: International Center for Diarrheal Disease and Research, Bangladesh; LDB: Light-dark box; MBT: Marble burying test; MECN: Methanol extract of C. nurvala leaves; OFT: Open field test; RRT: Rota-rod test; TS: Thiopental sodium

Acknowledgements

The authors are thankful to the Department of Pharmacy, Stamford University Bangladesh, for providing the basic facilities in the Pharmacology Laboratory.

Funding

This research received no grant from any funding agency in the public, commercial, or not-for-profit sectors.

Authors' contributions

MM conceived and designed the experiments. All authors were involved in conducting the experiments. MM and MA analyzed the data. MM wrote the manuscript and MAM, MFHK, ABA, and MA read and approved the final version of the manuscript.

Competing interests

The authors wish to confirm that there are no known competing interests associated with this publication and there has been no significant financial support for this work that could have influenced its outcome.

Author details

[1]Department of Pharmacy, Stamford University Bangladesh, 51 Siddeswari road, Dhaka 1217, Bangladesh. [2]Designated Reference Institute for Chemical Measurement (DRiCM), Bangladesh Council of Scientific & Industrial Research, Dhaka 1205, Bangladesh. [3]Mater Research Institute – UQ at Translational Research Institute, Faculty of Medicine, The University of Queensland, Brisbane QLD 4102, Australia.

References

1. Reynolds DS. The value of genetic and pharmacological approaches to understanding the complexities of GABA(a) receptor subtype functions: the anxiolytic effects of benzodiazepines. Pharmacol Biochem Behav. 2008;90: 37–42. https://doi.org/10.1016/j.pbb.2008.03.015.
2. Rickels K, Schweizer E. The clinical presentation of generalized anxiety in primary-care settings: practical concepts of classification and management. J Clin Psychiatry. 1997;58(Suppl 11):4–10.
3. Carlini EA. Plants and the central nervous system. Pharmacol Biochem Behav. 2003;75:501–12.
4. Zhang ZJ. Therapeutic effects of herbal extracts and constituents in animal models of psychiatric disorders. Life Sci. 2004;75:1659–99. https://doi.org/10.1016/j.lfs.2004.04.014.
5. Kirtikar KR, Basu BD. Indian medicinal plants. 2nd ed. India: International Book Publisher, Dehradun; 2005.
6. Bhattacharjee A, Shashidhara SC. Aswathanarayana. Phytochemical and ethno-pharmacological profile of Crataeva nurvala Buch-hum (Varuna): a review. Asian Pacific Journal of Tropical Biomedicine. 2012;2:S1162–8. https://doi.org/10.1016/S2221-1691(12)60379-7.
7. Ghani A. Medicinal Plant of Bangladesh with chemical constituents and uses. 2nd ed. Dhaka, Bangladesh: Asiatic Society of Bangladesh; 1998.
8. Moniruzzaman M, Imam MZ. Evaluation of antinociceptive effect of methanolic extract of leaves of Crataeva nurvala Buch.-ham. BMC Complement Altern Med. 2014;14:354. https://doi.org/10.1186/1472-6882-14-354.
9. Oliver-Bever B. Medicinal plants in tropical West Africa. II. Plants acting on the nervous system. J Ethnopharmacol. 1983;7:1–93.
10. Ali MS, Dey A, Abu Sayeed M, Rahman AA, Kuddus MR, Rashid MA. In vivo sedative and cytotoxic activities of methanol extract of leaves of Crataeva nurvala Buch-ham. Pak J Biol Sci. 2014;17:439–42.
11. Walker Cl, Trevisan G, Rossato MF, Franciscato C, Pereira ME, Ferreira J, Manfron MP. Antinociceptive activity of Mirabilis Jalapa in mice. J Ethnopharmacol. 2008;120:169–75. https://doi.org/10.1016/j.jep.2008.08.002.
12. Takagi K, Watanabe M, Saito H. Studies of the spontaneous movement of animals by the hole cross test; effect of 2-dimethyl-aminoethanol and its acyl esters on the central nervous system. Jpn J Pharmacol. 1971;21:797–810.
13. Gupta BD, Dandiya PC, Gupta ML. A psycho-pharmacological analysis of behaviour in rats. Jpn J Pharmacol. 1971;21:293–8.
14. Dunham NW, Miya TS. A note on a simple apparatus for detecting neurological deficit in rats and mice. J Am Pharm Assoc. 1957;46:208–9. https://doi.org/10.1002/jps.3030460322.
15. Fujimori H, Cobb DP. Central nervous system depressant activity of MA1337, 3-(3-(4-m-chlorophenyl-1-piperazyl)propyl)-2,4(1h,3h)quinazolinedione hydrochloride. J Pharmacol Exp Ther. 1965;148:151–7.
16. Pellow S, Chopin P, File SE, Briley M. Validation of open:closed arm entries in an elevated plus-maze as a measure of anxiety in the rat. J Neurosci Methods. 1985;14:149–67.
17. Bourin M, Hascoët M. The mouse light/dark box test. Eur J Pharmacol. 2003; 463:55–65. https://doi.org/10.1016/S0014-2999(03)01274-3.
18. Hascoët M, Bourin M. A new approach to the light/dark test procedure in mice. Pharmacol Biochem Behav. 1998;60:645–53.
19. Treit D, Pinel JP, Fibiger HC. Conditioned defensive burying: a new paradigm for the study of anxiolytic agents. Pharmacol Biochem Behav. 1981;15:619–26.
20. Ghani A. Medicinal plants of Bangladesh with chemical constituents and uses. Dhaka, Bangladesh: Asiatic Society of Bangladesh; 2003.
21. Johnson SW, North RA. Opioids excite dopamine neurons by hyperpolarization of local interneurons. J Neurosci. 1992;12:483–8.
22. Ginski MJ, Witkin JM. Sensitive and rapid behavioral differentiation of N-methyl-D-aspartate receptor antagonists. Psychopharmacology. 1994;114: 573–82.
23. López-Rubalcava C, Hen R, Cruz SL. Anxiolytic-like actions of toluene in the burying behavior and plus-maze tests: differences in sensitivity between 5-HT(1B) knockout and wild-type mice. Behav Brain Res. 2000;115:85–94.
24. Estrada-Reyes R, López-Rubalcava C, Rocha L, Heinze G, González Esquinca AR, Martinez-Vázquez M. Anxiolytic-like and sedative actions of Rollinia mucosa: possible involvement of the GABA/benzodiazepine receptor complex. Pharm Biol. 2010;48:70–5. https://doi.org/10.3109/13880200903046153.
25. Kulkarni SK, Reddy DS. Animal behavioral models for testing antianxiety agents. Methods Find Exp Clin Pharmacol. 1996;18:219–30.
26. Young R, Johnson DN. A fully automated light/dark apparatus useful for comparing anxiolytic agents. Pharmacol Biochem Behav. 1991;40:739–43.
27. Poling A, Cleary J, Monaghan M. Burying by rats in response to aversive and nonaversive stimuli. J Exp Anal Behav. 1981;35:31–44.
28. Whiting PJ. GABA-A receptor subtypes in the brain: a paradigm for CNS drug discovery? Drug Discov Today. 2003;8:445–50.
29. Fernández S, Wasowski C, Paladini AC, Marder M. Sedative and sleep-enhancing properties of linarin, a flavonoid-isolated from Valeriana officinalis. Pharmacol Biochem Behav. 2004;77:399–404.
30. de la Pena JB, Lee HL, Yoon SY, Kim GH, Lee YS, Cheong JH. The involvement of magnoflorine in the sedative and anxiolytic effects of Sinomeni caulis et Rhizoma in mice. J Nat Med. 2013;67:814–21. https://doi.org/10.1007/s11418-013-0754-3.
31. Hossain MF, Talukder B, Rana MN, Tasnim R, Nipun TS, Uddin SM, Hossen SM. In vivo sedative activity of methanolic extract of Stericulia villosa Roxb. Leaves. BMC Complement Altern Med. 2016;16:398. https://doi.org/10.1186/s12906-016-1374-8.
32. Ishihara Y, Katayama K, Sakabe M, Kitamura M, Aizawa M, Takara M, Itoh K. Antioxidant properties of rare sugar D-allose: effects on mitochondrial reactive oxygen species production in Neuro2A cells. J Biosci Bioeng. 2011; 112:638–42. https://doi.org/10.1016/j.jbiosc.2011.08.005.
33. Liu Y, Nakamura T, Toyoshima T, Shinomiya A, Tamiya T, Tokuda M, Keep RF, Itano T. The effects of D-allose on transient ischemic neuronal death and analysis of its mechanism. Brain Res Bull. 2014;109:127–31. https://doi.org/10.1016/j.brainresbull.2014.10.005.
34. Huang T, Gao D, Hei Y, Zhang X, Chen X, Fei Z. D-allose protects the blood brain barrier through PPARgamma-mediated anti-inflammatory pathway in the mice model of ischemia reperfusion injury. Brain Res. 2016;1642:478–86. https://doi.org/10.1016/j.brainres.2016.04.038.
35. Shinohara N, Nakamura T, Abe Y, Hifumi T, Kawakita K, Shinomiya A, Tamiya T, Tokuda M, Keep RF, Yamamoto T, Kuroda Y. D-Allose attenuates overexpression of inflammatory cytokines after cerebral ischemia/reperfusion injury in gerbil. J Stroke Cerebrovasc Dis. 2016;25:2184–8. https://doi.org/10.1016/j.jstrokecerebrovasdis.2016.01.030.
36. Costa JP, de Oliveira GA, de Almeida AA, Islam MT, de Sousa DP, de Freitas RM. Anxiolytic-like effects of phytol: possible involvement of GABAergic transmission. Brain Res. 2014;1547:34–42. https://doi.org/10.1016/j.brainres.2013.12.003.
37. de Almeida ER, Rafael KR, Couto GB, Ishigami AB. Anxiolytic and anticonvulsant effects on mice of flavonoids, linalool, and alpha-tocopherol presents in the extract of leaves of Cissus sicyoides L. (Vitaceae). J Biomed Biotechnol. 2009;2009:274740. https://doi.org/10.1155/2009/274740.
38. Häberlein H, Tschiersch KP, Schäfer HL. Flavonoids from Leptospermum scoparium with affinity to the benzodiazepine receptor characterized by structure activity relationships and in vivo studies of a plant extract. Pharmazie. 1994;49:912–22.
39. Thavasi V, Leong LP, Bettens RP. Investigation of the influence of hydroxy groups on the radical scavenging ability of polyphenols. J Phys Chem A. 2006;110:4918–23. https://doi.org/10.1021/jp057315r.
40. Wilkemeyer MF, Menkari CE, Charness ME. Novel antagonists of alcohol inhibition of l1-mediated cell adhesion: multiple mechanisms of action. Mol Pharmacol. 2002;62:1053–60.
41. Hossain MA, Izuishi K, Maeta H. Protective effects of D-allose against ischemia reperfusion injury of the rat liver. J Hepato-Biliary-Pancreat Surg. 2003;10:218–25. https://doi.org/10.1007/s00534-002-0785-8.
42. Hossain MA, Wakabayashi H, Goda F, Kobayashi S, Maeba T, Maeta H. Effect of the immunosuppressants FK506 and D-allose on allogenic orthotopic liver transplantation in rats. Transplant Proc. 2000;32:2021–3.
43. Murata A, Sekiya K, Watanabe Y, Yamaguchi F, Hatano N, Izumori K, Tokuda M. A novel inhibitory effect of D-allose on production of reactive oxygen species from neutrophils. J Biosci Bioeng. 2003;96:89–91.
44. Sui L, Dong Y, Watanabe Y, Yamaguchi F, Hatano N, Izumori K, Tokuda M. Growth inhibitory effect of D-allose on human ovarian carcinoma cells in vitro. Anticancer Res. 2005;25:2639–44.
45. Gong X, Zhou Q, Wang F, Wu W, Chen X. Efficacy and safety of ultrasound-guided percutaneous Polidocanol Sclerotherapy in benign cystic thyroid nodules: preliminary results. Int J Endocrinol. 2017;2017:8043429. https://doi.org/10.1155/2017/8043429.
46. Star P, Connor DE, Parsi K. Novel developments in foam sclerotherapy: focus on Varithena(R) (polidocanol endovenous microfoam) in the management of varicose veins. Phlebology. 2017;268355516687864. https://doi.org/10.1177/0268355516687864.

47. Chen SS, Zhang Y, Lu QL, Lin Z, Zhao Y. Preventive effects of cedrol against alopecia in cyclophosphamide-treated mice. Environ Toxicol Pharmacol. 2016;46:270–6. https://doi.org/10.1016/j.etap.2016.07.020.

48. Zhang SY, Li XB, Hou SG, Sun Y, Shi YR, Lin SS. Cedrol induces autophagy and apoptotic cell death in A549 non-small cell lung carcinoma cells through the P13K/Akt signaling pathway, the loss of mitochondrial transmembrane potential and the generation of ROS. Int J Mol Med. 2016; 38:291–9. https://doi.org/10.3892/ijmm.2016.2585.

49. Zhang Y, Han L, Chen SS, Guan J, Qu FZ, Zhao YQ. Hair growth promoting activity of cedrol isolated from the leaves of Platycladus orientalis. Biomed Pharmacother. 2016;83:641–7. https://doi.org/10.1016/j.biopha.2016.07.022.

50. Fang Z, Jeong SY, Jung HA, Choi JS, Min BS, Woo MH. Anticholinesterase and antioxidant constituents from Gloiopeltis furcata. Chem Pharm Bull (Tokyo). 2010;58:1236–9.

51. Guo J, Yuan Y, Lu D, Du B, Xiong L, Shi J, Yang L, Liu W, Yuan X, Zhang G, Wang F. Two natural products, trans-phytol and (22E)-ergosta-6,9,22-triene-3beta,5alpha,8alpha-triol, inhibit the biosynthesis of estrogen in human ovarian granulosa cells by aromatase (CYP19). Toxicol Appl Pharmacol. 2014; 279:23–32. https://doi.org/10.1016/j.taap.2014.05.008.

52. Saikia D, Parihar S, Chanda D, Ojha S, Kumar JK, Chanotiya CS, Shanker K, Negi AS. Antitubercular potential of some semisynthetic analogues of phytol. Bioorg Med Chem Lett. 2010;20:508–12. https://doi.org/10.1016/j.bmcl.2009.11.107.

53. Teal PE, Tumlinson JH, Heath RR. Chemical and behavioral analyses of volatile sex pheromone components released by callingHeliothis virescens (F.) females (Lepidoptera: Noctuidae). J Chem Ecol. 1986;12:107–26. https://doi.org/10.1007/bf01045595.

54. Himmelfarb J, Phinney S, Ikizler TA, Kane J, McMonagle E, Miller G. Gamma-tocopherol and docosahexaenoic acid decrease inflammation in dialysis patients. J Ren Nutr. 2007;17:296–304. https://doi.org/10.1053/j.jrn.2007.05.011.

55. Muid S, Froemming GR, Rahman T, Ali AM, Nawawi HM. Delta- and gamma-tocotrienol isomers are potent in inhibiting inflammation and endothelial activation in stimulated human endothelial cells. Food Nutr Res. 2016;60: 31526. https://doi.org/10.3402/fnr.v60.31526.

56. Traber MG, Atkinson J. Vitamin E, antioxidant and nothing more. Free Radic Biol Med. 2007;43:4–15. https://doi.org/10.1016/j.freeradbiomed.2007.03.024.

57. Adnan SN, Ibrahim N, Yaacob WA. Transcriptome analysis of methicillin-resistant Staphylococcus aureus in response to stigmasterol and lupeol. J Glob Antimicrob Resist. 2017;8:48–54. https://doi.org/10.1016/j.jgar.2016.10.006.

58. Aminu R, Umar IA, Rahman MA, Ibrahim MA. Stigmasterol retards the proliferation and pathological features of Trypanosoma congolense infection in rats and inhibits trypanosomal sialidase in vitro and in silico. Biomed Pharmacother. 2017;89:482–9. https://doi.org/10.1016/j.biopha.2017.02.068.

59. Antwi AO, Obiri DD, Osafo N. Stigmasterol modulates allergic airway inflammation in Guinea pig model of ovalbumin-induced asthma. Mediat Inflamm. 2017;2017:2953930. https://doi.org/10.1155/2017/2953930.

60. Gade S, Rajamanikyam M, Vadlapudi V, Nukala KM, Aluvala R, Giddigari C, Karanam NJ, Barua NC, Pandey R, Upadhyayula VS, Sripadi P, Amanchy R, Upadhyayula SM. Acetylcholinesterase inhibitory activity of stigmasterol & hexacosanol is responsible for larvicidal and repellent properties of Chromolaena odorata. Biochim Biophys Acta. 2017;1861: 541–50. https://doi.org/10.1016/j.bbagen.2016.11.044.

61. Ahn EK, Oh JS. Lupenone isolated from Adenophora triphylla var. japonica extract inhibits adipogenic differentiation through the downregulation of PPARgamma in 3T3-L1 cells. Phytother Res. 2013;27: 761–6. https://doi.org/10.1002/ptr.4779.

62. Villareal MO, Han J, Matsuyama K, Sekii Y, Smaoui A, Shigemori H, Isoda H. Lupenone from Erica multiflora leaf extract stimulates melanogenesis in B16 murine melanoma cells through the inhibition of ERK1/2 activation. Planta Med. 2013;79:236–43. https://doi.org/10.1055/s-0032-1328189.

63. Xu F, Wu H, Wang X, Yang Y, Wang Y, Qian H, Zhang Y. RP-HPLC characterization of lupenone and beta-sitosterol in rhizoma musae and evaluation of the anti-diabetic activity of lupenone in diabetic Sprague-Dawley rats. Molecules. 2014;19: 14114–27. https://doi.org/10.3390/molecules190914114.

64. Yoon YP, Lee HJ, Lee DU, Lee SK, Hong JH, Lee CJ. Effects of Lupenone, Lupeol, and Taraxerol derived from Adenophora triphylla on the gene expression and production of airway MUC5AC Mucin. Tuberc Respir Dis (Seoul). 2015;78:210–7. https://doi.org/10.4046/trd.2015.78.3.210.

13

An in vivo immunomodulatory and anti-inflammatory study of fermented *Dendropanax morbifera* Léveille leaf extract

Biruk Tesfaye Birhanu[1†], Jin-Yoon Kim[1†], Md. Akil Hossain[1,2], Jae-Won Choi[3], Sam-Pin Lee[3] and Seung-Chun Park[1*]

Abstract

Background: Medicinal plants represent a source of new drugs for the prevention and treatment of infectious diseases. *Dendropanax morbifera* Léveille is an economically and medicinally important subtropical tree that has various biological activities. However, its ability to affect immune responses in vivo is unknown. Hence, this study was designed to examine the immunomodulatory activity of fermented *D. morbifera* extract in BALB/c mice.

Methods: five-week-old female BALB/c mice were arranged in six groups and kept under a standard laboratory condition. Splenocyte counts were determined using the trypan blue dye exclusion method, and splenic lymphocyte proliferation was determined using concanavalin A and lipopolysaccharide (LPS). Flow cytometric analysis was performed to phenotype T-lymphocytes. Next, cytokine and immunoglobulin quantitation was performed using sandwich ELISA.

Results: The results showed an increase in spleen cells by 71 and 67% in mice treated with 125 and 250 mg/kg of *D. morbifera*, respectively. In addition, splenocyte proliferation was increased 58.7% in response to concanavalin A treatment, while LPS treatment induced a 73.3% increase in mice treated with 125 mg/kg. T-cell phenotypic analysis indicated that *D. morbifera*-treated groups showed higher CD8a+, CD11b and CD3+ T-cell expression. However, the treatment groups showed suppression of IL-1α, Il-1β and IL-4. In addition, the IgG super-family was downregulated in a dose-dependent manner by 4.5% up to 43.7%.

Conclusions: Taken together, we show that *D. morbifera* increases the number and proliferation of T- and B-lymphocytes. Moreover, these effects may play a role in boosting non-specific immunity, while suppressing proinflammatory cytokines and immunoglobulins after a single antigen exposure.

Keywords: *Dendropanax morbifera* Léveille, Immunomodulation, T-cell proliferation, Proinflammatory cytokines

Background

Medicinal plants play a vital role in the treatment of human and animal diseases. The application of these herbal medicines has contributed significantly to the search for a new drug for prevention and treatment of infectious agents. Recently, much interest has been directed to the use of natural compounds to enhance host immunity.

Plant extracts play a significant role in the prevention and curing of infections by modulating the immune system. As a result, their application and use has increased dramatically [1]. Herbal medicines act on the immune system by either suppressing or stimulating innate or adaptive immune cells/molecules [2]. Immune regulation is important in maintaining normal immunity, and the search for herbal immunomodulatory compounds to treat various infections by enhancing the body's natural resistance is of growing interest [3].

Dendropanax morbifera Léveille, also knowns as *Dendropanax trifidus*, is an economically and medicinally important subtropical broad-leaved tree that is endemic to Korea [4, 5]. The tree has been used in the treatment of different human infections and reported to have anti-thrombotic, anti-diabetic and anti-atherogenic components

* Correspondence: parksch@knu.ac.kr

†Biruk Tesfaye Birhanu and Jin-Yoon Kim contributed equally to this work.

[1]Laboratory of Veterinary Pharmacokinetics and Pharmacodynamics, College of Veterinary Medicine, Kyungpook National University, Bukgu, 80 Daehakro, Daegu 41566, South Korea

Full list of author information is available at the end of the article

[6–9]. Polyacetylene from plant leaves has been shown to have an anti-complement effect [10]. The plant is also known to increase the excretion of toxic elements, namely, cadmium from the kidney, and to reduce cadmium-induced oxidative stress in the hippocampus [11]. In addition, Hyun and his colleagues [4] reported the anti-cancer and anti-oxidant activity of the methanolic leaf and debarked stem extracts. The bioflavonoid extract, rutin, prevents rotenone-induced cell injury through inhibition of the JNK and p38 MAPK signaling pathways in a Parkinson's disease model [12]. Furthermore, the chloroform extract suppresses proinflammatory mediators and cytokines through inhibition of NF-κB [13].

Numerous studies have been conducted using fermented plant extracts with different techniques [14]. In our previous works [15], we optimized co-production of poly-γ-glutamic acid (γ-PGA) and γ-aminobutyric acid (GABA) in the presence of sodium-L-glutamate (MSG) in *Dendropanax morbifera* fermented by *Bacillus subtilis* HA (KCCM 10775P, patent strain) and *Lactobacillus plantarum* EJ2014 (KCCM 11545P, patent strain). The extract has shown to have an immunostimulatory activity in RAW 264.7 cells in in vitro experiment. A voucher of the specimen for the fermented extract was deposited at Keimyung Traditional center, Keimyung University.

To our knowledge, no studies have investigated the immunomodulatory activities of the fermented plant extract in vivo. Hence, the objective of this study was to determine the immunomodulatory activities of fermented *Dendropanax morbifera* Léveille leaf extract in BALB/c mice.

Methods

Dendropanax morbifera leaf extract preparation

Dendropanax morbifera leaf (Hambakjae Bio Farm Co., Ltd., Jeju Island, South Korea) was dried and 10 volume of water was added before macerated for 8 h at 98 °C. Fifty milliliter of the concentrated extract was supplemented with 5% (v/v) *Bacillus subtilis* and mixed with 3% monosodium glutamate (MSG) and 3% glucose and incubated for 3 days in shaking incubator with 160 rpm (SI-900R, Jeio Tech. Co., Ltd., Daejeon, Korea) at 42 °C for γ-PGA production. The first fermented product was mixed with *Lactobacillus plantarum* EJ2014 starter 1% (v/v) and incubated at 30 °C for 5 days in a constant temperature incubator (IS-971R, JeioTech, Kimpo, Korea) for GABA production through lactic acid fermentation. Finally, an additional 20% MSG, 20% glucose and 10% skim milk was supplemented to the solution and make the final volume 130 mL.

Animals and study design

All experimental protocols involving animals were approved by the Kyungpook National University Ethical Committee (KNU 2016–121). Five-week-old female

specific pathogen free (SPF) BALB/c mice were procured (ORIENT BIO, Republic of Korea) and acclimated to lab conditions for one week before the start of the study. The weight of the mice ranged from 18 to 20 g. The animal room was maintained at a relative humidity of 50–65% at 20 °C–24 °C temperature and equal 12 h light and dark time. Mice were provided with standard pellet diet and ad libitum filtered tap water access. After adaptation to laboratory conditions, the mice were arbitrarily divided into six groups, each consisting of ten mice (Table 1). The total number of mice used in the present study was calculated by the G*power program (3.1.9.2) based on effect size (0.5), α error probability (0.05), Power (1-β error probability) (0.8) and number of groups (6).

All mice in the treatment group received a daily oral dose of 200 μL of (125 mg/kg, 250 mg/kg and 500 mg/kg) *D. morbifera* extract for 14 days. The mice were immunized intraperitoneally with 5.0×10^8 sheep red blood cells (SRBCs) per milliliter on the 15th day, and treatment continued with the extract for an additional week. Body weight was measured regularly to adjust dosing volumes. After 21 days, mice were euthanized by carbon dioxide inhalation. Euthanasia lid was placed over the cage. CO_2 was delivered from the tank at a flow rate of 10–30% of the chamber per minute. Finally, animals were monitored for cessation of respiration and left in the chamber for at least 1 min after respiration has ceased, and blood and organs were collected (Fig. 1). Blood was collected in heparinized tubes and centrifuged at 10,000 RPM for 5 min. Plasma was separated and stored at – 70 °C until use in an ELISA. Moreover, the organs were weighed and processed accordingly.

Acute toxicity test

The test was carried out on six 5-week-old female rats with an average weight of 139 g. The rats were fasted overnight prior to dosing. A single administration of the fermented *Dendropanax morbifera* Léveille plant extract was given orally to 3 rats at a dose of 2000 mg/kg. In addition, 3 rats were left untreated to serve as negative controls. Rats were checked for physical and clinical symptoms. Body weight and abnormal behavior, if observed,

Table 1 Group arrangement and experimental design of mice

Groups	Treatment groups	Description
Group I	Normal control	Received only diet and water
Group II	Vehicle control	Received water and treated with SRBC
Group III	Positive control	Received Ginseng extract 200 mg/kg
Group IV	Low dosage treatment	Received 125 mg/kg of *D. morbifera*
Group V	Intermediate dosage treatment	Received 250 mg/kg of *D. morbifera*
Group VI	High dosage treatment	Received 500 mg/kg of *D. morbifera*

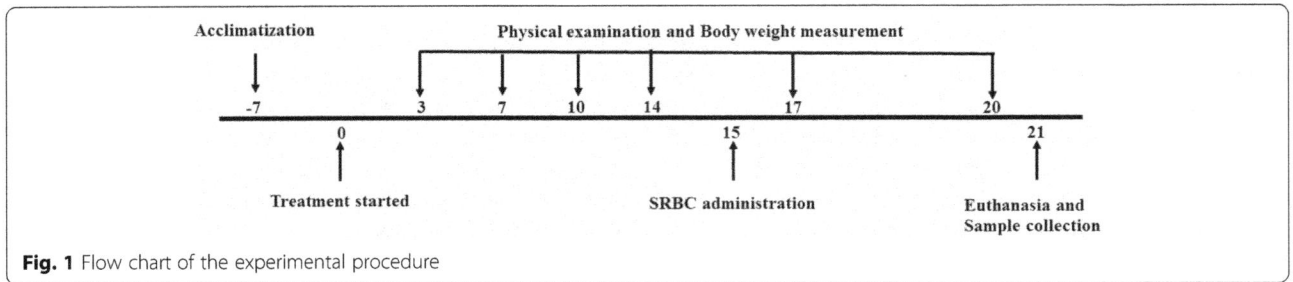

Fig. 1 Flow chart of the experimental procedure

were recorded on a daily basis. In addition, pathological examination was performed after 14 days of observation. Rats were euthanized by carbon dioxide inhalation. Euthanasia lid was placed over the cage. CO_2 was delivered from the tank at a flow rate of 10–30% of the chamber per minute. Finally, animals were monitored for cessation of respiration and left in the chamber for at least 1 min after respiration has ceased.

Preparation of splenocytes

Splenocyte preparation was performed as previously described (Ahmad et al., 2015). Briefly, after sacrifice, mouse spleen and other organs were removed aseptically from all experimental groups. The tissues were placed into a sterile tube with Hank's balanced salt solution (HBSS, Gibco Life Technologies, NY) on ice. The spleen was minced and pressed through a 70 μm fine nylon cell strainer (BD Biosciences, CA) using plunger at the end of a 3 mL syringe. The cells were washed with excess HBSS using the strainer. The cell suspensions were then centrifuged at 1600 rpm for 5 min. The supernatant was discarded, and the pellet was re-suspended in 1 mL pre-warmed Red Blood Cell Lysing Buffer solution (Sigma, UK). The cells were incubated at 37 °C for 1 min to lyse the RBCs before cold HBSS was added. Next, the cells were centrifuged for 5 min at 1600 rpm at 4 °C. The pelleted cells were washed three times with PBS after centrifugation. Afterwards, the supernatant was aspirated, and the pellet was re-suspended in RPMI-1640 medium (Sigma-Aldrich, MO) supplemented with 10% (v/v) FBS, 100 units/mL of penicillin and 100 μg/mL of streptomycin. The cell count was measured with a hemocytometer using the trypan blue dye exclusion method.

Splenic lymphocyte proliferation assay

Spleen cells (4×10^6 cells/mL) from the control and treatment groups were seeded (200 μL/well) into a 96-well plate in RPMI-1640 medium (10% FBS, 1% P/S). Cells from each group were cultured in the absence of any mitogen and in the presence of concanavalin A (5 μg/mL) or LPS (10 μg/mL) at 37 °C for 72 h. Results were read using an MTT (3-(4,5-Dimethylthiazol-2-yl)-2,5-Diphenyltetrazolium Bromide) reagent assay. The proliferation

index was calculated by dividing the sample OD readings to the control OD value.

$$\text{Proliferation index} = \frac{\text{OD of treated cells}}{\text{OD of control cells}}$$

Flow cytometric analysis for T-lymphocyte phenotyping

For T-lymphocyte phenotyping of spleen cells (1×10^6 cells/100 μL), they were harvested into FACS tubes. The cells were blocked with IgG blocking solution (1 μg IgG/10^6 cells) for 15 min at room temperature. The conjugating antibodies (10 μL/10^6 cells) were added and vortexed before the cells were incubated for 30 min in the dark. The cells were washed with Flow Cytometry Staining Buffer to remove the unbound antibody, and then suspended cells were centrifuged at 300 x g for 5 min. The cells were washed and re-suspended with 400 μL of the buffer solution for flow cytometric analysis. Finally, data were acquired and analyzed using multicolor FACS with FACSDiva version 6.1.3 software on BD FACSAria™ III (BD Biosciences, CA, US). Group comparisons were made among the different T-lymphocyte sub-populations, and the results were expressed as a percentage of expression.

Cytokine and immunoglobulin determination

Samples, standards and controls were incubated for 2 h (cytokines) and 30 min (immunoglobulins) at room temperature on a horizontal orbital microplate shaker after 50 μL of the microparticle cocktail was added to each well of the microplate, and 50 μL of the standard or sample was added to each well. After washing four times with a magnetic device, 50 μL of diluted Biotin Antibody Cocktail was added to each well for the cytokines and immunoglobulins and incubated for 1.5 h at room temperature on the shaker. Diluted Streptavidin-PE (50 μL) was added to each well and incubated for 30 or 15 min at room temperature on the shaker after washing. Finally, the microparticles were resuspended by adding 100 μL of Wash Buffer to each well and incubated for another 2 min before reading using a Luminex MAGPIX analyzer (Luminex, Austin, TX, USA). Each analyte in the sample reacted independently with the corresponding antibody attached to the specific number bead. The concentration of the samples was determined after a standard curve was generated using five parameters logistic curve-fit (MasterPlex QT 2010 (MiraiBio, Hitachi, CA, USA) and multiplied by the dilution factor.

Statistical analysis

Data were analyzed using a one-way and two-way analysis of variance followed by Dunnett's test and Tukey's test using GraphPad Prism 7 software. The results are expressed as the mean ± standard error of the mean. $P < 0.05$ was considered as statistically significant.

Results

The animal experiment was carried out for 21 days, and mice were supplemented with pelleted feed and water ad libitum. The amount of feed and water was measured twice a week, and a total of six measurements was carried out. The feed and water intake of the animals were reduced immediately after treatment with SRBC and increased towards the end of treatment. Although the results showed that mice treated with *D. morbifera* Léveille had gained more weight than the untreated groups, there is no significant difference observed between the treated and control groups for water and food intake.

The acute toxicity result showed that there were no physical or clinical signs observed in the treated rats from day zero to day fourteen. In addition, no apparent pathological lesions were found in the organs of the mice that received the treatment, and no mortality of rats was recorded.

In addition, the spleen, liver, thymus and both kidneys from each mouse were removed aseptically and measured accordingly at the end of the experiment (Table 2, Fig. 2b). A significant difference in the weight increase of spleens from mice receiving the ginseng extract or 125, 250 or 500 mg/kg of *D. morbifera* Léveille was observed compared with the other groups ($P < 0.05$). The spleen weight increased by 33.3, 30.8, 20.5 and 34.6% in mice treated with ginseng extract or 125, 250 or 500 mg/kg of *D. morbifera*, respectively.

Spleen cells were counted with a hemocytometer during the trypan Blue dye-exclusion assay. The total number of counted spleen cells was found to be increased in mice treated with the ginseng extract or 125 or 250 mg/kg of *D. morbifera* Léveille by 58, 71 and 67%, respectively ($P < 0.001$). However, spleen cell counts at the higher extract dosage of 500 mg/kg did not show any significant increase when compared with untreated control groups (Fig. 2a).

T- and B-cell lymphocyte proliferation assays were conducted using Con-A and LPS. Our in vivo and ex vivo (data not shown) results showed that splenocyte proliferation by con A and LPS treatment is four-fold higher than that of cells with no-mitogen activation (Fig. 2c). The OD value at 570 nm was significantly higher in mice treated with *D. morbifera* and in the positive control group for both the Con-A and LPS tests. Spleen cell proliferation after Con-A treatment was increased by 53.6, 58.7, 50.6 and 41% for mice treated with ginseng extract or 125, 250 or 500 mg/kg of *D. morbifera*, respectively. In addition, B cell proliferation by LPS was increased by 88.1, 73.3, 63.1 and 28% in mice treated with ginseng extract or 125, 250 or 500 mg/kg of *D. morbifera*, respectively.

Flow cytometry was performed for phenotyping the T-lymphocyte population. *D. morbifera* treated groups showed higher CD8a, CD3 and CD45RA T-cell expression than the control groups. The increase is significantly higher in those treated with 125 mg/kg of *D. morbifera* treatment, with percentages of 16.7, 5.7 and 7.1% for CD8a, CD3 and CD45RA T cells, respectively (Fig. 3). In addition, our results showed a dose-dependent reduction in the T-cell lymphocyte populations after the same treatment conditions as mentioned above (Fig. 3). Conversely, CD11b-expressing cells showed a significant reduction of 22% in low dosage (125 mg/kg)-treated mice.

Sandwich ELISA was performed to determine the effects of *D. morbifera* activity on Th1- and Th2- dependent cytokine release and adaptive immunity. The level of IL-1α, IL-1β and IL-4 was suppressed in mice treated with ginseng and *D. morbifera* extract (Fig. 4). The level of IL-4 was reduced in a dose-dependent manner by 53.2, 68.9 and 71.4% in mice treated with 125, 250 and 500 mg/kg *D. morbifera*, respectively. However, the levels of TNF-α, IL-2, IL-5, IL-6, IL-10, IL-12, IL-12p70 and IL-13 were below the detection limit of the ELISA kit. IFN-γ levels

Table 2 The average weight of the organs collected from treated and non-treated mice

	Spleen (Mean ± SEM)	Liver (Mean ± SEM)	Thymus (Mean ± SEM)	Left Kidney (Mean ± SEM)	Right Kidney (Mean ± SEM)
I	0.08 ± 0.002	0.854 ± 0.022	0.03 ± 0.0084	0.106 ± 0.006	0.110 ± 0.005
II	0.096 ± 0.008	0.824 ± 0.035	0.038 ± 0.0049	0.122 ± 0.007	0.116 ± 0.008
III	0.104 ± 0.007	0.894 ± 0.038	0.047 ± 0.0037	0.114 ± 0.007	0.12 ± 0.005
IV	0.102 ± 0.004	0.878 ± 0.024	0.059 ± 0.0086	0.112 ± 0.004	0.116 ± 0.004
V	0.103 ± 0.005	0.84 ± 0.028	0.049 ± 0.0031	0.114 ± 0.005	0.112 ± 0.002
VI	0.105 ± 0.005	0.863 ± 0.013	0.047 ± 0.0034	0.115 ± 0.006	0.128 ± 0.005

*Weight presented in grams. SEM; standard error of the mean

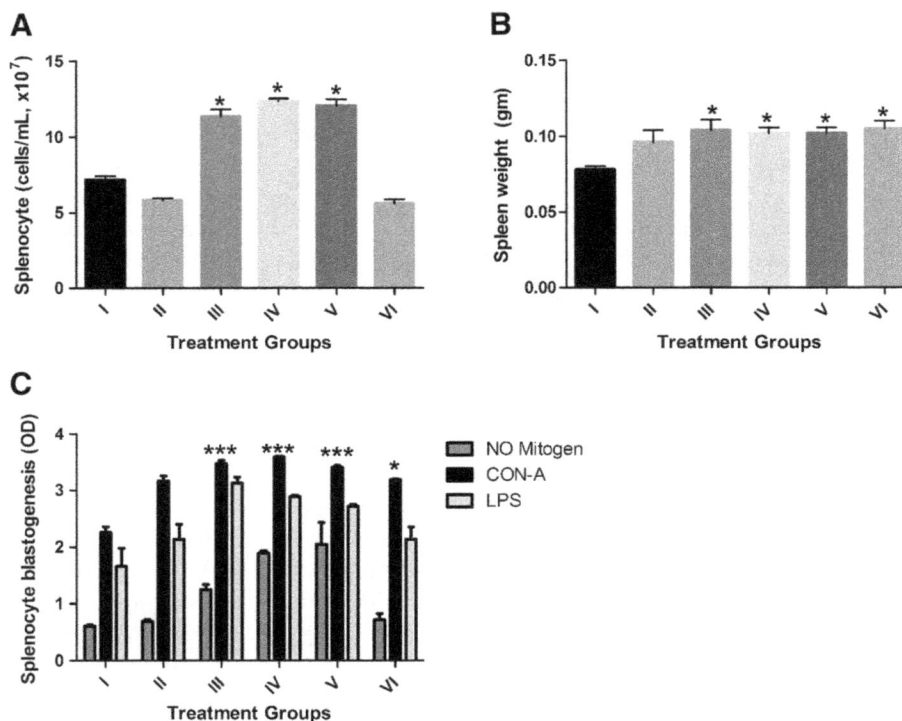

Fig. 2 Effect of *Denropanax morbifera* on the splenocytes of mice. **a** Total splenocyte count of different treatment groups. A significant increase in splenocyte counts was observed in mice among control groups and those that received ginseng extract or 125 and 250 mg/kg of *D. morbifera* Léveille. **b** Weight of spleen taken from each mouse group. **c** In vivo activation of splenocytes by Con A and LPS after 72 h of incubation. A significant difference was observed between group II and group III, as well as groups V and V treated with Con-A and LPS (*P value < 0.05; ***P < 0.001)

were elevated upon treatment with increasing *D. morbifera* treatment, although a significant difference was not observed among the groups.

D. morbifera Léveille results in the suppression of the tested immunoglobulins IgA, IgG (IgG1, IgG2A, IgG2B IgG3) and IgM in a dose-dependent manner (Fig. 5). The IgG super-family was increased when compared with normal control groups. However, immunoglobulins were reduced by 17.1, 31 and 43.7% for IgG1; 4.5, 15.4 and 35% for IgG2A; 9.5, 21.5 and 34.3% for IgG2B and 5.1, 6.8 and 15.6% for IgG3 in mice treated with 125, 250 and 500 mg/kg of *D. morbifera* compared to the antigen receiving control group.

Discussion

The immunomodulatory activity of plant extracts that stimulate or suppress the immune system, may be of paramount importance in regulating diseases that originate from immune cell disturbances. Moreover, plant extracts can provide a substitute for the currently available chemotherapies aimed at combating diseases such as autoimmune diseases. *D. morbifera* Léveille is a well-known Korean traditional medicine used for improvement of blood circulation that has anti-oxidant, anti-inflammatory, anti-complement, anti-thrombotic,

anti-diabetic and anti-atherogenic effects [7–10]. In this study, we used an in vivo approach to determine the effect of the plant extract on the immune system of mice.

In the current study, we have found that the *D. morbifera* Léveille extract was shown to increase the proliferation of both T- and B-lymphocytes. The number of splenocytes was increased in mice treated with the plant extract. The rising level of splenic B- and T-cells upon treatment with *D. morbifera* Léveille suggests an immunostimulatory effect of the plant extract on the innate immune system. Interestingly, higher T-cell proliferation was one of the more pronounced effects of plant extract treatment and has been explained by an increase in CD18 phenotypes.

Increasing levels of IFN-γ observed in a dose-dependent manner is indicative of Th1 cell activation by *D. morbifera* Léveille. Th1 immunity is known to defend against cancer development and several intracellular infectious diseases. These results agree with previous reports that suggest the anti-cancer activity of the plant extract [4].

Dose-dependent suppression of IL-4 results in the downregulation of immunoglobulins. These results show suppression of immunoglobulins, which may be an indicator of suppression of Th2 cells or antibody-mediated immunity [16, 17]. There is a chance of reducing purified

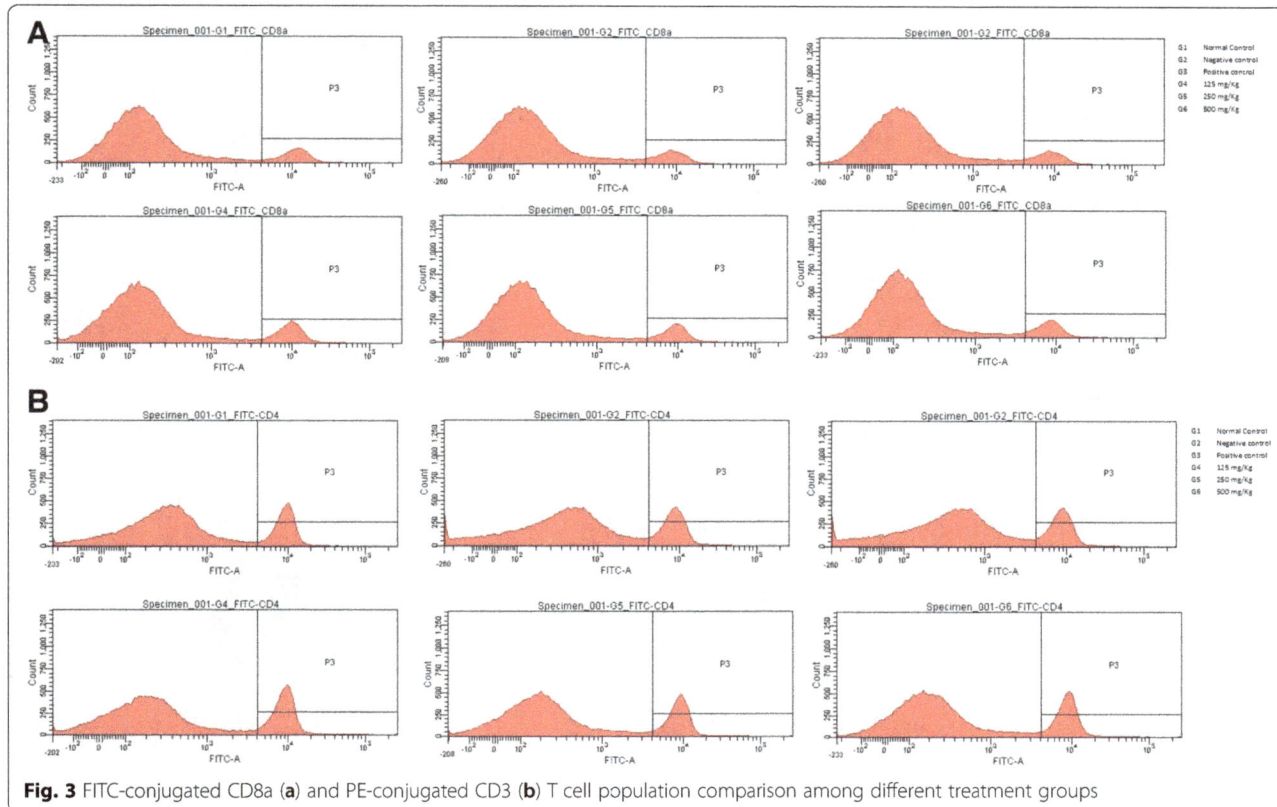

Fig. 3 FITC-conjugated CD8a (**a**) and PE-conjugated CD3 (**b**) T cell population comparison among different treatment groups

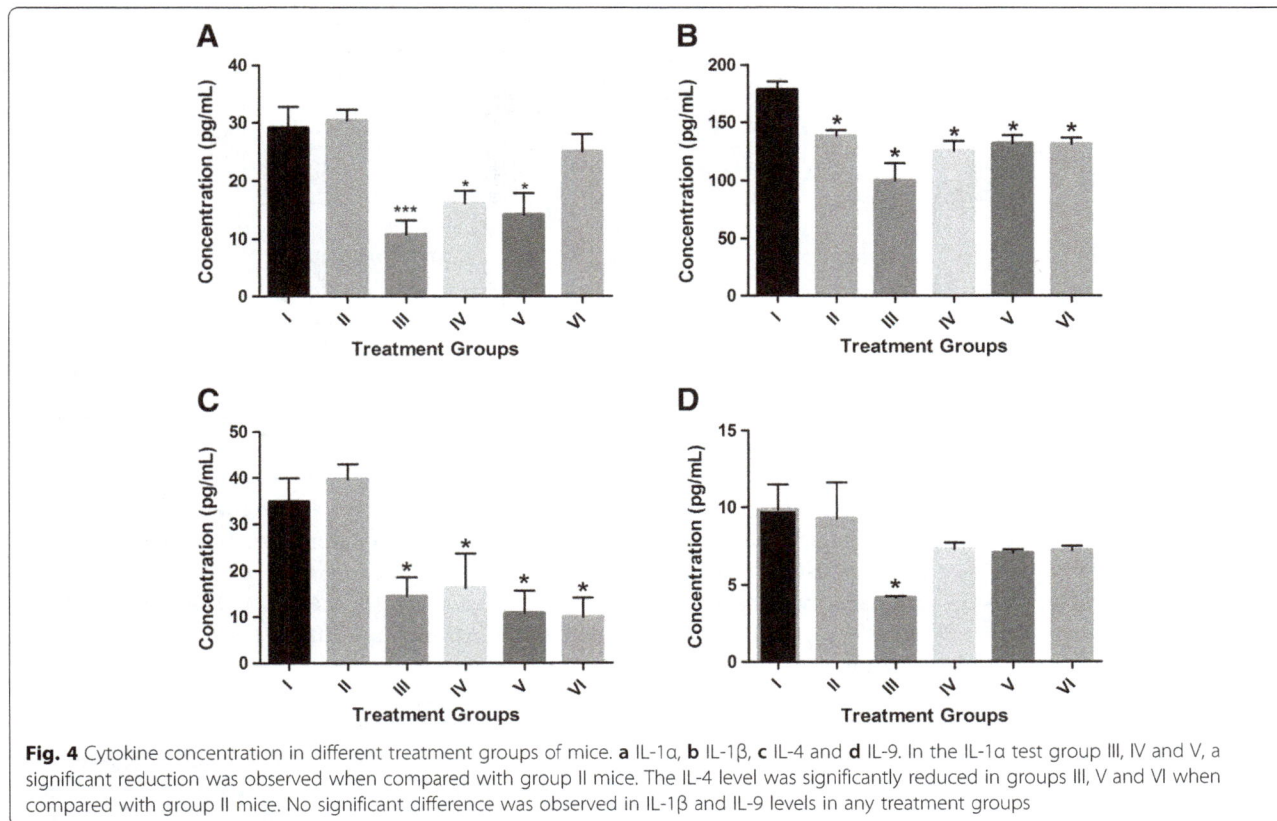

Fig. 4 Cytokine concentration in different treatment groups of mice. **a** IL-1α, **b** IL-1β, **c** IL-4 and **d** IL-9. In the IL-1α test group III, IV and V, a significant reduction was observed when compared with group II mice. The IL-4 level was significantly reduced in groups III, V and VI when compared with group II mice. No significant difference was observed in IL-1β and IL-9 levels in any treatment groups

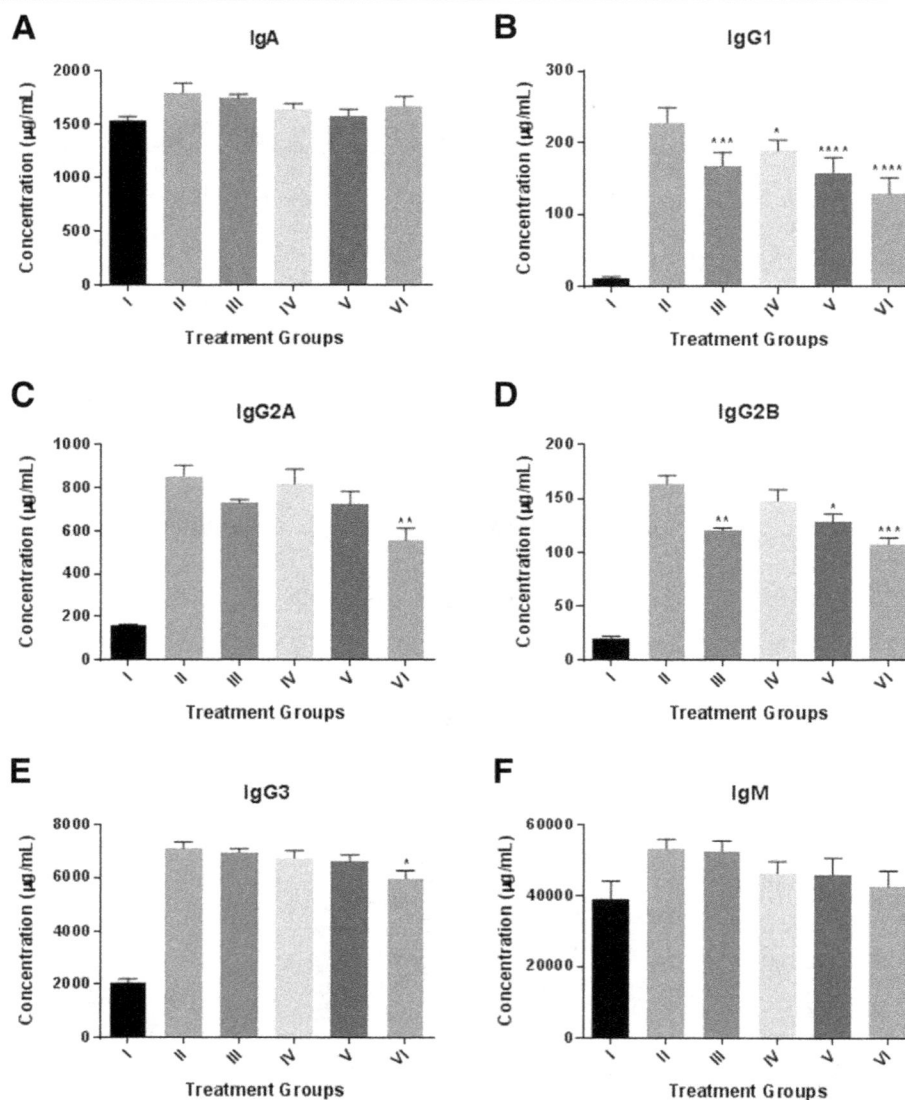

Fig. 5 Immunoglobulin levels of control and *D. morbifera* Léveille-treated mice. **a** IgA, **b** IgG1, **c** IgG2A, **d** IgG2B, **e** IgG3 and **f** IgM. All the tested immunoglobulins showed a dose-dependent reduction in treatment with *D. moribifera* Léveille, except for IgA. Group VI showed a significant reduction IgG2A levels. IgG2B was significantly reduced in groups III, V and VI. IgG3 showed significant suppression in group VI mice. No significant difference was observed between the IgM treatment groups. (* = P value < 0.05; ** = P value < 0.01; *** = P value< 0.001; **** = P value < 0.0001; all the comparisons were made using the untreated control groups)

B lymphocyte IgM and IgG synthesis in stimulated human peripheral blood mononuclear cells (PBMCs) without killing B cells [18]. This indicates the downregulation of the antibody-mediated immune system by the plant extract.

The levels of IL-1α were decreased in the plasma of mice treated with *D. morbifera* Léveille. The proinflammatory cytokine IL-1α is an initiator of immune responses via induction of neutrophil infiltration. Moreover, it stimulates the transcription and secretion of IL-1β, which is a known amplifier of inflammation [19]. Hence, the suppression of these cytokines shows the anti-inflammatory activity of the plant extract. This has been previously

indicated in the work of Akram and colleagues [13]. A compound in *D. morbifera* Léveille might inhibit the gene expression of proinflammatory cytokines, such as IL-1α, IL-1β, TNF-α and IL-6, in mice by decreasing COX-2 mRNA expression, as has been shown for the bioactive compound of citrus plants [20].

Conclusions

This study shows that *D. morbifera* Léveille treatment increases the number of lymphocytes and promotes proliferation of T and B lymphocytes. This can be indicative of boosting non-specific immunity by the plant extract.

However, the plant demonstrated suppressive effects in which it inhibited immunoglobulins by inhibiting synthesis/release of IL-4, a known stimulator of antibody-mediated immunity. In addition, the anti-inflammatory effects of the plant were shown through downregulation of the proinflammatory cytokine IL-1β. Although further mechanistic studies on the molecular mechanism of *D. morbifera* Léveille activity are needed, this study has demonstrated immunomodulatory effects of the plant extract in a murine model.

Abbreviations
CD: Cluster of differentiation; CON-A: concanavalin A; FBS: Fetal bovine serum; HBSS: Hank's balanced salt solution; IG: Immunoglobulins; IL: Interleukin; LPS: Lipopolysaccharide; PBMC: peripheral blood mononuclear cells; TNF: Tumor necrosis factor

Funding
This work was supported in part by the National Foundation of Korea (NRF) grant funded by the Korea government (2016R1A2B4013507), in part by the Technology Commercialization Support Program (314082–3), Ministry of Agriculture, Food and Rural Affairs and in part by a grant the Technology Development Program for Forestry (S111515 L050130), Korea forest service. The funding bodies have no role in designing the study, collection, analysis, and interpretation of data and in writing the manuscript.

Authors' contributions
BTB, designed and carried out the experiment, analyzed the results and wrote the manuscript. J-YK carried out the experiment and revised the manuscript. J-WC, prepared the plant extract and revised the manuscript. MAH, S-PL, S-CP designed the study and revised the manuscript. All authors read and approved the final manuscript.

Competing interests
The authors declare that there is no conflict of interests.

Author details
[1]Laboratory of Veterinary Pharmacokinetics and Pharmacodynamics, College of Veterinary Medicine, Kyungpook National University, Bukgu, 80 Daehakro, Daegu 41566, South Korea. [2]Veterinary drugs & Biologics Division, Animal and Plant Quarantine Agency (QIA), 177, Hyeoksin 8-ro, Gimcheon-si, Gyeongsangbuk-do 39660, South Korea. [3]The Center for Traditional Microorganism Resources (TMR), Keimyung University, Daegu 704-701, South Korea.

References
1. Shukla S, Bajpai V, Kim M. Plants as potential sources of natural immunomodulators. Rev Env Sci Biotechnol. 2014;13:17–33. https://doi.org/10.1007/s11157-012-9303-x.
2. Patwardhan B, Gautam M. Botanical immunodrugs: scope and opportunities. Drug Discov Today. 2005;10:495–502. https://doi.org/10.1016/S1359-6446(04)03357-4.
3. Brindha P. Role of phytochemicals as immunomodulatory agents: A review. Int J Green Pharm. 2016;10(1):1–18.
4. Hyun TK, Kim M, Lee H, Kim Y, Kim E, Kim J-S. Evaluation of anti-oxidant and anti-cancer properties of Dendropanax morbifera Léveille. Food Chem. 2013;141:1947–55. http://www.sciencedirect.com/science/article/pii/S0308814613006043
5. Moon MO, Ihm BS, Chung YC, Kang YJ, Kim CS, Kim MH. Taxonomic appraisal of Dendropanax morbifera Léveille and D. Trifidus (Thunb. Ex Murray) Makino based on morphological characters. Korean J Plant Taxon. 1999;29:231–48.
6. Chung I-M, Kim MY, Park W-H, Moon H-I. Antiatherogenic activity of Dendropanax morbifera essential oil in rats. Pharmazie. 2009;64:547–9. http://www.ncbi.nlm.nih.gov/pubmed/19746846
7. Moon H-I. Antidiabetic effects of dendropanoxide from leaves of Dendropanax morbifera Leveille in normal and streptozotocin-induced diabetic rats. Hum Exp Toxicol SAGE Publications. 2010;30:870–5. https://doi.org/10.1177/0960327110382131
8. Park B-Y, Min B-S, Oh S-R, Kim J-H, Kim T-J, Kim D-H, et al. Isolation and anticomplement activity of compounds from Dendropanax morbifera. J Ethnopharmacol [Internet]. 2004;90:403–8. http://www.sciencedirect.com/science/article/pii/S0378874103004112
9. Choi J-H, Kim D-W, Park S-E, Lee H-J, Kim K-MK-J, Kim K-MK-J, et al. Anti-thrombotic effect of rutin isolated from Dendropanax morbifera Leveille. J Biosci Bioeng [Internet]. 2015 [cited 2017 Feb 27];120:181–186. http://www.sciencedirect.com/science/article/pii/S1389172314004915
10. Chung I-M, Song H-K, Kim S-J, Moon H-I. Anticomplement activity of polyacetylenes from leaves of Dendropanax morbifera Leveille. Phyther res. John Wiley & sons, Ltd. 2011;25:784–6. https://doi.org/10.1002/ptr.3336
11. Kim W, Kim DW, Yoo DY, Jung HY, Nam SM, Kim JW, et al. Dendropanax morbifera L{é}veille extract facilitates cadmium excretion and prevents oxidative damage in the hippocampus by increasing antioxidant levels in cadmium-exposed rats. BMC Complement Altern Med. 2014;14:428. https://doi.org/10.1186/1472-6882-14-428
12. Park S-E, Sapkota K, Choi J-H, Kim M-K, Kim YH, Kim KM, et al. Rutin from Dendropanax morbifera Leveille protects human dopaminergic cells against rotenone induced cell injury through inhibiting JNK and p38 MAPK signaling. Neurochem Res. 2014;39:707–18. https://doi.org/10.1007/s11064-014-1259-5
13. Akram M, Kim K-A, Kim E-S, Syed AS, Kim CY, Lee JS, et al. Potent anti-inflammatory and analgesic actions of the chloroform extract of Dendropanax morbifera mediated by the Nrf2/HO-1 pathway. Biol Pharm Bull. 2016;39:728–36.
14. Park S-E, Seo S-H, Yoo S-A, Na C-S, Son H-S. Quality characteristics of Doenjang prepared with fermented Hwangchil (Dendropanax morbifera) extract. J Korean Soc Food Sci Nutr. 2016;45(3):372–9. https://doi.org/10.3746/jkfn.2016.45.3.372.
15. Choi J-W, Lim J-S, Lee S-P. Production of Dendropanax morbifera fortified with poly-γ-glutamic acid and γ-aminobutyric acid by co-fermentation using Bacillus subtilis and Lactobacillus plantarum. In: Proceedings of The Korean Society of Food Science and Nutrition. 2016. P06–21. PP 386. http://insight.dbpia.co.kr/article/related.do?nodeId=NODE07094558 accessed on 21 July 2017.
16. Ahmad W, Jantan I, Kumolosasi E, Bukhari SNA. Immunostimulatory effects of the standardized extract of Tinospora crispa on innate immune responses in Wistar Kyoto rats. Drug des Devel Ther. Dove Medical Press. 2015;9:2961–73. http://www.ncbi.nlm.nih.gov/pmc/articles/PMC4468953/
17. Kidd P. Th1/Th2 balance: the hypothesis, its limitations, and implications for health and disease. Altern Med Rev. 2003;8:223–46. http://www.ncbi.nlm.nih.gov/pubmed/12946237
18. Bancos S, Bernard MP, Topham DJ, Phipps RP. Ibuprofen and other widely used non-steroidal anti-inflammatory drugs inhibit antibody production in human cells. Cell Immunol. 2009;258:18–28. http://www.ncbi.nlm.nih.gov/pmc/articles/PMC2693360/
19. Rider P, Carmi Y, Guttman O, Braiman A, Cohen I, Voronov E, et al. IL-1α and IL-1β Recruit Different Myeloid Cells and Promote Different Stages of Sterile Inflammation. J Immunol. 2011;187:4835. LP-4843. http://www.jimmunol.org/content/187/9/4835.abstract
20. Lin N, Sato T, Takayama Y, Mimaki Y, Sashida Y, Yano M, et al. Novel anti-inflammatory actions of nobiletin, a citrus polymethoxy flavonoid, on human synovial fibroblasts and mouse macrophages. Biochem Pharmacol. 2003;65:2065–71. http://www.sciencedirect.com/science/article/pii/S000629520300203X

14

Antibacterial interactions, anti-inflammatory and cytotoxic effects of four medicinal plant species

Refilwe G. Kudumela[1], Lyndy J. McGaw[2] and Peter Masoko[1*]

Abstract

Background: The constant emergence of antibiotic resistant species and the adverse side effects of synthetic drugs are threatening the efficacy of the drugs that are currently in use. This study was aimed at investigating the possible antibacterial interactions, anti-inflammatory and cytotoxic effects of selected medicinal plants based on their traditional usage.

Methods: The acetone extracts of four plant species were assessed independently and in combination for antibacterial activity using microdilution assay and the sum of the fractional inhibitory concentration (FIC) was calculated. The ability of *Dombeya rotundifolia* and *Schkuhria pinnata* extracts to inhibit the production of reactive oxygen species (ROS) in LPS induced RAW 264.7 macrophage cells was evaluated using Dichloro-dihydro-fluorescein diacetate (H_2DCF-DA) assay to determine anti-inflammatory potential and the toxicity on African green monkey kidney (Vero) cells was evaluated using 3-(4,5-dimethylthiazol-2-yl)-2,5-diphenyl tetrazolium bromide (MTT) assay.

Results: The antibacterial efficacies of the different combinations of *Schkuhria pinnata* (A), *Commelina africana* (B), *Dombeya rotundifolia* (C) and *Elephantorrhiza elephantina* (D) plants varied from combination to combination. Synergistic effects were only exhibited against *P. aeruginosa*, while the antagonistic effects were only observed against *E. coli*. Both *S. pinnata* and *D. rotundifolia* demonstrated anti-inflammatory potential by inhibiting the production of ROS in a dose dependant manner. The cytotoxicity of the plants (LC_{50} values) ranged from < 25.0 to 466.1 μg/mL. *S pinnata* extract was the most toxic with the lowest LC_{50} value of < 25.0 μg/mL.

Conclusions: The synergistic interaction observed indicates that combinational therapy may improve biological activity. This report highlights the anti-inflammatory potential of *S. pinnata* and *D. rotundifolia*; which could be exploited in the search for anti-inflammatory agents. However, the cytotoxicity of *S. pinnata* highlights the importance of using this plant with caution.

Background

The extensive use and over reliance on antibiotics has caused the bacteria to develop resistant genes against the available antibiotics [1]. Some antibiotics have been associated with undesirable side effects, such as; nausea, depression of bone marrow, thrombocytopenic and agranulocytosis [2], therefore medicinal plants are researched as possible new sources of antimicrobial

agents with possibly novel mechanisms of action and fewer side effects since they have therapeutic relevance in folklore [3–7]. These medicinal plants are used in the form of herbal remedies which are prepared from one plant or a combination of different plant species [8]. Herbal mixtures containing a combination of different plant species have been reported to have better biological activities than isolated active compounds and herbal mixtures prepared from one plant species [8–10]. Therefore, these could be used to overcome the challenge of antimicrobial resistance [11].

The use of traditional medicine systems to treat various ailments has been in existence for years and

* Correspondence: Peter.Masoko@ul.ac.za
[1]Department of Biochemistry, Microbiology and Biotechnology, Faculty of Science and Agriculture, University of Limpopo, Turfloop Campus, Private Bag X1106, Sovenga, Limpopo 0727, South Africa
Full list of author information is available at the end of the article

continues to provide the human population with new medicines [12]. A single plant can be used for treatment of more than one type of disease and as a result have multiple medicinal properties. This justifies why it is important to screen for more than one biological activity when screening plants for biological activity. This approach explores and provides information on the overall medicinal properties of specific medicinal plants [11]. The current steroidal and non-steroidal anti-inflammatory drugs present adverse side effects, thus, exploring plants as an alternative has been increasing significantly [13].

Medicinal plants are assumed to be safe based on their long history of use in the treatment and management of diseases [14]. However, the use of these plants may be associated with irritation of the gastrointestinal tract, destruction of red blood cells, and damage of the heart and kidney [15]. Therefore, this necessitates the need for cytotoxicity evaluation of medicinal plants used in ethnopharmacology. The present study investigated the antibacterial interactions, anti-inflammatory and cytotoxic effects of the four selected plants. This was motivated by the results obtained in our previous work on phytochemical screening, antioxidant and antibacterial effects of the same plants [16]. The plants selected for this study include; *Commelina africana* L. var. *africana* (Commelinaceae) which is used traditionally for the treatment of venereal diseases [17]; *Dombeya rotundifolia* (Hochst.) Planch. var. (Sterculiaceae) used traditionally to treat diarrhoea [18]; *Elephantorrhiza elephantina* (Burch.) Skeels (Leguminosae) used for treatment of pneumonia and tick-borne diseases in cows [19] and *Schkuhria pinnata* (Lam.) Kuntze ex Thell (Asteraceae) which is used for treatment of stomach ache [20].

Methods
Chemicals
Acetone (Sigma Aldrich, SA), Ampicillin (Sigma Aldrich, SA), nutrient broth (Oxiod), Curcumin (Adcock-Ingram), Dichloro-dihydro-fluorescein diacetate (H_2DCF-DA) (ThermoFisher Scientific), Lipopolysaccharide (LPS) (Thermo-Fisher Scientific), RPMI-1640 medium (Whitehead Scientific), Phosphate Buffered Saline (PBS) (White Scientific), foetal bovine serum (FBS) (Hyclone, Thermo Scientific), Minimum Essential Medium (MEM, Whitehead Scientific) gentamicin (Virbac) 3-(4, 5-dimethylthiazol-2-yl)-2, 5-diphenyltetrazolium bromide (MTT) (Sigma Aldrich, SA), foetal calf serum (Highveld Biological).

Plant collection and preparations
The leaves of (*Commelina africana* L. var. *africana* (UNIN 12295), *Dombeya rotundifolia* (Hochst.) Planch. var. *rotundifolia* (UNIN 12296), *Elephantorrhiza elephantina* (Burch.) Skeels (UNIN 12297) and the whole plant excluding the roots of *Schkuhria pinnata* (Lam.)

Kuntze ex Thell (UNIN 12298) were collected in April 2015 at University of Limpopo, South Africa. The specimens were deposited at the Larry Leach Herbarium (UNIN) for authentication. Plant collection was based on ethnopharmacological information provided by traditional healers in Limpopo Province. The plants were dried at room temperature, protected from light and later ground to fine powder using a blender (Waring Laboratory Blender LB20ES). The plant materials (10 g) were extracted using acetone (100 mL) (Sigma-Aldrich, S.A) and the supernatants of each plant material were filtered through Whatman No.1 filter paper into pre-weighed vials and the filtrates were dried under a stream of air. The dried filtrates yielded 0.3 g, 0.7 g, 1.08 g and 0.5 g for *C. africana*, *D. rotundifolia*, *E. elephantina* and *S. pinnata* respectively.

Microorganisms used in this study
Two Gram-positive bacteria (*Staphylococcus aureus* ATCC 29213 and *Enterococcus faecalis* ATCC 29212) and 2 Gram-negative bacteria (*Escherichia coli* ATCC 28922 and *Pseudomonas aeruginosa* ATCC 27853) were used. These are major causes of nosocomial infections in hospitals [21] and are mainly the strains recommended for use by the National Committee for Clinical Laboratory Standards [22]. The bacterial species were maintained on nutrient agar at 4 °C. The cells were inoculated and incubated at 37 °C in nutrient broth for 12 h prior to screening tests.

Antibacterial interaction activity
The antibacterial activity interactions of the four selected plants were investigated by the determination of the minimum inhibitory concentration (MIC) of each plant independently and in combination using the micro-broth dilution assay described by Eloff [23]. Stock solutions (10 mg/mL) of acetone extracts of each plant were prepared by re-dissolving the extracts in acetone. For 1:1 test combinations, 50 μL of each of the two extracts were mixed to make up a volume of 100 μL in the first wells of a 96-well microtitre plate. Each extract contributed 33.3 μL and 25 μL for the 1:1:1 and 1:1:1:1 combinations respectively, to make up 100 μL in the first wells of a 96-well microtitre plate [8]. Two-fold serial dilutions of these extracts and ampicillin (positive control) (2.5 mg/mL to 0.02 mg/mL) were prepared in 96-well microtitre plates. The effects of the extracts were tested against 100 μL of each pathogen at the following densities of bacterial cultures: *S. aureus*, 2.6 X 10^{12} colony-forming units (CFU/mL); *E. faecalis*, 1.5 X 10^{10} CFU/mL; *P. aeruginosa*, 5.2 X 10^{13} CFU/mL; *E. coli*, 3.0 X 10^{11} CFU/mL. The microtitre plates were incubated at 37 °C overnight. Thereafter, 40 μL of 0.2 mg/mL iodonitrotetrazolium chloride (Sigma-Aldrich) was

added to each well and the plates were re-incubated for a further 30 min at 37 °C for *S. aureus* and *P. aeruginosa*, 1.5 h for *E. coli*, and 24 h for *E. faecalis*. The formation of a red-pink color signified microbial growth. All samples were assayed in triplicates and acetone was used as a negative control. The synergistic or antagonistic interactions between the plants were investigated by determining the Fractional inhibitory concentrations (FIC). These were calculated for 1:1 combinations of the plants with the equation below, where (i) and (ii) represented the different 1:1 plant combinations [24]. The FIC index was expressed as the sum of FIC $_{(i)}$ and FIC $_{(ii)}$ and this was used to classify the interaction as either synergistic (≤0.50), additive (0.50–1.00), indifferent (> 1.00–4.00) or antagonistic (> 4.00) [25].

$$\text{FIC(i)} \frac{\text{MIC of (a)in combination with (b)}}{\text{MIC of (a)independently}}$$

$$\text{FIC(ii)} \frac{\text{MIC of (b)in combination with (a)}}{\text{MIC of (b)independently}}$$

Anti-inflammatory activity assay using Dichloro-dihydro-fluorescein diacetate H₂DCF-DA assay

Based on the reported high antioxidant and antibacterial activities of *D. rotundifolia* and *S. pinnata* respectively [16] the anti-inflammatory activity assay of the two plants were investigated using the H$_2$DCF-DA assay as described by Sekhar et al., [26] with slight modifications. This assay uses stimulants such as lipopolysaccharide (LPS) to induce oxidative stress and Dichloro-dihydro-fluorescein diacetate (H$_2$DCF-DA) to detect the presence of reactive oxygen species.. In the presence of reactive oxygen species H$_2$DCF-DA is oxidized to fluorescent 2, 7-dichlorofluorescein (DCF). Two hundred microliters of cells (RAW 264.7 macrophages) obtained from the American Type Culture Collection (ATCC) in RPMI-1640 was seeded in a 96-well plate. The cells were incubated at 37 °C, 5% CO$_2$ overnight to attain confluency. The medium was removed and the cells were washed with Phosphate Buffered Saline (PBS). Cells were exposed to 100 µL of acetone extracts (8 mg/mL, 0.64 mg/mL, and 0.32 mg/mL) of *D. rotundifolia* and *S. pinnata* and 20 µL of LPS for 24 h. Following incubation, the medium was aspirated and fresh medium without Foetal Bovine Serum (FBS) was added and the cells were stained with 100 µL of 20 µM of H$_2$DCF-DA and incubated for 30 min in the dark. The fluorescence was measured at an excitation wavelength of 480 nm. Curcumin (50 µM) and untreated cells were used as positive and negative controls respectively.

Cytotoxicity assay

The toxic effects of the selected plants on African green monkey kidney (Vero) cells obtained from the culture collection of the Department of Veterinary Tropical Diseases (University of Pretoria) was determined by the 3-(4, 5-dimethylthiazol-2-yl)-2, 5-diphenyltetrazolium bromide (MTT) assay [27]. The cells were maintained in Minimum Essential Medium (MEM, Whitehead Scientific) supplemented with 0.1% gentamicin (Virbac) and 5% foetal calf serum (Highveld Biological). The cell suspension (5×10^4 cells/mL) was seeded in a sterile 96-well microtitre plate and incubated for 24 h at 37 °C in 5% CO$_2$ for the cells to attach. The MEM was aspirated and the cells were washed with 150 µL phosphate buffered saline (PBS, Whitehead Scientific). The cells were treated with different concentrations of the extracts (1–0.025 mg/mL) prepared in MEM. The microtitre plates were incubated for 48 h with the extracts in the same conditions as described earlier. Untreated cells were included as a negative control. After treatment, the treatment medium was aspired and replaced with 200 µL of fresh MEM and then 30 µL of MTT (5 mg/ mL) in PBS (Sigma) and the plates were incubated further for 4 h at 37 °C. The medium was removed and replaced with 50 µL of DMSO to dissolve the MTT formazan crystals. The absorbance was measured in a microplate reader (BioTek Synergy) at 570 nm. Cytotoxicity was expressed as the concentration of test sample resulting in a 50% reduction of absorbance compared to untreated cells (LC$_{50}$ values). All the analysis was made in quadruplicate. The selectivity index (SI) was expressed as LC$_{50}$/ MIC value.

Statistical analysis

Each experiment was performed in triplicates and the results were expressed as mean values. Linear regression analysis was used to calculate LC$_{50}$ values. Microsoft Excel® was used to enter and capture data. Various graphs and tables were extracted from this data. Data was then exported to SPSS for further analysis. The MIC for each microorganism was analyzed using one-way analysis of variance (ANOVA). P value < 0.05 was considered as significant. SPSS 25.0 was employed for statistical analysis.

Results

Antibacterial interaction activity assay

When the plants were combined in a 1:1:1 combination potent activities were observed when *S. pinnata* was combined with *C. africana* and *D. rotundifolia* (combination A + B + C) against *E. coli* (0.09 ± 0.04 mg/mL) and *P. aeruginosa* (0.06 ± 0.02 mg/mL). Meanwhile, the combination with *D. rotundifolia*, *S. pinnata*, and *E. elephantina* (C + A + D) exhibited potent activities against *P. aeruginosa* (0.07 ± 0.04 mg/mL) only (Table 1). When all

Table 1 Antibacterial interaction effects with standard deviation of the acetone extracts of the different combinations of the selected plants against selected bacterial species

Combinations	Minimum Inhibitory Concentration (mg/ml)			
	Escherichia coli	*Pseudomonas aeruginosa*	*Enterococcus faecalis*	*Staphylococcus aureus*
A	0.84 ± 0.21	0.27 ± 0.05	1.67 ± 0.83	1.67 ± 0.83
A + B	0.16 ± 0.00	0.04 ± 0.00	0.63 ± 0.00	0.53 ± 0.10
A + B + C	0.09 ± 0.04	0.06 ± 0.02	0.63 ± 0.00	0.32 ± 0.00
A + B + C + D	0.13 ± 0.03	0.07 ± 0.04	0.63 ± 0.00	0.27 ± 0.53
B	0.03 ± 0.01	0.53 ± 0.10	1.67 ± 0.83	0.84 ± 0.00
B + C	0.13 ± 0.03	0.67 ± 0.59	0.63 ± 0.00	0.32 ± 0.00
B + C + D	0.13 ± 0.03	0.76 ± 0.59	0.63 ± 0.00	0.21 ± 0.05
C	0.52 ± 0.36	0.42 ± 0.10	1.25 ± 0.00	0.63 ± 0.00
C + A	0.73 ± 0.27	0.04 ± 0.00	1.25 ± 0.00	0.84 ± 0.21
C + A + D	0.52 ± 0.36	0.07 ± 0.04	1.04 ± 0.21	0.84 ± 0.21
D	1.04 ± 0.21	0.42 ± 0.10	1.67 ± 0.83	0.84 ± 0.21
D + C	0.63 ± 0.00	0.04 ± 0.00	1.67 ± 0.83	0.84 ± 0.21
D + A + B	0.16 ± 0.00	0.67 ± 0.59	0.63 ± 0.00	0.27 ± 0.5
Ampicillin	0.03	0.02	0.03	0.08

Keywords
A = *Schkuhria pinnata* B = Commelina africana C = Dombeya rotundifolia D = Elephantorrhiza elephantina

the selected plants were combined (combination A + B + C + D) the efficacy against all the tested bacteria except for *E. coli* was enhanced with average MIC values lower than the MIC values of the plants independently. Ampicillin was used as positive control and its MIC values ranged from 0.02 to 0.08 mg/mL. Using ANOVA test (one way ANOVA), the mean difference between the MIC values of some of the acetone extracts combination (A + B; A + B + C; A + B + C + D and C + A against all tested pathogens was statistically significant ($p < 0.05$).

The Fractional Inhibitory Concentration (FIC) values were calculated as outlined above for the 1:1 combinations to establish any synergistic or antagonistic interactions. Synergistic effects were only exhibited against *P. aeruginosa* with 0.22, 0.24, and 0.19 FIC index values for the A + B, C + A and C + D combinations, respectively. Meanwhile, the antagonistic effects were only observed against *E. coli* with 5.52 and 4.58 FIC index values for combinations A + B and B + C respectively (Table 2).

Anti-inflammatory activity
The plant extracts inhibited ROS generation in a dose dependant manner. The inhibition was higher in *D. rotundifolia* than in *S. pinnata* (Fig. 1). Curcumin (50 μM) was used as a positive control and all the plants had better anti-inflammatory potential than curcumin at the highest concentration tested. Potent activities were observed in *D. rotundifolia* even at the lowest concentration tested.

Cytotoxicity assay
The cytotoxicity of the acetone extracts of the selected plants ranged from < 25 to 466.1 μg/mL. The American National Cancer Institute (NCI) described an $LC_{50} < 30$ μg/mL for plant extracts as a cut off point for cytotoxicity after 72 h of exposure [28]. Therefore, *S. pinnata* extract was highly toxic to the Vero cells with the lowest LC_{50} (< 25 μg/mL) that is outside the cut-off point (Table 3).

Discussion
Most traditional healers in South Africa often combine different plants in herbal mixtures. This method has been proposed to be a better way of approaching antimicrobial resistance problem [11]. Plants used in this study, have been reported to have antibacterial activities independently against the tested bacteria [16], hence we here evaluated the possible antibacterial interactions between the plants to see if such combination will potential their antimicrobial activity. To achieve this, the

Table 2 Fractional inhibitory concentration indexes of the 1:1 combinations of the selected plants

Microorganisms	A + B	B + C	C + A	C + D
Escherichia coli	5.52	4.58	2.27	1.82
Pseudomonas aeruginosa	0.22	2.86	0.24	0.19
Enterococcus faecalis	0.75	0.88	1.75	2.34
Staphylococcus aureus	0.95	0.89	1.84	2.33

Keywords
A = *Schkuhria pinnata* B = Commelina africana C = Dombeya rotundifolia D = Elephantorrhiza elephantina

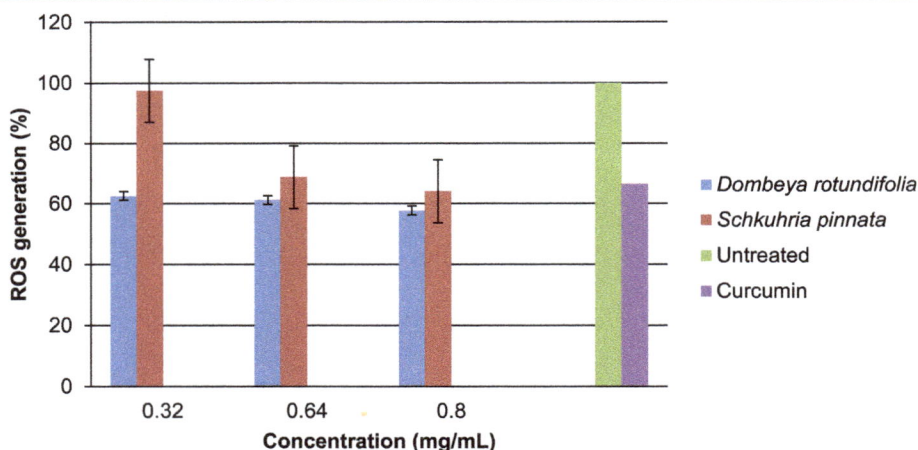

Fig. 1 The effect of two of the selected plants on ROS generation inhibition activity in LPS induced RAW 264.7 macrophage cells

Minimum Inhibitory Concentration (MIC) values of acetone extracts of the selected plants individually and in combination were determined (Table 1). As suggested by Ríos and Recio [29] this study highlights only the MIC values of less or equal to 0.1 mg/mL as these are said to be noteworthy.

Overall the Gram-negative bacteria were more sensitive to the combinations than the Gram-positive bacteria. The difference in sensitivity for these bacteria may be attributed to the difference in membrane morphology [30]. This suggests that the problem of antimicrobial resistance of the Gram-negative strains may be addressed with combinational therapy of these plants. In most cases it is assumed that when two plants are combined synergism is likely to occur [31]. The plants contained in the combinations in this study are used for treatment of various infections and they have been screened for antimicrobial properties individually [16, 32–35]. Mpofu [31] also reported on the synergistic interactions of the 1:1 combinations of *Elephantorrhiza elephantina* and *Pentanisia prunelloides* aqueous extracts against *E. coli* and *E. faecalis*. As such, one could advice on the combination of these plants since combination of plant extracts often offer a wide range of biological activities [36].

There are substantial numbers of reports linking ROS production to inflammation and related diseases [26,

37]. As such, the effects of *S. pinnata* and *D. rotundifolia* acetone extracts on the inhibition of ROS production were investigated in LPS induced RAW 264.7 macrophage cells. This plant was reported to have high free radical scavenging and ferric reducing antioxidant properties [16]. Therefore, the observed anti-inflammatory effect may be attributed to these antioxidant properties. Nevertheless, *S. pinnata* also exhibited ROS inhibition activity at higher concentrations. Therefore, the anti-inflammatory efficacy should be evaluated in vivo before the plant is recommended for any use. Reid et al. [33] also reported on the high inflammatory activity of the ethanol and dichloromethane leaf and bark extracts of *D. rotundifolia*. Meanwhile, Luseba et al. [38] reported that DCM extracts of *S. pinnata* had high inhibitory activity against cyclooxgenase-1 enzyme (COX-1). More often farmers use the same plants to treat different degrees of inflammation and stages of infections [38]. This statement was supported by the potent antibacterial and anti-inflammatory activities of both *S. pinnata* and *D. rotundifolia*.

Many of the plants used in ethnopharmacology to treat various ailments are used with no knowledge of their toxic effect [15]. As such, the toxic effects of the selected plants were evaluated on African green monkey (Vero) cells using MTT assay. This assay is based on the

Table 3 Cytotoxicity, Minimum Inhibitory Concentrations (MIC), and selectivity index (SI) of the acetone extracts of the selected plants

Plant species	LC$_{50}$ (µg/mL)	MIC values (µg/mL)				Selectivity index (SI)			
		E. coli	P. aeruginosa	E. faecalis	S. aureus	E. coli	P. aeruginosa	E. faecalis	S. aureus
Schkuhria pinnata	< 25.0	320	640	1250	1250	0.08	0.04	0.02	0.02
Dombeya rotundifolia	466.1	320	1250	1250	1250	1.46	0.37	0.37	0.37
Elephantorrhiza elephantina	416.4	640	2500	2500	2500	0.17	0.17	0.17	0.17
Commelina africana	441.1	20	2500	2500	2500	22.06	0.18	0.18	0.18

conversion of MTT to an insoluble purple formazan by the mitochondrial succinate dehydrogenase of viable cells [39]. The concentrations of the extracts which resulted in 50% reduction of absorbance compared to untreated cells (LC_{50}) are presented in Table 3. Deutschländer et al. [40] also reported the toxicity of the acetone and ethanol extracts of *S. pinnata* on 3 T3-L1 preadipocytes and Chang liver cells. However, McGaw et al. [41] reported that plants containing toxic compounds may have useful biological activities, since toxicity at low doses can be associated with pharmacological activity. Nevertheless, the rest of the plants were less toxic with high LC_{50} values.

Selectivity index was used to relate cytotoxicity and antibacterial activities of plant extracts. These values ranged from 0.02 to 22.06 (Table 3). The plant extracts had low selectivity with an exception of *C. africana* (22.06). The efficacy of biological activity is considered not to be due to toxicity if the selectivity index is ≥10 [42]. Therefore the observed antibacterial activity of acetone leaf extracts of *C. africana* was not due to toxicity. Meanwhile, those of the other plants were probably due to toxicity because of their low selectivity index values. It should be noted that cytotoxicity observed in vitro is not always encountered in vivo. This is probably because when in the biological system, some toxic compounds have the ability to undergo metabolic transformations which leads to the formation of less toxic end products [43].

Conclusions
This study demonstrated that combinational therapy may be used to address antimicrobial resistance of Gram-negative strains. Furthermore, this report highlights the anti-inflammatory potential of *S. pinnata* and *D. rotundifolia* acetone extracts which could be exploited in the search for plant-based anti-inflammatory agents. However, the cytotoxicity of *S. pinnata* highlights the importance of using this plant with caution.

Abbreviations
COX: cyclooxygenases; DCFHD-A: dichlorofluorescein diacetate assay; FIC: fractional inhibitory concentration; iNOS: inducible nitric oxide synthase; MEM: Minimum Essential Medium; RNS: Reactive nitrogen species; ROS: Reactive oxygen species

Acknowledgements
The authors thanks Ms. Mangokoana for assistance with anti-inflammatory studies.

Funding
We would like to thank the NRF (Reference: IFR1203260814; SFH150709124813; Grant No: 81341 and University of Limpopo (Grant no: 624) for financial support.

Authors' contributions
RGK, carried out the experiments, analysed the data and drafting of the manuscript. LJM: Toxicity studies and proof reading. PM, study design, data collection, analysis and interpretation of data and drafting of the manuscript. All authors read and approved the final manuscript.

Author details
[1]Department of Biochemistry, Microbiology and Biotechnology, Faculty of Science and Agriculture, University of Limpopo, Turfloop Campus, Private Bag X1106, Sovenga, Limpopo 0727, South Africa. [2]Department of Paraclinical Sciences, Phytomedicine Programme, Faculty of Veterinary Science, University of Pretoria, Private Bag X04, Onderstepoort 0110, South Africa.

References
1. Mundy L, Pendry B, Rahman M. Antimicrobial resistance and synergy in herbal medicine. J Herb Med. 2016;6:53–8.
2. Marchese A, Schito GC. Resistance patterns of lower respiratory tract pathogens in Europe. Int J Antimicrob Agents. 2000;16:25–9.
3. Machado TB, Pinto AV, Pinto MCFR, Leal ICR, Silva MG, Amaral ACF, Kuster RM, Netto-dosSantos KR. In vitro activity of Brazilian medicinal plants, naturally occurring naphthoquinones and their analogues, against methicillin-resistant Staphylococcus aureus. Int J Antimicrob Agents. 2003;21:279–84.
4. Motsei ML, Lindsey KL, van Staden J, Jäger AK. Screening of traditionally used south African plants for antifungal activity against Candida albicans. J Ethnopharmacol. 2003;86:235–41.
5. Barbour EK, Al Sharif M, Sagherian VK, Habre AN, Talhouk RS, Talhouk SN. Screening of selected indigenous plants of Lebanon for antimicrobial activity. J Ethnopharmacol. 2004;93:1–7.
6. Parekh J, Chanda S. In vitro antibacterial activity of the crude methanol extract of Woodfordia fruticosa Kurz. Flower (Lythraceae). Braz J Microbiol. 2007b;38:204–7.
7. Ncube B, Finnie JF, van Staden J. In vitro antimicrobial synergism within plant extracts combinations from three south African medicinal bulbs. J Ethnopharmacol. 2012;139:81–9.
8. Chung PY, Navaratnam P, Chung LY. Synergistic antimicrobial activity between pentacyclic triterpenoids and antibiotics against Staphylococcus aureus strains. Ann Clin Microbiol Antimicrob. 2011;10:25–30.
9. Nahrstedt A, Butterweck V. Lessons learned from herbal medicinal products: the example of St. John's wort. J Nat Prod. 2010;73:1015–21.
10. Wagner H. Synergy research: approaching a new generation of phytopharmaceuticals. Fitoterapia. 2011;82:34–7.
11. van Vuuren S, Holl D. Antimicrobial natural product research: a review from a south African perspective for the years 2009–2016. J Ethnopharmacol. 2017;208:236–52.
12. Serpeloni JM, Barcelos GRM, Mori MP, Yanagui K, Vilegas W, Varanda EA, de Syllos Colus IM. Cytotoxic and mutagenic evaluation of extracts from plant species of the Miconia genus and their influence on doxorubicin-induced mutagenicity: an in vitro analysis. Exp Toxicol Pathol. 2011;63:499–504.
13. de Oliveira RG, Mahon CPAN, Ascêncio PGM, Ascêncio SD, Balogun SO, de Oliveira Martins DT. Evaluation of anti-inflammatory activity of hydroethanolic extract of Dilodendron bipinnatum Radlk. J Ethnopharmacol. 2014;155:387–95.
14. Fennell CW, Lindsey KL, McGaw LJ, Sparg SG, Stafford GI, Elgorashi EE, Grace OM, van Staden J. Assessing African medicinal plants for efficacy and safety: pharmacological screening and toxicology. J. Ethnopharmacol. 2004;94:205–17.
15. Nondo RS, Moshi MJ, Erasto P, Zofou D, Njouendou AJ, Wanji S, Ngemenya MN, Kidukuli AW, Masimba PJ, Titanji VP. Evaluation of the cytotoxic activity of extracts from medicinal plants used for the treatment of malaria in Kagera and Lindi regions, Tanzania. J Appl Pharm Sci. 2015;5:007–12.
16. Kudumela RG, Masoko P. In vitro assessment of selected medicinal plants used by the Bapedi Community in South Africa for treatment of bacterial infections. J Evid Based Integr Med. 2018;23:2515690X18762736.

17. Leistner OA, editor. Seeds plants of Southern Africa: families and genera. In: Southern African Botanical Diversity Network Report No 26. Pretoria: Southern African Botanical Diversity Network; 2000.

18. Brink M. *Dombeya rotundifolia* (Hochst) planch. In: Louppe D, Oteng-Amoako AA, Brink M, editors. Plant resources of tropical Africa. Vol. 7. Totnes, England: Earthprint limited; 2008. p. 223–4.

19. Maphosa V, Masika PJ, Moyo B. Investigation of the anti-inflammatory and antinociceptive activities of *Elephantorrhiza elephantina* (Burch.) Skeels root extract in male rats. Afr J Biotechnol. 2009;8:7068–72.

20. Sandoval P, Choque J, Uriona P. Cartilla popular sobre las plantas utiles de los Alten*os de Mizque-Cochabamba. Cochabamba, Bolivia: FONAMA-CIBE-UMSA; 1996.

21. Sacho H, Schoub BD. Current Properties on Nosocomial Infections. (Glaxo Wellcome sponsored pamphlet). Natal, South Africa: The Natal Witness Printing and Publishing Company; 1993.

22. National Committee for Clinical Laboratory Standards. Performance Standards for Antimicrobial Disk Susceptibility Tests. 4th ed. Villanora: Approved Standard NCCLS Document M2-A4; 1992.

23. Eloff JN. A sensitive and quick microplate method to determine the minimal inhibitory concentration of plant extracts for bacteria. Planta Med. 1998;64:711–3.

24. Mabona U, Viljoen A, Shikanga E, Marston A, van Vuuren S. Antimicrobial activity of southern African medicinal plants with dermatological relevance: from an ethnopharmacological screening approach, to combination studies and the isolation of a bioactive compound. J Ethnopharmacol. 2013;148:45–55.

25. van Vuuren SF, Viljoen AM. In vitro evidence of phyto-synergy for plant part combinations of Croton gratissimus (Euphorbiaceae) used in African traditional healing. JEthnopharmacol. 2008;119:700–4.

26. Sekhar S, Sampath-Kumara KK, Niranjana SR, Prakash HS. Attenuation of reactive oxygen/nitrogen species with suppression of inducible nitric oxide synthase expression in RAW 264.7 macrophages by bark extract of Buchanania lanzan. Pharmacogn Mag. 2015;11:283–91.

27. Mosmann T. Rapid colorimetric assay for cellular growth and survival: application to proliferation and cytotoxicity assays. J Immunol Methods. 1983;65:55–63.

28. Itharat A, Houghton PJ, Eno-Amooquaye E, Burke PJ, Sampson JH, Raman A. In vitro cytotoxic activity of Thai medicinal plants used traditionally to treat cancer. J Ethnopharmacol. 2004;90:33–8.

29. Ríos JL, Recio MC. Medicinal plants and antimicrobial activity. J Ethnopharmacol. 2005;100:80–4.

30. Masoko P, Gololo SS, Mokgotho MP, Eloff JN, Howard RL, Mampuru LJ. Evaluation of the antioxidant, antibacterial and antiproliferatory activities of the acetone extracts of the roots of *Senna italica* (Fabaceae). Afri J Trad Compl Altern Med. 2010;7(2):138–48.

31. Mpofu S, Ndinteh DT, van Vuuren S, Olivier D, Krause R. Interactive efficacies of *Elephantorrhiza elephantina* and *Pentanisia prunelloides* extracts andisolated compounds against gastrointestinal bacteria. S Afr J Bot. 2014; 94:224–30.

32. Aaku E, Dharani SP, Majinda RRT, Motswaiedi MS. Chemical and antimicrobial studies on *Elephantorrhiza elephantina*. Fitoterapia. 1998;69:464–5.

33. Reid KA, Jäger AK, van Staden J. Pharmacological and phytochemical properties of *Dombeya rotundifolia*. S Afr J Bot. 2001;67:349–53.

34. Mathabe MC, Nikolova RV, Lall N, Nyazema NZ. Antibacterial activities of medicinal plants used for the treatment of diarrhoea in Limpopo Province, South Africa. J Ethnopharmacol. 2006;105:286–93.

35. Mupfure A, GHM M, Imbayarwo-Chikosi VE, Nyamushamba GB, Marandure T, Masama E. Potential use of *Schkuhria Pinnata* in the control of *Mastitis* pathogens. Int J Innov Res Dev. 2014;3:ISSN 2278–0211.

36. Wambugu SN, Mathiu PM, Gakuya DW, Kanui TI, Kabasa JD, Kiama SG. Medicinal plants used in the management of chronic joint pains in Machakos and Makueni counties, Kenya. J Ethnopharmacol. 2011;137: 945–55.

37. Ames BN, Shigenaga MK, Hagen TM. Oxidants, antioxidants, and the degenerative diseases of aging. Proc Natl Acad Sci U S A. 1993;90:7915–22. [PMC free article] [PubMed]

38. Luseba D, Elgorashi EE, Ntloedibe DT, van Staden J. Antibacterial, anti-inflammatory and mutagenic effects of some medicinal plants used in South Africa for the treatment of wounds and retained placenta in livestock. S Afri J of Bot. 2007;73:378–83.

39. Fotakis G, Timbrell JA. *In vitro* cytotoxicity assays: comparison of LDH, neutral red, MTT, and protein assay in hepatoma cell lines following exposure to cadmium chloride. Toxicol Lett. 2006;160:171–7.

40. Deutschländer MS, van de Venter M, Roux S, Louw J, Lall N. Hypoglycaemic activity of four plant extracts traditionally used in South Africa for diabetes. J Ethnopharmacol. 2009;124:619–24.

41. McGaw LJ, van der Merwe D, Eloff JN. In vitro anthelmintic, antibacterial and cytotoxic effects of extracts from plants used in south African ethnoveterinary medicine. Vet J. 2007;173:366–72.

42. Caamal-Fuentes E, Torres-Tapia LW, Simá-Polanco P, Peraza-Sánchez SR, Moo-Puc R. Screening of plants used in Mayan traditional medicine to treat cancer-like symptoms. J Ethnopharmacol. 2011;135:719–24.

43. Nchu F, Githiori JB, McGaw LJ, Eloff JN. Anthelmintic and cytotoxic activities of extracts of Markhamia obtusifolia Sprague (Bignoniaceae). Vet Parasitol. 2011;183:184–8.

15

Weipixiao attenuate early angiogenesis in rats with gastric precancerous lesions

Jinhao Zeng[1], Ran Yan[1], Huafeng Pan[2*], Fengming You[1*] (iD), Tiantian Cai[2], Wei Liu[2], Chuan Zheng[1], Ziming Zhao[3], Daoyin Gong[1], Longhui Chen[4] and Yi Zhang[1]

Abstract

Background: Angiogenesis is a pathobiological hallmark of gastric cancer. However, rare studies focus on angiogenesis in gastric precancerous lesions (GPL). Weipixiao (WPX), a Chinese herbal preparation, is proved clinically effective in treating GPL. Here, we evaluated WPX's anti-angiogenic potential for GPL, and also investigated the possibility of its anti-angiogenic mechanisms.

Methods: HPLC analysis was applied to screen the major chemical components of WPX. After modeling N-methyl-N '-nitro-N-nitrosoguanidine (MNNG)-induced GPL in male Sprague-Dawley rats, different doses of WPX were administrated orally for 10 weeks. Next, we performed histopathological examination using routine H&E staining and HID-AB-PAS staining. In parallel, we assessed angiogenesis revealed by microvessel density (MVD) using CD34 immunostaining, and subsequently observe microvessel ultrastructure in gastric mucosa under Transmission Electron Microscope. Finally, we detect expression of angiogenesis-associated markers VEGF and HIF-1α using immunohistochemistry. Moreover, mRNA expressions of ERK1, ERK2, Cylin D1 as well as HIF-1α in gastric mucosa were determined by quantitative real-time reverse transcription- polymerase chain reaction.

Results: We observed the appearance of active angiogenesis in GPL rats, and demonstrated that WPX could reduce microvascular abnormalities and attenuate early angiogenesis in most of GPL specimens with a concomitant regression of most intestinal metaplasia (IM) and a portion of gastric epithelial dysplasia (GED). In parallel, WPX could suppress HIF-1α mRNA expression ($P < 0.01$) as well as protein expression (although without statistical significance), and could markedly inhibit VEGF protein expression in GPL rats. Mechanistically, WPX intervention, especially at low dose, caused a significant decrease in the ERK1 and Cylin D1 mRNA levels. However, WPX might probably have no regulatory effect on ERK2 amplification.

Conclusions: WPX could attenuate early angiogenesis and temper microvascular abnormalities in GPL rats. This might be partly achieved by inhibiting on the angiogenesis-associated markers HIF-1α and VEGF, and on the ERK1/Cylin D1 aberrant activation.

Keywords: Gastric precancerous lesions, ERK signaling, VEGF, HIF-1α, Herbal medicine, Weipixiao

Background

Gastric precancerous lesions (GPL) are generally defined as intestinal metaplasia (IM) and gastric epithelial dysplasia (GED). A direct link has been sought between gastric cancer and high prevalence of GPL worldwide [1–3], especially in Asia. Thus, blocking of gastric precancerosis toward malignant transformation is crucial to reducing the gastric cancer incidence. Nowadays, endoscopic mucosal resection is clinically applied only to severe GED and definite intramucosal carcinoma, yet most cases of GPL are not amenable to the endoscopic resection [4]. Moreover, vitacoenzyme tablet, a chemopreventive agent used in China, has been reported to be beneficial in treating atrophic gastritis and metaplasia lesion [5, 6]. Its therapeutic effect against GPL, however, was not completely confirmed. Therefore, the pursuit to discover alternative therapies to treat GPL is of high concern. In China, early

* Correspondence: gzphf@gzucm.edu.cn; yfmdoc@163.com
[2]Guangzhou University of Chinese Medicine, Guangzhou 510405, China
[1]Chengdu University of Traditional Chinese Medicine, Chengdu 610075, China
Full list of author information is available at the end of the article

herbal intervention has proved to be effective in halting and even reversing the majority of GPL [7, 8].

Angiogenesis, the sprouting of new capillaries from pre-existing vessels, is a fundamental process accelerating gastric cancer progression. Considerable evidence has demonstrated that excessive angiogenesis is significantly correlated with enhanced migratory and invasive activity, and therefore with poor prognosis [9–11]. Hence, targeting angiogenesis has been a central focus in gastric cancer treatment [12]. Angiogenesis is generally resulted from hypoxia orchestrated by multiple transcriptional activators, aiming at restoring intratumoral O_2 delivery to hypoxic regions, thereby sustaining tumor growth [13]. Hypoxia inducible factor-1α (HIF-1α) has been proved to be a key regulator of cellular adaptation to hypoxia involved in angiogenesis process, and the process is frequently accompanied by a concomitant aberrant activation of vascular endothelial growth factor (VEGF) [14], which is essential for vascular development and can induce proliferation, differentiation and apoptosis of endothelial cells. Extracellular signal-regulated kinase (ERK), which may serve as specific effectors of VEGF signaling, play a vital role in sprouting endothelial cells during vascular development [15]. Aberrant activation of ERK signaling is closely linked to the carcinogenesis and development of gastric cancer [16]. ERK1 has been reported to overexpressed in 52.98% (231/436) cases of human gastric tumor, and high level of ERK1 protein expression was significantly correlated with age, tumor location, depth of invasion, Lauren's classification, lymph node metastasis and tumor node metastasis (TNM) stage [17]. ERK2 is similarly important for predicting the prognosis of gastric cancer. The positive occurrence of ERK2 mRNA expression is 64.0% (32/50) in tumor tissues from patients with gastric cancer, which is markedly higher than that in non-cancerous tissues showing 18.0% (9/50) [18]. Furthermore, ERK2 expression level is significantly increased from TNM stage II to stage IV, suggesting a closely relationship between elevated ERK2 level and tumor invasion and TNM stage [18]. Cyclin D1 is involved in G1-S point of cell cycle, and thus induces cell proliferation and migration coexisted with angiogenesis. Cyclin D1 is frequently overexpressed in a substantial proportion of gastric cancer, and its expression may be governed by the ERK signaling [19, 20]. Although studies reported in recent years have addressed the pro-angiogenic role of the molecules in gastric cancer, it is unclear what role the molecules may play in gastric precancerosis.

Weipixiao (WPX) is a Chinese herbal prescription consisting of six herbs including *Astragalus Membranaceus, Pseudostellaria Heterophylla, Atractylodis Macrocephalae, Curcuma zedoaria, Salvia Miltiorrhiza* and *Hedyotis Diffusa Willd*. WPX prescription has been widely used in

clinical for more than 15 years, and it shows satisfactory effects against "non-progressive GPL". In previous clinical trials, different teams demonstrated that WPX possesses excellent abilities at relieving the clinical symptoms, reducing the precursor lesions (through gastroscopic and pathohistological examination), as well as partially eradicating *Helicobacter pylori* in GPL patients, and shows no toxic or side effects [21–23]. Experimentally, some WPX individuals exhibited potential anti-angiogenesis activities in several solid tumors. Extracts from *Astragalus membranaceus*, a "Yi Qi Hua Yu" herb (function to tonify qi and activate blood) belonging to WPX, could reduce angiogenesis-related molecules vascular endothelial growth factor and cyclooxygenase-2 in ovarian tumor-bearing mice [24]. Another active compound of *Astragalus membranaceus*, named formononetin, has been reported to repress hypoxia-induced retinal angiogenesis via the HIF-1α/VEGF signaling pathway [25]. Essential oil from another member *Curcuma zedoaria*, a widely used "Hua Yu Tong Luo" herb (function to dissipate blood stasis and free the collateral vessels), presented the anti-angiogenic activity, which therefore contributed to suppressing melanoma growth and lung metastasis [26]. A recent study suggested that Danshensu, a major water-soluble compound from *Salvia miltiorrhiza*, could improve microcirculation and remodel tumor vasculature, thereby enhancing the radioresponse for Lewis lung carcinoma xenografts in mice [27]. The aforementioned researchers revealed the anti-angiogenesis properties of several herbs from WPX. However, the anti-angiogenic potential of WPX in GPL treating, and the possibility of its anti-angiogenic mechanisms still remain unclear.

In this study, we tested whether early angiogenesis existed in N-methyl-N′-nitro-N-nitrosoguanidine (MNNG)-induced GPL rats. Also, we determined whether WPX had the ability against hyper- angiogenesis. In parallel, we screened potential anti-GPL constituents of WPX. More importantly, the hypothesis we wished to test was that the anti-angiogenesis property of WPX was associated with its regulatory effects on the angiogenesis-associated markers HIF-1α and VEGF, and on the ERK/Cylin D1 signal transduction pathway.

Methods
Animals
Male Sprague-Dawley rats weighting 150–170 g were obtained from Experimental Animal Center of Sun Yat-sen University (certificate No. 0111909). Animals were housed in a specific pathogen-free animal room, kept under optimal condition at 23 ± 1 °C and 40–60% humidity with a 12 h light-dark cycle, and fed with standard rat chow. All procedures relating to animal care and the animal research protocols conformed to the guidelines for the Care and Use of Laboratory Animal, issued by the Ministry of Science and Technology of China. This experiment was conducted in Guangdong

Provincial Institute of Traditional Chinese Medicine, and was presented to the institutional ethical review board for approval (Ethic No. GDPITCM111018).

Drugs and reagents

WPX comprises the following components: Huangqi (*Astragalus Membranaceus*)30 g, Taizishen (*Pseudostellaria Heterophylla*)15 g, Baishu (*Atractylodis Macrocephalae*)15 g, Eshu (*Curcuma zedoaria*)10 g, Danshen (*Salvia Miltiorrhiza*)10 g and Baihuasheshecao (*Hedyotis Diffusa Willd*)30 g. The herbs were provided and authenticated by the First Affiliated Hosipital of Guangzhou University of Chinese Medicine. The medical herbs were boiled with distilled water, and concentrated into a mixture containing crude drugs 1.5 g/mL. MNNG was supplied by Tokyo Kabushiki Kaisha, Japan (No. ZG4T1-FP). CD34 antibody was abtained from R&D Systems, USA (lot ZDP0112111); VEGF antibody was supplied by Abcam, UK (lot GR-116031-1); HIF-1α antibody was purchased from Santa Cruz Biotechnology, USA (lot L1212). Maxima™ SYBR Green/Fluorescein qPCR Master Mix (2X) was supplied by Fermentas, USA.

High performance liquid chromatography (HPLC) analysis

HPLC analysis was performed to screen the potential chemical constituents of WPX preparation. Condition optimization of fingerprint: JADE-PAK ODS-AQ column (250 × 4.6 mm, 5 μm) and Inertsil ODS-SP column (4.6 × 150 mm, 5 μm) were utilized, with acetonitrile 0.1% phosphoric acid solution and acetonitrile 0.4% phosphoric acid solution as the mobile phase respectively, under full wavelength detection. The following chromatographic analysis conditions were determined: the separation was determined on Inertsil ODS-SP column (4.6 × 150 mm, 5 μm) with a mobile phase of acetonitrile (solvent A) 0.4% phosphoric acid solution (solvent B). For HPLC analysis, a 10 μL sample was injected into the column and eluted at a flow rate of 1.0 ml/min under room temperature. The detective wavelength was 203 nm.

Grouping, modeling and treatment

SD rats were randomly divided into six experimental groups: control group ($n = 9$), model group ($n = 11$), model + vitacoenzyme group (VIT, $n = 9$, 0.2 g/kg/d), model + high-dose WPX group (H-WPX, $n = 9$, 15 g/kg/d), model + medium-dose WPX group (M-WPX, $n = 9$, 7.5 g/kg/d), and model + low-dose WPX group (L-WPX, $n = 9$, 3.75 g/kg/d). Based on the literatures [8, 28, 29], the GPL rat model was set up with minor modifications. Briefly, All the rats, except for control rats, were allowed to drink MNNG solution (200 μg·ml^{-1}) ad libitum, and underwent hunger-satiety shift every other day. At the end of 15th week, 2 random rats in the model group were humanely terminated with sodium pentobarbital (140 mg/kg i.p.) and examined for IM/GED. At the beginning of 16th week, the treated rats were administered WPX or VIT by gastrogavage for 10 consecutive weeks, while the control and the model rats were given 2 mL distilled water by gastrogavage once daily.

Pathological examination

Animals were humanely euthanized with sodium pentobarbital (140 mg/kg i.p.) after 12 h fasting, and the stomachs were removed immediately, incised along the greater curvature, and fixed in 10% neutralized formalin solution. Then, each sample was embedded in paraffin wax and serially sectioned at 3 μm thick. The sections were stained with hematoxylin and eosin (H-E staining), and with high-iron diamine-alcian blue-periodic acid Schiff (HID-AB-PAS staining). Gastric tissues were examined macroscopically to identify IM and GED lesions in rats.

Evaluation of microvessel density

To evaluate microvessel density (MVD) in gastric mucosa, CD34 expression was determined using EnVision immunohistochemistry. Quantification of MVD was specified by Weidner et al. [30]. Briefly, area of highest angiogenesis (also called hot-spot) were identified under low-power magnification (40× and 100×), and stained microvessels in three random views of the 'hot-spot' area were counted under high-power magnification (200×). The mean value of the three 200× field counts was recorded as MVD for each case. Any brown staining endothelial cell or cell cluster that was clearly separated from adjacent microvessels or other connective tissue was considered a single countable microvessel.

Microvessel ultrastructure

The gastric mucosa tissue were sliced into 1 mm^3 pieces and fixed with 2.5% glutaraldehyde in phosphate buffer for 2.5 h, and then re-fixed in 1% osmium tetroxide in phosphate buffer for 2 h. The tissues were dehydrated in a graded series of ethanol solutions and then immersion in a mixture of acetone and epoxy resin twice (2:1 for 3 h in the first time, 1:2 for overnight in the second time). Finally, the tissues were embedded in epoxy resin-filled capsules and heated at 70 °C overnight, ultrathin sections (60–80 nm) were sliced with LKB microtome. The sections were viewed and photographed under a transmission electron microscope (JEOL 100C, JEOL, Tokyo, Japan).

Levels of ERK1, ERK2, Cyclin D1 and HIF-1α by RT-qPCR

The mRNA levels of ERK1, ERK2, Cyclin D1 and HIF-1α were determined by quantitative real-time reverse transcription-polymerase chain reaction (RT-qPCR) method using Maxima™ SYBR Green/Fluorescein qPCR Master Mix

(Fermentas, USA) via IQ™5 real-time PCR detection system (Bio-Rad, USA). The PCR primers used were as follows: ERK1 (GenBank accession no. NM_011952; 104 bp) forward, 5′-CGGATTGCTGACCCT-3′ and reverse 5′-GTGTAGCC CTTGGAGTT-3′; ERK2 (GenBank accession no. NM_053842; 113 bp) forward, 5′-CAACCTCCTGCTGAA C-3′ and reverse 5′-GCGTGGCTACATACTC-3′; Cyclin D1 (GenBank accession no. NM_171992; 191 bp) forward, 5′-GCAGAAGTGCGAAGAGG-3′ and reverse 5′-GGCG GATAGAGTTGTCAGT-3′; HIF-1α (GenBank accession no. NM_024359; 132 bp) forward, 5′-CAACTGCCACCAC TGATG-3′ and reverse 5′-CACTGTATGCTGATGCCTT AG-3′; 18S (GenBank accession no. M11188; 204 bp) forward, 5′-TCAGCCACCCGAGATT-3′ and reverse 5′-GCT TATGACCCGCACTTA-3′. The level of 18 s mRNA transcript was used to normalize all reported gene expression levels, and the data were analyzed using $2^{-\triangle\triangle Ct}$ method.

Expression of VEGF and HIF-1α by immunohistochemistry

Formalinfixed and paraffin-embedded gastric tissues were cut at 3 μm thick. The EnVision immunohistochemical technology was utilized, VEGF protein immunoreactivity was shown as brown color in the cytosolic and perinuclear regions of gastric epithelial cells. HIF-1α positive staining was brown or brown yellow and was detected predominantly in the cytoplasm and nucleus. To access the protein expression levels of VEGF and HIF-1α, three visual fields were randomly selected from each slice under light microscope (100×), and then images were acquired and analyzed by Image Pro Plus 6.0 software. Quantification of VEGF and HIF-1α levels was determined using mean of integrated optical density (IOD).

Statistical analysis

Data were presented as mean ± standard deviation (SD). Statistical analysis was performed using IBM SPSS 19.0 software (SPSS, Chicago, IL). One-way analysis of variance (ANOVA) was applied to analyze the comparisons among multiple groups. The comparison between two groups was performed with SNK method for the homogeneous variances, while the variances were heterogeneous, Dunnett's T3 method should be adopted. A P value of less than 0.05 was considered as significant.

Results

HPLC profile

WPX possessed an excellent ability against GPL revealed by our previous clinical trials and animal testing, so we are curious about the major constituents of WPX polyherbal mixture. Figure 1 shows the HPLC chromatograms of WPX test sample (A) and reference sample (B). The retention times of the major chemical constituents were 20.5 min (Calycosin-7- glucoside), 34.8 min (ginsenoside-Rg1), 48.3 min (ginsenoside-Rb1), 49.5 min (astragaloside IV), 59.0 min (atractylenolide III), 71.7 min (atractylenolide II), and 81.7 min (atractylenolide I) (Fig. 1).

WPX efficiently blocked and even reversed gastric intestinal metaplasia

We evaluated the degree of IM lesion in gastric tissues by HID-AB-PAS staining. As depicted in Fig. 2, neutral mucins present in normal mucosa were stained red, gastric specimens from controls didn't exhibit IM lesion. In model rats, sialomucins expressed only in small intestinal-type metaplasia (S-IM) were stained blue, and sulfomucins present in colonic-type metaplasia (C-IM) were stained brown, indicating that both S-IM and C-IM were widespread. In treated rats, IM lesion was regressed slightly in VIT-treated rats. Comparatively, IM lesion was regressed visibly in WPX-treated rats. Our observation revealed that WPX has a potent anti-IM capacity in GPL rats (Fig. 2).

WPX partly ameliorated gastric epithelial dysplasia

To further investigate the anti-GPL effect of WPX, we also examined the GED lesion in H&E stained sections of gastric tissues. Histologically, the control gland and cell structure of gastric epithelium remained intact. By contrast, almost all model rats displayed GED pathology. In detail, gastric epithelium was characterized by architectural abnormalities showing splitting, elongated, crowded glands and back-to-back tubular structure, and also by cytological atypia with hyperchromatic nuclei, increased nuclear-cytoplasmic ratio, loss of nuclear polarity and occasional binucleation. Inflammatory infiltration was variable, and sometimes extensive. Occasionally, two model rats exhibited mild dysplasia, due to the multifocal nature of the dysplastic lesion. In most cases of WPX-treated rats, GED lesion alterations, especially tubular structure irregularities and inflammatory infiltration, were regressed in varying degrees. However, the treatment was not able to restore the GED pathology near to the normal tissues. In contrast, this GED-rescuing effect was not presented in most VIT-treated rats. These observations suggested that WPX could partly halt and even reverse dysplastic process, especially the "non-progressive GED" (Fig. 3).

WPX reduced the CD34+ MVD level in GPL tissues

In order to identify whether early angiogenesis occur in GPL, we examined the angiogenic state in gastric tissues using CD34-labelled sections. As visualized by light microscopy, an increased number of CD34+ microvessels, which were suggestive of active angiogenesis, could be found in most cases of GPL tissues, whereas those in control tissues were minimal. Moreover, we found more GEDs with a higher number of microvessels than IMs, and more severe GEDs than mild or moderate GEDs.

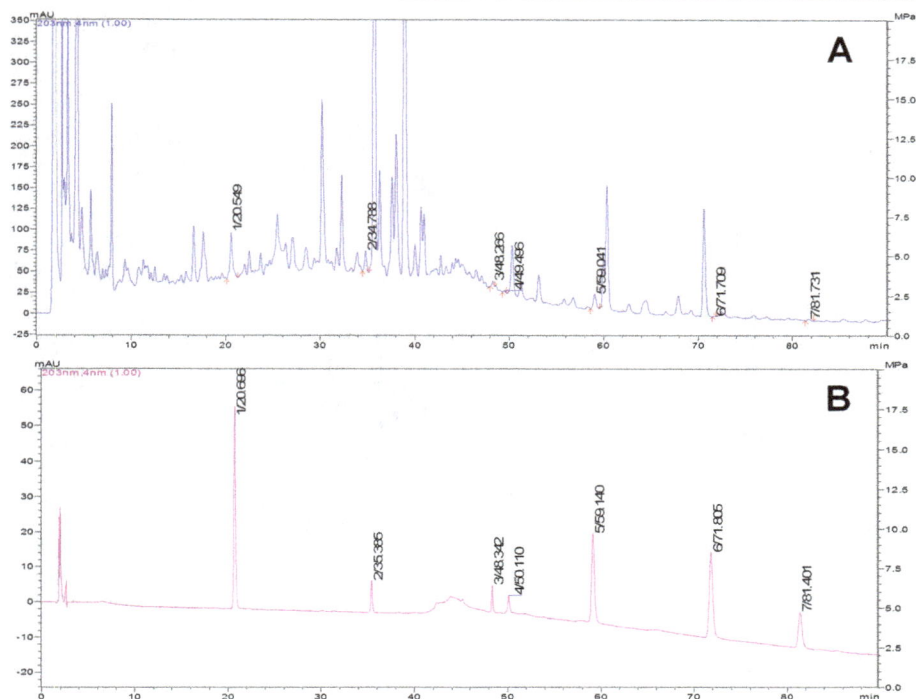

Fig. 1 HPLC chromatogram of WPX test sample (**a**) and reference sample (**b**). Notes: Peak: 1, Calycosin-7-glucoside; 2, ginsenoside-Rg1; 3, ginsenoside-Rb1; 4, astragaloside IV; 5–7, atractylenolide III, II, and I, respectively

Occasionally, CD34+ microvessels were apparently abundant and distributed diffusely in two model rats all diagnosed with severe GED. By contrast, we observed a clear decreased CD34+ microvessel count in many cases of WPX-treated rats. Our data showed a statistic significant increase of CD34+ MVD level in model rats comparing to controls. But it dropped by at least half after WPX intervention, when in comparison to the non-treatment rats. Thus, WPX could effectively inhibit active angiogenesis in GPL rats (Fig. 4).

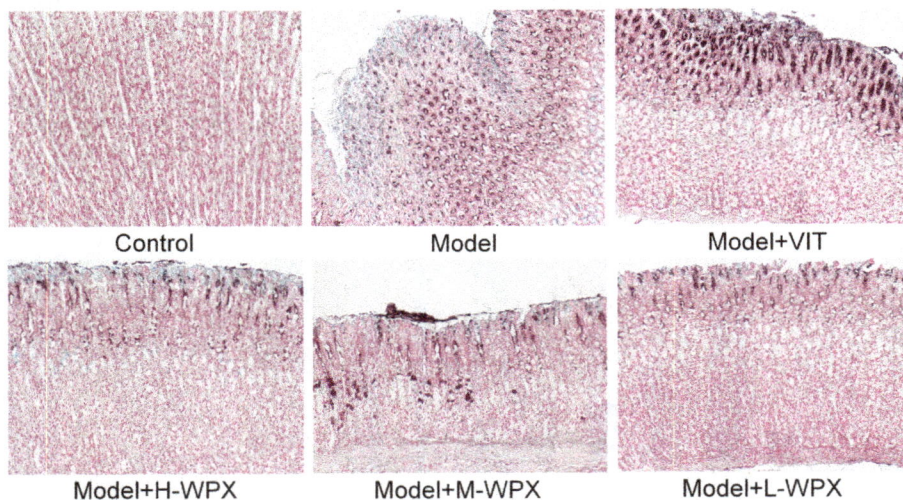

Fig. 2 Histological evaluation of gastric intestinal metaplasia. Neutral mucins present in normal mucosa were stained red. Sialomucins expressed only in small intestinal-type metaplasia (S-IM) were stained blue, and sulfomucins present in colonic-type metaplasia (C-IM) were stained brown. Images of model gastric epithelium depicted prominent S-IM and C-IM lesions, which were dramatically reduced after WPX administration. $n = 9$ in each group. (HID-AB-PAS staining, 100×)

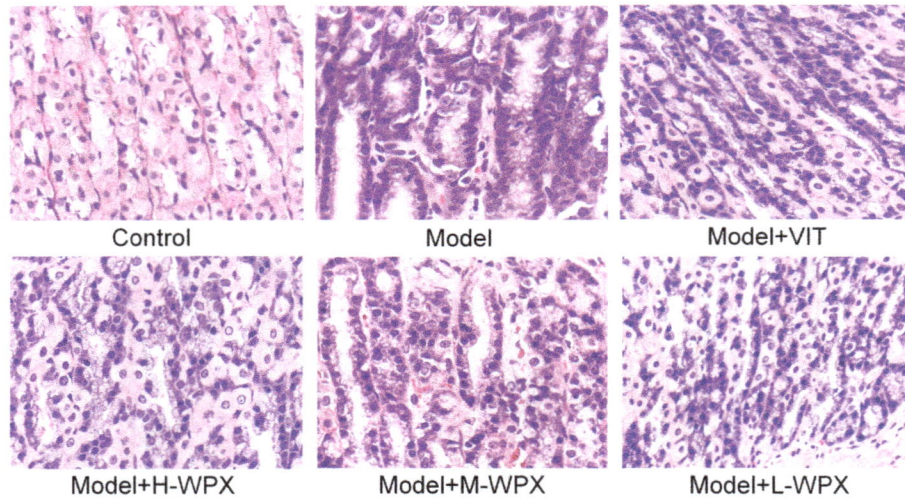

Fig. 3 Histological evaluation of gastric epithelial dysplasia. Model gastric epithelium displayed GED pathology characterized by glandular architectural abnormalities such as splitting, elongated and crowded glands, back to back formation, as well as by cytological atypia with rounded, pleomorphic nuclei that display prominent nucleoli and loss of polarity. After WPX intervention, these GED pathological alterations, especially irregularities of glandular structure, were regressed in varying degrees. $n = 9$ in each group. (H&E staining, 100×)

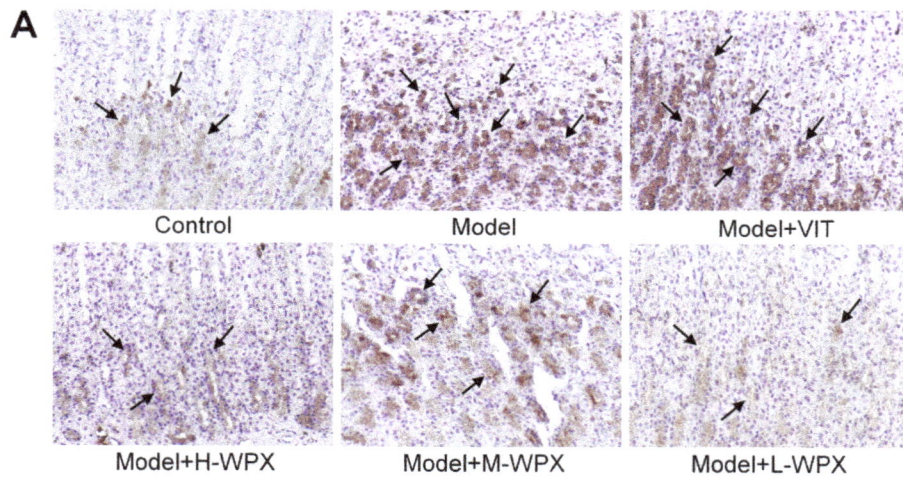

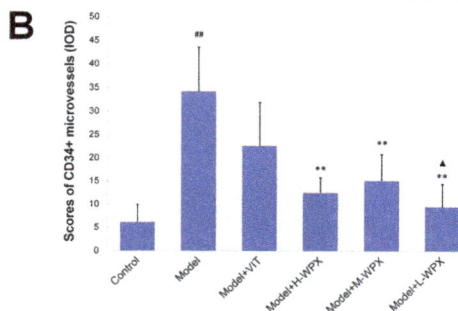

Fig. 4 Evaluation of CD34-labelled microvessel density in gastric mucosa. **a** CD34-labelled microvessels in gastric mucosa from various groups. Some representative microvessels are indicated by black arrows. **b** Scores of CD34+ MVD levels. The results are expressed as mean ± SD ($n = 9$ in each group). Note: ##$P < 0.01$, vs Control; **$P < 0.01$, vs Model; ▲$P < 0.05$, vs VIT. (IHC, 200×)

WPX tempered microvascular abnormalities in GPL tissues

We further examined the morphological changes of microvessels in gastric mucosa under transmission electron microscope. In control rats, microvessels were clearly demarcated from the surrounding connective tissues. The microvessels appeared a normal vascular inner diameter, smooth basal lamina with uniform thickness, and also showed a complete and clear structure of basal lamina with homogeneous electron-density. Endothelial cell bordering the basal lamina was morphologically flat or elongated, with smooth and clear nuclear membrane and normal chromatin distribution.

In model rats, intervascular boundaries were ill-defined or invisible. Remodeled microvessels showed dilated vascular lumen but with a markedly decreased inner diameter, accompanied with clearly thickened, rough basal lamina which was often coated by abundant high-density granules aggregation. Some vascular lumens were partly or completely occluded by erythrocytes and neutrophils. Apart from these, features such as segmental breakup of basal lumina and increased vascular permeability also existed. Furthermore, endothelial cells displayed severe swelling and were shaped like grapes,

with debased cytoplasm electron-density, nucleus chromatin condensation, as well as abundant pinocytotic vesicles. Abnormalitiesof vascular lumen, basal lamina and endothelial cell were still prominent in VIT-treated rats.

In WPX-treated rats, vascular lumen showed a mild-moderate decrease in inner diameter. Basal lamina coated by some high-density granule aggregation was still a little rough, and also with occasional breakup. Endothelial cells exhibited slight swelling and mild vacuolisation. Most of the nuclear membrane became clear and complete, and nucleus chromatin distribution also became normalized. Accordingly, WPX intervention could normalize ultrastructural alterations of vascular lumen, basal lamina and endothelial cell, thus showing the potent rescuing effect of WPX on microvascular abnormalities in GPL rats (Fig. 5).

Effect of WPX on HIF-1α mRNA levels

HIF-1α plays an important role in hypoxic responses and induces the transcription of various genes responsible for tumor angiogenesis, invasion and metastasis. Thus, we texted whether WPX possessed a regulatory ability on hypoxic responses in GPL rats through classic HIF-1α marker detection. Figure 6 clearly showed that

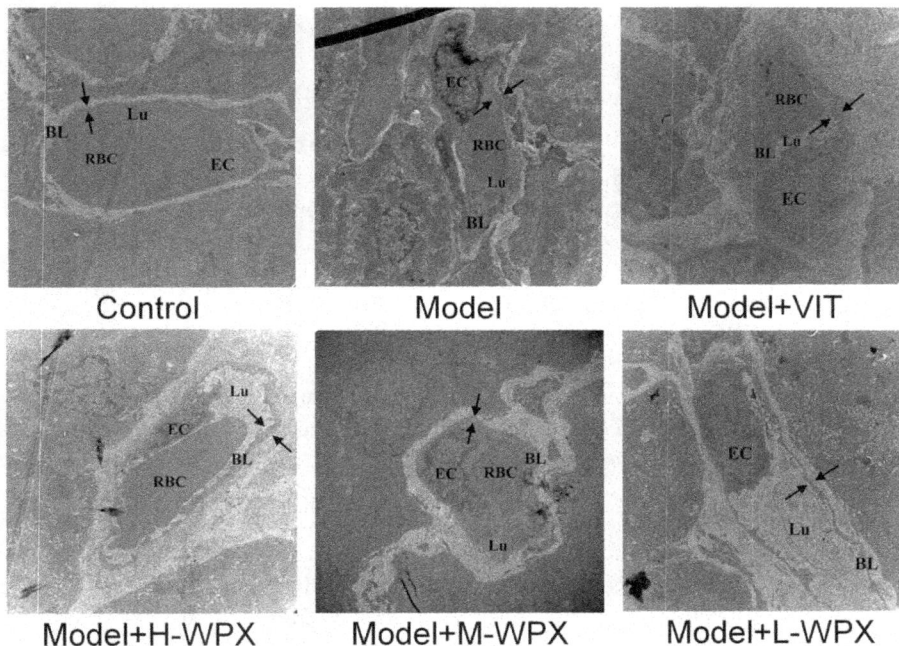

Fig. 5 Representative electron micrographs of microvessels in gastric mucosa. **Control group**: TEM observation of control microvessel ultrastructures appeared intact, in terms of vascular lumen, basal lamina and endothelial cell. **Model group**: Microvessels lost their typical structures. Vascular lumen, frequently plugged by erythrocytes, was dilated but with a markedly decreased inner diameter. Clearly thickened, rough basal lamina was coated by abundant high-density granules aggregation. Segmental breakup of basal lumina and increased vascular permeability were also existed. Endothelial cells were conglobated and shaped as grapes, characterized by debased cytoplasm electron-density, nucleus chromatin condensation, as well as numerous pinocytotic vesicles. **Treatment group**: Microvascular abnormalities were still prominent in VIT-treated tissues. However, the abnormalities reversed markedly in WPX-treated tissues, especially in terms of vascular lumen and basal lamina. Even in a few cases, the microvessels were detected to ultrastructurally resemble the normal ones. Note: Opposing arrows mark the thickness of basal lamina; EC, endothelial cell; BL, basal lamina; Lu, lumen; RBC, red blood cell. $n = 9$ in each group. (10000×)

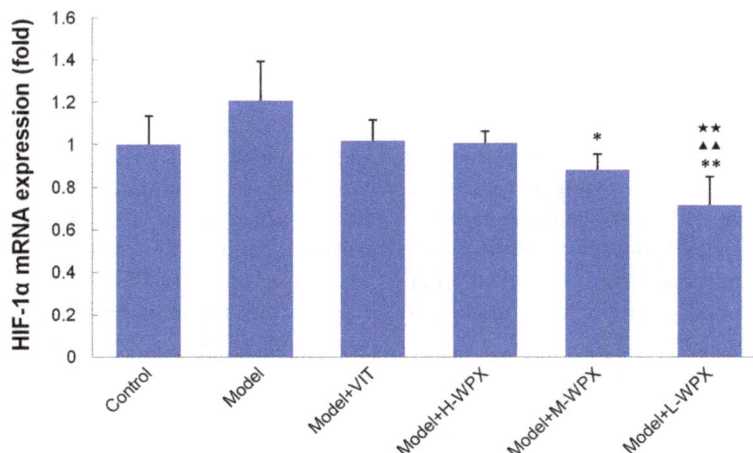

Fig. 6 Effect of WPX on HIF-1α mRNA levels in gastric epithelial cells. The results are expressed as mean ± SD ($n = 9$ in each group). Note: $^{**}P < 0.01$, $^{*}P < 0.05$, vs Model; ▲▲$P < 0.01$, vs VIT; ★★$P < 0.01$, vs H-WPX

HIF-1α mRNA level was elevated in GPL rats when compared with those of controls (although without statistical significance). Compared with model rats, HIF-1α mRNA levels in rats were significantly diminished by medium and low doses of WPX. By comparison, treatment with low dose of WPX led to a marked reduction in HIF-1α mRNA level. The data suggest that WPX, especially at low dose, could efficiently inhibit HIF-1α mRNA expression in GPL rats (Fig. 6).

Effect of WPX on HIF-1α protein expressions

We subsequently applied immunohistochemistry to visualize activation of presumptive HIF-1α marker in gastric mucosa. By immunostaining, HIF-1α was sparsely expressed in normal gastric mucosa, whereas HIF-1α positive cells were found relatively abundant in most GPL tissues. Moreover, we found that WPX could visually reduce the number of HIF-1α positive cells in majority of GPL tissues, as shown in Fig. 7a. Semiquantitatively, elevated HIF-1α protein expression was observed in GPL mucosa as compared to normal mucosa. After WPX intervention, we found a clearly downtrend, although without statistical significance, of HIF-1α levels in gastric mucosa. Our results indicated that WPX treatment may produce regulatory effects on hypoxic responses in GPL gastric mucosa (Fig. 7).

Effect of WPX on VEGF protein expressions

VEGF is generally considered as a vital driving force behind the angiogenesis process, thus we next tested whether VEGF inhibition was of relevance for WPX's anti-angiogenic capacity. As shown in Fig. 8a, normal gastric mucosa did not or barely express VEGF marker, while diffuse and intense cytoplasmic labeling, found in most cases of GPL rats, could be markedly diminished by WPX. Statistically, GPL rats displayed an increased

VEGF protein expression compared with negative controls, whereas WPX treatment reduced the over-expression. In addition, we observed a stronger inhibition effect of L-WPX on VEGF over-expression than that of VIT treatment. Intriguingly, we found HIF-1α and VEGF reduction was frequently along with the attenuation of CD34+ angiogenesis in GPL tissues, indicating that HIF-1α and VEGF inhibition may play a beneficial role in WPX-alleviated angiogenesis (Fig. 8).

Effect of WPX on ERK1, ERK2 and Cyclin D1 mRNA levels

To identify the possible mechanism underlying the anti-angiogenesis activity of WPX on GPL rats, we examined the key targets ERK1, ERK2 and Cyclin D1, which are closely related to the HIF-1α and EVGF signals. As described above, ERK is a specific effector of VEGF signaling and plays a pro-angiogenic role in sprouting [12], thereby instrumental in the progression of gastric cancer. As shown in Fig. 9, we found the gastric precancerous tissues with dramatically elevated ERK1 mRNA levels, which could be reversed by varying concentrations of WPXs. In addition, low dose WPX was found to be markedly superior to VIT in reducing mucosal ERK1 levels. We also noted an elevated ERK2 mRNA levels in GPL tissues, when in comparison to normal gastric tissues. However, in most cases of WPX-treated rats, upregulated ERK2 mRNA levels remained.

We then analyzed mRNA levels of Cyclin D1, a downstream molecule related to ERK signals. Real-time PCR results revealed that GPL rats exhibited notably elevated Cyclin D1 levels compared with the controls. Importantly, WPX treatment caused a marked drop of Cyclin D1 levels in GPL tissues. Similar to ERK1, the inhibitory activity on Cyclin D1 by WPX was more distinct at low dose. Taken together, our findings implicated that the

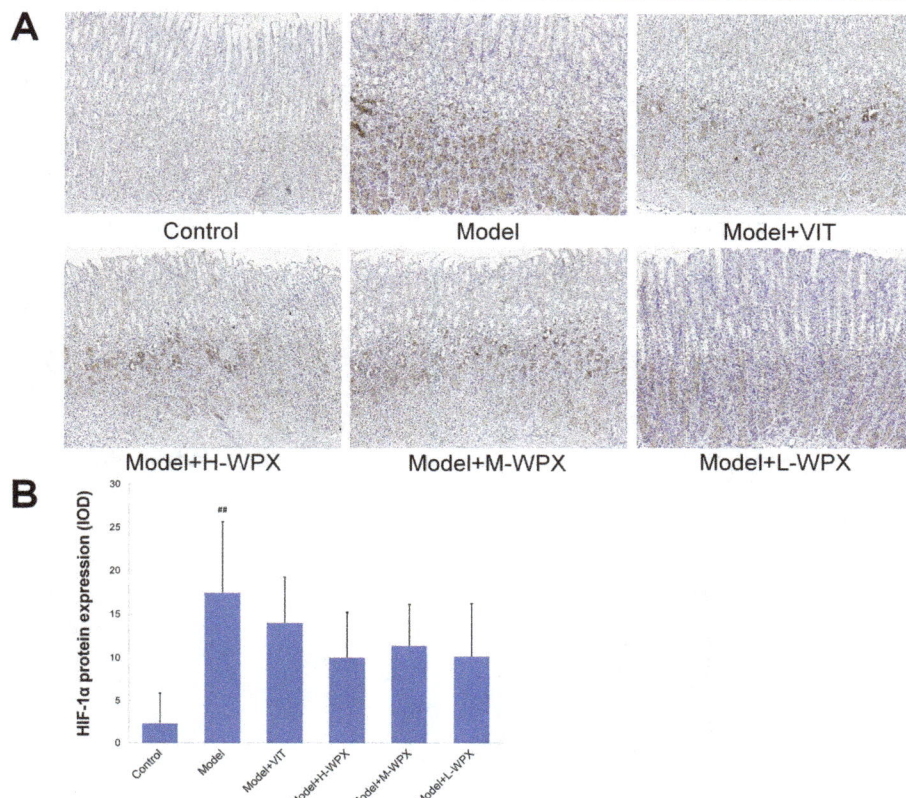

Fig. 7 Effect of WPX on HIF-1α protein expressions in gastric epithelium. **a** HIF-1α protein expressions in gastric epithelium from different groups. **b** IOD scores of HIF-1α protein levels. The results are expressed as mean ± SD ($n = 9$ in each group). Note: $^{##}P < 0.01$, vs Control. (IHC, 100×)

anti-angiogenesis effect of WPX was achieved partly by suppressing ERK1 and Cyclin D1 activation, and its inhibitory effect was identified to be more potent than that of VIT. However, WPX may have little effect on ERK2 amplification (Fig. 9).

Discussion

It is well established that gastric carcinogenesis is a complex and multifactorial process, in which accumulation of multiple genetic changes may be implicated. The recognized human model [31] of gastric carcinogenesis comprises the following precancerous steps: superficial gastritis → multifocal atrophic gastritis → intestinal metaplasia → dysplasia. Based on differences in the magnitude of the malignant risk, GPL could be categorized into (1) "non-progressive GPL" (mainly contains S-IM, mild and moderate dysplasia), remaining a comparatively stable status and with a reduced risk of evolving into gastric carcinoma [32, 33], and (2) "progressive GPL" (comprises some cases of C-IM and severe dysplasia), which is more ominous due to a relatively high risk of malignant transformation and requires advisably interval endoscopic and histologic controls [34, 35]. The vast majority of GPL represents a stage within a

prolonged process and remains stable, thereby providing an opportunity to block and even reverse the precursors. WPX is a typical Chinese herbal prescription proved clinically effective in treating GPL.

In this project, almost all model rats exhibited GPL pathology, which ranged from moderate IM to severe GED lesion. After WPX administration, IM lesion (including S-IM and C-IM) were markedly regressed in most cases of GPL rats. We also found that WPX could halt and even reverse the majority of mild and moderate dysplasia. However, 4 WPX-treated rats (two M-WPX rats, one H-WPX rat, one L-WPX rat) displayed moderate or severe GED pathology, suggesting that a refractory state to WPX administration might have developed in a certain percentage of "progressive GPL". Our observations reinforce the view that a few advanced GED and early gastric cancer are partly similar, in terms of cell proliferative activity and cell atypia. Thus, some cases of "progressive GPL" might be difficult to block and reverse.

Microvasculature serves to circulate and transport oxygen and nutrients, which is imperative to various tissues including gastric mucosa. In contrast to the normal microvasculature, cancer-related angiogenesis, which is continually activated and unregulated [36], is a fundamental

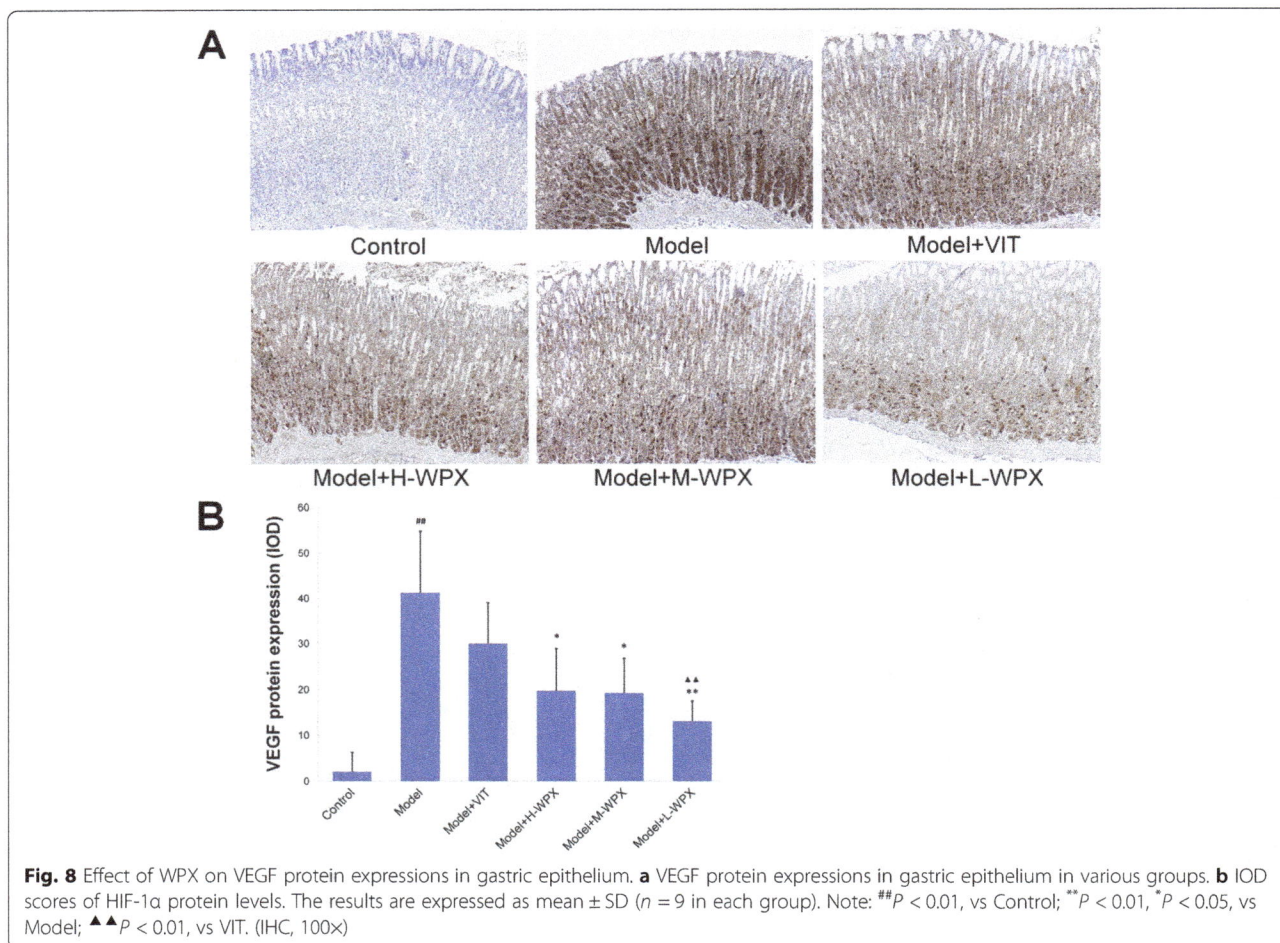

Fig. 8 Effect of WPX on VEGF protein expressions in gastric epithelium. **a** VEGF protein expressions in gastric epithelium in various groups. **b** IOD scores of HIF-1α protein levels. The results are expressed as mean ± SD ($n = 9$ in each group). Note: $^{##}P < 0.01$, vs Control; $^{**}P < 0.01$, $^{*}P < 0.05$, vs Model; $^{▲▲}P < 0.01$, vs VIT. (IHC, 100×)

pathobiological process. It develops a new but malfunctional microvasculature [37], aiming at facilitating oxygen and nutrients supply, and thereby fuels tumor fast-growth. However, the occurrence of angiogenic activity in GPL, and microvessel morphological changes still remain unclear. In this study, we found that CD34+ microvessels were distributed sparsely in normal gastric mucosa, while their number increased significantly in GPL tissue, supporting the hypothesis that early angiogenesis is existed in GPL rats. Interestingly, in more advanced lesions, gastric mucosa frequently exhibited a higher CD34+ microvessel count. We found more GEDs with a higher number of microvessels than IMs, and more severe GEDs than mild or moderate GEDs. Notably, the most numerous CD34+ microvessels were detected in two model rats with severe GED. The above mentioned phenomena may reveal that gastric precancerosis were frequently heterogeneous in angiogenic behavior, and that a significant higher angiogenic state may imply an increased potential biological attitude towards malignancy, which is in agreement with a previous study [38]. Micromorphologically, the microvessel ultrastructural alterations found in GPL tissue were

mainly characterized by dilated vascular lumen, clearly thickened and rough basal lamina, and also by conglobated, degenerated endothelial cell. These characteristics suggest that microvascular abnormalities and hypoxia vasodilation often co-existed in GPL rats. This subsequently induces hypoxia stress together with the activation of hypoxia-inducible factors [39], which stimulate secretion of VEGF and angiogenesis. Hence, angiogenesis may be an adaptive pathobiological response, often accompanying with microvascular abnormalities, triggered by microenvironmental hypoxia in gastric mucosa, aiming at restoring O_2 delivery to hypoxic regions. We speculated that chronic inflammation is a prominent inducer, which could result in microvascular injury [40] and also render gastric tissues more hypoxic [41], and therefore drive angiogenesis [42]. (inflammatory infiltration and altered expressions of inflammatory cytokines TNF-α and IL-4 were observed in GPL rats revealed by our previous study [43]). Nonetheless, these were just our preliminary findings, detailed information concerning microcirculation blood flow, inflammation-induced hypoxia and angiogenesis in GPL tissues became our next focus.

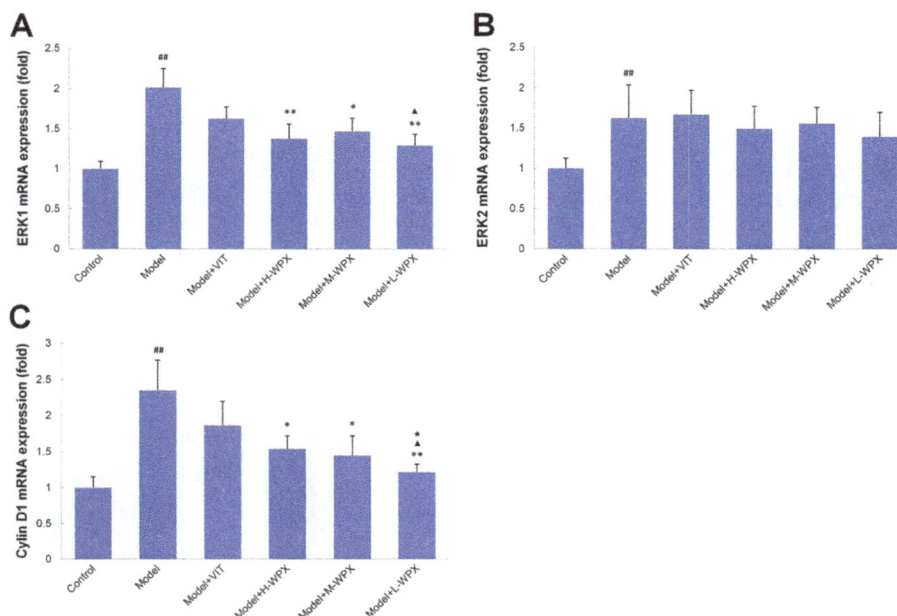

Fig. 9 Effect of WPX on the mRNA levels of ERK1, ERK2 and Cyclin D1 in gastric epithelial cells. **a** ERK1 mRNA levels of gastric epithelium in various groups. **b** ERK2 mRNA levels of gastric epithelium in various groups. **c** Cyclin D1 mRNA levels of gastric epithelium in various groups. The results are expressed as mean ± SD ($n = 9$ in each group). Note: $^{##}P < 0.01$, vs Control; $^{**}P < 0.01$, $^{*}P < 0.05$, vs Model; $^{▲}P < 0.05$, vs VIT; $^{★}P < 0.05$, vs H-WPX

Interestingly, WPX administration could rescue microvascular abnormalities and attenuate early angiogenesis in most of the specimens with a concomitant regression of IM and GED lesions. These findings suggested that WPX might possess multi-functions in blocking the GPL aggravation, not only by its anti-angiogenesis ability revealed by a marked drop of MVD level, but also, probably the most important, by ameliorating the microvascular abnormalities and the subsequent microcirculatory dysfunction. HIF-1α and VEGF have been implicated as classic factors controlling multiple proangiogenic processes hijacked by hypoxic tumors, aimed at normalizing blood flow [13]. In this study, we noted that early angiogenesis observed in GPL tissue is paralleled by HIF-1α and VEGF activation. More importantly, WPX could suppress the hypoxia-triggered accumulation of HIF-1α and the VEGF activation, this result supports the hypothesis that HIF-1α and VEGF inhibition plays a beneficial role in WPX-alleviated angiogenesis. While HIF-1α mRNA levels were elevated in GPL tissues, and the number of HIF-1α positive cells was visually reduced after WPX treatment, we archived no statistically significant differences. Given the hypoxia was a heterogeneous concept with uneven oxygen tensions in localized regions [44], spatial maldistribution of HIF-1α activation in GPL tissues may factor in these non-significant differences. Besides, sample size limitation may be another possible contributor.

Angiogenesis is a complex multistep process regulated by compounding factors. It is proposed that ERK/Cyclin

D1 could act as specific effectors of VEGF signaling to elicit excessive angiogenesis behavior, and thus facilitated cell proliferation, suggesting a crucial role of the molecules in the initiation and progression of gastric cancer. However, what role the molecules may play in GPL is less clear. In this study, as expected, up-regulated mRNA expressions of ERK1, ERK2 and Cyclin D1 were observed in gastric mucosa from GPL rats as compared to normal mucosa. Our results bring a crucial contribution by evidencing that hyper-angiogenesis observed in GPL is driven, in part, through aberrant activation of ERK-related molecules, suggesting their involvement in the malignant transformation. We were also curious as to whether inhibition of ERK signals is involved in the underlying mechanisms of WPX-mediated attenuation of angiogenesis. Interestingly, after WPX intervention, a decrease in ERK1levels was frequently concurrent with the reduction of CD34+ microvessels. Hence, this ERK mitigating effect might be contributed to the anti-angiogenic activity of WPX against precursor lesions. In addition, no significant decrease in ERK2 levels was observed in WPX-treated rats, which might be due to sample size limitation, or to the speculation that ERK2 might not be the potential therapeutic target for GPL with WPX.

Previously, we have found that H-WPX and M-WPX were more superior to L-WPX in ameliorating gastric precancerosis [45], as well as suppressing cell proliferation and promoting apoptosis [46]. In this study, conversely, L-WPX showed a relatively better anti-GPL activity by attenuating early angiogenesis, and by regulating ERK-related molecules as compared to those of H-WPX and M-WPX. We speculate that different treatment duration (10 weeks in the present study, 4 weeks in the previous studies) might be responsible for the inconsistency. It remains possible that WPX, at low dose, might be more efficient for long-term intervention of GPL when compared with that at high and medium doses. However, due to the small sample size, the speculation need to be further validated in larger scale studies. Our HPLC analysis revealed that Calycosin-7-glucoside, ginsenoside-Rg1, ginsenoside-Rvb1, astragaloside IV, as well as atractylenolide III, II and I might be the potential anti-angiogenic candidates of WPX. Ginsenoside Rg1 has been reported to suppress the vascular neointimal hyperplasia by inhibiting on ERK2 signaling [47]. Ginsenoside Rb1 displayed anti-angiogenesis through suppressing the formation of endothelial tube-like structures [48]. Besides, atractylenolide I displayed a potent inhibitory effect on angiogenesis driven by chronic inflammation in vivo and vitro [49]. Although the aforementioned reports likely support the anti-angiogenesis capacity of WPX, there are some caveats. For instance, there have been conflicting reports regarding the pro-angiogenic role [50, 51] or anti-angiogenic role [52] of astragaloside IV. Thus, much more work remains to be addressed in order to fully exploit anti-angiogenic potential of the compounds in MNNG-induced GPL rats and other GPL models in the future.

Conclusion

In summary, WPX could attenuate the angiogenic response and temper microvascular abnormalities in GPL rats. The anti-angiogenesis property might be related to inhibition on the angiogenesis-associated markers HIF-1α and VEGF, and on the ERK1/Cylin D1 aberrant activation. Additional files 1, 2, 3, 4, 5, 6 and 7.

Abbreviations
ANOVA: Analysis of variance; ERK: Extracellular signal-regulated kinase; GED: Gastric epithelial dysplasia; GPL: Gastric precancerous lesions; H&E: Hematoxylin and eosin; HID-AB-PAS: High-iron diamine- alcian blue-periodic acid schiff; HIF-1α: Hypoxia inducible factor-1α; HPLC: High performance liquid chromatography; IM: Intestinal metaplasia; IOD: Integrated optical density.; MNNG: N-methyl-N'-nitro-N-nitrosoguanidine; MVD: Microvessel density; RT-qPCR: Quantitative real-time reverse transcription-polymerase chain reaction; TEM: Transmission electron microscope; TNM: Tumor node metastasis; VEGF: Vascular endothelial growth factor; VIT: Vitacoenzyme; WPX: Weipixiao

Funding
This work was supported by National Natural Science Foundation of China (Nos. 81473620, 81673946, 81774284), and by Science and Technology Developmental Foundation of Affiliated Hospital of Chengdu University of TCM (2016-D-YY-34).

Authors' contributions
JHZ and TTC carried out the experiments. HFP and FMY designed the work. ZMZ and WL prepared for WPX and preformed the HPLC analysis. DYG and RY performed histopathological examination. CZ, LHC and YZ provided helpful advice for the manuscript. All authors agree to be accountable for all aspects of the work.

Competing interests
The authors declare that they have no competing interests.

Author details
[1]Chengdu University of Traditional Chinese Medicine, Chengdu 610075, China. [2]Guangzhou University of Chinese Medicine, Guangzhou 510405, China. [3]Guangdong Provincial Institute of Chinese Medicine, Guangzhou 510095, China. [4]Guangzhou Institutes of Biomedicine and Health, Chinese Academy of Sciences, Guangzhou 510530, China.

References
1. Joo YE, Park HK, Myung DS, Baik GH, Shin JE, Seo GS, Kim GH, Kim HU, Kim HY, Cho SI, Kim N. Prevalence and risk factors of atrophic gastritis and intestinal metaplasia: a nationwide multicenter prospective study in Korea. Gut Liver. 2013;7(3):303–10.
2. de Vries AC, van Grieken NC, Looman CW, Casparie MK, de Vries E, Meijer GA, Kuipers EJ. Gastric cancer risk in patients with premalignant gastric lesions: a nationwide cohort study in the Netherlands. Gastroenterology. 2008;134(4):945–52.
3. Sun SB, Chen ZT, Zheng D, Huang ML, Xu D, Zhang H, Wang P, Wu J. Clinical pathology and recent follow-up study on gastric intraepithelial neoplasia and gastric mucosal lesions. Hepatogastroenterology. 2013; 60(127):1597–601.
4. Srivastava A, Lauwers GY. Gastric epithelial dysplasia: the Western perspective. Dig Liver Dis. 2008;40(8):641–9.
5. Zhang RF, Li JT, He SB, Xiao ZD. Effects of vitacoenzyme on atrophic and intestinal metaplastic lesions in chronic atrophic gastritis—pathologic and histochemical studies of 94 cases. Acad J Sun Yat-Sen Univ Med Sci. 1987;8(2):1–5.

6. Chen XT, Jiang YH, Chen LH, Li XQ, Kuang ZS, Xie YH, Fang YQ. Effects of Weiyankang plus vitacoenzyme on gastric precancerous lesions and its possible mechanism. Acad J Tradit Chin Med. 2004;22(9):1703–4.

7. Deng X, Liu ZW, Wu FS, Li LH, Liang J. A clinical study of weining granules in the treatment of gastric precancerous lesions. J Tradit Chin Med. 2012; 32(2):164–72.

8. Li HZ, Wang H, Wang GQ, Liu J, Zhao SM, Chen J, Song QW, Gao W, Qi XZ, Gao Q. Treatment of gastric precancerous lesions with Weiansan. World J Gastroenterol. 2006;12(33):5389–92.

9. Zhang X, Zheng Z, Shin YK, Kim KY, Rha SY, Noh SH, Chung HC, Jeung HC. Angiogenic factor thymidine phosphorylase associates with angiogenesis and lymphangiogenesis in the intestinal-type gastric cancer. Pathology. 2014;46(4):316–24.

10. Gao LM, Wang F, Zheng Y, Fu ZZ, Zheng L, Chen LL. Roles of fibroblast activation protein and hepatocyte growth factor expressions in angiogenesis and metastasis of gastric cancer. Pathol Oncol Res. 2017; https://doi.org/10.1007/s12253-017-0359-3.

11. Maeda K, Chung YS, Takatsuka S, Ogawa Y, Onoda N, Sawada T, Kato Y, Nitta A, Arimoto Y, Kondo Y. Tumour angiogenesis and tumour cell proliferation as prognostic indicators in gastric carcinoma. Br J Cancer. 1995; 72(2):319–23.

12. Pinto MP, Owen GI, Retamal I, Garrido M. Angiogenesis inhibitors in early development for gastric cancer. Expert Opin Investig Drugs. 2017; 26(9):1007–17.

13. Rey S, Schito L, Wouters BG, Eliasof S, Kerbel RS. Targeting hypoxia-inducible factors for antiangiogenic cancer therapy. Trends Cancer. 2017;3(7):529–41.

14. Arany Z, Foo SY, Ma Y, Ruas JL, Bommi-Reddy A, Girnun G, Cooper M, Laznik D, Chinsomboon J, Rangwala SM, Baek KH, Rosenzweig A, Spiegelman BM. HIF-independent regulation of VEGF and angiogenesis by the transcriptional coactivator PGC-1alpha. Nature. 2008;451(7181):1008–12.

15. Shin M, Beane TJ, Quillien A, Male I, Zhu LJ, Lawson ND. Vegfa signals through ERK to promote angiogenesis, but not artery differentiation. Development. 2016;143(20):3796–805.

16. Yang JJ, Cho LY, Ma SH, Ko KP, Shin A, Choi BY, Han DS, Song KS, Kim YS, Chang SH, Shin HR, Kang D, Yoo KY, Park SK. Oncogenic CagA promotes gastric cancer risk via activating ERK signaling pathways: a nested case-control study. PLoS One. 2011;6(6):e21155.

17. Luo ZY, Wang YY, Zhao ZS, Li B, Chen JF. The expression of TMPRSS4 and Erk1 correlates with metastasis and poor prognosis in Chinese patients with gastric cancer. PLoS One. 2013;8(7):e70311.

18. Yang D, Fan X, Yin P, Wen Q, Yan F, Yuan S, Liu B, Zhuang G, Liu Z. Significance of decoy receptor 3 (Dcr3) and external-signal regulated kinase 1/2 (Erk1/2) in gastric cancer. BMC Immunol. 2012;13:28.

19. Modi PK, Komaravelli N, Singh N, Sharma P. Interplay between MEK-ERK signaling, cyclin D1, and cyclin-dependent kinase 5 regulates cell cycle reentry and apoptosis of neurons. Mol Biol Cell. 2012;23(18):3722–30.

20. Weber JD, Raben DM, Phillips PJ, Baldassare JJ. Sustained activation of extracellular-signal- regulated kinase 1 (ERK1) is required for the continued expression of cyclin D1 in G1 phase. Biochem J. 1997;326(Pt 1):61–8.

21. Guo YL, Rao J, Pan HF, Fang J. Effect of the treatment of Jianpi Huayu Jiecu for patients with chronic atrophic gastritis and its influence on cyclin E protein expression. Chin J Exp Tradit Med Form. 2013;19(11):292–5.

22. He JJ, Zhang BP, Zhao XY. Clinical efficacy of Weipixiao in treating chronic atrophic gastritis. J Guangzhou Univ Tradit Chin Med. 2017;34(6):823–7.

23. Zhang SL. Clinical efficacy of Weipixiao in treating chronic atrophic gastritis (spleen-stomach weakness, syndrome type of TCM): a randomized clinical trial. J Pr Tradit Chin Intern Med. 2017;31(9):12–4.

24. Yin G, Tang D, Dai J, Liu M, Wu M, Sun YU, Yang Z, Hoffman RM, Li L, Zhang S, Guo X. Combination efficacy of Astragalus membranaceus and Curcuma wenyujin at different stages of tumor progression in an imageable orthotopic nude mouse model of metastatic human ovarian cancer expressing red fluorescent protein. Anticancer Res. 2015;35(6):3193–207.

25. Wu J, Ke X, Ma N, Wang W, Fu W, Zhang H, Zhao M, Gao X, Hao X, Zhang Z. Formononetin, an active compound of Astragalus membranaceus (Fisch) Bunge, inhibits hypoxia-induced retinal neovascularization via the HIF-1alpha/VEGF signaling pathway. Drug Des Devel Ther. 2016;10:3071–81.

26. Chen W, Lu Y, Gao M, Wu J, Wang A, Shi R. Anti-angiogenesis effect of essential oil from Curcuma zedoaria in vitro and in vivo. J Ethnopharmacol. 2011;133(1):220–6.

27. Cao HY, Ding RL, Li M, Yang MN, Yang LL, Wu JB, Yang B, Wang J, Luo CL, Wen QL. Danshensu, a major water-soluble component of Salvia miltiorrhiza, enhances the radioresponse for Lewis lung carcinoma xenografts in mice. Oncol Lett. 2017;13(2):605–12.

28. Saito T, Inokuchi K, Takayama S, Sugimura T. Sequential morphological changes in N-methyl-N'-nitro-N-nitrosoguanidine carcinogenesis in the glandular stomach of rats. J Natl Cancer Inst. 1970;44(4):769–83.

29. Tatematsu M, Aoki T, Inoue T, Mutai M, Furihata C, Ito N. Coefficient induction of pepsinogen 1-decreased pyloric glands and gastric cancers in five different strains of rats treated with N-methyl-N'-nitro-N-nitrosoguanidine. Carcinogenesis. 1988;9(3):495–8.

30. Weidner N, Semple JP, Welch WR, Folkman J. Tumor angiogenesis and metastasis-correlation in invasive breast carcinoma. N Engl J Med. 1991; 324(1):1–8.

31. Correa P. A human model of gastric carcinogenesis. Cancer Res. 1988;48(13): 3554–60.

32. Dinis-Ribeiro M, Lopes C, da Costa-Pereira A, Guilherme M, Barbosa J, Lomba-Viana H, Silva R, Moreira-Dias L. A follow up model for patients with atrophic chronic gastritis and intestinal metaplasia. J Clin Pathol. 2004;57(2):177–82.

33. Li D, Bautista MC, Jiang SF, Daryani P, Brackett M, Armstrong MA, Hung YY, Postlethwaite D, Ladabaum U. Risks and predictors of gastric adenocarcinoma in patients with gastric intestinal metaplasia and dysplasia: a population-based study. Am J Gastroenterol. 2016;111(8):1104–13.

34. Di Gregorio C, Morandi P, Fante R, De Gaetani C. Gastric dysplasia. A follow-up study. Am J Gastroenterol. 1993;88(10):1714–9.

35. Gonzalez CA, Sanz-Anquela JM, Companioni O, Bonet C, Berdasco M, López C, Mendoza J, Martín-Arranz MD, Rey E, Poves E, Espinosa L, Barrio J, Torres MÁ, Cuatrecasas M, Elizalde I, Bujanda L, Garmendia M, Ferrández Á, Muñoz G, Andreu V, Paules MJ, Lario S, Ramírez MJ, Gisbert JP. Incomplete type of intestinal metaplasia has the highest risk to progress to gastric cancer: results of the Spanish follow-up multicenter study. J Gastroenterol Hepatol. 2016;31(5):953–8.

36. Tarnawski AS, Ahluwalia A, Jones MK. Angiogenesis in gastric mucosa: an important component of gastric erosion and ulcer healing and its impairment in aging. J Gastroenterol Hepatol. 2014;29(Suppl 4):112–23.

37. Carmeliet P, Jain RK. Principles and mechanisms of vessel normalization for cancer and other angiogenic diseases. Nat Rev Drug Discov. 2011; 10(6):417–27.

38. Spina D, Vindigni C, Presenti L, Schürfeld K, Stumpo M, Tosi P. Cell proliferation, cell death, E-cadherin, metalloproteinase expression and angiogenesis in gastric cancer precursors and early cancer of the intestinal type. Int J Oncol. 2001;18(6):1251–8.

39. Walshe TE, D'Amore PA. The role of hypoxia in vascular injury and repair. Annu Rev Pathol. 2008;3:615–43.

40. Lentsch AB, Ward PA. Regulation of inflammatory vascular damage. J Pathol. 2000;190(3):343–8.

41. Colgan SP, Campbell EL, Kominsky DJ. Hypoxia and mucosal inflammation. Annu Rev Pathol. 2016;11:77–100.

42. Whiteford JR, De Rossi G, Woodfin A. Mutually supportive mechanisms of inflammation and vascular remodeling. Int Rev Cell Mol Biol. 2016; 326:201–78.

43. Li HW, Pan HF, Zhao ZM, Shi YF, Yan Y, Yuan YM, Zeng JH, Lin ZY, Zhao JY. Effect of Weipixiao on plasma tumor necrosis factor alpha and interleukin-4 expression in rats with gastric precancerous lesions. J Guangzhou Univ Tradit Chin Med. 2015;32(2):271–4.

44. Span PN, Bussink J. Biology of hypoxia. Semin Nucl Med. 2015;45(2):101–9.

45. Pan HF, Zhao ZM, Ren JL, Shi YF. Effect of Weipixiao on gastric epithelial intestinal metaplasia in chronic atrophic gastritis rats. Tradit Chin Drug Res Clin Pharmacol. 2012;23(1):55–7.

46. Pan HF, Ren JL, Zhao ZM, Liu J. Effect of Weipixiao on cell generation cycle distribution and apoptosis-related gene expression in gastric mucosal epithelial cells of gastric precancerous lesion rats with spleen-deficiency chronic atrophic gastritis. J Guangzhou Univ Tradit Chin Med. 2010;27(5):488–91.

47. Gao Y, Deng J, Yu XF, Yang DL, Gong QH, Huang XN. Ginsenoside Rg1 inhibits vascular intimal hyperplasia in balloon-injured rat carotid artery by down-regulation of extracellular signal-regulated kinase 2. J Ethnopharmacol. 2011;138(2):472–8.

48. Leung KW, Cheung LW, Pon YL, Wong RN, Mak NK, Fan TP, Au SC, Tombran-Tink J, Wong AS. Ginsenoside Rb1 inhibits tube-like structure formation of endothelial cells by regulating pigment epithelium-derived factor through the oestrogen beta receptor. Br J Pharmacol. 2007; 152(2):207–15.

49.   Wang C, Duan H, He L. Inhibitory effect of atractylenolide I on angiogenesis in chronic inflammation in vivo and in vitro. Eur J Pharmacol. 2009;612(1–3):143–52.

50.   Wang SG, Xu Y, Chen JD, Yang CH, Chen XH. Astragaloside IV stimulates angiogenesis and increases nitric oxide accumulation via JAK2/STAT3 and ERK1/2 pathway. Molecules. 2013;18(10):12809–19.

51.   Wang S, Chen J, Fu Y, Chen X. Promotion of astragaloside IV for EA-hy926 cell proliferation and angiogenic activity via ERK1/2 pathway. J Nanosci Nanotechnol. 2015;15(6):4239–44.

52.   Zhang S, Tang D, Zang W, Yin G, Dai J, Sun YU, Yang Z, Hoffman RM, Guo X. Synergistic inhibitory effect of traditional Chinese medicine astragaloside IV and curcumin on tumor growth and angiogenesis in an orthotopic nude-mouse model of human hepatocellular carcinoma. Anticancer Res. 2017;37(2):465–73.

16

Effects of a hydroalcoholic extract of *Juglans regia* (walnut) leaves on blood glucose and major cardiovascular risk factors in type 2 diabetic patients: a double-blind, placebo-controlled clinical trial

Khadijeh Rabiei[1], Mohammad Ali Ebrahimzadeh[2], Majid Saeedi[2], Adele Bahar[3], Ozra Akha[3] and Zahra Kashi[3,4*] (iD)

Abstract

Background: We aimed to evaluate the effects of a hydroalcoholic extract of *Juglans regia* L. leaves on blood glucose level and cardiovascular risk factors in type 2 diabetic patients.

Methods: In this randomized, double-blind, placebo-controlled, parallel-group (2 arms) clinical trial, 50 diabetic patients were divided into two groups: treatment group (receive the capsules containing 100 mg *J. regia* leaf extract) and control group (receive the capsules containing placebo, microcrystallin cellulose). Baseline participant data were matched between the two arms of the study. We administered the prepared capsules to the patients twice daily for 8 weeks. Blood glucose level, glycosylated hemoglobin (HbA1c) level, body weight, body mass index, blood pressure, lipid profile, serum insulin, and insulin resistance were compared between the two groups before and after the intervention. $P < 0.05$ was considered significant.

Results: After excluding eleven patients, 20 received *J. regia* leaf extract and 20 patients received placebo. The *J. regia* leaf extract did not significantly change the blood glucose and insulin resistance condition. However, in this group, body weight, body mass index, and systolic blood pressure significantly decreased compared with the baseline measurements ($P = 0.028$, $P = 0.030$, and $P = 0.005$, respectively). The lipid profile did not change significantly compared with the baseline measurements. In the control group, postprandial glucose and HbA1c levels significantly decreased after the intervention ($P = 0.030$ and $P = 0.028$, respectively). The other variables were not significantly different in this group. At the end of the study, the variables were not significantly different between the two groups.

Conclusion: In this double-blind study, 200 mg/d of *J. regia* leaf extract had no significant effect on blood glucose level and HOMA-IR score in patients with type 2 diabetes. However, the *J. regia* leaf extract was effective in reducing body weight and blood pressure. An accidental finding of our study was that microcrystalline cellulose, a widely used placebo in clinical trials, led to a reduction in blood glucose level.

Keywords: Diabetes mellitus, *Juglans regia*, Walnut leaves, Herbal medicine, Weight, Blood glucose, Blood pressure, Cardiovascular, Microcrystalline cellulose, Avicel

* Correspondence: kashi_zahra@yahoo.com
[3]Diabetes Research Center, Mazandaran University of Medical Sciences, Sari, Iran
[4]Traditional and Complementary Medicine Research Center, Addiction Institute, Mazandaran University of Medical Sciences, Sari, Iran
Full list of author information is available at the end of the article

Background

Diabetes mellitus is an important metabolic disease and the most prevalent chronic illness around the world with a high financial burden. According to the World Health Organization report, 422 million people have diabetes worldwide, and this rate is rising rapidly [1].

Diet, exercise, and medications are used to manage the disease. However, most patients are reluctant to use chemical drugs, and sometimes, they do not achieve adequate disease control despite the use of multiple medications [2]. The management of cardiovascular risk factors, including weight, lipid levels, and blood pressure, in addition to blood glucose, is very important in patients with type 2 diabetes mellitus [3]. The available anti-diabetic drugs have different effects on the cardiovascular risk factors in diabetic patients, with some of them having a positive effect and some a negative effect. Currently, researchers are giving special attention to the use of medicinal herbs for the treatment of various diseases. The leaves of *Juglans regia L.* (*J. regia*) have been used in traditional medicines as an antimicrobial, anthelmintic, keratolytic, and antidiarrheal and are rich in polyphenolic compounds and flavonoids [4] Amongst the several categories of phytochemicals, polyphenols are the most attractive ones, especially for medicinal purposes [5]. Polyphenols are an important class of secondary metabolites of the plant, possessing a variety of pharmacological activities. Plant phenolics are multifunctional and can act as reducing agents, metal chelators, and singlet oxygen quenchers [6]. Several polyphenols have been shown to have significant antioxidant activities through in vitro and in vivo studies [5]. Studies have shown that consumption of foods and beverages rich in phenolic content is correlated with a reduced risk of atherosclerosis and cardiovascular disease [7]. Literature review shows that polyphenols have demonstrated beneficial effects in animal models of several cardiovascular disorders like hypertension, atherosclerosis, endothelial dysfunction, dyslipidemia, and diabetes-related cardiovascular complications [5] Flavonoids form a ubiquitous group of polyphenolic substances typically produced by plants. Flavonoids are of great interest because of their bioactivities, which are basically related to their antioxidant properties [8]. It has been recognized that flavonoids show antioxidant activity, and their effects on human nutrition and health are considerable. Flavonoids may slow the pathogenesis of atherosclerosis and cardiovascular diseases by their ROS scavenging effects. The mechanism of action of flavonoids involves a scavenging or chelating process [8].

Some studies have reported the anti-diabetic effects of *J. regia* leaves in rats [9–11]; nevertheless, the number of human studies is few. The present study was designed to evaluate the effect of a hydroalcoholic extract of *J. regia* leaves on hyperglycemia and cardiovascular risk factors in patients with type 2 diabetes mellitus.

Methods

This study was a randomized, double-blind, placebo-controlled, parallel group clinical trial. We evaluated the effect of a hydroalcoholic extract of *J. regia* leaves on blood glucose as the primary outcome and insulin resistance, lipid profile, blood pressure, and body weight, the cardiac risk factors, as the secondary outcomes in type 2 diabetic patients.

Preparation of the formulations plant material

J. regia (Juglandaceae) leaf was collected from Dashtenaz area, Sari, Iran. After identification by Dr. Bahman Eslami (Assistance professor of plant systematic, Islamic Azad University, Branch of Ghaemshahr, Iran), Voucher specimen (No 629) was deposited in the Sari School of Pharmacy. The sample was dried at room temperature on the ground before extraction. One kilogram of the sample was extracted by percolation with 70% ethanol (2.5 L × 3) for 24 h [12–14]. The resultant extracts were concentrated in a rotary evaporator until a solid crude extract was obtained, which was freeze-dried to remove the solvent (15.5%) completely. The dried extracts were powdered and mixed with microcrystalline cellulose (Avicel) and then were encapsulated. Avicel was purchased from Sigma-Aldrich (USA). Each capsule contained 100 mg extract and 400 mg Avicel. Avicel itself was used as placebo. Each placebo capsule contained 500 mg Avicel. The final formulations were controlled microbiologically based on the United States Pharmacopeia (USP) method [15].

Standardization of extract

The extract was standardized based on the phenol content. The total phenolic content was determined using the Folin–Ciocalteu method [16] . Each capsule contained 40 mg ± 1.3 mg gallic acid equivalent per gram extract.

Study design

The participants in the study were selected from among those referred to the diabetes outpatient academic clinic in Imam Khomeini Hospital, Sari, Iran (2012–2013). The inclusion criteria were an age of 30–80 years and glycosylated hemoglobin (HbA1c) level more than 7% in spite of receiving the maximal dose of two anti-diabetic drugs (metformin and glibenclamide). Patients were not included in the study if they had immunodeficiency, uncontrolled thyroid dysfunction, cardiovascular disease, proliferative retinopathy, acute hepatitis or cirrhosis, acute infection, history of diabetic ketoacidosis, severe weight loss (at least 10% during the past 6 months), current corticosteroid or thiazide consumption, and serum creatinine (Cr) level > 1.5 mg/dl in males and > 1.4 mg/dl in females. The exclusion criteria also included pregnancy, lactation, changes in anti-diabetic drug type, and lack of follow-up.

Fifty eligible type 2 diabetic patients were enrolled in the study. The minimum sample size was determined to be 20 patients in each group for a statistical power of 0.8 and 95% confidence level and treatment effect size of 0.5–0.8 decrease in the HbA1C following the intervention. After being explained about the trial, the patients signed an informed consent form and were randomly (manual methods and sequentially numbered envelopes) divided into two groups (by a trained general physician who was blind to the content of the capsules), *J. regia* leaves group or the placebo capsule group. The fasting blood sugar (FBS), postprandial glucose (PPG), HbA1c, HOMA-IR, body weight, and blood pressure (BP) were not different between the two groups at baseline. (Table 1) All the patients were advised not to change their previous medications and standard diet during the study period.

The drug or placebo was administered by a trained physician once per day for 1 week and then twice per day for 7 weeks. Body weight, body mass index (BMI), BP, FBS, serum insulin, HbA1c, PPG, serum lipid profile, and liver function were measured at baseline and after treatment. A general physician, who was blinded to the treatment type, examined the patients after 2 weeks and 8 weeks and counted the number of the remaining capsules for the assessment of the participants' adherence to

the interventions. Insulin resistance was calculated using the homeostasis model assessment-estimated insulin resistance (HOMA-IR) method [17].

$$HOMA_{IR} = fasting\ plasma\ insulin\ ^{mIU}\!/\!_{L} \times fasting\ plasma\ glucose\ \frac{mmol/_L}{22.5}$$

Statistical analysis

The analysis was according to the original assigned groups. Student's t-test and paired t-test were used to compare the quantitative variables between the two groups and the before-after values of each group, respectively. The qualitative variables were compared between the two groups using Chi-square test and Fisher exact test, if necessary. In all calculations, $P < 0.05$ was considered to be significant.

Results

In this study, 25 patients were assigned to the intervention group, and 25 patients were assigned to the control group (2012 until 2013). However, because of the changes in the anti-diabetic drug type or lack of follow-up, five patients in the extract group and six patients in the control group were excluded from the study. Fig 1.

Table 1 Baseline participant data in two arms, *Juglans regia* leaves group and control group ($n = 50$)

Variable	*Juglans regia* leaves group n ($N = 25$) Mean ± SD	placebo group ($N = 25$) Mean ± SD	P value
Weight (kg)	74.5 ± 15.4	73.1 ± 9.2	0.744
BMI (kg/cm²)	29.7 ± 5.8	30.2 ± 3.8	0.738
Systolic blood pressure (mm Hg)	126.4 ± 9.1	121.7 ± 10.5	0.153
Diastolic blood pressure (mm Hg)	79.7 ± 6.7	76.7 ± 9.8	0.275
Fasting blood glucose (mg/dl)	195.2 ± 38.2	205 ± 51.9	0.500
Postprandial blood glucose (mg/dl)	283.8 ± 45.5	303.2 ± 68.1	0.323
HbA1C (%)	9.6 ± 1.1	9.8 ± 0.8	0.421
Insulin level	7.2 ± 5	6.4 ± 3.2	0.598
HOMA IR	3.6 ± 2.9	2.9 ± 1.6	0.451
Creatinine (mg/dl)	0.8 ± 0.1	0.9 ± 0.2	0.671
Hemoglobin (mg/dl)	12.8 ± 1.8	12.4 ± 1.3	0.458
Cholesterol (mg/dl)	176.4 ± 39.7	183.4 ± 31.5	0.547
Triglyceride (mg/dl)	180 ± 81.7	167.8 ± 76.6	0.631
HDL Cholesterol (mg/dl)	49.3 ± 8.9	46 ± 12.8	0.336
LDL Cholesterol (mg/dl)	92.5 ± 30.1	102.2 ± 22.3	0.257
AST (U/L)	18.9 ± 4	24.4 ± 9.7	0.022
ALT (U/L)	20 ± 6.2	25.2 ± 13	0.114
ALP (IU/L)	196.9 ± 59.1	214.1 ± 55.1	0.347
TSH (IU/L)	2.2 ± 1.2	2.4 ± 0.9	0.716

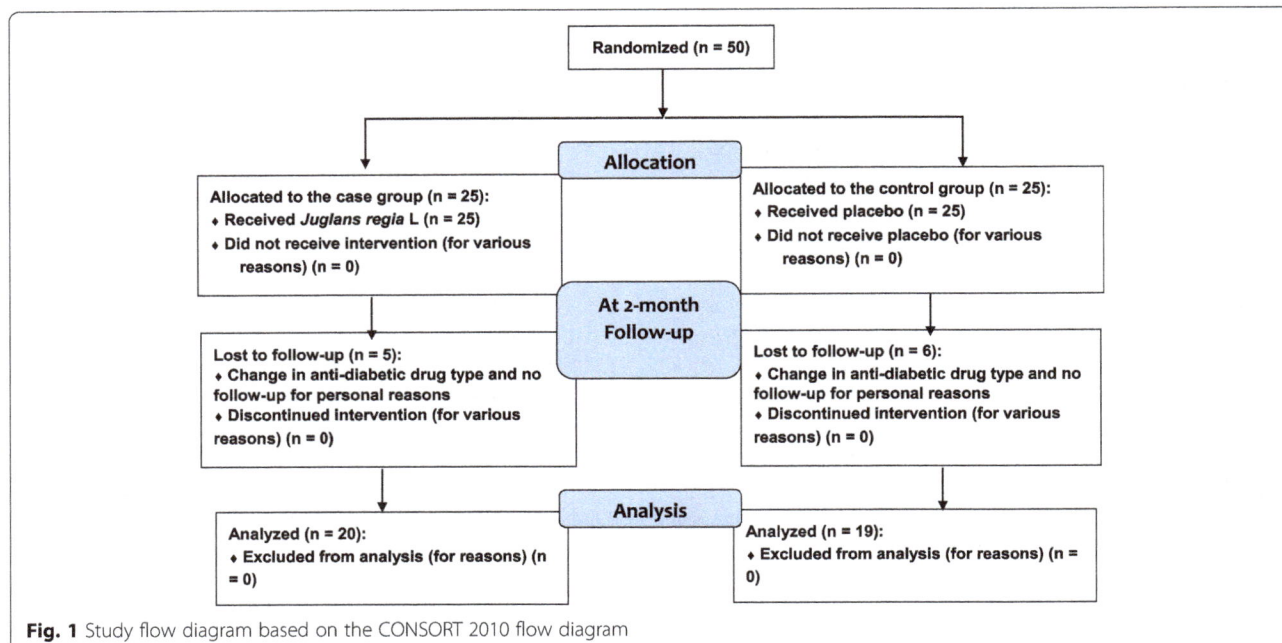

Fig. 1 Study flow diagram based on the CONSORT 2010 flow diagram

The mean age of the patients was not significantly different between the intervention group (50.5 ± 8.3 years) and the control group (49.9 ± 8.6 years) ($P = 0.84$). There was a history of hypertension and dyslipidemia in 52.4 and 85.7% of the participants in the intervention group, respectively, and 42.1 and 84.2% in the control group, respectively ($P = 0.5$ for hypertension and $P = 0.9$ for dyslipidemia). Most of the participants were female; there were 18 females in the control group and 19 females in the intervention group ($P = 0.08$).

The *J. regia* leaves extract had no significant effect on the FBS, PGG, HbA1c level, insulin resistance, and lipid profile, but *J. regia* leaves extract significantly decreased the body weight, BMI, and systolic BP compared with the baseline measurements ($P = 0.028$, $P = 0.030$, and $P = 0.005$, respectively). In the control group, the PGG, HbA1c, and alanine transaminase (ALT) levels decreased significantly after the intervention ($P = 0.030$, $P = 0.028$ and $P = 0.044$, respectively). Although the aspartate transaminase (AST) level was higher in the placebo group at baseline, there were no significant differences in any of the variables between the two groups at the end of the study (Table 2). The participants in the treatment and control group reported no side effects.

Discussion

The use of *J. regia* leaves for the management of diabetes mellitus has been described in the Iranian traditional medicine [18].

In the present study, the *J. regia* leaves had no significant effect on the blood glucose and HOMA-IR levels in the diabetic patients. However, the leaf extract significantly decreased the body weight and systolic BP without any adverse effects on the liver and kidney function.

According to the literature on traditional medicines, the herbal medicines and their extracts are useful in the treatment of chronic disorders, including diabetes mellitus. The herbal medicines have a protective and therapeutic effect in diabetes mellitus via regeneration of the pancreatic β cell, glycogen degradation, decreased gluconeogenesis, α-glucosidase enzyme inhibitor activity, and antioxidative stress [19, 20].

Some previous studies investigated the effect of *J. regia* leaves in rats and showed that it had a positive effect on the blood glucose level. They reported that the hypercellularity of the pancreatic islet tissue was associated with increased hyperchromic nucleus of the islet cells. This finding may be indicative of regeneration of the beta cells [9]. According to the study by Kamyab et al. [21] in mice, oral walnut leaf and ridge extracts significantly reduced liver pyruvate carboxykinase activity and increased liver glycogen phosphorylase activity. They concluded that walnut could reduce the blood glucose level by inhibiting hepatic gluconeogenesis and stimulating secretion of pancreatic insulin.

There are a few scientific studies on the anti-diabetic effect of *J. regia* leaves in humans. We found only two human studies that looked at the effect of *J. regia* leaves in patients with type 2 diabetes [13, 22]. Both studies were done in Iran and reported the significant effect of this plant on blood glucose and insulin levels. However, in the study by Hosseini et al. [13], the plant extract was not standardized, and it was not clear what the placebo was. Also, the researchers

Table 2 Participant data before and after intervention in the case group (extract of *Juglans regia* leaves) and the placebo group (Avicel)

Variable	Juglans regia leaves group✝ (N = 20)		P value	placebo group (N = 19)		P value
	Before intervention Mean ± SD	After intervention Mean ± SD		Before intervention Mean ± SD	After intervention Mean ± SD	
Weight (kg)	73.0 ± 15.1	**71.7 ± 13.8**	**0.028**	73.2 ± 9.2	72.3 ± 8.7	0.303
BMI (kg/cm²)	29.2 ± 6.0	**28.7 ± 5.3**	**0.030**	30.3 ± 3.9	29.9 ± 4.0	0.336
Systolic blood pressure (mm Hg)	126.1 ± 9.5	**121.1 ± 8.8**	**0.005**	121.8 ± 10.6	120.6 ± 9.7	0.637
Diastolic blood pressure (mm Hg)	79.2 ± 6.7	77.4 ± 4.8	0.185	76.8 ± 9.8	79.7 ± 4.8	0.116
Fasting blood glucose (mg/dl)	191.7 ± 36.6	179.5 ± 49.0	0.309	205.1 ± 51.9	194.6 ± 64.8	0.447
Postprandial blood glucose (mg/dl)	283.2 ± 46.8	307.7 ± 99.0	0.249	303.2 ± 68.2	**255.4 ± 53.7**	**0.030**
HbA1C (%)	9.6 ± 1.1	9.5 ± 1.8	0.646	9.90 ± 0.9	**9.1 ± 1.3**	**0.028**
Insulin level	6.4 ± 3.7	7.3 ± 3.9	0.447	6.2 ± 3.3	4.5 ± 3.1	0.139
HOMA IR	3.3 ± 2.7	2.9 ± 2.2	0.186	3.0 ± 1.7	2.7 ± 1.4	0.395
Creatinine (mg/dl)	0.9 ± 0.2	0.8 ± 0.2	0.474	0.9 ± 0.2	0.8 ± 0.2	0.270
Hemoglobin (mg/dl)	12.8 ± 1.9	13.2 ± 2.0	0.119	12.5 ± 1.3	12.3 ± 1.2	0.601
Cholesterol (mg/dl)	176.5 ± 41.8	169.0 ± 30.5	0.413	183.4 ± 31.6	176.5 ± 35.8	0.495
Triglyceride (mg/dl)	179.7 ± 86.1	170.6 ± 81.9	0.622	167.8 ± 76.7	184.1 ± 105.6	0.276
HDL Cholesterol (mg/dl)	49.0 ± 9.3	51.1 ± 9.1	0.337	44.9 ± 12.2	46.2 ± 13.6	0.710
LDL Cholesterol (mg/dl)	93.2 ± 31.6	83.5 ± 16.0	0.151	102.3 ± 22.3	93.0 ± 15.7	0.187
AST (U/L)	19.1 ± 4.2	19.2 ± 6.2	0.902	23.9 ± 9.6	19.4 ± 6.7	0.056
ALT (U/L)	20.7 ± 6.5	20.2 ± 8.1	0.803	24.7 ± 12.4	**18.3 ± 5.7**	**0.044**
ALP (IU/L)	200.7 ± 61.3	197.4 ± 68.0	0.817	202.9 ± 51.1	194..6 ± 64.2	0.594
TSH (IU/L)	2.2 ± 1.2	–	–	2.4 ± 0.9	–	–

✝ There were no significant differences in any of the variables between the two groups at the end of the study

These entries are in boldface because these variables significantly changed after internention (p value <0.05)

prepared the plant extract and placebo in a tablet form, which can affect the double blinding of the study because of the smell of walnut. In a study by Abdoli et al. [22], the aqueous extract of *J. regia* leaves had significant blood glucose lowering effect in patients with type 2 diabetes. The baseline fasting plasma glucose was significantly lower than that in the control group in the study by Abdoli et al. Also, toast powder was used as the placebo in this study, which may itself increase the blood glucose levels [23].

In the present study, we used microcrystalline cellulose (Avicel) as the placebo. Microcrystalline cellulose is an insoluble fiber. When given orally, the agent is not absorbed and has no toxicity; therefore, it is widely used as a placebo in clinical trials [24, 25]. Surprisingly, in our study, low dose of Avicel taken orally (1000 mg/day) significantly lowered the PPG and HbA1c. We did not find any published article on the effect of microcrystalline cellulose (Avicel) on blood glucose in humans. In the study by Takahashi et al. [23] in rats, the consumption of cellulose with meals increased the digestive viscosity and modulated the postprandial plasma glucose.

In our study, the extract of *J. regia* leaves had a significant effect on the body weight and BP. Neither Hosseini et al. [13] nor Abdoli et al. [22] reported about the effect of the extract of *J. regia* leaves on the body weight or BP. Ma et al. [26]. evaluated the effects of a walnut-enriched diet on the endothelial function in patients with type 2 diabetes and reported a significant improvement in the endothelial function and BP. However, the walnut-enriched diet had no significant effect on the blood glucose, HbA1c, and insulin sensitivity. In our study, the consumption of *J. regia* leaves extract led to a significant reduction in the body weight. This effect was also reported by Rock et al. [27] in obese men and women who were given a walnut-enriched diet. We did not find a positive or negative effect of *J. regia* leaves on the lipid profile. Though Hosseini et al. [13] reported the hypolipidemic effects of *J. regia* leaves, Abdoli et al. [22] did not find a positive effect similar to our study. In the study by Ma et al., the walnut-enriched diet had no significant effect on lipid profile.

One of the limitations of our study was that most of the patients were female, although gender did not

appear to have a significant effect on the participants'
response to the plant extract [28]. Another limitation
was the short duration of our study.

Conclusion

The main finding of our study is that the *J. regia* leaves extract is effective in decreasing some major cardiovascular
risk factors including body weight and BP in patients with
type 2 diabetes. However, the extract had no significant effect on the blood glucose, HOMA-IR, and lipid profile. An
accidental finding of our study was that microcrystalline cellulose, which is widely used as a placebo in clinical trials, led
to a reduction in the blood glucose level, particularly the
PPG. The *J. regia* leaves had no side effects and were safe in
low dose (200 mg/d) in our study. These results can be important for researchers who want use this agent as a placebo
in clinical trials. On the other hand, this finding may be the
first step for future studies to use this substance as a
hypoglycemic drug.

Abbreviations
ALT: Alanine transaminase; AST: Aspartate aminotransferase; BMI: body mass
index; BP: blood pressure; Cr: Creatinine; FBS: Fasting blood sugar;
HbA1c: glycosylated hemoglobin; HOMA-IR: homeostasis model assessment
method–insulin resistance; *J. regia*: *Juglans regia* L.; PPG: postprandial blood
glucose; USP: United States pharmacopeia

Acknowledgements
This paper is derived from a research proposal approved by research
committee Traditional and Complementary Medicine Research Center. We
sincerely thank the patients who trusted us to perform the study. We
sincerely thank Dr. Mohhamadpour for statistical analysis helping.

Funding
This research was supported by the Mazandaran University of Medical
Sciences.

Authors' contributions
ZK, KHR: Designer and project manager, Sample collection, Article writing.
AB, OA: Designer, Sample collection, Article writing. MAE, MS: designer and
preparing the drug and placebo, Article writing. All authors read and
approved the final manuscript.

Competing interests
None.

Author details
[1]World Federation of Acupuncture-Moxibustion Societies (WFAS), Scientific
Studies Institute of Nadali Esmaeili, Acupuncture Center, Sari, Iran.
[2]Pharmaceutical Sciences Research Center, Hemoglobinopathy Institute,
Mazandaran University of Medical Sciences, Sari, Iran. [3]Diabetes Research
Center, Mazandaran University of Medical Sciences, Sari, Iran. [4]Traditional and
Complementary Medicine Research Center, Addiction Institute, Mazandaran
University of Medical Sciences, Sari, Iran.

References
1. Mathers CD, Loncar D. Projections of global mortality and burden of disease
   from 2002 to 2030. PLoS Med. 2006;3(11):e442.
2. Schmieder RE, Tschope D, Koch C, Ouarrak T, Gitt AK. Individualised
   treatment targets in patients with type-2 diabetes and hypertension.
   Cardiovasc Diabetol. 2018;17(1):18.
3. Kurukulasuriya LR, Sowers JR. Therapies for type 2 diabetes: lowering HbA1c
   and associated cardiovascular risk factors. Cardiovasc Diabetol. 2010;9:45.
4. Qureshi MN, Stecher G, Bonn GK. Determination of total polyphenolic
   compounds and flavonoids in Juglans regia leaves. Pak J Pharm Sci. 2014;
   27(4):865–9.
5. Bahramsoltani R, Ebrahimi F, Farzaei MH, Baratpourmoghaddam A, Ahmadi P,
   Rostamiasrabadi P, Rasouli Amirabadi AH, Rahimi R. Dietary polyphenols for
   atherosclerosis: a comprehensive review and future perspectives. Crit Rev
   Food Sci Nutr. 2017;11:1–19.
6. Rabiei K, Bekhradnia S, Nabavi SM, Nabavi SF, Ebrahimzadeh MA.
   Antioxidant activity of polyphenol and ultrasonic extracts from fruits of
   Crataegus pentagyna subsp. elburensis. Nat Prod Res. 2012;26(24):2353–7.
7. Manach C, Mazur A, Scalbert A. Polyphenols and prevention of
   cardiovascular diseases. Curr Opin Lipidol. 2005;16(1):77–84.
8. Naginezhad A, Nabavi SM, Nabavi SF, Ebrahimzadeh MA. Antioxidant and
   antihemolytic activities of flavonoid rich fractions of Artemisia
   tschernieviana Besser. Eur Rev Med Pharmacol Sci. 2012;16(Suppl 3):88–94.
9. Jelodar G, Mohsen M, Shahram S. Effect of walnut leaf, coriander and
   pomegranate on blood glucose and histopathology of pancreas of alloxan
   induced diabetic rats. Afr J Tradit Complement Altern Med. 2007;4(3):299–305.
10. Gholamreza K, Hossein B. Effects of walnut leaf aqueous extract on blood
    sugar and lipids in male diabetic rats. Saudi Med J. 2008;29(9):1350–2.
11. Asgary S, Parkhideh S, Solhpour A, Madani H, Mahzouni P, Rahimi P. Effect
    of ethanolic extract of Juglans regia L. on blood sugar in diabetes-induced
    rats. J Med Food. 2008;11(3):533–8.
12. Akhondzadeh S, Sabet MS, Harirchian MH, Togha M, Cheraghmakani H,
    Razeghi S, Hejazi S, Yousefi MH, Alimardani R, Jamshidi A, et al. Saffron
    in the treatment of patients with mild to moderate Alzheimer's disease:
    a 16-week, randomized and placebo-controlled trial. J Clin Pharm Ther.
    2010;35(5):581–8.
13. Hosseini S, Huseini HF, Larijani B, Mohammad K, Najmizadeh A, Nourijelyani
    K, Jamshidi L. The hypoglycemic effect of Juglans regia leaves aqueous
    extract in diabetic patients: a first human trial. Daru. 2014;22(1):19.
14. Cui Y, Tao Y, Jiang L, Shen N, Wang S, Wen H, Liu Z. Antihypoxic activities
    of constituents from Arenaria kansuensis. Phytomedicine : Int J
    Phytotherapy and Phytopharmacology. 2018;38:175–82.
15. The United States Pharmacopeia (USP 39). In. USA. Baltimore: United Book
    Press Inc; 2016. p. 111–42.
16. Ghasemi K, Ghasemi Y, Ebrahimzadeh MA. Antioxidant activity, phenol and
    flavonoid contents of 13 citrus species peels and tissues. Pak J Pharm Sci.
    2009;22(3):277–81.
17. Wallace TM, Matthews DR. The assessment of insulin resistance in man.
    Diabet Med. 2002;19(7):527–34.
18. Zargari A. Medical plants. Tehran: Tehran University Press; 1990.
19. Farzaei F, Morovati MR, Farjadmand F, Farzaei MH. A mechanistic review on
    medicinal plants used for diabetes mellitus in traditional Persian medicine.
    J Evid Based Complementary Altern Med. 2017;22(4):944–55.
20. Farzaei MH, Rahimi R, Farzaei F, Abdollahi M. Traditional medicinal herbs for
    the Management of Diabetes and its complications: an evidence-based
    review. Int J Pharmacol. 2015;11(7):14.
21. Kamyab H, Hejrati S, Khanavi M, Malihi F, Mohammadirad A, Baeeri M,
    Esmaily H, Abdollahi M. Hepatic mechanisms of the walnut antidiabetic
    effect in mice. Central Eur J Biol. 2010;5(3):304–9.
22. Abdoli M, Dabaghian FH, Goushegir A, Shirazi MT, Nakhjavani M, Shojaii A,
    Rezvani S, Mahlooji K. Anti-hyperglycemic effect of aqueous extract of

Juglans regia L. leaf (walnut leaf) on type 2 diabetic patients: a randomized controlled trial. Advances in Integrative Med. 2017;4(3): 98-102.

23. Takahashi T, Karita S, Ogawa N, Goto M. Crystalline cellulose reduces plasma glucose concentrations and stimulates water absorption by increasing the digesta viscosity in rats. J Nutr. 2005;135(10):2405–10.

24. Arnaud M. Chronic venous disorders: pharmacological and clinical aspects of micronized purified flavonoid fraction. Phlebolymphology. 2016;23(2):8.

25. Rowe RC, Sheskey PJ, Quinn ME, Association AP. In: Rowe RC, Sheskey PJ, Quinn ME, editors. Handbook of pharmaceutical excipients. 6th ed. EDN England: London; Chicago : Washington, DC: Pharmaceutical Press; American Pharmacists Association; 2009.

26. Ma Y, Njike VY, Millet J, Dutta S, Doughty K, Treu JA, Katz DL. Effects of walnut consumption on endothelial function in type 2 diabetic subjects: a randomized controlled crossover trial. Diabetes Care. 2010;33(2):227–32.

27. Rock CL, Flatt SW, Barkai HS, Pakiz B, Heath DD. Walnut consumption in a weight reduction intervention: effects on body weight, biological measures, blood pressure and satiety. Nutr J. 2017;16(1):76.

28. Gale EAM, Gillespie KM. Diabetes and gender. Diabetologia. 2001;44(1):3–15.

Acanthus ebracteatus leaf extract provides neuronal cell protection against oxidative stress injury induced by glutamate

17

Anchalee Prasansuklab[1] and Tewin Tencomnao[2*]

Abstract

Background: *Acanthus ebracteatus* (AE), an herb native to Asia, has been recognized in traditional folk medicine not only for its antioxidant properties and various pharmacological activities but also as an ingredient of longevity formulas. However, its anti-neurodegenerative potential is not yet clearly known. This work aimed to evaluate the protective effect of AE leaf extract against glutamate-induced oxidative damage in mouse hippocampal HT22 cells, a neurodegenerative model system due to a reduction in glutathione levels and an increase in reactive oxygen species (ROS).

Methods: Cell viability, apoptosis, and ROS assays were performed to assess the protective effect of AE leaf extract against glutamate-induced oxidative toxicity in HT22 cells. The antioxidant capacity of AE was evaluated using in vitro radical scavenging assays. The subcellular localization of apoptosis-inducing factor (AIF) and the mRNA and protein levels of genes associated with the nuclear factor erythroid 2–related factor 2 (Nrf2) antioxidant system were determined to elucidate the mechanisms underlying the neuroprotective effect of AE leaf extract.

Results: We demonstrated that AE leaf extract is capable of attenuating the intracellular ROS generation and HT22 cell death induced by glutamate in a concentration-dependent manner. Co-treatment of glutamate with the extract significantly reduced apoptotic cell death via inhibition of AIF nuclear translocation. The increases in Nrf2 levels in the nucleus and gene expression levels of antioxidant-related downstream genes under Nrf2 control were found to be significant in cells treated with the extract.

Conclusions: The results suggested that AE leaf extract possesses neuroprotective activity against glutamate-induced oxidative injury and may have therapeutic potential for the treatment of neurodegenerative diseases associated with oxidative stress.

Keywords: *Acanthus ebracteatus*, HT22 cells, Glutamate toxicity, Oxidative stress, Oxytosis, Neuroprotection, Antioxidant, Nrf2/ARE pathway

Background

Oxidative stress is classically described as an imbalance of redox homeostasis, resulting from the overproduction of free radicals relative to the innate ability of cells to scavenge them. This detrimental event causes damage to cellular components and alterations in cellular function that ultimately contribute to cell death [1, 2]. Reactive oxygen species (ROS) are the most common type of free radicals produced in the human body and play an important role in cellular injury in various tissues, particularly the central nervous system (CNS), which is highly sensitive to oxidative damage due to its large dependence on oxygen consumption [3, 4]. In fact, oxidative stress is associated with aging and is a common pathological feature of age-related neurodegenerative diseases, such as Alzheimer's disease (AD), Parkinson's disease (PD), and amyotrophic lateral sclerosis (ALS), in which ROS accumulation is implicated in the mechanism of neuronal loss [5–7]. Currently, many researchers believe that compounds or drugs possessing powerful antioxidant activity could be effective in treating such ROS-related diseases [8–10].

* Correspondence: tewin.t@chula.ac.th
[2]Age-Related Inflammation and Degeneration Research Unit, Department of Clinical Chemistry, Faculty of Allied Health Sciences, Chulalongkorn University Bangkok 10330, Thailand
Full list of author information is available at the end of the article

Glutamate, the principal excitatory neurotransmitter in the brain, has been suggested as a critical trigger of neuronal cell death in several CNS disorders and neurodegenerative diseases [11]. In addition to its involvement in many aspects of normal brain functions, glutamate can also act as a neurotoxin when it is present in excessively high concentrations in the brain extracellular space, causing cellular damage in the context of neurodegeneration. One of the main mechanisms underlying the neurotoxic effects of glutamate is an oxidative stress-induced programmed cell death pathway called oxytosis [12]. In this cell death paradigm, glutamate at pathological levels induces inhibition of cystine uptake via the cystine/glutamate antiporter (system Xc^-), leading to impaired production of the endogenous antioxidant glutathione (GSH) and thereby enhancing accumulation of ROS as well as oxidative stress. Subsequently, the elevated ROS level disrupts mitochondrial membrane integrity and results in the release of apoptosis-inducing factor (AIF), which eventually triggers neuronal death via a caspase-independent pathway [13, 14]. Therefore, suppression of glutamate-induced oxidative stress-mediated neuronal cell death may have the potential to provide a beneficial therapeutic approach for the treatment of neurodegenerative diseases.

At the present time, there is growing worldwide use of herbal medicines for preventive and therapeutic applications based on historical knowledge. In connection with the aforementioned mechanism of glutamate-induced oxidative toxicity, medicinal plants or naturally derived compounds with antioxidant and antiapoptotic effects are currently being researched as neuroprotective agents [15–19]. *Acanthus ebracteatus* Vahl. (AE), commonly known as "Sea Holly", is a medicinal mangrove plant in the family Acanthaceae and is widely distributed in Southeast Asia, including China, India, and Australia [20, 21]. All parts of this plant have been used historically for a variety of medicinal purposes, such as hair root nourishment, reduction of cough and fever, expulsion of kidney stones, relief of rheumatoid arthritis pain and inflammation, and treatment of hypertension, cancer, skin diseases such as rash, chronic wounds and snakebites [22–26]. Interestingly, AE is also used as an important ingredient in traditional Thai longevity and neurotonic remedies for improving brain and body functions [23, 27]. Moreover, previous chemical investigations on this plant revealed the presence of some bioactive components possessing considerable antioxidant activity, neuromodulatory function or memory-improving effects [28–32]. However, currently, there is no conclusive evidence to substantiate its brain and neural health promotion properties. Thus, the present study was conducted to investigate, for the first time, the neuroprotective effect of AE leaf extract against glutamate-induced oxidative cytotoxicity and to further elucidate its underlying protective mechanisms using the mouse hippocampal neuronal HT22 cell line as a cellular model of neurodegeneration.

Methods
Plant material and preparation of the extracts
The plant material used in this study is the leaves of *A. ebracteatus* collected from the Princess Maha Chakri Sirindhorn Herbal Garden (Rayong Province, Thailand). The plant was authenticated by Professor Dr. Thaweesakdi Boonkerd and deposited with voucher specimen number A013422(BCU) at the herbarium of Kasin Suvatabhandhu (Department of Botany, Faculty of Science, Chulalongkorn University, Thailand). The extraction was carried out twice using hexane and absolute ethanol as extracting solvents. Briefly, the leaves were dried in a ventilated incubator at a temperature of at 40 °C and ground into a fine powder. Then, the extracts were prepared by macerating 35 g of the dried leaf powder in 350 mL of each solvent for 48 h under agitation at room temperature (RT), followed by filtration. The residue powder was re-extracted by a similar process, and all filtrates were subsequently combined before removing the solvent by vacuum evaporation. The yield of hexane extract (AEH) and ethanolic extract (AEE) of *A. ebracteatus* leaves was found to be 2.14% and 7.98% (w/w), respectively. Each resulting extract was dissolved in dimethyl sulfoxide (DMSO) as a stock solution of 100 mg/mL, stored at − 20 °C, and protected from light until further analysis.

Determination of total flavonoid content
The total flavonoid content was determined using the aluminum chloride colorimetric method modified for a microplate format as described previously [33]. In brief, 50 µL of the extract sample (1 mg/mL) was made up to 200 µL with 95% ethanol, and mixed well with 10 µL of 10% (v/v) $AlCl_3$ solution and 10 µL of 1 M NaOAc solution. After the reaction was allowed to stand for 40 min in the dark, the absorbance of the reaction mixture was measured at 415 nm using a microplate reader (Perkin-Elmer). Quercetin (Sigma-Aldrich) was used as a standard to construct the calibration curve for quantification, and the content of total flavonoids was reported as mg of quercetin equivalent (QE) per g of dry weight extract.

Determination of total phenolic content
The total phenolic content was determined using the Folin-Ciocalteu method adapted for analysis with a microplate reader, as previously described [33]. Briefly, 50 µL of the extract sample (1 mg/mL) was mixed thoroughly with 50 µL of 10-fold diluted Folin-Ciocalteu's phenol reagent (Sigma-Aldrich). After 20 min of incubation, the mixture was neutralized by addition of 50 µL of a 7.5% (w/v) Na_2CO_3 solution and then kept in the dark at RT for a further 20 min. Finally, the absorbance was measured at 760 nm using an EnSpire® Multimode Plate Reader (Perkin-Elmer). The content of total phenolics was calculated from a standard calibration curve using gallic acid (TCI

America, Portland, OR, USA), and the results are expressed as mg of gallic acid equivalent (GAE) per g of dry weight extract.

LC-MS analysis

The extract was submitted to Institute of Systems Biology (Universiti Kebangsaan Malaysia, Malaysia) for screening of phytochemical constituents using Liquid Chromatography-Mass Spectrometry (LC-MS) analysis. The analytical system used was a Dionex™ UltiMate 3000 UHPLC system (Thermo Fisher Scientific) coupled with a high-resolution micrOTOF-Q III (Bruker Daltonik GmbH, Bremen, Germany). The chromatographic separation was performed on an Acclaim™ Polar Advantage II C18 column (3 μm, 3 mm × 150 mm) (Thermo Fisher Scientific) with a gradient mobile phase consisting of 0.1% formic acid in water (A) and 100% acetonitrile (B). The elution program was as follows: 5% B (0-3 min); 80% B (3-10 min); 80% B (10-15 min) and 5% B (15-22 min). The flow rate was 400 μL/min and the injection volume was 1 μL. The MS instrument was operated in the positive electrospray ionization (ESI) mode with the parameters setting as follows: drying gas flow at 8 L/min, drying gas temperature at 200 °C, nebulizer pressure at 1.2 bar, capillary voltage at 4500 V, and m/z scan range of 50 to 1000. For identification of putative compounds, the observed (experimental) m/z values were compared with the METLIN and the KNApSAcK databases as well as with the calculated (theoretical) mass values of previously reported compounds in *A. ebracteatus*, with an accepted difference of less than 30 parts-per-million (ppm). Relative amount is expressed as the percentage of peak area relative to total area of all peaks observed in the chromatogram.

Cell culture

The immortalized mouse hippocampal HT22 cell line, which served as an in vitro model of neurodegeneration, was a generous gift from Prof. David Schubert at the Salk Institute (San Diego, CA, USA). The HT22 cell line was originally a glutamate-sensitive subclone of the HT-4 cell line, which was derived from the immortalization of primary mouse hippocampal neuronal tissues with a temperature-sensitive SV40 T-antigen [34]. These cells were cultured in Dulbecco's modified Eagle's medium (DMEM) (Sigma-Aldrich, St. Louis, MO, USA) supplemented with 10% (*v*/v) fetal bovine serum (Sigma-Aldrich), 100 units/mL penicillin, and 100 μg/mL streptomycin (Gibco, Waltham, MA, USA) in a humidified atmosphere of 5% CO_2 at 37 °C. The culture medium was replaced every two days. Upon reaching approximately 80% confluency, the cells were passaged by trypsinization and subcultured into fresh medium to maintain their exponential growth.

MTT reduction assay

The MTT assay measures cell viability based on the metabolic activity of viable cells to reduce the yellow tetrazolium salt, 3-(4,5-dimethylthiazol-2-yl)-2,5-diphenyltetrazolium bromide (MTT), to a purple formazan product. HT22 cells were seeded at a density of 6×10^3 cells/well in a 96-well plate and incubated overnight prior to treatment with 5 mM glutamate (Sigma-Aldrich) alone or glutamate in combination with different concentrations of the extracts for 24 h. After the exposure period, the MTT solution (Biobasic, Markham, Ontario, Canada) was added to each well at a final concentration of 0.5 mg/mL and incubated for an additional 4 h in the dark. The generated formazan crystals were dissolved in a DMSO-ethanol mixture (1:1, *v*/v) after the supernatants were carefully removed from the wells. Finally, the absorbance was determined at 550 nm by using an EnSpire® Multimode Plate Reader (Perkin-Elmer, Waltham, MA, USA). The results are expressed as a percentage relative to control (untreated) cells.

LDH leakage assay

The LDH assay determines cell viability based on the release of cytoplasmic lactate dehydrogenase (LDH) from damaged cells, which converts the colorless tetrazolium salt, 2-(*p*-iodophenyl)-3-(*p*-nitrophenyl)-5-phenyl tetrazolium chloride (INT), into a red formazan product. HT22 cells were seeded at a density of 6×10^3 cells/well in a 96-well plate and incubated overnight prior exposure to 5 mM glutamate alone or glutamate in combination with different concentrations of the extracts for 24 h. After treatment, the amount of LDH released into the culture medium was measured using the CytoTox 96® assay (Promega, Madison, WI, USA) according to the manufacturer's instructions. In brief, the culture supernatant was incubated with reconstituted substrate mix in the dark for 30 min at RT, followed by addition of the stop solution before measurement. The absorbance was then recorded at 490 nm by a microplate reader (Perkin-Elmer). The results are expressed as a percentage of maximum LDH release obtained by complete lysis of control (untreated) cells.

Flow cytometric determination of apoptotic cells

Apoptotic cell death was determined based on the externalization of phosphatidylserine to the outer cell surface and increased plasma membrane permeability to dye by using an FITC Annexin V apoptosis detection kit with propidium iodide (PI) (BioLegend, San Diego, CA, USA) according to the manufacturer's protocol. Briefly, HT22 cells were seeded onto a 6-well plate at a density of 1.5×10^5 cells/well and incubated overnight prior to treatment with 5 mM glutamate alone or glutamate in combination with the extracts for 18 h. At the end of the exposure period, the harvested cells were washed twice with phosphate-buffered saline (PBS), re-suspended in the binding buffer, and stained by the solution of FITC-conjugated annexin V and PI for 15 min in the dark. The fluorescence intensity of stained cells, at least 10,000 cells per group, was immediately analyzed by a BD FACS-Calibur™ flow cytometer (BD Bioscience, Heidelberg, Germany). The results are expressed as a percentage of annexin V-positive/PI-negative cells (early apoptosis) plus annexin V/PI-positive cells (late apoptosis).

In vitro radical scavenging assay

The radical scavenging assay was performed using the DPPH and ABTS methods for evaluation of antioxidant activity of the sample based on its hydrogen atom- or electron-donating capacity to neutralize the free radicals. A working solution of stable free radical 2,2-diphenyl-1--picrylhydrazyl (DPPH•) (Sigma-Aldrich) was dissolved in ethanol to a final concentration of 0.2 mg/mL. The cation radical ABTS•+ working solution was generated by the oxidation of 7 mM 2,2′-azinobis-(3-ethylbenzothiazoline-6-sulfonic acid) (ABTS) (Sigma-Aldrich) with 2.45 mM potassium persufhate at a 1:1 (v/v) ratio. The reaction mixture was allowed to stand for 16–18 h in the dark prior to dilution with ethanol until the absorbance reached between 0.7 and 0.8 at 734 nm. For the assay protocol, the DPPH• or ABTS•+ working solution was added to the extract sample (1 mg/mL) at a ratio of 9:1 (v/v). The reaction mixture was incubated in the dark at RT for 15 min or 30 min, and the absorbance was recorded using a microplate reader (Perkin-Elmer) at 517 nm or 734 nm for the DPPH or ABTS assay, respectively. Ascorbic acid (vitamin C) (Calbiochem, San Diego, CA, USA) was used as a reference standard in both assays. Radical scavenging activity was expressed as the percent inhibition of free radicals calculated by the following equation: % Inhibition = 100 - [(Abs of sample - Abs of blank) × 100/ Abs of control]. The antioxidant capacity is expressed as vitamin C equivalent antioxidant capacity (VCEAC) in mg per g of dry weight extract.

Assay for intracellular ROS level

Measurement of the intracellular ROS level was performed using oxygen-sensitive 2′,7′-dichloro-dihydrofluoroscein diacetate (H_2DCFDA) (Molecular Probes, Eugene, OR, USA) based on the ability of ROS to oxidize the cell-permeant, non-fluorescent H_2DCFDA molecule into a highly fluorescent 2′,7′-dichlorofluorescein (DCF) molecule. HT22 cells were seeded at a density of 1×10^4 cells/well in a 96-well plate and incubated overnight prior to exposure to 5 mM glutamate alone or glutamate in combination with different concentrations of the extracts for 14 h. After treatment, the cells were loaded with 5 µM H_2DCFDA, incubated at 37 °C for another 30 min, and

then washed three times with Hank's balanced salt solution (HBSS) (Gibco). Fluorescence was immediately determined using an EnSpire® Multimode Plate Reader (Perkin-Elmer), and photographs were obtained using an Axio Observer A1 fluorescence microscope (Carl Zeiss, Jena, Germany), with an excitation wavelength of 485 nm and an emission wavelength of 535 nm. Data are expressed as the percentage of fluorescence intensity relative to control (untreated) cells.

Quantitative real-time PCR analysis

At the end of treatments, the total RNA from HT22 cells in each group was extracted with Trizol reagent (Invitrogen, Carlsbad, CA, USA) according to the manufacturer's instructions. The amount of RNA was quantified by measuring absorbance at 260 nm, and then 1 µg of total RNA was reverse transcribed to cDNA using oligo(dT)17 primer and AccuPower RT PreMix (Bioneer, Daejeon, South Korea). The cDNA was used as a template for subsequent real-time PCR reactions performed on an Exicycler™ 96 real-time quantitative thermal block (Bioneer) by using the GreenStar™ qPCR PreMix (Bioneer) and the specific primers listed in Table 1. The thermal cycling conditions included an initial denaturation step at 95 °C for 10 min, followed by 40 cycles, each consisting of 15 s of denaturation at 95 °C, 15 s at 55 °C for primer annealing, and 30 s at 72 °C for chain elongation. A melting curve analysis was performed after amplification to verify the accuracy of the amplicon. The relative expression level of each target gene was normalized to β-actin expression and analyzed using the $2^{-\Delta\Delta CT}$ method.

Western blot analysis

Protein expression of target genes was determined by Western blotting. After the treatments, HT22 cells were

Table 1 Primers used for real-time PCR

Gene	Accession number	Sequence (5' → 3')	Product length (bp)
EAAT3	NM_009199.2	Forward: ATGATCTCG TCCAGTTCGGC	202
		Reverse: TGACGATCT GCCCAATGCTT	
NQO1	NM_008706.5	Forward: CGACAACG GTCCTTTCCAGA	253
		Reverse: CTCCCAGA CGGTTTCCAGAC	
GCLM	NM_008129.4	Forward: GGAGCTTC GGGACTGTATCC	236
		Reverse: CAACTCCAA GGACGGAGCAT	
ACTB	NM_007393.5	Forward: GGCTGTATT CCCCTCCATCG	154
		Reverse: CCAGTTGGT AACAATGCCATGT	

harvested, washed, and prepared for whole cell lysates as well as cytoplasmic and nuclear fractions. Whole cell lysates were obtained by lysing the cells on ice in NP-40 lysis buffer (50 mM Tris pH 8.0, 150 mM NaCl, 1% NP-40, 1 mM PMSF, 1 mM DTT). Cytoplasmic and nuclear fractions were isolated using the NE-PER nuclear and cytoplasmic extraction reagents (Thermo Fisher Scientific, Rockford, IL, USA) according to the manufacturer's protocol. Total protein concentrations were measured by the Bradford reagent (Bio-Rad, Hercules, CA, USA) with bovine serum albumin (BSA) as a standard. Equal amounts of proteins were separated by electrophoresis on 10% (v/v) SDS-polyacrylamide gels and electrotransferred to polyvinylidene difluoride (PVDF) membranes. The membranes were blocked for 1 h with 5% skim milk in TBS-T (Tris-buffered saline, 0.1% Tween 20) and allowed to incubate overnight at 4 °C with primary antibodies specific for nuclear factor erythroid 2-related factor 2 (Nrf2) (1:2000; Santa Cruz Biotechnology, Dallas, Texas, USA), excitatory amino acid transporter 3 (EAAT3) (1:8000; Abcam, Cambridge, UK), apoptotic-inducing factor (AIF) (1:2000; Cell Signaling Technology, Danvers, MA, USA), Lamin B1 (1:2000; Cell Signaling Technology) or β-actin (1:16000; Cell Signaling Technology) and subsequently incubated for an additional 45 min at RT with horseradish peroxidase (HRP)-conjugated secondary antibodies (1:10000; Cell Signaling Technology). Specific protein bands were visualized with an enhanced chemiluminescence (ECL) detection reagent (GE Healthcare, Marlborough, MA, USA). Densitometric analysis of the bands was performed with an image analysis system (Syngene, Cambridge, UK).

Immunofluorescence microscopy

HT22 cells were seeded in 12-well plate at a density of 4×10^4 cells/well prior exposure to 5 mM glutamate alone or glutamate in combination with the extract for 16 h. After treatments, an immunofluorescence technique was performed to determine nuclear translocation of AIF. In brief, the cells were fixed with cold 4% (w/v) paraformaldehyde solution for 20 min, permeabilized in 0.1% (w/v) Triton X-100 for 10 min, and blocked with 5% (w/v) BSA for 30 min. Then, the cells were incubated overnight with anti-AIF antibody (1:400; Cell Signaling Technology) at 4 °C, followed by incubation for 1 h with Alexa Fluor 555-conjugated goat anti-rabbit (1:2000; Sigma-Aldrich) at RT. Nuclei were counterstained with 4′,6-diamidino-2-phenylindole (DAPI) solution for 10 min at RT. Following mounting with ProLong Gold antifade mountant (Thermo Fisher Scientific), stained cells were imaged using an LSM 700 confocal laser scanning microscope (Carl Zeiss, Jena, Germany).

Statistical analysis

All experiments were performed in at least triplicate and the data are represented as means ± standard deviation (SD) or means ± standard error of mean (SEM) as indicated in figures. All of the calculations were performed using SPSS software version 17.0 (SPSS Inc., Chicago, IL, USA). The differences between groups were analyzed using one-way analysis of variance (ANOVA), followed by the post hoc Tukey HSD multiple comparison test. The results were considered statistically significant when $P < 0.05$.

Results

Analysis of phytochemical compounds in AEE

To identify putative phytochemical components in AE leaf extract that may be responsible for neuroprotection against glutamate-induced oxidative toxicity, we carried out LC-MS analysis as well as quantitative determination of total flavonoids and phenolics in AEE. Our results revealed a total of 95 ion chromatographic peaks of AEE detected in the positive ion mode (Fig. 1). After identification of each molecular ion peak $[M + H]^+$ by comparison of observed m/z values with the calculated (theoretical) values recorded in databases and the literature, we proposed 11 phytochemical compounds that could have beneficial effects for antioxidant defense or neurological function, of which 5 have been previously reported for *A. ebracteatus* (Fig. 1 and Table 2). The identified peaks were annotated by number and are detailed in Table 2 as follows: peak number, retention time (Rt), observed m/z, peak area, compound name, theoretical mass, and mass error. Furthermore, the total flavonoid content and total phenolic content of AEE were found to be 20.22 ± 3.69 mg QE and 84.86 ± 3.69 mg GAE per g of dry weight extract, respectively.

AE leaf extracts attenuate glutamate-induced cytotoxicity in HT22 cells

To examine the neuroprotective effect of AE leaf extracts against glutamate-induced oxidative cytotoxicity, HT22 cells were exposed to various concentrations of either AEE or AEH (3.125, 6.25, 12.5, 25, and 50 μg/mL) in the presence or absence of 5 mM glutamate, and then cell viability was assessed. We first evaluated the toxic effects of AEH and AEE on HT22 cells and found that neither extract caused noticeable cell death, as shown in Fig. 2a. Treatment of glutamate alone at 5 mM caused a reduction in cell viability of approximately 50%; however, this effect could be rescued in the presence of AE leaf extracts. Our results showed that both AEH and AEE exhibited a significant protective effect by restoring the viability of glutamate-treated HT22 cells in a dose-dependent manner, as determined by the MTT reduction (Fig. 2b) and LDH leakage (Fig. 2c) assays. Morphological examination under a microscope showed normal morphology of HT22 cells upon glutamate treatment combined with AEH or

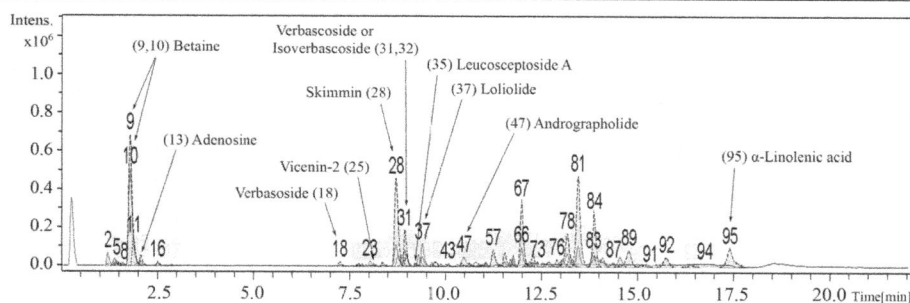

Fig. 1 LC-MS total ion chromatogram of AEE obtained in positive ESI mode. All indicated peak numbers of proposed compounds are detailed in Table 2

AEE (Fig. 2d). These results indicate that AE leaf extracts protect against neuronal damage caused by glutamate. The concentration of 50 μg/mL AEH and AEE was chosen for subsequent experiments, as it resulted in maximal protection among the concentrations tested.

AE leaf extracts suppress glutamate-induced apoptosis in HT22 cells

As it is known that the toxicity caused by excessive glutamate contributes to neuronal cell death via the apoptotic pathway [12], we therefore tested whether the AE leaf extracts could suppress glutamate-induced apoptotic cell death by using Annexin V-FITC/PI staining and flow cytometric analysis to further confirm the neuroprotective effect of the extracts. Our results demonstrated the induction of apoptosis in HT22 cells following glutamate exposure and that the percentage of apoptotic cell death in 5 mM glutamate-treated cells was dramatically increased to approximately 40% compared to that of the control, in which the majority of apoptotic cells were in late stage (Fig. 3a). However, co-treatment of the cells with 50 μg/mL AEH or AEE could significantly reduce the apoptotic rate of glutamate-treated cells to an extent comparable to that observed in the control cells (Fig. 3b),

indicating the cytoprotective and antiapoptotic effects of AE leaf extracts against glutamate toxicity in neurons.

AE leaf extract inhibits glutamate-induced AIF nuclear translocation in HT22 cells

Previous studies have demonstrated that the main mechanism of glutamate-induced apoptotic cell death in HT22 cells is mediated by AIF translocation into the nucleus [35]. Thus, we performed immunocytochemistry and Western blot analysis to determine the effect of AE leaf extract on the subcellular distribution of AIF. Our results revealed that AIF proteins, which are mainly distributed throughout the cytosol under control conditions, were translocated into neuronal nuclei of the HT22 cells following treatment with 5 mM glutamate (Fig. 4a). Moreover, the AIF expression detected by Western blotting was found to be significantly increased in the nucleus but decreased in the cytoplasm (Fig. 4b), confirming that glutamate caused the nuclear translocation of AIF. However, exposure of glutamate-treated cells to 50 μg/mL of AEE significantly restored both nuclear and cytoplasmic expression of AIF proteins to a level similar to those of untreated cells (Fig. 4a and b). These results suggest that the protective effect of AE leaf extract against neuronal cell

Table 2 Proposed phytochemical constituents in AEE

Peak No.	Rt (min)	[M + H]$^+$ (m/z)	Area (%)	Proposed compound	Theoretical mass	Mass error (ppm)	Database/ Reference
9	1.8	118.088	10.5	Betaine	117.079	14	METLIN
10	1.8	118.087	7.7	Betaine	117.079	6	METLIN
13	2.1	268.104	0.7	Adenosine	267.097	0	METLIN, [23]
18	7.3	463.181	0.4	Verbasoside	462.174	0	METLIN
25	8.1	595.165	0.2	Vicenin-2	594.158	1	METLIN, [23]
28	8.7	325.091	6.9	Skimmin	324.085	2	METLIN, KNApSAcK
31	9.0	625.212	2.3	Verbascoside, Isoverbascoside	624.205	1	METLIN, [23]
32	9.0	625.210	1.2	Verbascoside, Isoverbascoside	624.205	4	METLIN, [23]
35	9.2	639.228	0.2	Leucosceptoside A	638.221	1	[23]
37	9.4	197.117	1.7	Loliolide	196.110	1	METLIN, KNApSAcK
47	10.5	351.214	1.1	Andrographolide	350.209	7	METLIN
95	17.4	279.231	2.9	α-Linolenic Acid	278.225	3	METLIN

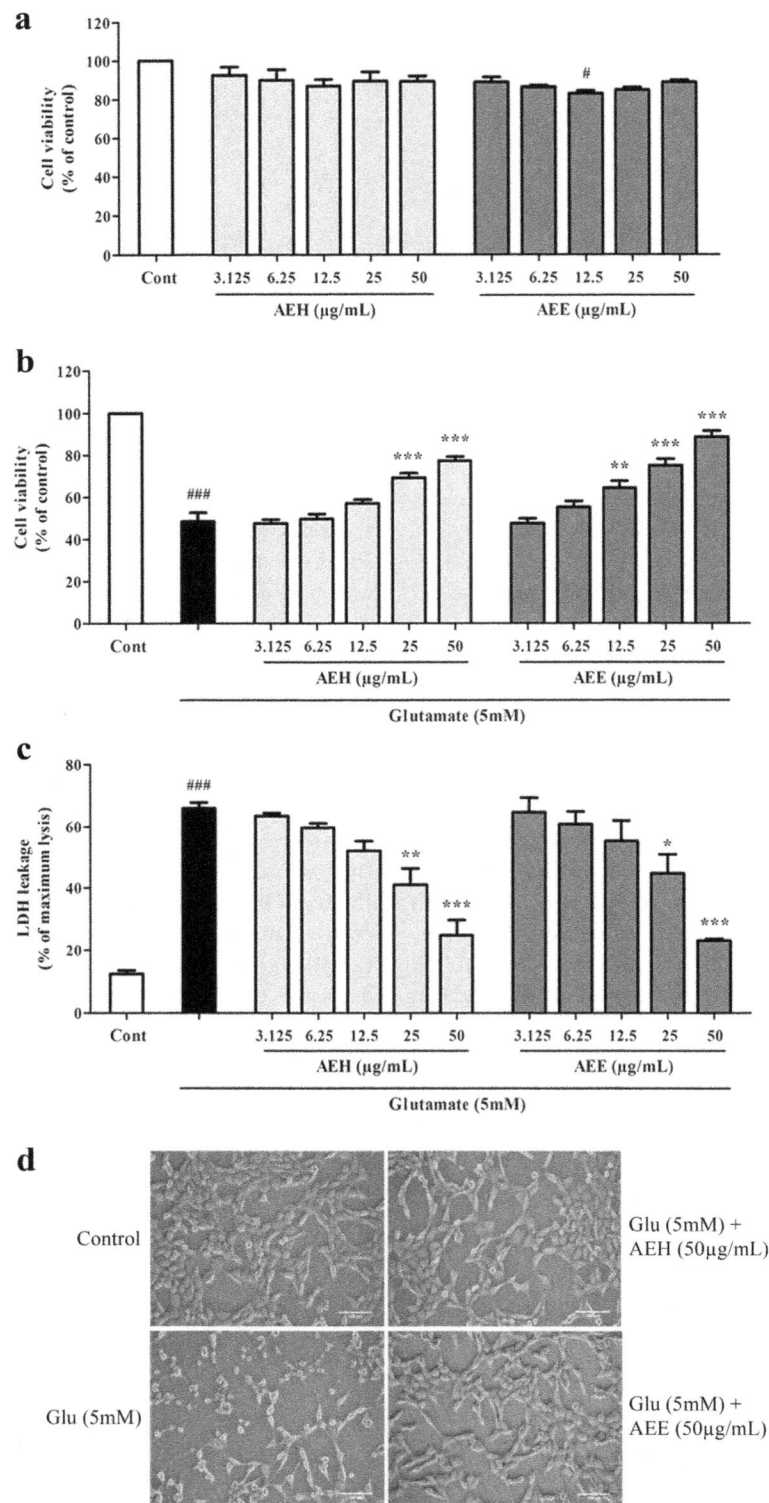

Fig. 2 (See legend on next page.)

(See figure on previous page.)

Fig. 2 Protective effect of AE leaf extracts against glutamate-induced cytotoxicity in HT22 cells. (**a**) Relative MTT viability of HT22 cells exposed to various concentrations of AEH or AEE. (**b**) Relative MTT viability of HT22 cells exposed to 5 mM glutamate alone or glutamate combined with different concentrations of extracts for 24 h. (**c**) Relative LDH release from HT22 cells exposed to similar treatment conditions as in (**b**). (**d**) Representative morphological images at 5X magnification of untreated HT22 cells (control), or cells treated with glutamate alone or with glutamate plus either AEH or AEE at 50 μg/mL. Data are expressed as the means ± SEM, $^#P < 0.05$, $^{###}P < 0.001$ vs. control; $^*P < 0.05$, $^{**}P < 0.01$, $^{***}P < 0.001$ vs. glutamate alone

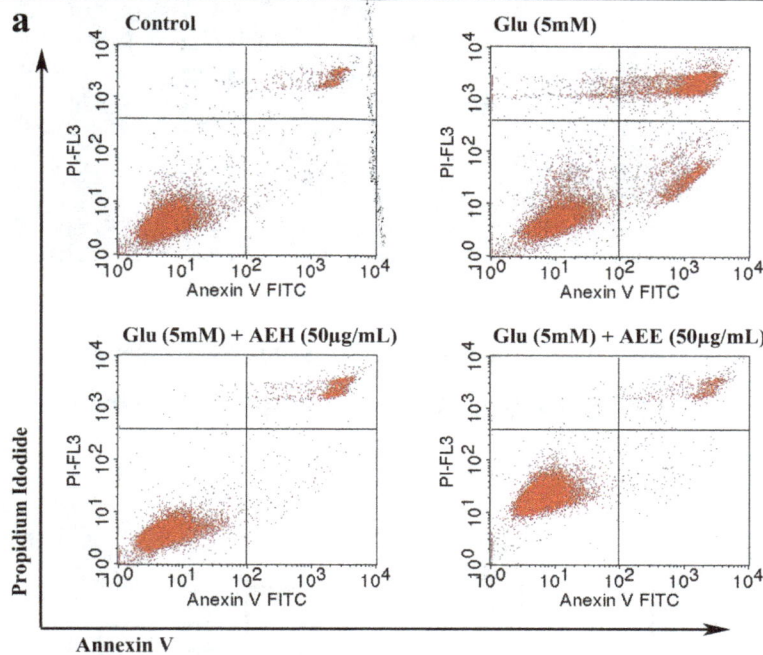

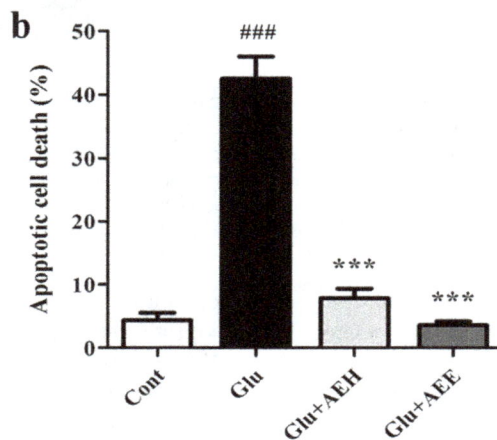

Fig. 3 Protective effect of AE leaf extracts against glutamate-induced apoptotic cell death in HT22 cells. (**a**) Representative flow cytometric scatter plots of annexin V-FITC and PI staining in untreated HT22 cells (control), or cells exposed to 5 mM glutamate alone or glutamate combined with either AEH or AEE at 50 μg/mL for 18 h. (**b**) The percentages of apoptotic cells in each treatment group calculated as the sum of annexin V-positive/PI-negative cells (early-stage apoptosis, lower right quadrant) plus annexin V/PI double-positive cells (late-stage apoptosis, upper right quadrant). Data are expressed as the means ± SD, $^{###}P < 0.001$ vs. control; $^{***}P < 0.001$ vs. glutamate alone

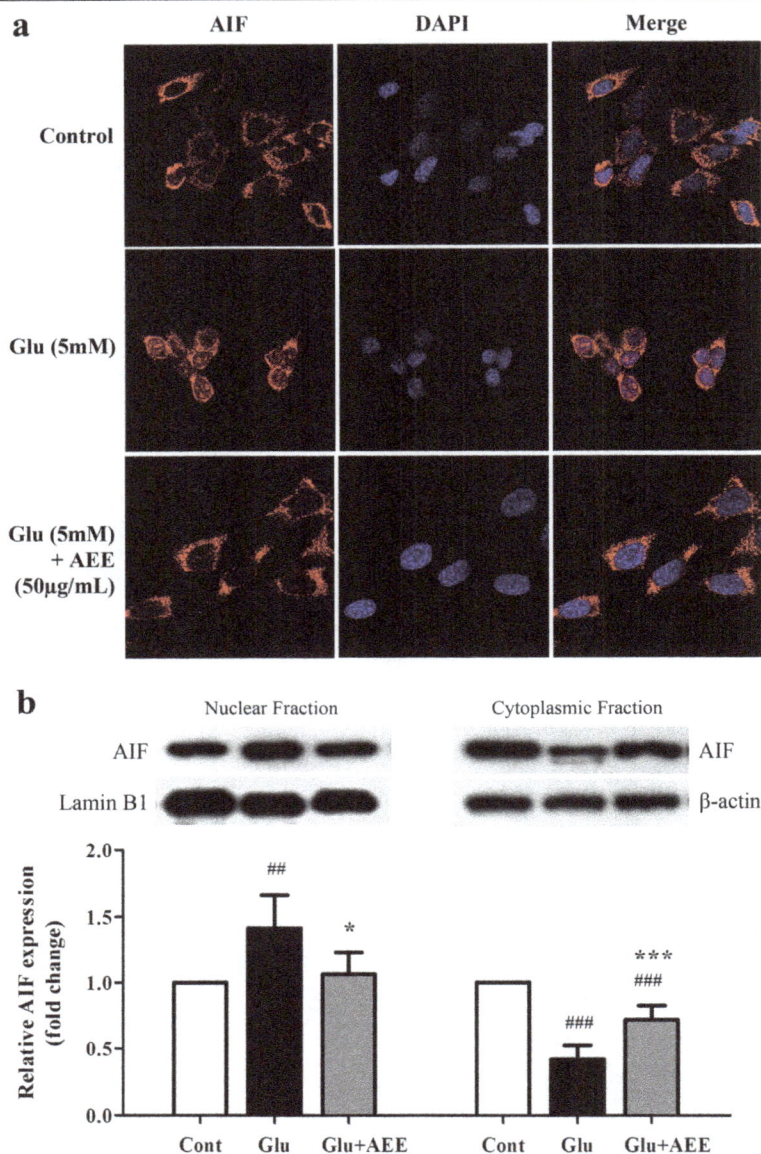

Fig. 4 Effect of AE leaf extract on subcellular distribution of AIF in glutamate-treated HT22 cells. (**a**) Representative confocal photographs of immunofluorescence staining with an antibody specific for AIF (red) and nuclei counterstaining with DAPI (blue) of untreated HT22 cells (control; top panel) or cells exposed to 5 mM glutamate alone (middle panel) or glutamate combined with 50 μg/mL AEE (bottom panel) for 16 h. (**b**) Western blot analysis of AIF protein in nuclear and cytoplasmic fractions isolated from HT22 cells exposed to the similar treatment conditions as in (**a**). Lamin B1 and β-actin were used as endogenous loading controls to normalize the expression level of AIF protein from nuclear and cytoplasmic fractions, respectively. Data are expressed as the means ± SD, $^{\#\#}P < 0.01$, $^{\#\#\#}P < 0.001$ vs. control; $^{*}P < 0.05$, $^{***}P < 0.001$ vs. glutamate alone

death may be mediated by the inhibition of glutamate-induced translocation of AIF to the nucleus.

AE leaf extracts protects neurons against glutamate-induced oxidative stress

We further explored the mechanism by which AE leaf extracts protected neurons from glutamate-induced cytotoxicity. Since enhanced oxidative stress has been considered a pivotal mechanism underlying the neurotoxic action of glutamate and it is well known that increases in oxygen

free radical formation trigger an AIF-mediated pathway of apoptotic cell death [14], we thus investigated whether the AE leaf extracts could attenuate ROS accumulation induced by glutamate and evaluated the antioxidant activities of the extracts in vitro. The results of the DCFH-DA assay showed that 5 mM glutamate treatment caused significantly increased intracellular ROS formation in HT22 cells, as represented by an approximately twofold higher DCF-derived fluorescence intensity relative to untreated cells (Fig. 5a and b). However, co-treatment of the cells with 50 µg/mL of either AEH or AEE was able to restore ROS production in glutamate-treated cells to a level comparable to that observed in the control cells in a dose-dependent manner (Fig. 5b). In contrast, the DPPH and ABTS assays revealed different antioxidant activities of the extracts, as shown in Table 3. The AEE exhibited a much greater capacity for radical scavenging than AEH. These data demonstrate that AE leaf extracts possess antioxidant properties and are capable of attenuating glutamate-mediated neuronal death, possibly by lowering ROS production.

Role of Nrf2 in AE leaf extract-mediated neuroprotection against glutamate-induced oxidative toxicity

We further elucidated the mechanism of AE leaf extract in antioxidant-mediated neuroprotection against glutamate-induced toxicity. It is well known that the induction of the Nrf2/antioxidant response element (ARE) signaling pathway is a major mechanism of cellular protection against oxidative stress by controlling the expression of antioxidant-related genes whose protein products are involved in the elimination of free radicals [36, 37]. Therefore, we examined the effect of AE leaf extracts on the Nrf2 signaling pathway by using real-time reverse transcription (RT) PCR and Western blot analysis. Our results revealed that 50 µg/mL AEE significantly increased the mRNA expression levels of antioxidant-related genes under Nrf2 regulation, including excitatory amino acid transporter 3 (EAAT3), NAD(P)H:quinone oxidoreductase (Nqo1), and

glutamate-cysteine ligase modifier subunit (Gclm), by approximately 2- to 4-fold over controls and samples treated with 5 mM glutamate, whereas exposure to glutamate and AEH or to glutamate alone did not result in a significant difference in their expression (Fig. 6a). These findings were also correlated with a significant increase in protein expression of EAAT3, which was confirmed by Western blots of AEE-treated cells (Fig. 6b). Thus, we next investigated whether AEE could activate transcription factor Nrf2. We found that AEE treatment caused rapid Nrf2 accumulation in the nucleus of glutamate-exposed HT22 cells, while there was no alteration in the cytoplasmic level. After an hour-long exposure of HT22 cells to 5 mM glutamate and 50 µg/mL of AEE, the nuclear Nrf2 level was significantly elevated by 3- and 2-fold the level of the control and glutamate alone groups, respectively (Fig. 6c), indicating activation of Nrf2 by AEE. Taken together, the above results suggest that AE leaf extract protected neurons from the cytotoxic effect of glutamate, possibly by effective activation of transcription factor Nrf2, promoting the expression of downstream antioxidant-related genes of the Nrf2/ARE signaling pathway.

Discussion

Neurodegenerative diseases are a group of disorders that occur as a result of chronic and progressive degeneration of neurons in the brain areas specific for each disorder, such as Alzheimer's disease (AD), Parkinson's disease (PD), Huntington's disease (HD), multiple sclerosis (MS), and

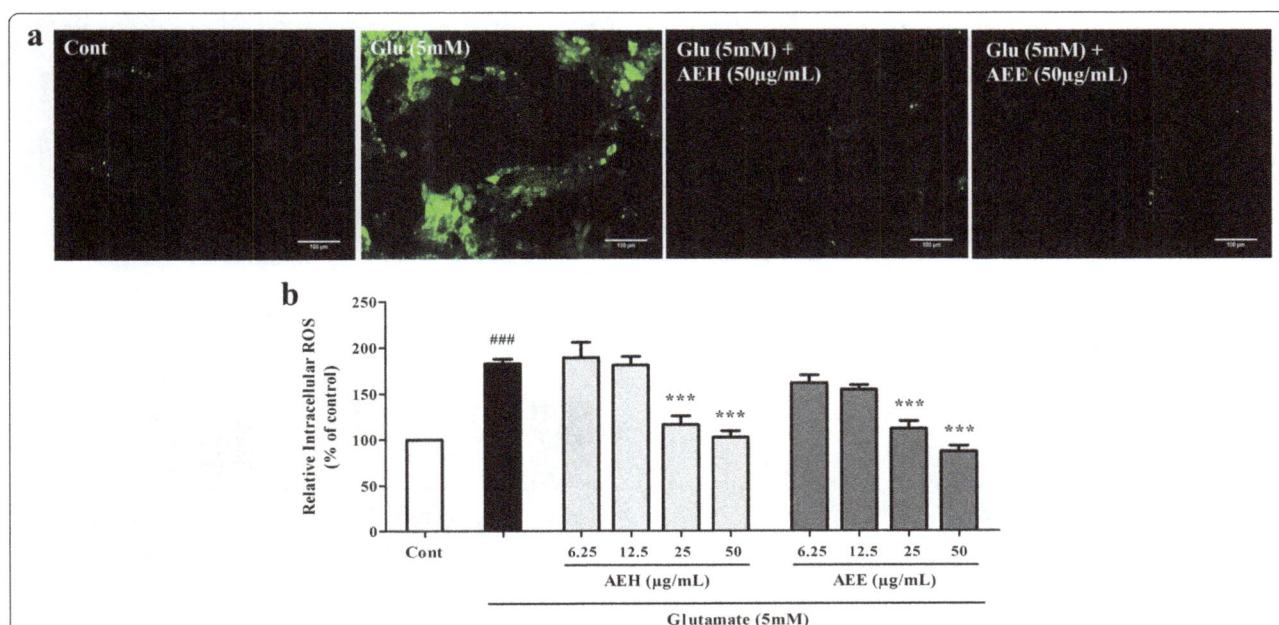

Fig. 5 Effect of AE leaf extracts on glutamate-induced ROS accumulation in HT22 cells. (**a**) Representative confocal micrographs of DCF-derived fluorescence in untreated HT22 cells (control), or cells exposed to 5 mM glutamate alone or glutamate combined with either AEH or AEE at 50 µg/mL for 14 h. (**b**) Relative intracellular ROS levels of HT22 cells treated with 5 mM glutamate alone or with different concentrations of either AEH or AEE for 14 h, determined using a microplate reader. Data are expressed as the means ± SEM, $^{###}P < 0.001$ vs. control; $^{***}P < 0.001$ vs. glutamate alone

Table 3 Free radical scavenging activities of AE leaf extracts

Sample	DPPH scavenging assay		ABTS scavenging assay	
	%Radical Scavenging activity (of 1 mg/mL extract)	mg VCEAC/g dry weight sample	%Radical Scavenging activity (of 1 mg/mL extract)	mg VCEAC/g dry weight sample
Leaf Hexane (AEH)	1.65 ± 0.17	2.44 ± 0.31	7.29 ± 1.36	4.54 ± 0.87
Leaf Ethanol (AEE)	58.46 ± 0.76	65.60 ± 1.21	89.98 ± 6.83	72.01 ± 1.02

Values are expressed as mean ± SD ($n = 3$)

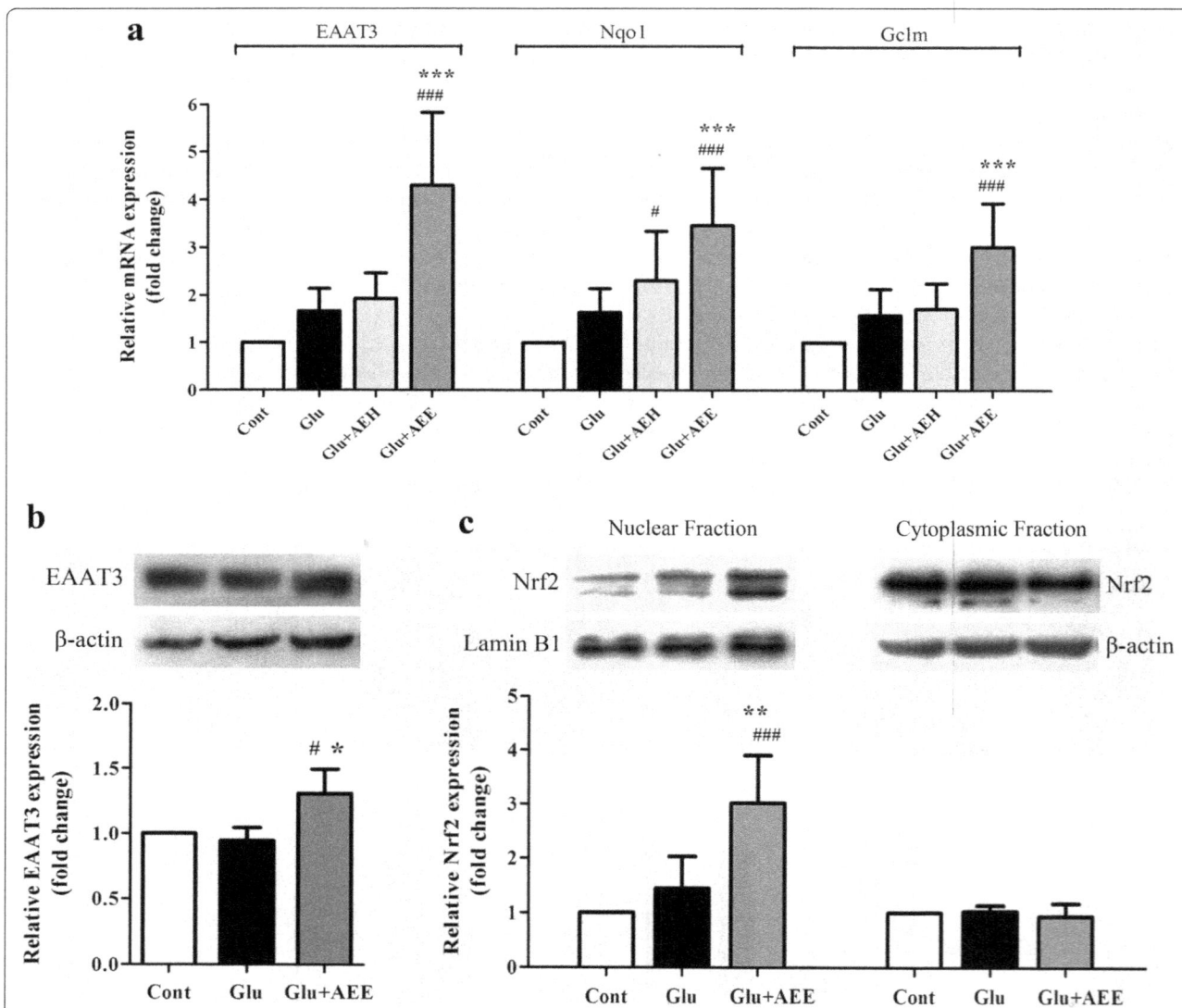

Fig. 6 Effect of AE leaf extracts on expression of Nrf2-regulated antioxidant genes in glutamate-treated HT22 cells. (**a**) Quantitative real-time RT PCR analysis of EAAT3, Nqo1, and Gclm mRNA expression in untreated HT22 cells (control) or cells exposed to 5 mM glutamate alone or glutamate combined with either AEH or AEE at 50 μg/mL for 20 h. β-actin served as an internal control to normalize the mRNA expression levels. (**b**) Western blot analysis of EAAT3 protein in whole cell lysates isolated from untreated HT22 cells (control) or cells exposed to 5 mM glutamate alone or glutamate combined with 50 μg/mL AEE for 22 h. (**c**) Western blot analysis of Nrf2 protein in nuclear and cytoplasmic fractions isolated from HT22 cells exposed for 1 h to the similar treatment conditions as in (**b**). Lamin B1 and β-actin were used as endogenous loading controls to normalize the protein expression levels from nuclear and cytoplasmic fractions/whole cell lysates, respectively. Data are expressed as the means ± SD, $^{\#}P < 0.05$, $^{\#\#\#}P < 0.001$ vs. control; $^{*}P < 0.05$, $^{**}P < 0.01$, $^{***}P < 0.001$ vs. glutamate alone

amyotrophic lateral sclerosis (ALS). Among a variety of neurodegenerative diseases, AD is the most prevalent disorder in the elderly. AD accounts for approximately 60–80% of all dementia cases and is now in the top 10 causes of death in the United States (U.S.) [38]. Moreover, the number of AD patients is rising dramatically every year, partly owing to a growing aging population worldwide [39]. The therapeutic action of most of the U.S. Food and Drug Administration (FDA)-approved AD drugs is to inhibit the enzyme acetylcholinesterase (AChE), which may not be effective in preventing or curing this kind of disease. Therefore, the development of an alternative treatment strategy for AD by focusing on other targets is promising and urgently needed for the management of neurodegenerative diseases in the near future. Currently, traditional plant-based remedies, especially in the Ayurveda system, have attracted the attention of society as well as the scientific world for their potential to treat several chronic and uncured illnesses, including neurodegenerative disorders [40–43]. The benefits of plant-derived compounds over synthetic drugs include the ease of availability at low cost and the comparative safety, especially for patients with long-term medication treatment.

Dysregulation of glutamatergic neurotransmission has been implicated as a critical contributor to various neurodegenerative diseases [11, 44–47]. Thus, several recent studies have drawn on the search of new drugs for neurodegenerative disorders by targeting this neurotransmitter. In the central nervous system (CNS), glutamate neurotoxicity is commonly mediated by two major pathways; receptor-dependent (excitotoxicity) and non-receptor-mediated (oxidative toxicity or oxytosis) pathways [35, 48]. Indeed, oxidative stress is involved not only in oxytosis but also in the mechanism of excitotoxicity, in which high intracellular Ca^{2+} influx caused by overstimulation of glutamate receptors could eventually contribute to excessive ROS production [48]. However, directly inhibiting glutamate receptors may not be a suitable approach as these receptors are important for maintaining normal brain functions [49]. Unsuccessful treatment of AD patients with mild to moderate symptoms by memantine, an antagonist of the N-methyl-D-aspartate (NMDA)-type glutamate receptor, further supports that oxidative stress, rather than receptor stimulation, plays a key role in the pathogenesis of neurodegenerative diseases [50]. Interestingly, a previous clinical trial has shown a significant beneficial efficacy of the well-known, powerful antioxidant vitamin E in comparison with memantine for mild to moderate AD cases [51]. Therefore, in this present study, we exclusively focused on the oxidative toxicity pathway in examining the cytotoxic responses to glutamate.

In researching glutamate-mediated toxicity, various cell lines have been used as model systems, each originating from different brain areas and exhibiting distinct responses

to glutamate [52]. In comparison with other models, the HT22 cell line serves as an appropriate model system for mechanistic studies of oxidative stress-mediated neuronal injury induced by glutamate. Since the HT22 cells do not express the NMDA type of glutamate receptor, toxicity in this model occurs mainly through oxytosis. In this work, our experiments were performed using a high concentration of glutamate (5 mM), which caused a 50% reduction in cell viability relative to a previous report [33]. The present study also confirmed increased ROS generation and AIF nuclear translocation as the mechanism of cell death in this model. Furthermore, the majority of dead cells observed in this study, likely in the late stage of apoptosis after glutamate treatment for 18 h, is consistent with the previous finding that glutamate-induced apoptotic cell death was relatively late, ranging from 16 to 24 h post-treatment [35].

Although AE has long been used in traditional remedies, there are unexpectedly few scientific reports regarding its therapeutic usages, particularly for anti-aging and anti-neurodegeneration. This study provides the first scientific evidence on its neuroprotective activity. In this present work, we found that both AE hexane (AEH) and ethanol (AEE) leaf extracts ameliorated the cytotoxic effects of glutamate in neurons, supporting the historical use of AE as a neurotonic agent [27]. The protective mechanism of AEE against glutamate-induced neuronal cell death could be through lowering intracellular ROS levels, inhibition of nuclear AIF translocation, and activation of the Nrf2/ARE pathway. Moreover, the alteration in Nrf2 levels was observed only in the nucleus after treatment (Fig. 6c), indicating that there might be an increase in both Nrf2 expression and nuclear translocation processes. Unlike AEE, AEH showed lower free radical scavenging activity and did not increase transcription levels of Nrf2-regulated antioxidant genes. The exact mechanism of AEH to mediate neuronal protection is still unclear, and requires further investigation. A limitation of this study is that the effect of AEE upon Nrf2 activation was not directly elucidated by suppressing Nrf2 transcriptional activity using either small interfering RNA or an inhibitor. However, as Nrf2 is a central controlling factor required for mediating positive regulation of NQO1 and GCLM gene expression [53, 54], the observation that elevated mRNA levels of NQO1 and GCLM occurred upon AEE treatment support possible involvement of Nrf2 in the protective effect of AEE.

The majority of previously reported phytochemical components in AE are polyphenolic in structure [23, 28], which is generally known to possess strong antioxidant activity [55, 56]. In agreement with those previous studies, our results of total flavonoids and phenolic contents support the presence of those compounds in AE leaf extract. Additionally, the LC-MS analysis (Table 2) revealed 5 bioactive components previously reported in this plant, which includes adenosine, vicenin-2, verbascoside, isoversbacoside, and leucosceptoside

A. Among these compounds, verbascoside (or acteoside) is a molecule of interest, as it has been shown to have antioxidant functions and protective activities in different cell models of neurodegeneration [30, 31, 57–61]. It is noteworthy that this compound also exerts a beneficial effect on cognition and memory enhancement [32, 62, 63]. Furthermore, we proposed 6 additional compounds, namely, betaine, verbacoside, skimmin, loliolide, andrographolide, and α-linolenic acid, which were identified according to m/z values against the database and selected due to either earlier reports of their antioxidant defense function or their potential neuroprotection roles [64–72]. Nevertheless, due to the complexity of crude extracts and limitations of the single mass analysis, all compounds proposed here need to be confirmed using other identification techniques, such as quantitative HPLC or liquid chromatography-tandem mass

spectrometry (LC-MS/MS). In addition, the neuroprotective activity of the AE components should be re-evaluated later both individually and in combination.

Conclusion

In summary, our results demonstrated for the first time that the extract of AE leaves protects hippocampal neurons from glutamate-induced oxidative toxicity. We showed that the mechanism of neuroprotective action of AE is mediated by inhibition of the AIF-mediated apoptotic pathway and by attenuation of ROS accumulation, likely through the activation of Nrf2 antioxidant system (Fig. 7). Thus, AE may have a protective effect against neurodegenerative diseases, as well as other oxidative stress-associated disorders, due to its profound effect on the Nrf2/ARE pathway.

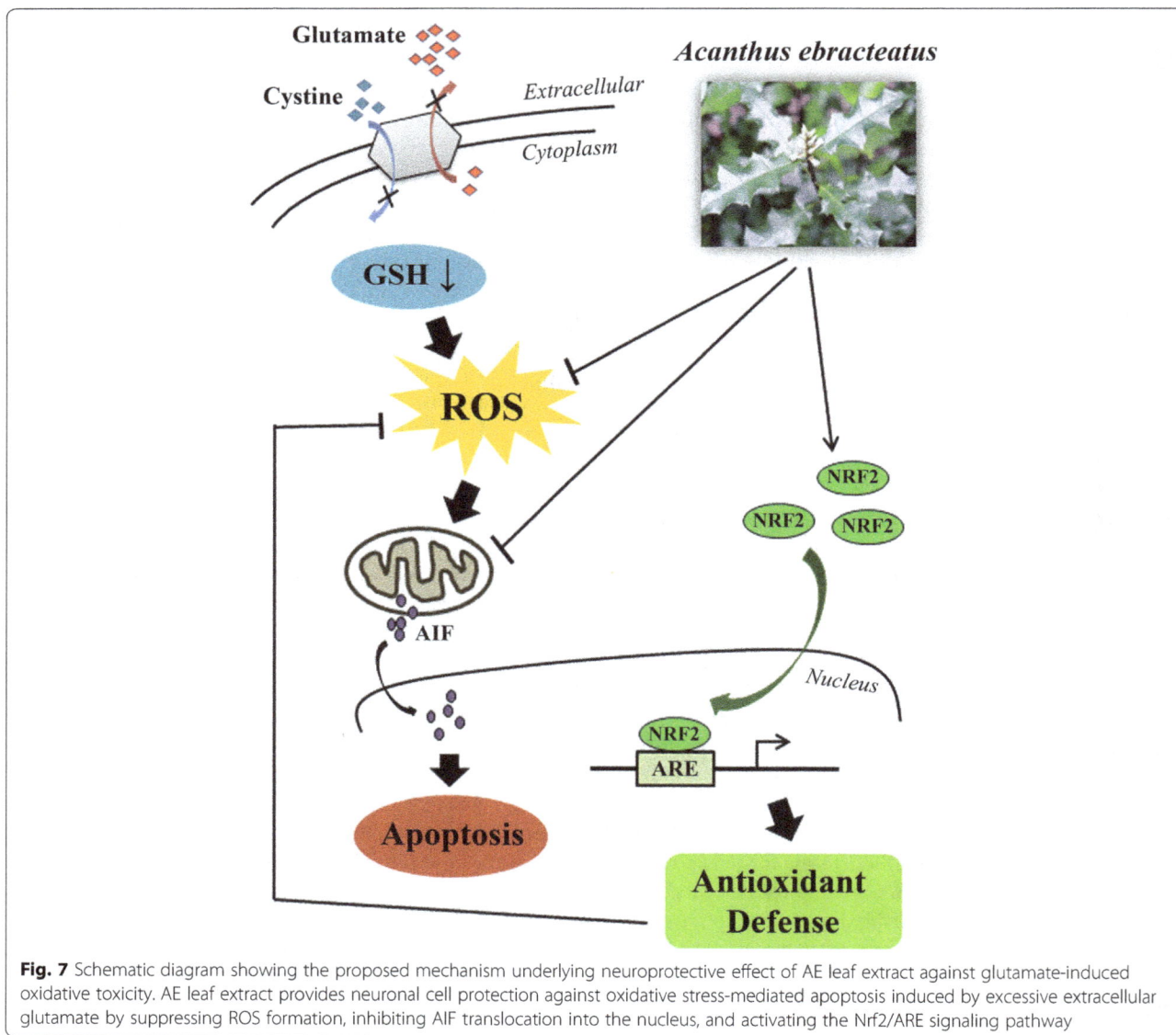

Fig. 7 Schematic diagram showing the proposed mechanism underlying neuroprotective effect of AE leaf extract against glutamate-induced oxidative toxicity. AE leaf extract provides neuronal cell protection against oxidative stress-mediated apoptosis induced by excessive extracellular glutamate by suppressing ROS formation, inhibiting AIF translocation into the nucleus, and activating the Nrf2/ARE signaling pathway

Abbreviations

ABTS: 2,2'-Azino-bis(3-ethylbenzothiazoline-6-sulfonic acid) diammonium salt; AD: Alzheimer's disease; AE: *Acanthus ebracteatus* Vahl; AEE: Ethanolic extract of *A. ebracteatus* leaves; AEH: Hexane extract of *A. ebracteatus* leaves; AIF: Apoptotic-inducing factor; DAPI: 4',6-diamidino-2-phenylindole; DMSO: Dimethyl sulfoxide; DPPH: 2,2-Diphenyl-1-picrylhydrazyl; EAAT3: Excitatory amino acid transporter 3; GAE: Gallic acid equivalent; GCLM: Glutamate cysteine ligase complex modifier subunit; GSH: Glutathione; H_2DCFDA: 2', 7'-dichlorodihydrofluorescein diacetate; LC-MS: Liquid Chromatography-Mass Spectrometry; LDH: Lactate dehydrogenase; MTT: 3-(4,5-dimetylthiazol-2-yl)-2,5-diphenyltetrazoliumbromide; NMDA: N-methyl-D-aspartate; NQO1: NAD(P)H:quinone oxidoreductase 1; Nrf2: nuclear factor erythroid 2-related factor 2; PI: Propidium iodide; QE: Quercetin equivalent; ROS: Reactive oxygen species; System Xc⁻: Cystine/Glutamate antiporter

Acknowledgments

The authors are very grateful to the Princess Maha Chakri Sirindhorn Herbal Garden (Rayong Province, Thailand) for providing plant material and to Prof. David Schubert (The Salk Institute, San Diego, CA, USA) for his generous gift of HT22 cells. We also thank Varaporn Rakkhitawatthana for her help in plant extraction as well as to Noppadol Sa-Art-lam for his technical assistance in flow cytometry.

Funding

This work was financially supported by the National Research University Project, Office of the Higher Education Commission (NRU-59-057-AS) and the 90th anniversary of Chulalongkorn University fund. AP was supported by a Chulalongkorn University Graduate Scholarship to commemorate the 72nd Anniversary of His Majesty King Bhumibol Adulyadej, an Overseas Research Experience Scholarship for Graduate Student by the Graduate School, Chulalongkorn University, and a Grant for Joint Funding, Ratchadaphiseksomphot Endowment Fund.

Authors' contributions

AP and TT conceived and designed the research study. AP performed the experiments, analyzed data, and wrote the manuscript. TT supervised and corrected the manuscript. All authors approved the final version of the manuscript.

Competing interests

The authors declared that they have no competing interests.

Author details

¹Graduate Program in Clinical Biochemistry and Molecular Medicine, Department of Clinical Chemistry, Faculty of Allied Health Sciences, Chulalongkorn University, Bangkok 10330, Thailand. ²Age-Related Inflammation and Degeneration Research Unit, Department of Clinical Chemistry, Faculty of Allied Health Sciences, Chulalongkorn University Bangkok 10330, Thailand.

References

1. Ryter SW, Kim HP, Hoetzel A, Park JW, Nakahira K, Wang X, Choi AM. Mechanisms of cell death in oxidative stress. Antioxid Redox Signal. 2007;9(1):49–89.
2. Storr SJ, Woolston CM, Zhang Y, Martin SG. Redox environment, free radical, and oxidative DNA damage. Antioxid Redox Signal. 2013;18(18):2399–408.
3. Raichle ME, Gusnard DA. Appraising the brain's energy budget. Proc Natl Acad Sci U S A. 2002;99(16):10237–9.
4. Raichle ME. Neuroscience. The brain's dark energy. Science. 2006;314(5803): 1249–50.
5. Emerit J, Edeas M, Bricaire F. Neurodegenerative diseases and oxidative stress. Biomed Pharmacother. 2004;58(1):39–46.
6. Gandhi S, Abramov AY: Mechanism of oxidative stress in neurodegeneration. Oxidative Med Cell Longev 2012, 2012:428010.
7. Kim GH, Kim JE, Rhie SJ, Yoon S. The role of oxidative stress in neurodegenerative diseases. Exp Neurobiol. 2015;24(4):325–40.
8. Liu Z, Zhou T, Ziegler AC, Dimitrion P, Zuo L. Oxidative stress in neurodegenerative diseases: from molecular mechanisms to clinical applications. Oxidative Med Cell Longev. 2017;2017:2525967.
9. Niedzielska E, Smaga I, Gawlik M, Moniczewski A, Stankowicz P, Pera J, Filip M. Oxidative stress in neurodegenerative diseases. Mol Neurobiol. 2016;53(6):4094–125.
10. Uttara B, Singh AV, Zamboni P, Mahajan RT. Oxidative stress and neurodegenerative diseases: a review of upstream and downstream antioxidant therapeutic options. Curr Neuropharmacol. 2009;7(1):65–74.
11. Lewerenz J, Maher P. Chronic glutamate toxicity in neurodegenerative diseases-what is the evidence? Front Neurosci. 2015;9:469.
12. Tan S, Schubert D, Maher P. Oxytosis: a novel form of programmed cell death. Curr Top Med Chem. 2001;1(6):497–506.
13. Landshamer S, Hoehn M, Barth N, Duvezin-Caubet S, Schwake G, Tobaben S, Kazhdan I, Becattini B, Zahler S, Vollmar A, et al. Bid-induced release of AIF from mitochondria causes immediate neuronal cell death. Cell Death Differ. 2008;15(10):1553–63.
14. Tobaben S, Grohm J, Seiler A, Conrad M, Plesnila N, Culmsee C. Bid-mediated mitochondrial damage is a key mechanism in glutamate-induced oxidative stress and AIF-dependent cell death in immortalized HT-22 hippocampal neurons. Cell Death Differ. 2011;18(2):282–92.
15. Hugel HM. Brain food for Alzheimer-free ageing: focus on herbal medicines. Adv Exp Med Biol. 2015;863:95–116.
16. Abushouk AI, Negida A, Ahmed H, Abdel-Daim MM. Neuroprotective mechanisms of plant extracts against MPTP induced neurotoxicity: future applications in Parkinson's disease. Biomed Pharmacother. 2017;85:635–45.
17. Dey A, Bhattacharya R, Mukherjee A, Pandey DK. Natural products against Alzheimer's disease: Pharmaco-therapeutics and biotechnological interventions. Biotechnol Adv. 2017;35(2):178–216.
18. Elufioye TO, Berida TI, Habtemariam S: Plants-derived neuroprotective agents: cutting the cycle of cell death through multiple mechanisms. Evid Based Complement Alternat Med 2017, 2017:3574012.
19. Tewari D, Stankiewicz AM, Mocan A, Sah AN, Tzvetkov NT, Huminiecki L, Horbanczuk JO, Atanasov AG. Ethnopharmacological approaches for dementia therapy and significance of natural products and herbal drugs. Front Aging Neurosci. 2018;10:3.
20. Ragavan P, SAXENA A, Mohan P, JAYARAJ RS, Ravichandran K. Taxonomy and distribution of species of the genus Acanthus (Acanthaceae) in mangroves of the Andaman and Nicobar Islands, India. Biodiversitas Journal of Biological Diversity. 2015;16(2).
21. Bora R, Adhikari PP, Das AK, Raaman N, Sharma GD. Ethnomedicinal, phytochemical, and pharmacological aspects of genus Acanthus. Int J Pharm Pharm Sci. 2017;9(12):8.
22. Bandaranayake WM. Traditional and medicinal uses of mangroves. Mangrove Salt Marshes. 1998;2(3):133–48.
23. Kanchanapoom T, Kasai R, Picheansoonthon C, Yamasaki K. Megastigmane, aliphatic alcohol and benzoxazinoid glycosides from Acanthus ebracteatus. Phytochemistry. 2001;58(5):811–7.
24. Laupattarakasem P, Houghton P, Hoult J, Itharat A. An evaluation of the activity related to inflammation of four plants used in Thailand to treat arthritis. J Ethnopharmacol. 2003;85(2):207–15.
25. Charoonratana T, Songsak T, Monton C, Saingam W, Bunluepuech K, Suksaeree J, Sakunpak A, Kraisintu K. Quantitative analysis and formulation development of a traditional Thai antihypertensive herbal recipe. Phytochem Rev. 2014;13(2):511–24.
26. Poonthananiwatkul B, Lim RH, Howard RL, Pibanpaknitee P, Williamson EM. Traditional medicine use by cancer patients in Thailand. J Ethnopharmacol. 2015;168:100–7.
27. Ingkaninan K, Temkitthawon P, Chuenchom K, Yuyaem T, Thongnoi W. Screening for acetylcholinesterase inhibitory activity in plants used in Thai traditional rejuvenating and neurotonic remedies. J Ethnopharmacol. 2003; 89(2–3):261–4.

28. Li MY, Xiao Q, Pan JY, Wu J. Natural products from semi-mangrove flora: source, chemistry and bioactivities. Nat Prod Rep. 2009;26(2):281–98.

29. Gomes CV, Kaster MP, Tome AR, Agostinho PM, Cunha RA. Adenosine receptors and brain diseases: neuroprotection and neurodegeneration. Biochim Biophys Acta. 2011;1808(5):1380–99.

30. Sgarbossa A, Dal Bosco M, Pressi G, Cuzzocrea S, Dal Toso R, Menegazzi M. Phenylpropanoid glycosides from plant cell cultures induce heme oxygenase 1 gene expression in a human keratinocyte cell line by affecting the balance of NRF2 and BACH1 transcription factors. Chem Biol Interact. 2012;199(2):87–95.

31. Alipieva K, Korkina L, Orhan IE, Georgiev MI. Verbascoside--a review of its occurrence, (bio)synthesis and pharmacological significance. Biotechnol Adv. 2014;32(6):1065–76.

32. Shiao YJ, Su MH, Lin HC, Wu CR. Acteoside and Isoacteoside protect amyloid beta peptide induced cytotoxicity, cognitive deficit and neurochemical disturbances in vitro and in vivo. Int J Mol Sci. 2017;18(4).

33. Prasansuklab A, Meemon K, Sobhon P, Tencomnao T. Ethanolic extract of Streblus asper leaves protects against glutamate-induced toxicity in HT22 hippocampal neuronal cells and extends lifespan of Caenorhabditis elegans. BMC Complement Altern Med. 2017;17(1):551.

34. Davis JB, Maher P. Protein kinase C activation inhibits glutamate-induced cytotoxicity in a neuronal cell line. Brain Res. 1994;652(1):169–73.

35. Fukui M, Song JH, Choi J, Choi HJ, Zhu BT. Mechanism of glutamate-induced neurotoxicity in HT22 mouse hippocampal cells. Eur J Pharmacol. 2009;617(1–3):1–11.

36. Nguyen T, Nioi P, Pickett CB. The Nrf2-antioxidant response element signaling pathway and its activation by oxidative stress. J Biol Chem. 2009; 284(20):13291–5.

37. Ma Q. Role of nrf2 in oxidative stress and toxicity. Annu Rev Pharmacol Toxicol. 2013;53:401–26.

38. Alzheimer's Association: 2017 Alzheimer's Disease Facts and Figures 2017. https://www.alz.org/documents_custom/2017-facts-and-figures.pdf. Accessed 11 Dec 2017.

39. United Nations, Department of Economic and Social Affairs, Population Division: World Population Prospects: The 2017 Revision, Key Findings and Advance Tables. 2017. https://esa.un.org/unpd/wpp/Publications/Files/WPP2017_KeyFindings.pdf. Accessed 11 Dec 2017.

40. Pistollato F, Battino M. Role of plant-based diets in the prevention and regression of metabolic syndrome and neurodegenerative diseases. Trends Food Sci Technol. 2014;40(1):62–81.

41. Iriti M, Vitalini S, Fico G, Faoro F. Neuroprotective herbs and foods from different traditional medicines and diets. Molecules. 2010;15(5):3517–55.

42. Rasool M, Malik A, Qureshi MS, Manan A, Pushparaj PN, Asif M, Qazi MH, Qazi AM, Kamal MA, Gan SH, et al. Recent updates in the treatment of neurodegenerative disorders using natural compounds. Evid Based Complement Alternat Med. 2014;2014:979730.

43. Prasansuklab A, Tencomnao T: Amyloidosis in Alzheimer's disease: the toxicity of amyloid Beta (a beta), mechanisms of its accumulation and implications of medicinal plants for therapy. Evid Based Complement Alternat Med 2013, 2013:413808.

44. Butterfield DA, Pocernich CB. The glutamatergic system and Alzheimer's disease: therapeutic implications. CNS Drugs. 2003;17(9):641–52.

45. Sheldon AL, Robinson MB. The role of glutamate transporters in neurodegenerative diseases and potential opportunities for intervention. Neurochem Int. 2007;51(6–7):333–55.

46. Dong XX, Wang Y, Qin ZH. Molecular mechanisms of excitotoxicity and their relevance to pathogenesis of neurodegenerative diseases. Acta Pharmacol Sin. 2009;30(4):379–87.

47. Kostic M, Zivkovic N, Stojanovic I. Multiple sclerosis and glutamate excitotoxicity. Rev Neurosci. 2013;24(1):71–88.

48. Wang Y, Qin ZH. Molecular and cellular mechanisms of excitotoxic neuronal death. Apoptosis. 2010;15(11):1382–402.

49. Meldrum BS. Glutamate as a neurotransmitter in the brain: review of physiology and pathology. J Nutr. 2000;130(4S Suppl):1007s–15s.

50. Schneider LS, Dagerman KS, Higgins JP, McShane R. Lack of evidence for the efficacy of memantine in mild Alzheimer disease. Arch Neurol. 2011; 68(8):991–8.

51. Dysken MW, Sano M, Asthana S, Vertrees JE, Pallaki M, Llorente M, Love S, Schellenberg GD, McCarten JR, Malphurs J, et al. Effect of vitamin E and memantine on functional decline in Alzheimer disease: the TEAM-AD VA cooperative randomized trial. Jama. 2014;311(1):33–44.

52. Kritis AA, Stamoula EG, Paniskaki KA, Vavilis TD. Researching glutamate - induced cytotoxicity in different cell lines: a comparative/collective analysis/study. Front Cell Neurosci. 2015;9:91.

53. Nioi P, Hayes JD. Contribution of NAD(P)H:quinone oxidoreductase 1 to protection against carcinogenesis, and regulation of its gene by the Nrf2 basic-region leucine zipper and the arylhydrocarbon receptor basic helix-loop-helix transcription factors. Mutat Res. 2004;555(1–2):149–71.

54. Ferguson G, Bridge W. Glutamate cysteine ligase and the age-related decline in cellular glutathione: the therapeutic potential of gamma-glutamylcysteine. Arch Biochem Biophys. 2016;593:12–23.

55. Pereira D, Valentão P, Pereira J, Andrade P. Phenolics: from chemistry to biology. Molecules. 2009;14(6):2202.

56. Ghasemzadeh A, Ghasemzadeh N. Flavonoids and phenolic acids: role and biochemical activity in plants and human. J Med plants Res. 2011;5(31): 6697–703.

57. Sheng GQ, Zhang JR, Pu XP, Ma J, Li CL. Protective effect of verbascoside on 1-methyl-4-phenylpyridinium ion-induced neurotoxicity in PC12 cells. Eur J Pharmacol. 2002;451(2):119–24.

58. Koo KA, Sung SH, Park JH, Kim SH, Lee KY, Kim YC. In vitro neuroprotective activities of phenylethanoid glycosides from Callicarpa dichotoma. Planta Med. 2005;71(8):778–80.

59. Koo KA, Kim SH, Oh TH, Kim YC. Acteoside and its aglycones protect primary cultures of rat cortical cells from glutamate-induced excitotoxicity. Life Sci. 2006;79(7):709–16.

60. Wang H, Xu Y, Yan J, Zhao X, Sun X, Zhang Y, Guo J, Zhu C. Acteoside protects human neuroblastoma SH-SY5Y cells against beta-amyloid-induced cell injury. Brain Res. 2009;1283:139–47.

61. Esposito E, Dal Toso R, Pressi G, Bramanti P, Meli R, Cuzzocrea S. Protective effect of verbascoside in activated C6 glioma cells: possible molecular mechanisms. Naunyn Schmiedeberg's Arch Pharmacol. 2010;381(1):93–105.

62. Gao L, Peng XM, Huo SX, Liu XM, Yan M. Memory enhancement of Acteoside (Verbascoside) in a senescent mice model induced by a combination of D-gal and AlCl3. Phytother Res. 2015;29(8):1131–6.

63. Peng XM, Gao L, Huo SX, Liu XM, Yan M. The mechanism of memory enhancement of Acteoside (Verbascoside) in the senescent mouse model induced by a combination of D-gal and AlCl3. Phytother Res. 2015;29(8):1137–44.

64. Alirezaei M, Khoshdel Z, Dezfoulian O, Rashidipour M, Taghadosi V. Beneficial antioxidant properties of betaine against oxidative stress mediated by levodopa/benserazide in the brain of rats. J Physiol Sci. 2015; 65(3):243–52.

65. Knight LS, Piibe Q, Lambie I, Perkins C, Yancey PH. Betaine in the brain: characterization of betaine uptake, its influence on other Osmolytes and its potential role in neuroprotection from osmotic stress. Neurochem Res. 2017;42(12):3490–503.

66. Mazimba O. Umbelliferone: sources, chemistry and bioactivities review. Bulletin of Faculty of Pharmacy, Cairo University. 2017.

67. Yang X, Kang M-C, Lee K-W, Kang S-M, Lee W-W, Jeon Y-J. Antioxidant activity and cell protective effect of loliolide isolated from Sargassum ringgoldianum subsp. coreanum. Algae. 2011;26(2):201–8.

68. Vasu S, Palaniyappan V, Badami S. A novel microwave-assisted extraction for the isolation of andrographolide from Andrographis paniculata and its in vitro antioxidant activity. Nat Prod Res. 2010;24(16):1560–7.

69. Serrano FG, Tapia-Rojas C, Carvajal FJ, Hancke J, Cerpa W, Inestrosa NC. Andrographolide reduces cognitive impairment in young and mature AbetaPPswe/PS-1 mice. Mol Neurodegener. 2014;9:61.

70. Blondeau N, Lipsky RH, Bourourou M, Duncan MW, Gorelick PB, Marini AM: Alpha-linolenic acid: an omega-3 fatty acid with neuroprotective properties-ready for use in the stroke clinic? Biomed Res Int 2015, 2015:519830.

71. Shashikumar S, Pradeep H, Chinnu S, Rajini PS, Rajanikant GK. Alpha-linolenic acid suppresses dopaminergic neurodegeneration induced by 6-OHDA in C. elegans. Physiol Behav. 2015;151:563–9.

72. Pan H, Piermartiri TC, Chen J, McDonough J, Oppel C, Driwech W, Winter K, McFarland E, Black K, Figueiredo T, et al. Repeated systemic administration of the nutraceutical alpha-linolenic acid exerts neuroprotective efficacy, an antidepressant effect and improves cognitive performance when given after soman exposure. Neurotoxicology. 2015;51:38–50.

18

Meripilus giganteus ethanolic extract exhibits pro-apoptotic and anti-proliferative effects in leukemic cell lines

Monia Lenzi[1†], Veronica Cocchi[1†], Aleksandra Novaković[2], Maja Karaman[3], Marijana Sakač[2], Anamarija Mandić[2], Milica Pojić[2], Maria Cristina Barbalace[4], Cristina Angeloni[5], Patrizia Hrelia[1], Marco Malaguti[4*†] [ID] and Silvana Hrelia[4†]

Abstract

Background: The interest towards botanicals and plant extracts has strongly risen due to their numerous biological effects and ability to counteract chronic diseases development. Among these effects, chemoprevention which represents the possibility to counteract the cancerogenetic process is one of the most studied. The extracts of mushroom *Meripilus giganteus* (MG) (Phylum of Basidiomycota) showed to exert antimicrobic, antioxidant and antiproliferative effects. Therefore, since its effect in leukemic cell lines has not been previously evaluated, we studied its potential chemopreventive effect in Jurkat and HL-60 cell lines.

Methods: MG ethanolic extract was characterized for its antioxidant activity and scavenging effect against different radical species. Moreover, its phenolic profile was evaluated by HPLC-MS-MS analyses. Flow cytometry (FCM) analyses of Jurkat and HL-60 cells treated with MG extract (0–750 μg/mL) for 24–72 h- allowed to evaluate its cytotoxicity, pro-apoptotic and anti-proliferative effect. To better characterize MG pro-apoptotic mechanism ROS intracellular level and the gene expression level of FAS, BAX and BCL2 were also evaluated. Moreover, to assess MG extract selectivity towards cancer cells, its cytotoxicity was also evaluated in human peripheral blood lymphocytes (PBL).

Results: MG extract induced apoptosis in Jurkat and HL-60 cells in a dose- and time- dependent manner by increasing BAX/BCL2 ratio, reducing ROS intracellular level and inducing FAS gene expression level. In fact, reduced ROS level is known to be related to the activation of apoptosis in leukemic cells by the involvement of death receptors. MG extract also induced cell-cycle arrest in HL-60 cells. Moreover, IC_{50} at 24 h treatment resulted 2 times higher in PBL than in leukemic cell lines.

Conclusions: Our data suggest that MG extract might be considered a promising and partially selective chemopreventive agent since it is able to modulate different mechanisms in transformed cells at concentrations lower than in non-transformed ones.

Keywords: Meripilus giganteus, Cytotoxicity, Apoptosis, Chemoprevention, Flow-cytometry, Leukemic cell lines

Background

Mushrooms have been used for centuries as food all over the world, due to their unique taste and flavour [1]. Archaeological knowledge shows that humans have been using mushrooms since the Palaeolithic [2] and traditional uses in the treatment of infectious diseases have been previously described especially in Asian countries [3]. Over the last few years the interest in therapeutic potential of different species of lignicolous mushrooms has increased, justified by the traditional use of these organisms in the folk medicine of many countries [4, 5].

Meripilus giganteus (MG) is a lignicolous saprobiontic or parasite mushroom, which fructifies from summer to autumn at the base of broad-leaved trees, on stumps and roots, especially on beech wood. It derives its name

* Correspondence: marco.malaguti@unibo.it
†Monia Lenzi, Veronica Cocchi, Marco Malaguti and Silvana Hrelia contributed equally to this work.
⁴Department for Life Quality Studies, University of Bologna, Corso d'Augusto 237, 47921 Rimini, Italy
Full list of author information is available at the end of the article

from the remarkable dimensions that it is able to reach: up to a meter in diameter, protruding from the guest trunk for more than 30 cm, with a weight up to 10 kg. The upper portion is zoned, furrowed radially and concentrically by streaks of light brown to dark colour, wrinkled and covered with numerous scales. The tissue is initially soft and tenacious, and then becomes fibrous, leathery and whitish, blackening on contact or rubbing.

Although the young tops are edible after cooking, the completely grown mushroom is considered not edible due to its hard and tough consistency. For these reasons it is considered a species of little value in the culinary field.

Recently MG has drawn the attention of several scientists on its pharmacological properties such as antioxidant, antimicrobial, and anti-proliferative activities.

Karaman et al. [5, 6] investigated the antioxidant and antimicrobial activity of numerous lignicolous mushroom extracts. They demonstrated that MG extract exerts both DPPH radical (DPPH˙) and hydroxyl radical (OH˙) scavenging activity. Moreover, they demonstrated that the antioxidant activity of lignicolous mushroom extracts directly correlate with their phenolic content, that in MG are mainly represented by gallic and protocatechuic acids.

More recently, Maity et al. [7] isolated from the fruiting body of MG a polysaccharide (MGPS), which seems to possess an antioxidant capacity. In detail, it has been shown that increasing concentrations of MGPS are well correlated with the ability to scavenge OH˙ and superoxide anion radical ($O_2^{˙-}$). In order to have a more complete understanding of MGPS antioxidant mechanisms, the researchers also investigated its potential as a chelating agent of ferrous ions (Fe^{2+}). Also in this case the ability of MGPS to chelate Fe^{2+} ions was demonstrated [7].

The results obtained from this study seem to confirm what was previously demonstrated by Rai et al. [8], who investigated the antioxidant properties of different MG extracts, finding a similar antiradical action against OH˙ and $O_2^{˙-}$.

Researchers investigated the antimicrobial potential of several fungal species, including MG, against five species of gram-positive bacteria, and four of gram-negative bacteria. The methanolic extracts of MG were shown to have a narrow spectrum of action against gram-negative bacteria, while strongly inhibit the growth of gram-positive species [6]. These data implement results previously obtained by Rai and co-workers [9], who described a moderate antibacterial action of MG against *E. coli* and *P. aeruginosa*.

Many substances with anti-proliferative effect have been isolated from fungi. Tomasi. et al. [10] analysed the effects of numerous methanolic mushroom extracts and demonstrated that MG exerts antiproliferative activity

on 3LL murine lung cancer cell line. Previously Narbe et al. [11] isolated ergosterol peroxide from MG extract, which is known for its antiproliferative properties on both solid and liquid cancer models [12, 13].

Aim of the study

Considering the numerous biological and pharmacological properties of MG extracts, it is possible to hypothesize its application as a chemopreventive agent in leukaemia. Therefore, the aim of this study was to evaluate the antitumor potential of MG ethanolic extract, fully characterized in its phenolic profile and antioxidant properties, in two different leukaemic cell lines. More specifically, its pro-apoptotic and anti-proliferative effects were analysed in human lymphoblastic leukaemia cells (Jurkat cells) and in human promyelocytic leukaemia cells (HL-60 cells). Moreover, expression level of genes involved in apoptotic pathways was evaluated. In addition to evaluating its selectivity towards cancer cells, its cytotoxic effect on non-transformed human peripheral blood lymphocytes (PBL) was also tested.

Methods
Materials

Sodium carbonate, Aluminium trichloride, Sodium acetate, Quercetin, Formic acid, FRAP reagent, Sodium nitroprusside (SNP), Griess reagent, TBA-reagent, Nitro Blue Tetrazolium (NBT), Ethylenediaminetetraacetic acid (EDTA), Ascorbic acid (AA), Gallic acid (GA), DPPH solution, Thiobarbituric acid (TBA), Trichloroacetic acid (TCA), Dimethyl sulfoxide (DMSO), Fetal Bovine Serum (FBS), Formaldehyde, Hanks' balanced salt solution (HBSS), Histopaque-1077, Hoechst 33342, L-Glutamine (L-GLU), Penicillin-Streptomicin (PS), Phitohemagglutinin (PHA), Phosphate buffered saline (PBS), Primers (BAX, BCL2, FAS, GADPH, 18S rRNA), Roswell Park Memorial Institute (RPMI)1640 medium, Triton X-100, 2'-7'-dichlorodihydrofluorescin diacetate (DCFH-DA) were obtained from Sigma Co. (St. Louis, MO). Folin-Ciocalteu reagent (FC) was obtained from Merck (Darmstadt, Germany). Methanol (MeOH), Ethanol (EtOH) were purchased from Zorka (Šabac, Serbia). Guava Cell Cycle Reagent, Guava Nexin Reagent, Guava ViaCount Reagent (all from Merck, Darmstadt, Germany). RNeasy Mini Kit (from QIAGEN GmbH, Hilden, Germany), SsoAdvanced Universal SYBR Green Supermix, iScript cDNA Synthesis Kit (both from BIO-RAD, Hercules, CA, USA).

Meripilus giganteus extract preparation

The extract was provided by the Institute of Food Technology (FINS) (Novi Sad, Republic of Serbia) as a part of the collaborative activities included in the Horizon 2020 project, FOODSTARS.

Mushrooms were collected in 2012 in the Sikole area (Serbia), fungal material was identified by Professor Maja Karaman (University of Novi Sad), expert in mycology. A voucher specimen of the fungal material has been deposited at "Buns herbarium" (Department of Biology and Ecology, University of Novi Sad, Serbia) with voucher number: 12–00697. After the exact determination of specie, mushrooms were stored at – 20 °C, freeze dried (Martin Christ GmbH, Germany) and ground to a fine powder. The extraction was obtained by macerating the powder (1 g) with 10 mL of 80% ethanol (EtOH) for 24 h in a shaker at room temperature (25 °C). The extract was filtered through Whatman No. 4 filter paper and, subsequently, the solvent was evaporated to dryness in a Rotavapor at 40 °C (Büchi, Switzerland) and stored. For further analysis the dried extract was dissolved in ethanol to obtain 5% (w/w) solution.

Total phenolic content

Total phenolic content (TP) was determined in the ethanolic extract according to the method by Singleton et al. [14] and modified by Novaković et al. [15]. Briefly, 125 µL of Folin–Ciocalteu (0.1 M) reagent were added to 25 µL of the extract. After 10 min incubation, 100 µL of 7.5% sodium carbonate was added and the reaction mixture was incubated for 2 h. Absorbance was read at 690 nm in a plate reader (Multiskan Ascent, Thermo Electron Corporation). A standard curve was constructed using gallic acid in the range of 0 to 1000 µmol/L. Total phenolic content was expressed as mg gallic acid equivalents (GAE)/g of extract on dry weight basis.

Total flavonoid content

The total flavonoid (TF) content of the ethanolic extract was determined by Chang et al. [16] modified for the measurements in a 96-well plate reader [15]. Briefly, 90 µL of methanol, 6 µL of aluminium trichloride (0.75 M), 6 µL of sodium acetate (1 M) and 170 µL of distilled water were added to 30 µL of the extract. After 30 min incubation absorbance was measured at 414 nm. A standard curve was constructed using quercetin in the range of 1.25–100 µg/mL. Results were expressed as mg quercetin equivalents (QE)/g of extract dry weight.

HPLC–MS/MS determination of the phenolic compounds

Phenolic compounds were determined in the ethanolic extract according to the method of Orčić et al. [17], using an Agilent 1200 series liquid chromatograph equipped with a Zorbax Eclipse XDB-C18 RR 4.6 mm × 50 mm × 1.8 mm column (Agilent Technologies) at 40 ° C. The separated compounds were detected by an Agilent series 6410A triple-quadrupole mass spectrometer with electrospray ionization (ESI). MassHunter ver.

B.03.01. Software (Agilent Technologies) was used for instrument control and data analysis. The mobile phase consisted of 0.05% formic acid (A) and methanol (B) with a flow rate of 1 mL/min. The following gradient elution was used: at 0 min, 30% B, at 6.00 min reaching 70% B, then at 9.00 min 100% B, holding until 12.00 min, followed by equilibration time of 3 min to the starting mixture of 30% B. Samples were injected automatically, the injection volume for all samples was 5 µL. ESI parameters were: drying gas (N_2) at 350 °C, flow of 9 L/min, nebulizer gas pressure of 40 psi, capillary voltage of 4 kV with negative polarity. All compounds were quantified in dynamic MRM mode (multiple reaction monitoring mode). The stock solution was prepared by mixing the solutions of 44 individual phenolic acids and flavonoids at concentration of 100 µg/mL each. Working standard solutions were prepared by dilution of stock solution in methanol–water (1:1, v/v) to obtain final concentrations in the range of 0.0015 to 25.0 µg/mL. Concentrations of compounds in the extract were determined from the peak areas using the equation for linear regression obtained from the calibration curves ($r^2 > 0.995$) and expressed as µg/g dry weight.

DPPH radical (DPPH˙) scavenging activity

Free radical scavenging activity based on the monitoring of DPPH˙ radical transformation in the presence of the ethanolic extract was determined as previously described by Espin et al. [18]. Briefly, the reaction mixture in the wells consisted of the extract (10 µL), DPPH solution (60 µL) and methanol (180 µL). The reaction mixture was incubated in the dark for 60 min at 25 °C. The absorbance was measured at 540 nm using a plate reader (Multiskan Ascent, Thermo Electron Corporation). Each sample was tested at five different concentrations in the range of 7.5–200 µg/mL to obtain IC_{50}. The IC_{50} value (µg/mL) was defined as the concentration of an antioxidant extract which was required to quench 50% of the initial amount of DPPH˙ under the experimental conditions given.

Ferric reducing antioxidant power (FRAP)

FRAP assay was performed on the ethanolic extract according to modified procedure of Benzie et al. [19]. The FRAP reagent is a mixture of 300 mM acetate buffer (pH 3.6): 10 mM 2,4,6-tris(2-pyridyl)-s-triazine (TPTZ) in 40 mM HCl: 20 mM $FeCl_3$ (10:1:1, v/v/v). The reaction mixture in the wells consisted of the extract (10 µL), FRAP reagent (225 µL) and distilled water (22.5 µL). Absorbance was measured at 620 nm, after 6 min of incubation. Ascorbic acid was used to construct the standard curve and results were expressed as mg ascorbic acid equivalents (AAE)/g of extract on dry weight basis.

Nitric oxide radical (NO⋅) scavenging capacity

NO scavenging capacity was determined according to the procedure of Green et al. [20]. Briefly, the reaction mixture in the test tubes consisted of the extract (30 μL), sodium nitroprusside (SNP) (500 μL) and 0.067 mol/L phosphate buffer at pH 7.4 (500 μL). Test tubes were incubated under light exposure at 25 °C for 90 min. After incubation, Griess reagent consisting of 0.2% solution of N-(1-naphthyl) ethylenediamine dihydrochloride (NEDA): 2% solution of sulphanilamide in 4% of phosphoric acid (1:1, v/v) was added (1 mL). Aliquots of the reaction mixture (250 μL) were transferred to the plate, and their absorbances were measured using a plate reader at 540 nm (Multiskan Ascent, Thermo Electron Corporation). Samples were tested at five different concentrations in the range of 74–591 μg/mL to obtain IC_{25}, defined as the concentration of the extract which scavenges 25% of the initial amounts of NO⋅.

Hydroxyl radical (OH⋅) scavenging capacity

Determination of scavenging activity on OH⋅, generated in Fenton reaction, was performed from the reaction of 2-deoxyribose degradation [21]. The reaction mixture contained 100 μL of 2-deoxyribose, 100 μL of $FeSO_4$ (127 mg $FeSO_4 \cdot 7 \, H_2O$ in 50 mL of phosphate buffer, pH 7.4) and 10 μL of the tested extract. Phosphate buffer was added to the mixture to the final volume of 3 mL and incubated at 37 °C for 1 h. Two millilitres of TBA-reagent (10.4 mL of 10% $HClO_4$, 3 g of thiobarbituric acid (TBA) and 120 g of 20% trichloroacetic acid (TCA) dissolved in 800 mL of distilled H_2O) and 0.2 mL of 0.1 M EDTA were added to terminate the reaction. The absorbance was measured at 532 nm using a UV-Vis spectrophotometer (Agilent Technologies, Santa Clara, CA). To obtain IC_{50} value, the range of concentrations of 0.7–4.7 μg/mL MG extract was tested.

Superoxide anion radical (O₂⋅⁻) scavenging activity

Superoxide anion radical scavenging activity of the ethanolic extract was determined by measuring its ability to neutralize superoxide anion radicals generated during aerobic reduction of nitro blue tetrazolium (NBT) by NADH, mediated by 5-methylphenazin-5-ium methyl sulphate (PMS) [22]. The reaction mixture in a test tube was composed by 677 μM NADH (100 μL), 60 μM PMS (100 μL), 144 μM NBT (200 μL), 0.017 mol/L phosphate buffer at pH 8.3 (1,1 mL) and the extract (10 μL). After 5 min of incubation, aliquots (250 μL) were transferred to the plate wells (Multiskan Ascent, Thermo Electron Corporation), and their absorbances were measured at 540 nm. Five different concentrations of each sample in the range of 2.4–33.1 μg/mL were tested to obtain IC_{50}, defined as the concentration of the extract able to scavenge 50% of $O_2 \cdot^-$.

Jurkat and HL-60 cell culture and treatments

Jurkat cells (acute T-cell lymphoblastic leukaemia) and HL-60 cells (acute promyelocytic leukaemia) were purchased at the "Istituto Zooprofilattico" of Lombardia and Emilia-Romagna (Brescia, Italy). Both cell lines were cultured at 37 °C and 5% CO_2 in Roswell Park Memorial Institute (RPMI)1640 medium supplemented with 1% Penicillin-Streptomicin (PS), 1% L-Glutamine (L-GLU) and 10% of Fetal Bovine Serum (FBS) for Jurkat cells and 20% of FBS for HL-60 cells (all from Sigma Aldrich, Saint Luis, MO, USA).

The MG extract was dissolved in RPMI at 20% of DMSO (v/v), in order to obtain a Working Solution 50 mg/mL. The solution thus prepared has been stored for a maximum of 72 h at − 20 °C and protected from light. The concentrations of the different extracts tested ranged from 0 to 750 μg/mL and the concentration of DMSO was always within the 0.05–1% range in all experimental conditions.

In particular, 3.75×10^5 of Jurkat cells were treated with increasing concentrations of extract from 0 to 500 μg/mL and incubated for 24, 48 and 72 h. The cell density never exceeded the critical value of 3.00×10^6 cells/mL of medium. One hundred twenty-five thousand of HL-60 cells were treated with increasing concentrations of extracts from 0 to 750 μg/mL and incubated for 24, 48 and 72 h. The cell density never exceeded the critical value of 1.00×10^6 cells/mL of medium.

PBL culture and treatments

Authorization to the use of human blood samples (Buffy coat), for research purposes, was obtained from AUSL of Bologna, Italy, S. Orsola-Malpighi Hospital -PROT GEN No. 0051937, and written informed consent was obtained by AUSL of Bologna, Italy, S. Orsola-Malpighi Hospital from donors for the use of their blood for scientific research purposes. PBL were isolated from the whole peripheral blood of 5 AVIS healthy donors (Association of Italian Blood Volunteers), by density gradient centrifugation with Histopaque-1077 (Sigma Aldrich, Saint Luis, MO, USA) [23].

PBL were cultured at 37 °C and 5% CO_2 in RPMI-1640 supplemented with 1% PS, 1% L-GLU, 15% FBS and in the presence of 0.5% Phitohemagglutinin (PHA) (Sigma Aldrich, Saint Louis, MO, USA) for 48 h to stimulate cell proliferation. Two hundred thousand PBL were than treated with increasing concentrations of extract from 0 to 1000 μg/mL and incubated for 24 h.

Flow cytometry (FCM)

All FCM analyzes reported below were performed using a Guava easyCyte 5HT flow cytometer equipped with a class IIIb laser operating at 488 nm (Merck, Darmstadt, Germany).

Cytotoxicity analysis by FCM

The cytotoxicity induced by MG was evaluated by the *Guava ViaCount Assay protocol*. In particular, the percentage of viable cells was assessed by FMC using the Guava ViaCount Reagent (Merck, Darmstadt, Germany) that contains the dye Propidium Iodide (PI) and analyzed by Guava ViaCount software [24].

The results obtained in the samples treated with different concentrations of extracts were normalized on those obtained in control cultures and used to calculate the IC_{50} by interpolation from the dose-response curve. In the subsequent experiments concentrations $\leq IC_{50}$ were used.

Analysis of apoptosis by FCM and optical microscopy

The discrimination of the death mechanism was assessed by the *Guava Nexin Assay Protocol*. In particular, the percentage of live, apoptotic and necrotic cells was assessed by FCM using the Guava Nexin Reagent (Merck, Darmstadt, Germany) that containing 7-aminoactinomycin D (7-AAD) and Annexin-V-PE and analyzed by Guava Nexin software as previously reported [24, 25].

Moreover, the nuclear condensation and fragmentation associated with the apoptotic process was evaluated by fluorescence microscopy with 100X magnification. After treatment, 1.00×10^6 cells were loaded into cytospin chamber and centrifuged ad 450 rpm for 10 min. Cells were than fixed in formaldehyde 3.7%, washed in PBS pH 7.2, permeabilized in 0.15% triton X-100 (all Sigma-Aldrich, Saint Louis, MO, USA) and nuclei were stained using Hoechst 33342 500 nM as previously reported [26].

Cell-cycle analysis by FCM

The effect of MG on the cancer cells replication was evaluated by *GUAVA Cell-Cycle Assay protocol*. In particular, the percentage of cells in the different phases of the cell-cycle (G_0/G_1, S, G_2/M) was assessed by FCM using the Cell-Cycle Reagent (Merck, Darmstadt, Germany) that containing PI and analysed by Guava Cell-Cycle software [24].

RNA extraction

After 16 h treatments, total RNA was extracted from Jurkat and HL-60 cells by using RNeasy Mini Kit (QIAGEN GmbH, Hilden, Germany), following the manufacturer's protocol. The yield and purity of the RNA were measured using NanoVue Spectrophotometer (GE Healthcare, Milan, Italy).

Analysis of FAS, BAX and BCL2 mRNA expression levels by reverse transcriptase polymerase chain reaction

cDNA was obtained by reverse transcribing mRNA starting from 1 µg of total RNA using iScript cDNA Synthesis Kit (BIO-RAD, Hercules, CA, USA), following the manufacturer's protocol. The subsequent polymerase chain reaction (PCR) was performed in a total volume of 10 µl containing 2.5 µl (12.5 ng) of cDNA, 5 µl SsoAdvanced Universal SYBR Green Supermix (BIO-RAD, Hercules, CA, USA) and 0.5 µl (500 nM) of each primer. The primers used are reported in Table 1 18S rRNA and GAPDH were used as reference genes.

Intracellular ROS level

After 24 h treatment Jurkat and HL-60 cells (1.00×10^6 cells/mL), were washed twice in HBSS, and incubated with 5 µM 2'-7'-dichlorodihydrofluorescin diacetate (DCFH-DA) (Sigma-Aldrich, Saint Louis, MO, USA), for 20 min at 37 °C. When inside the cell, DCFH-DA is deacetylated and can be oxidized by ROS to the highly fluorescent 2',7'-dichlorofluorescein (DCF). DCF fluorescence was measured using a multi-well plate reader (Wallac Victor2, PerkinElmer) at excitation and emission wavelengths of 485 and 535 nm, respectively [27]. Fluorescence values were reported as percentage of intracellular ROS with respect to control.

Statistical analysis

Results on TP and TF content, on DPPH·, OH·, $O_2^{·-}$, NO· scavenging activity and FRAP are expressed as mean ± standard deviation (SD). All results on cell viability, analysis of apoptosis, cell-cycle, gene expression and intracellular ROS are expressed as mean ± standard error mean (SEM) of at least five independent experiments. For the statistical analysis of apoptosis, cell-cycle and gene expression level we used the Analysis of Variance for paired data (repeated ANOVA), followed by Bonferroni as the post-test. For statistical analyses of ROS intracellular level we used the t-test for paired data. All the statistical analyses

Table 1 Both forward and reverse primer sequences for BAX, BCL2, FAS, GAPDH and 18S rRNA genes are reported

Gene	5'-Forward-3'	5'-Reverse-3'
BAX	AACTGGACAGTAACATGGAG	TTGCTGGCAAAGTAGAAAAG
BCL2	GATTGTGGCCTTCTTTGAG	GTTCCACAAAGGCATCC
FAS	CTGTCCTCCAGGTGAAAG	TGTACTCCTTCCCTTCTTG
GAPDH	ACAGTTGCCATGTAGACC	TTGAGCACAGGGTACTTTA
18S rRNA	CAGAAGGATGTAAAGGATGG	TATTTCTTCTTGGACACACC

were performed using GraphPad Software Prism 6 (GraphPad Software LLC, La Jolla, CA, USA).

Results

MG phenolic composition
TP content of MG ethanolic extract resulted in 106.33 ± 11.27 mg GAE/g extract, while TF content resulted in 13.84 ± 1.11 mg QE/g extract. HPLC-MS/MS analyses revealed the presence of *p*-OH-benzoic acid, protocatechuic acid, *p*-coumaric acid and caffeic acid. Quantitative determination is reported in Table 2.

Antioxidant activity of MG extract
Since different mechanisms are involved in the neutralization of different radical species Table 3 reports the antioxidant activity of MG extract measured according to five methods, DPPH·, NO·, OH· and O_2^{-} scavenging capacity and FRAP.

Cytotoxicity analysis on Jurkat and HL-60 cells
After 24 h treatment the IC_{50} for MG was found to be 385 μg/mL in Jurkat cells and equal to 461 μg/mL in HL-60 (Fig. 1).

Apoptosis analysis on Jurkat and HL-60 cells
In order to evaluate the involvement of a specific cell death mechanism in the demonstrated cytotoxic action, the analysis of apoptosis possibly induced at different concentrations on Jurkat and HL-60 cells was performed, after 24, 48 and 72 h, in order to determine if the event was dose and/or time-dependent.

Specifically, the cells were treated with concentrations ≤ IC_{50} and the double staining Annexin V-PE / 7-AAD allowed to measure the percentage of live, apoptotic and necrotic cells.

In Jurkat cells, MG showed a dose- and time-dependent induction of apoptosis. In fact after 24 h there was a statistically significant increase of apoptotic cells percentage at the concentration 125 μg/mL equal to 2 times compared to the control (7.3% vs 3.1%) and an increase equal to 3 times at 250 μg/mL (8.4% vs 3.1%). After 48 h, on the other hand, a doubling of the fraction of apoptotic cells compared to 24 h was

Table 2 Content of phenolic compounds in MG extract

Phenolic compounds	μg/g dry weight
p-OH-benzoic acid	23.9 ± 3.66
Protocatechuic acid	1.26 ± 0.13
p-coumaric acid	0.2 ± 0.05
Caffeic acid	1.3 ± 0.11

Values are expressed as means ± SD of triplicate measurements. Phenolic acid contents were determined by HPLC-MS/MS as described in the Methods section

Table 3 Antioxidant activity of MG extract

DPPH· $(IC_{50})^a$ μg/mL	57.77 ± 2.48
NO· $(IC_{25})^b$ μg/mL	148.04 ± 4.98
OH· $(IC_{50})^a$ μg/mL	1.74 ± 0.2
O_2^{-} $(IC_{50})^a$ μg/mL	24.28 ± 2.06
$FRAP^c$ mg (AAE)/g	22.54 ± 3.51

Values are expressed as means ± SD of triplicate measurements. Antioxidant activity was determined as described in the Methods section
[a]IC_{50} (μg/mL), concentration of extract that neutralized 50% of DPPH·, OH· and O_2^{-}
[b]IC_{25} (μg/mL), concentration of extracts that neutralized 25% of NO·
[c]Ferric reducing antioxidant power (FRAP) is expressed as mg ascorbic acid equivalents/g extract dry weight (mg AAE/g d.w)

observed at both concentrations tested. Specifically there was a 4 times increase at 125 μg/mL (13.3% vs 3.5%) and a 6 times increase at 250 μg/mL (21.2% vs 3.5%). At 72 h the trend is comparable (Fig. 2a, b, c).

In HL-60 (Fig. 3) after 24 h there was evidence at the concentration of 125 μg/mL, a statistically significant increase in the fraction of apoptotic cells, equal to 3 times compared to control (11.3% vs. 3.8%), parallel to an

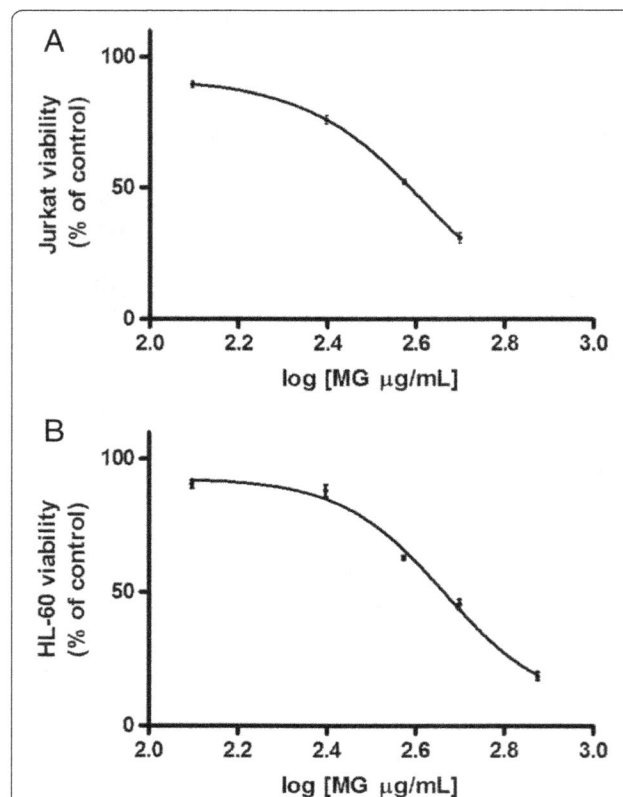

Fig. 1 Effect of MG on viability of Jurkat and HL-60 cells. Cell viability was determined as described in Methods section. IC_{50} obtained by curve fitting of viable cells after 24 h treatment with MG for Jurkat cells (**a**) and HL-60 cells (**b**). Data are presented as means ± SEM of five independent experiments

increase of 3 and 4 times, for 250 μg/mL and 375 μg/mL, respectively (11.1% vs. 3.8, 16.2% vs 3.8%). After 48 h, the trend remained comparable to 24 h for the 125 μg/mL concentration (11.6% vs 3.7%), while for 250 μg/mL a further increase in the number of apoptotic cells was observed, equal to at 4 times the control (15.2% vs. 3.7%); the same concentration, at the longest treatment time (72 h), was instead associated with an increase equal to 6 times (8.6% vs 1.4%). Therefore, these data demonstrate a dose- and time-correlated trend at all times analysed, particularly evident for the concentration of 250 μg/mL.

Considering the demonstrated pro-apoptotic effect, we wanted to confirm the results obtained by FCM, also by fluorescence microscopy analysis, visualizing the morphological changes characteristic of apoptosis, such as nuclear condensation and fragmentation (Fig. 4).

Cell-cycle analysis on Jurkat and HL-60 cells

In order to evaluate whether the induction of apoptosis caused by MG was an independent event or subsequent a slowing/blocking of the cell-cycle, the Jurkat and HL-60 cells were treated with the concentration selected on the basis of the results obtained from the apoptosis analysis and incubated at the same treatment times. The PI staining allowed to highlight that MG does not show any activity on the cell-cycle of Jurkat cells, at the tested concentration (250 μg/mL), at any treatment time (Fig. 5a, b, c).

Conversely, on HL-60 cells, after 24 h a slowing of the cell-cycle is observed in the G_2/M phase, underlined by an increase in the cell fraction equal to a 33.1% vs 25.2% in the control cultures. At 48 h instead, there was an increase in the number of cells in the G_0/G_1 phase (47.7% vs 35.1%), with a consequent reduction in S phases (30.0% vs 40.4%) and G_2/M (21.8% vs 24.5%); the same behaviour is observed at 72 h (Fig. 6a, b, c).

FAS, BAX and BCL2 expression analysis on Jurkat and HL-60 cells

mRNA expression analysis of three genes involved in apoptotic pathways regulation such as FAS, BAX, BCL2 were performed.

Figure 7 shows that MG extract after 16 h treatment significantly induced, in both Jurkat and HL-60, FAS mRNA expression level (Fig. 7a, c) and increases the ratio between BAX and BCL2 mRNA expression (Fig. 7b, d).

Intracellular ROS level

To characterize the mechanism behind MG capability to induce apoptosis in leukaemia cells its potential modulatory effect on intracellular ROS level was investigated in both Jurkat and HL-60 cells by the DCFH-DA assay. As

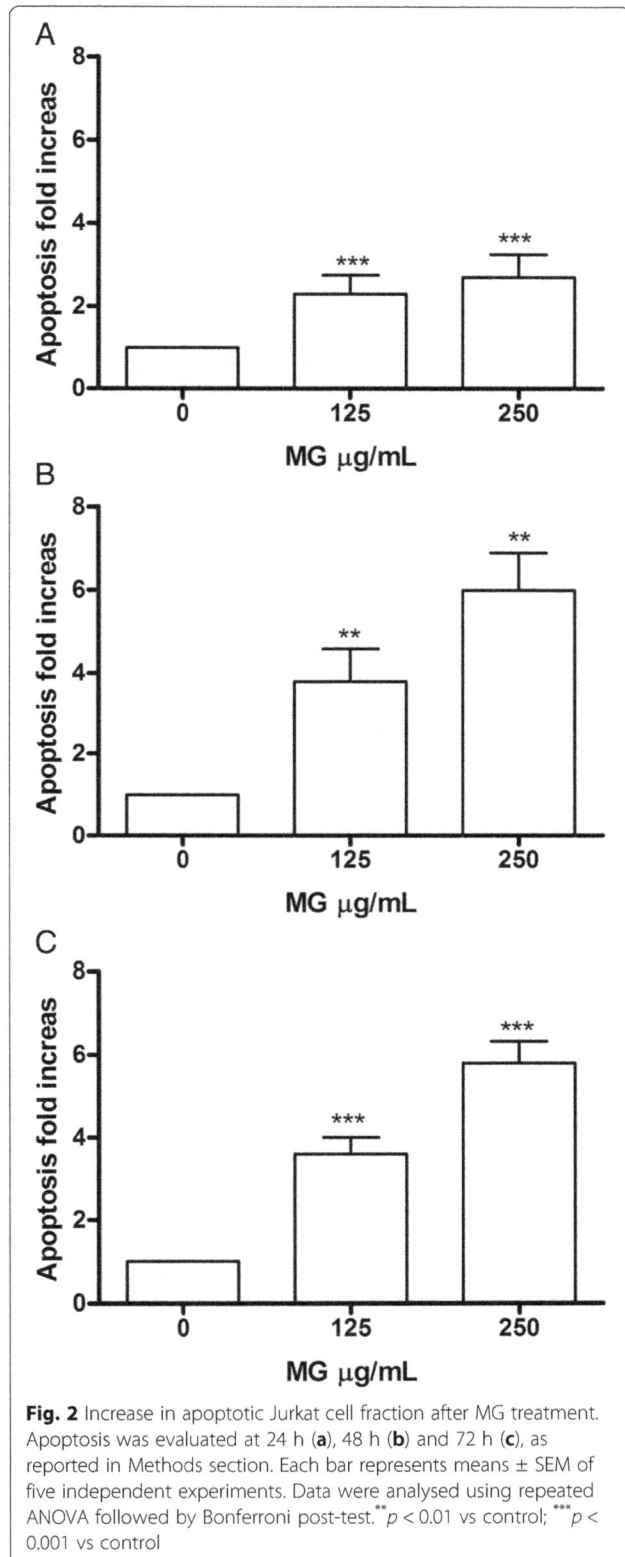

Fig. 2 Increase in apoptotic Jurkat cell fraction after MG treatment. Apoptosis was evaluated at 24 h (a), 48 h (b) and 72 h (c), as reported in Methods section. Each bar represents means ± SEM of five independent experiments. Data were analysed using repeated ANOVA followed by Bonferroni post-test. [**] $p < 0.01$ vs control; [***] $p < 0.001$ vs control

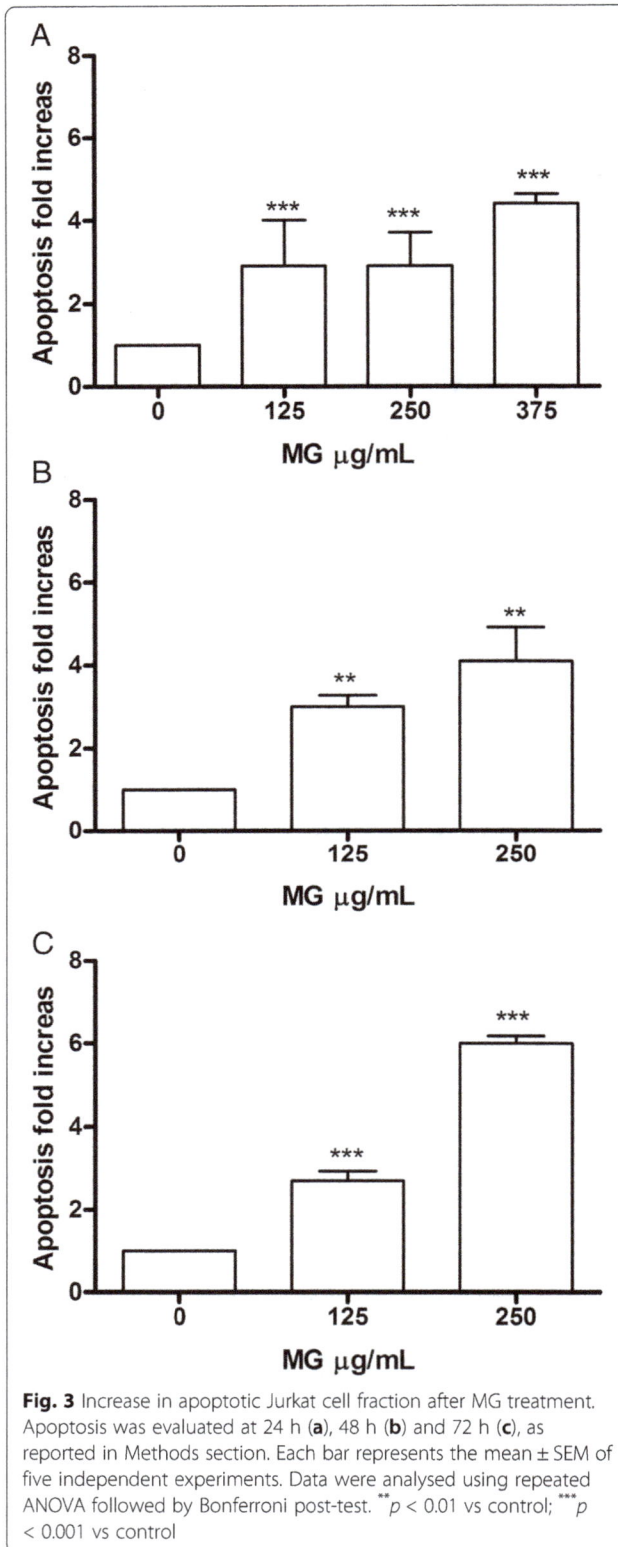

Fig. 3 Increase in apoptotic Jurkat cell fraction after MG treatment. Apoptosis was evaluated at 24 h (**a**), 48 h (**b**) and 72 h (**c**), as reported in Methods section. Each bar represents the mean ± SEM of five independent experiments. Data were analysed using repeated ANOVA followed by Bonferroni post-test. $^{**}p < 0.01$ vs control; $^{***}p < 0.001$ vs control

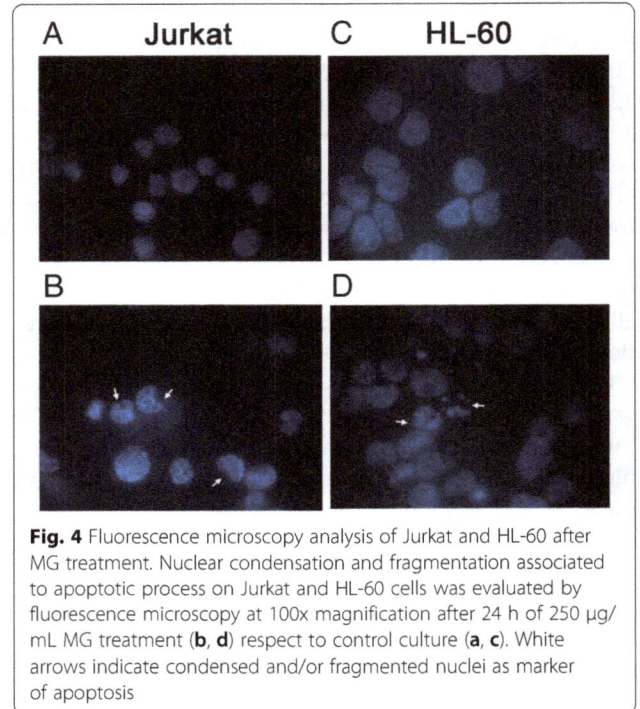

Fig. 4 Fluorescence microscopy analysis of Jurkat and HL-60 after MG treatment. Nuclear condensation and fragmentation associated to apoptotic process on Jurkat and HL-60 cells was evaluated by fluorescence microscopy at 100x magnification after 24 h of 250 µg/mL MG treatment (**b**, **d**) respect to control culture (**a**, **c**). White arrows indicate condensed and/or fragmented nuclei as marker of apoptosis

shown in Fig. 8, ROS intracellular level was significantly decreased respect to control by MG 250 µg/mL after 24 h treatment in both cell-lines.

Cytotoxicity analysis on PBL
The analysis of the viability of PBL following MG treatment for 24 h allowed to obtain an IC_{50} value of 761 µg/mL, which demonstrated a cytotoxicity lower than that manifested on the two leukaemia cell lines (Fig. 9).

Discussion
Great attention has been dedicated to the potential of many extracts and naturally occurring compounds in the prevention/counteraction of chronic diseases [28–30]. Numerous studies have demonstrated that molecules that exhibit antioxidant properties such as polyphenols, isothiocyanates and other compounds counteract cardio-vascular, neurodegenerative diseases and the carcino-genic process at various levels by acting through multiple mechanisms [31–34]. Extracts from plant origin may contain various compounds with useful biological properties, thus configuring themselves as complex mixtures with multi-target activities, capable of inhibiting or modulating simultaneously numerous critical targets [25, 35, 36].

Edible mushrooms, including MG, possess antioxidant, antimicrobial and anti-inflammatory properties [7, 37–39], suggesting their potential application as chemopreventive agents. The purpose of this work was, therefore,

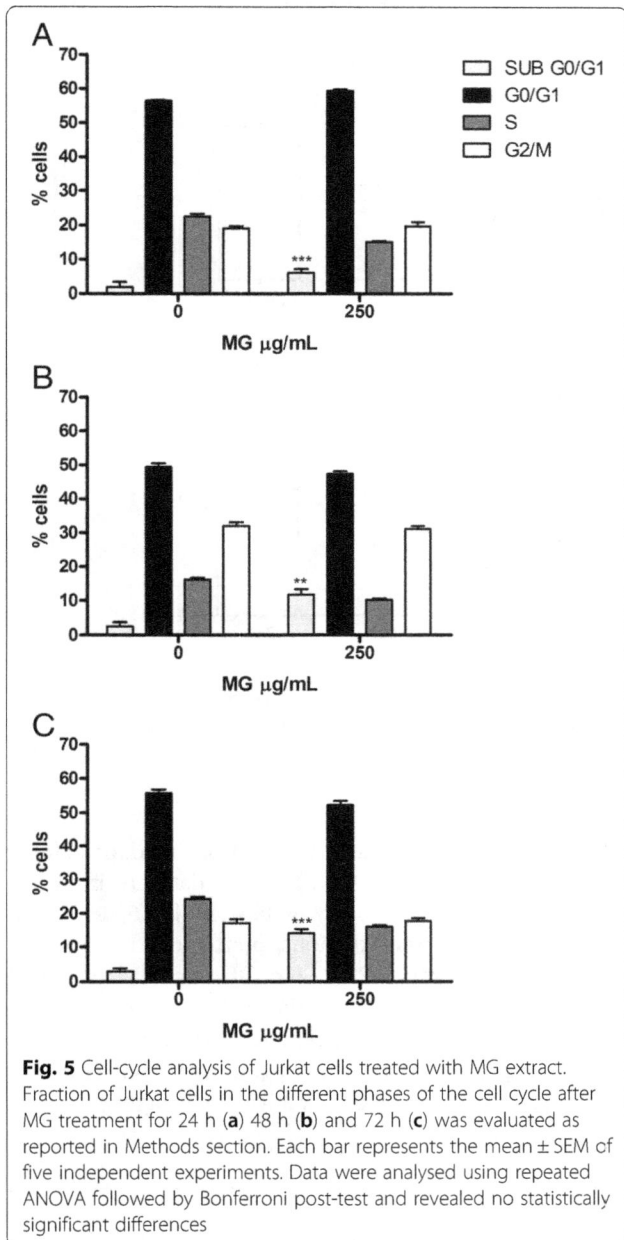

Fig. 5 Cell-cycle analysis of Jurkat cells treated with MG extract. Fraction of Jurkat cells in the different phases of the cell cycle after MG treatment for 24 h (**a**) 48 h (**b**) and 72 h (**c**) was evaluated as reported in Methods section. Each bar represents the mean ± SEM cf five independent experiments. Data were analysed using repeated ANOVA followed by Bonferroni post-test and revealed no statistically significant differences

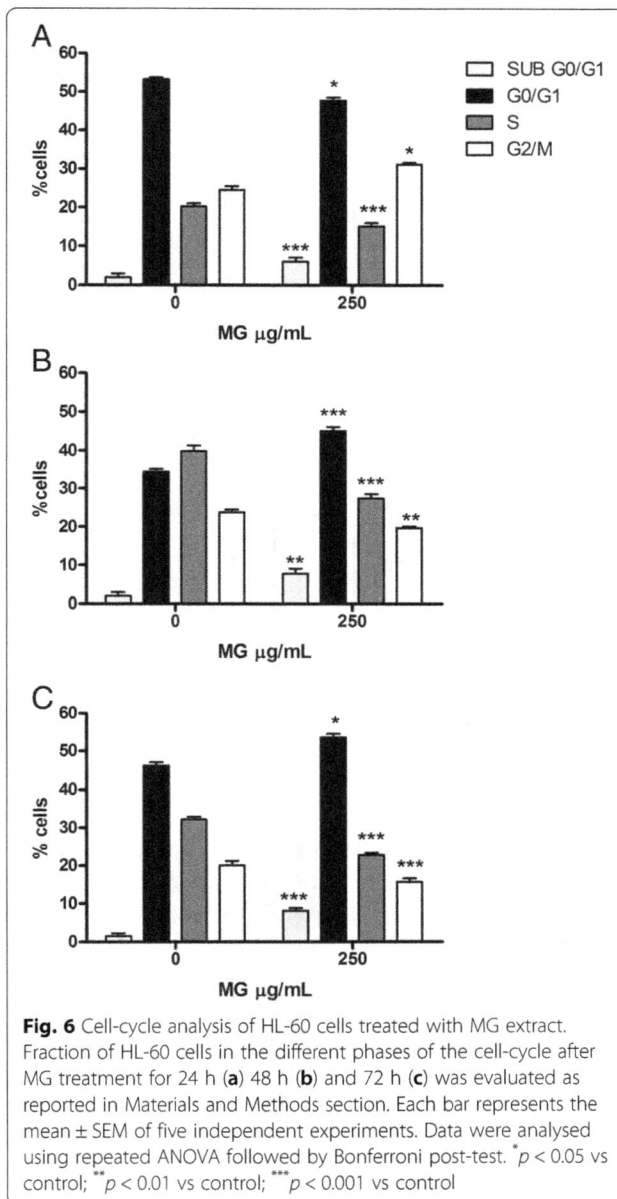

Fig. 6 Cell-cycle analysis of HL-60 cells treated with MG extract. Fraction of HL-60 cells in the different phases of the cell-cycle after MG treatment for 24 h (**a**) 48 h (**b**) and 72 h (**c**) was evaluated as reported in Materials and Methods section. Each bar represents the mean ± SEM of five independent experiments. Data were analysed using repeated ANOVA followed by Bonferroni post-test. $^{*}p < 0.05$ vs control; $^{**}p < 0.01$ vs control; $^{***}p < 0.001$ vs control

to evaluate whether MG extract is able, thanks to its antioxidant activity to exhibit chemopreventive activities. The research focused on the evaluation of numerous in vitro end-points in two leukemic cell lines (Jurkat and HL-60 cells) and subsequently in healthy lymphocytes (PBL).

Among scientific literature, strong discrepancies can be observed when comparing TP and TF content of MG extracts., These differences are probably due to extraction methods, mushroom provenance and the fact that TP and TF might be expressed in different ways. Papers reporting the TP of wild edible mushrooms other than MG differ in a very wide range in the order of mg/mL [6, 40–42].

HPLC-MS/MS analysis of MG ethanolic extract resulted in quantification of four phenolic acids, giving the total sum of 26.66 µg/g. Dominant phenolic acid was p-hydroxybenzoic acid, in accordance with previously published data on MG [6]. All the differences that can be observed when comparing the previously published data for MG and other wild mushrooms should be attributed to the changes that occur during the mushrooms harvest and postharvest period of time, due to the enzymatic and oxidative processes [43, 44].

It has been shown that the strong antiradical activity of mushroom extracts on different radical species is due to the presence of different phenolic compounds and flavonoids [45, 46].

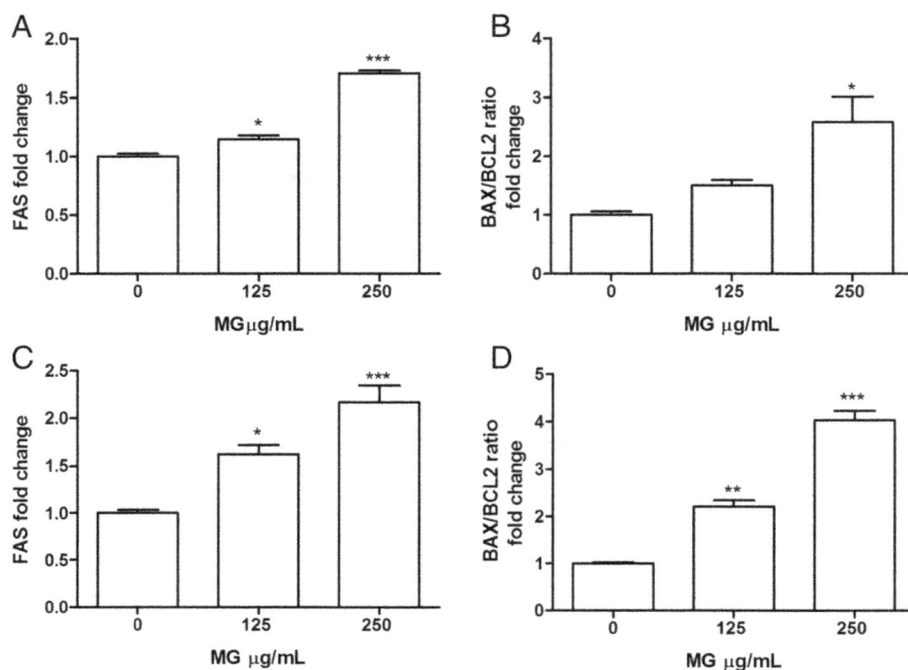

Fig. 7 Effect of MG extract treatment on FAS, BAX and BCL2 expression level in Jurkat (**a, b**) and HL-60 (**c, d**) cells. Total RNA was isolated, and the mRNA level of target genes was quantified using RT-PCR normalized to 18S rRNA and GAPDH as reference genes. Triplicate reactions were performed for each experiment. Each bar represents the mean ± SEM of three independent experiments. Data were analysed by one-way ANOVA followed by Bonferroni's test. $^*p < 0.05$ vs control; $^{**}p < 0.01$ vs control; $^{***}p < 0.001$ vs control

Determination of DPPH˙ scavenging capacity is a commonly employed assay in antioxidant studies, Ferreira et al. [47] analysed DPPH˙ scavenging capacity of different mushroom methanolic extracts finding that DPPH EC_{50} was in the range of 8–50 mg/mL. Similarly, Puttaraju et al. [48] analysed methanolic and water extracts of 23 different edible mushrooms and found that DPPH EC_{50} values were in the same order of magnitude.

Only few studies have previously evaluated MG extracts antioxidant activity. Our data show MG ethanolic extract ability to scavenge different radicals such as DPPH˙, $O_2^{˙-}$, OH˙, NO and to exert antioxidant activity by reducing Fe^{3+} ions (FRAP). These data are in agreement with those previously published [5, 6, 8] which found that MG water, ethanolic, methanolic and chloroformic extracts exert DPPH˙ and OH˙ radical scavenging activity with EC_{50} values in the order of μg/mL. Similarly, FRAP result is in agreement with previous report [6]. All together, these data suggest that MG extract is characterized by a strong radical scavenging activity

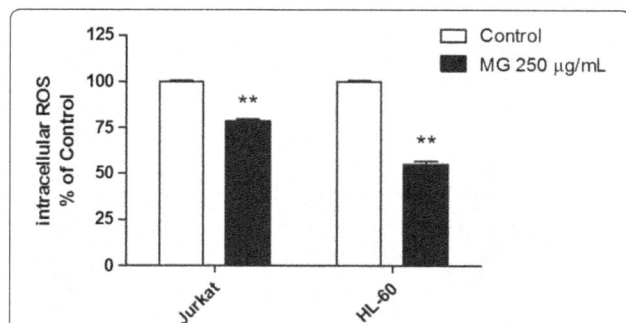

Fig. 8 Intracellular ROS level in Jurkat and HL-60 cells treated with MG at 250 μg/mL for 24 h. Each bar represents the mean ± SEM of three independent experiments. Data were analysed by t-test, $^{**}p < 0.01$ vs control

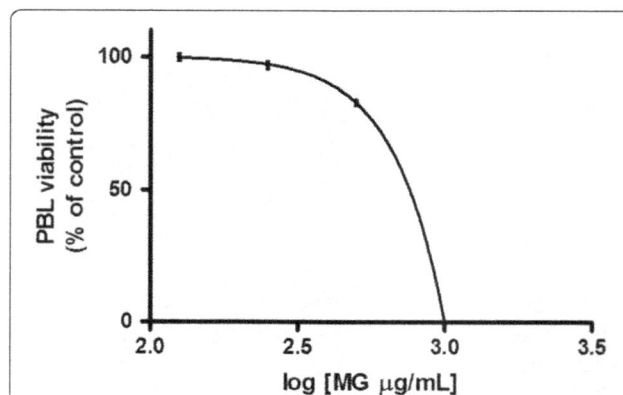

Fig. 9 Effect of MG on viability of PBL. IC_{50} was obtained by curve fitting of viable cells after 24 h treatment. Data are presented as mean ± SEM of five independent experiments

mainly related to its phenols content as previously reported by Karaman et al. [6].

Due to the strong antioxidant activity, it was possible to hypothesize a chemopreventive role for MG ethanolic extract.

A chemopreventive agent can act in different ways: by modulating the biotransformation enzymes involved in the activation/detoxification processes of carcinogens or by stimulating apoptosis and inhibiting the proliferation of transformed cells [49].

Even though some studies reporting pro-apoptotic and anti-proliferative effects of mushroom extract have already been published [50, 51], to our knowledge no data on MG effects in leukemic cell lines are available. Therefore, specific mechanisms of cell death, apoptosis and/or necrosis and MG ability to modulate cell-cycle were investigated.

Results show that MG is able to significantly induce apoptosis in a dose- and time- related manner in both leukemic cell lines. Moreover, it does not modulate, in any way, Jurkat cell-cycle while it inhibits HL-60 proliferation by causing a slowdown in G_2/M phase after 24 h treatment, which results in a real block after 48 h in G_0/G_1 phase with a corresponding decrease in the percentage of cells in phase S and G_2/M. This effect is confirmed after 72 h of treatment. These data are in agreement with previous reports showing that different flavonoids and polyphenols exert cell-cycle arrest in HL-60 [52]. A possible hypothesis to explain the differences between MG treatment effect on Jurkat and HL-60 cell cycle resides in the substantial differences that exist between these two cell lines. Jurkat cells are a lymphocyte cell line in an advanced state of maturation and differentiation, while HL-60 are a highly undifferentiated immature promyelocytic cell line. Future studies are needed to clarify whether these differences are responsible for the different effect of MG on the cell cycle [53].

In order to elucidate which mechanism is responsible for the pro-apoptotic effect we evaluated the expression level of genes such as FAS, BAX and BCL2.

FAS receptor belongs the family of death receptors, it is located on the cell membrane and the binding to its ligand leads to apoptosis through caspase-8 activation which directly activates caspase 3 and simultaneously promote Bid cleavage leading to mitochondrial membrane potential loss [54]. Moreover, it has been demonstrated that FAS over-expression induces apoptosis in Jurkat cell and other malignant T-cell lines [55]. In our study, 16 h treatment with MG induced FAS mRNA expression in both Jurkat and HL-60 cells. Bax and Bcl-2 are mitochondrial proteins, while Bax exhibits pro-apoptotic activity, Bcl-2 is considered an anti-apoptotic and is often overexpressed in different cancers [56, 57]. In order to induce apoptosis in

cancer cells, most therapies are based on stimulating the expression of Bax and/or suppressing Bcl-2 protein. In this study we contemporaneously observed, in Jurkat cells, an increase of BAX and a decrease of BCL2 gene expression level after 250 μg/mL MG treatment. Otherwise, in HL-60 cells a reduction of BCL2 level was found, while BAX was not affected. Our data demonstrate that BAX/BCL2 mRNA expression ratio significantly increased in both cell lines suggesting the involvement of these two proteins in the progression of the apoptotic cascade induced by MG.

It is known, that high ROS intracellular level is a common characteristic of leukaemic and other cancer cells [58]. This feature has been observed in numerous

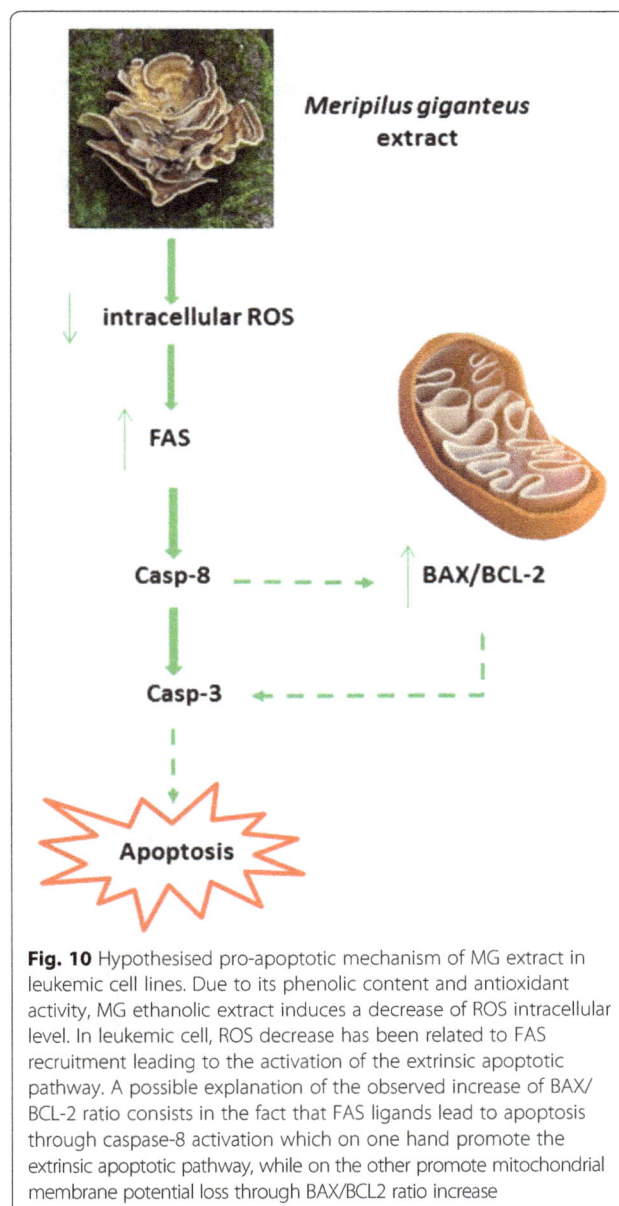

Fig. 10 Hypothesised pro-apoptotic mechanism of MG extract in leukemic cell lines. Due to its phenolic content and antioxidant activity, MG ethanolic extract induces a decrease of ROS intracellular level. In leukemic cell, ROS decrease has been related to FAS recruitment leading to the activation of the extrinsic apoptotic pathway. A possible explanation of the observed increase of BAX/BCL-2 ratio consists in the fact that FAS ligands lead to apoptosis through caspase-8 activation which on one hand promote the extrinsic apoptotic pathway, while on the other promote mitochondrial membrane potential loss through BAX/BCL2 ratio increase

leukaemic cell lines and also in cells from patients with different types of leukaemia [59]. Therefore, it is generally accepted that increased ROS production is important for the proliferation of hematological malignancies [60, 61]. Due to ROS importance in sustaining leukemic cell proliferation and survival, the reduction of their levels could represent an effective strategy to reduce leukemic cells proliferation [59]. Moreover, Aronis et al. [62] demonstrated that a reduced ROS level could induce apoptosis by the involvement of death receptor in Jurkat cells.

In this context, our data show MG ability to exert scavenging and antioxidant activity leading to a significant reduction of ROS intracellular level which contributes to explain the pro-apoptotic effect induced by the activation of the extrinsic apoptotic pathway as indicated by FAS increased expression level.

The hypothesised pro-apoptotic mechanism of MG extract is summarized in the scheme shown in Fig. 10.

A fundamental feature of a good chemopreventive agent is the low toxicity towards healthy cells and the relative selectivity of action against tumor cells [63]. Therefore, the study was completed by evaluating MG cytotoxicity on PBL after 24 h of treatment.

MG demonstrated good selectivity as shown by the IC_{50}, calculated for PBL by interpolation of the dose response curve, that resulted 2 and 1.7 times higher than those obtained on Jurkat and HL-60 cells respectively.

Conclusions

MG demonstrated good pro-apoptotic capacity in both Jurkat and HL-60 cell lines, with a predominant antiproliferative effect in HL-60 and to be partially selective towards leukemic cells. These findings allow to propose MG extracts as possible candidate as chemopreventive agents.

Abbreviations

7-AAD: 7-aminoactinomycin D; AAE/g: mg ascorbic acid equivalents; DCF: 2′,7′-dichlorofluorescein; DCFH-DA: 2′-7′-dichlorodihydrofluorescin diacetate; DMSO: Dimethyl sulfoxide; DPPH: DPPH radical; EtOH: Ethanol; FBS: Fetal bovine serum; FCM: Flow cytometry; Fe^{2+}: Ferrous ions; FRAP: Ferric reducing antioxidant power; GAE/g: mg gallic acid equivalents; HL-60 cells: Acute promyelocytic leukemia; Jurkat cells: Acute T-cell lymphoblastic leukemia; L-GLU: L-Glutamine; MG: *Meripilus giganteus*; MGPS: MG a polysaccharide; MRM mode: Multiple reaction monitoring mode; NBT: Nitro blue tetrazolium; NEDA: N-(1-naphthyl) ethylenediamine dihydrochloride; NO˙: Nitric oxide; O_2^-: Superoxide anion radical; OH˙: Hydroxyl radical; PBL: Human peripheral blood lymphocytes; PHA: Phitohemagglutinin; PI: Propidium iodide; PMS: 5-methylphenazin-5-ium methyl sulfate; PS: Penicillin-strptomicin; QE/g: mg quercetin equivalents; RPMI 1640 medium: roswell park memorial institute; SNP: Sodium nitroprusside; TBA: Tiobarbituric acid; TCA: Trichloroacetic acid; TF: Total flavonoid; TP: Total phenolic content; TPTZ: 2,4,6-tris(2-pyridyl)-s-triazine

Acknowledgements
Not applicable.

Funding
The work on this paper is supported by project that has received funding from the European Union's Horizon 2020 Spreading Excellence and Widening Participation programme under grant agreement No 692276, and by the Ministry of Education, Science and Technological Development of the Republic of Serbia (Project No III 46001).

Authors' contributions
ML, MM, AM, SH designed the study. ML, VC, AN, MK, MS, AM, MCB, performed the experiments. ML, MM, VC, AN, AM, MK, MS, MP, AC, PH, SH analyzed and discussed the data. ML, VC, MM, AN, MS, AM, SH wrote the manuscript. All authors read and approved the final version of the manuscript.

Competing interests
The authors declare that they have no competing interests.

Author details
[1]Department of Pharmacy and Biotechnology, University of Bologna, Via San Donato 15, 40127 Bologna, Italy. [2]Institute of Food Technology, University of Novi Sad, Bul. Cara Lazara 1, Novi Sad 21000, Serbia. [3]Faculty of Sciences, Department of Biology and Ecology, University of Novi Sad, Trg Dositeja Obradovića 2, Novi Sad 21000, Serbia. [4]Department for Life Quality Studies, University of Bologna, Corso d'Augusto 237, 47921 Rimini, Italy. [5]School of Pharmacy, University of Camerino, Via Madonna delle Carceri, 9 - 62032 Camerino, MC, Italy.

References
1. Tsai SY, Tsai HL, Mau JL. Antioxidant properties of *Agaricus blazei*, *Agrocybe cylindracea*, and *Boletus edulis*. LWT Food Sci Technol. 2007;40:1392–402.
2. Stamets P. Growing gourmet and medicinal mushrooms. New York: Ten Speed Press; 2000.
3. Kalyoncu F, Oskay M, Saglam H, Erdogan TF, Tamer AU. Antimicrobial and antioxidant activities of mycelia of 10 wild mushroom species. J Med Food. 2010;13(2):415–9.
4. Lindequist U, Niedermeyer TH, Julich WD. The pharmacological potential of mushrooms. Evid Based Complement Alternat Med. 2005;2(3):285–99.
5. Karaman M, Jovin E, Malbasa R, Matavuly M, Popovic M. Medicinal and edible lignicolous fungi as natural sources of antioxidative and antibacterial agents. Phytother Res. 2010;24(10):1473–81.
6. Karaman M, Stahl M, Vulic J, Vesic M, Canadanovic-Brunet J. Wild-growing lignicolous mushroom species as sources of novel agents with antioxidative and antibacterial potentials. Int J Food Sci Nutr. 2014;65(3):311–9.
7. Maity P, Nandi AK, Manna DK, Pattanayak M, Sen IK, Bhanja SK, Samanta S, Panda BC, Paloi S, Acharya K, et al. Structural characterization and antioxidant activity of a glucan from *Meripilus giganteus*. Carbohydr Polym. 2017;157:1237–45.
8. Acharya K, Rai M. Proximate composition, free radical scavenging and NOS activation properties of a wild edible mushroom. Int J Pharm Pharm Sci. 2013;5(1):67–72.

9. Rai M, Sen S, Acharya K. Antimicrobial activity of four wild edible mushrooms from Darjeeling hills, West Bengal, India. Int J PharmTech Res. 2013;5(3):949–56.

10. Tomasi S, Lohezic-Le Devehat F, Sauleau P, Bezivin C, Boustie J. Cytotoxic activity of methanol extracts from Basidiomycete mushrooms on murine cancer cell lines. Pharmazie. 2004;59(4):290–3.

11. Narbe G, Lindequist U, Teuscher E, Franke P, Vainiotalo P, Basner R. The chemistry of immunosuppressive acting fractions of Meripilus giganteus (PERS ex. FR.) KARST., the giant spore. Pharmazie. 1991;46(10):738–40.

12. Nam KS, Jo YS, Kim YH, Hyun JW, Kim HW. Cytotoxic activities of acetoxyscirpenediol and ergosterol peroxide from Paecilomyces tenuipes. Life Sci. 2001;69(2):229–37.

13. Kahlos K, Kangas L, Hiltunen R. Ergosterol peroxide, an active compound from Inonotus radiatus. Planta Med. 1989;55(4):389–90.

14. Singleton VL, Orthofer R, Lamuela-Raventós RM. Analysis of total phenols and other oxidation substrates and antioxidants by means of folin-ciocalteu reagent. Methods Enzymol. 1999;299:152–78.

15. Novaković AR, Karaman MA, Milovanović IL, Belović MM, Rašeta MJ, Radusin TI, Ilić NM. Edible mycorrhizal species Lactarius controversus Pers. 1800 as a source of antioxidant and cytotoxic agents. Hemijska Industrija. 2016;70(2): 113–22.

16. Chang CC, Yang MH, Wen HM, Chern JC. Estimation of total flavonoid content in propolis by two complementary colorimetric methods. J Food Drug Anal. 2002;10(3):178–82.

17. Orcic D, Franciskovic M, Bekvalac K, Svircev E, Beara I, Lesjak M, Mimica-Dukic N. Quantitative determination of plant phenolics in Urtica dioica extracts by high-performance liquid chromatography coupled with tandem mass spectrometric detection. Food Chem. 2014;143:48–53.

18. Espin JC, Soler-Rivas C, Wichers HJ. Characterization of the total free radical scavenger capacity of vegetable oils and oil fractions using 2,2-diphenyl-1-picrylhydrazyl radical. J Agric Food Chem. 2000;48(3):648–56.

19. Benzie IF, Strain JJ. Ferric reducing/antioxidant power assay: direct measure of total antioxidant activity of biological fluids and modified version for simultaneous measurement of total antioxidant power and ascorbic acid concentration. Methods Enzymol. 1999;299:15–27.

20. Green LC, Wagner DA, Glogowski J, Skipper PL, Wishnok JS, Tannenbaum SR. Analysis of nitrate, nitrite, and [15N]nitrate in biological fluids. Anal Biochem. 1982;126(1):131–8.

21. Cheeseman KH, Beavis A, Esterbauer H. Hydroxyl-radical-induced iron-catalysed degradation of 2-deoxyribose. Quantitative determination of malondialdehyde. Biochem J. 1988;252(3):649–53.

22. Nishikimi M, Appaji N, Yagi K. The occurrence of superoxide anion in the reaction of reduced phenazine methosulfate and molecular oxygen. Biochem Biophys Res Commun. 1972;46(2):849–54.

23. Fimognari C, Berti F, Cantelli-Forti G, Hrelia P. Effect of sulforaphane on micronucleus induction in cultured human lymphocytes by four different mutagens. Environ Mol Mutagen. 2005;46(4):260–7.

24. Lenzi M, Cocchi V, Malaguti M, Barbalace MC, Marchionni S, Hrelia S, Hrelia P. 6-(Methylsulfonyl) hexyl isothiocyanate as potential chemopreventive agent: molecular and cellular profile in leukaemia cell lines. Oncotarget. 2017;8(67):111697–714.

25. Lenzi M, Malaguti M, Cocchi V, Hrelia S, Hrelia P. Castanea sativa Mill. bark extract exhibits chemopreventive properties triggering extrinsic apoptotic pathway in Jurkat cells. BMC Complement Altern Med. 2017;17(1):251.

26. Henry CM, Hollville E, Martin SJ. Measuring apoptosis by microscopy and flow cytometry. Methods. 2013;61(2):90–7.

27. Angeloni C, Malaguti M, Rizzo B, Barbalace MC, Fabbri D, Hrelia S. Neuroprotective effect of sulforaphane against methylglyoxal cytotoxicity. Chem Res Toxicol. 2015;28(6):1234–45.

28. Angeloni C, Hrelia S, Malaguti M. Neuroprotective effects of Glucosinolates. In: Mérillon JM, Ramawat KG, editors. Glucosinolates, reference series in phytochemistry. Switzerland: Springer International Publishing; 2016. p. 1–25.

29. Jurikova T, Mlcek J, Skrovankova S, Sumczynski D, Sochor J, Hlavacova I, Snopek L, Orsavova J. Fruits of black chokeberry Aronia melanocarpa in the prevention of chronic diseases. Molecules. 2017;22(6):944.

30. Fimognari C, Ferruzzi L, Turrini E, Carulli G, Lenzi M, Hrelia P, Cantelli-Forti G. Metabolic and toxicological considerations of botanicals in anticancer therapy. Expert Opin Drug Metab Toxicol. 2012;8(7):819–32.

31. Zhang H, Tsao R. Dietary polyphenols, oxidative stress and antioxidant and anti-inflammatory effects. Curr Opin Food Sci. 2016;8:33–42.

32. Zhang C, Shu L, Kim H, Khor TO, Wu R, Li W, Kong AN. Phenethyl isothiocyanate (PEITC) suppresses prostate cancer cell invasion epigenetically through regulating microRNA-194. Mol Nutr Food Res. 2016; 60(6):1427–36.

33. Angeloni C, Malaguti M, Barbalace MC, Hrelia S. Bioactivity of olive oil phenols in neuroprotection. Int J Mol Sci. 2017;18(11):E2230.

34. Malaguti M, Angeloni C, Hrelia S. Nutraceutical bioactive compounds promote healthspan counteracting cardiovascular diseases. J Am Coll Nutr. 2015;34(Suppl 1):22–7.

35. Chiarini A, Micucci M, Malaguti M, Budriesi R, Ioan P, Lenzi M, Fimognari C, Gallina Toschi T, Comandini P, Hrelia S. Sweet chestnut (Castanea sativa Mill.) bark extract: cardiovascular activity and myocyte protection against oxidative damage. Oxidative Med Cell Longev. 2013; 2013:471790.

36. Micucci M, Malaguti M, Toschi TG, Di Lecce G, Aldini R, Angeletti A, Chiarini A, Budriesi R, Hrelia S. Cardiac and vascular synergic protective effect of Olea europea L. Leaves and Hibiscus sabdariffa L. Flower Extracts. Oxidative Med Cell Longev. 2015;2015:318125.

37. Klaus A, Kozarski M, Niksic M, Jakovljevic D, Todorovic N, Stefanoska I, Van Griensven LJ. The edible mushroom Laetiporus sulphureus as potential source of natural antioxidants. Int J Food Sci Nutr. 2013;64(5):599–610.

38. Zhang S, Liu X, Yan L, Zhang Q, Zhu J, Huang N, Wang Z. Chemical compositions and antioxidant activities of polysaccharides from the sporophores and cultured products of Armillaria mellea. Molecules. 2015; 20(4):5680–97.

39. Trumbeckaite S, Benetis R, Bumblauskiene L, Burdulis D, Janulis V, T A, Viskelis P, Jakstas V. Achillea millefolium L.s.l. herb extract: antioxidant activity and effect on the rat heart mitochondrial functions. Food Chem. 2011;127:1540–8.

40. Keles A, Koca I, Genççelep H. Antioxidant properties of wild edible mushrooms. J Food Process Technol. 2011;2(6):130.

41. Yildiz O, Can Z, Laghari AQ, Ahin SH, Malkoç M. Wild edible mushrooms as a natural source of Phenolics and antioxidants. J Food Biochem. 2015;39: 148–54.

42. Alvarez-Parrilla E, de la Rosa LA, Martínez NR, Aguilar-González GA. Total phenols and antioxidant activity of commercial and wild mushrooms from Chihuahua, Mexico. CYTA J Food. 2007;5(5):329–34.

43. Ribeiro B, Valentao P, Baptista P, Seabra RM, Andrade PB. Phenolic compounds, organic acids profiles and antioxidative properties of beefsteak fungus (Fistulina hepatica). Food Chem Toxicol. 2007;45(10):1805–13.

44. Vaz JA, Barros L, Martins A, Morais JS, Vasconcelos MH, Ferreira IC. Phenolic profile of seventeen Portuguese wild mushrooms. LWT Food Sci Technol. 2011;44(1):343–6.

45. Barros L, Cruz T, Baptista P, Estevinho LM, Ferreira IC. Wild and commercial mushrooms as source of nutrients and nutraceuticals. Food Chem Toxicol. 2008;46(8):2742–7.

46. Heleno SA, Martins A, Queiroz MJ, Ferreira IC. Bioactivity of phenolic acids: metabolites versus parent compounds: a review. Food Chem. 2015;173:501–13.

47. Ferreira ICFR, Baptista P, Vilas-Boas M, Barros L. Free-radical scavenging capacity and reducing power of wild edible mushrooms from Northeast Portugal: individual cap and stipe activity. Food Chem. 2007;100(4):1511–6.

48. Puttaraju NG, Venkateshaiah SU, Dharmesh SM, Urs SM, Somasundaram R. Antioxidant activity of indigenous edible mushrooms. J Agric Food Chem. 2006;54(26):9764–72.

49. Lenzi M, Fimognari C, Hrelia P. Sulforaphane as a promising molecule for fighting cancer. Cancer Treat Res. 2014;159:207–23.

50. Arora S, Tandon S. Mushroom extracts induce human colon cancer cell (COLO-205) death by triggering the mitochondrial apoptosis pathway and go/G1-phase cell cycle arrest. Arch Iran Med. 2015;18(5):284–95.

51. Leon F, Quintana J, Rivera A, Estevez F, Bermejo J. Lanostanoid triterpenes from Laetiporus sulphureus and apoptosis induction on HL-60 human myeloid leukemia cells. J Nat Prod. 2004;67(12):2008–11.

52. Abubakar MB, Abdullah WZ, Sulaiman SA, Suen AB. A review of molecular mechanisms of the anti-leukemic effects of phenolic compounds in honey. Int J Mol Sci. 2012;13(11):15054–73.

53. Fimognari C, Lenzi M, Cantelli-Forti G, Hrelia P. Induction of differentiation in human promyelocytic cells by the isothiocyanate sulforaphane. In Vivo. 2008;22(3):317–20.

54. Harrington HA, Ho KL, Ghosh S, Tung KC. Construction and analysis of a modular model of caspase activation in apoptosis. Theor Biol Med Model. 2008;5:26.

55. Li L, Zhang R, Chen Z, Xue S, Wang X, Ruan C. Over-expressed Fas improves the apoptosis of malignant T-cells in vitro and vivo. Mol Biol Rep. 2011;38(8):5371–7.
56. Autret A, Martin SJ. Emerging role for members of the Bcl-2 family in mitochondrial morphogenesis. Mol Cell. 2009;36(3):355–63.
57. Wang Z, Tang X, Zhang Y, Qi R, Li Z, Zhang K, Liu Z, Yang X. Lobaplatin induces apoptosis and arrests cell cycle progression in human cholangiocarcinoma cell line RBE. Biomed Pharmacother. 2012;66(3):161–6.
58. Szatrowski TP, Nathan CF. Production of large amounts of hydrogen peroxide by human tumor cells. Cancer Res. 1991;51(3):794–8.
59. Prieto-Bermejo R, Romo-Gonzalez M, Perez-Fernandez A, Ijurko C, Hernandez-Hernandez A. Reactive oxygen species in haematopoiesis: leukaemic cells take a walk on the wild side. J Exp Clin Cancer Res. 2018; 37(1):125.
60. Sallmyr A, Fan J, Rassool FV. Genomic instability in myeloid malignancies: increased reactive oxygen species (ROS), DNA double strand breaks (DSBs) and error-prone repair. Cancer Lett. 2008;270(1):1–9.
61. Hole PS, Darley RL, Tonks A. Do reactive oxygen species play a role in myeloid leukemias? Blood. 2011;117(22):5816–26.
62. Aronis A, Melendez JA, Golan O, Shilo S, Dicter N, Tirosh O. Potentiation of Fas-mediated apoptosis by attenuated production of mitochondria-derived reactive oxygen species. Cell Death Differ. 2003;10(3):335–44.
63. Fimognari C, Lenzi M, Hrelia P. Apoptosis induction by sulfur-containing compounds in malignant and nonmalignant human cells. Environ Mol Mutagen. 2009;50(3):171–89.

19

Spontaneous spinal epidural hematoma of the thoracic spine after herbal medicine: a case report

Eo Jin Kim[1], Joonghyun Ahn[2] and Seung-Ju Kim[1*]

Abstract

Background: Spontaneous spinal epidural hematoma (SSEH) is an uncommon disease, but it can lead to acute cord compression with disabling consequences. Identifiable reasons for spontaneous hemorrhage are vascular malformations and bleeding disorders. However, SSEH after taking herbal medicines has not been described yet.

Case presentation: A 60-year-old female experienced sudden back pain combined with numbness and weakness in the lower limbs for several hours with no trauma, drug use, family history or any disease history. Her deep tendon reflexes were normoactive, and Babinski was negative. An emergent MRI showed a spinal epidural hematoma extending from T3 to T5. She was taken to surgery after immediate clinical and laboratory evaluations had been completed. Emergency decompression with laminectomy was performed and the patient recovered immediately after the surgery. Additional history taken from the patient at outpatient clinic after discharge revealed that she had been continuously taking herbal medicine containing black garlic for 8 weeks.

Conclusion: To our knowledge, no report has been previously issued on SSEH after taking herbal medicines. Although contradictory evidence is present on bleeding risks with herbal uses, we believe that it's reasonable to ascertain if patients with SSEP are taking herbal medication before or during spinal surgery.

Keywords: Spontaneous spinal epidural hematoma, Surgical treatment, Herbal medicines, Black garlic, Spinal cord

Background

Spinal epidural hematoma (SEH) is an idiopathic aggregation of blood in epidural space which can be as acute, chronic, spontaneously, post traumatic, or iatrogenic [1]. SEH occurring without a trauma is called as spontaneous SEH (SSEH) and it is an uncommon neurosurgical emergency which can lead to acute cord compression with disabling consequences [2]. The incidence of SSEH was estimated to be 0.1 patients per 100,000 populations per year [3]. As SSEH is one of the potentially reversible pressure lesions on the spinal cord and roots, its prompt diagnosis and treatment have a vital importance [1]. Although some nonsurgical treatments have been reported in cases that neurologic deficit improves in the early phase of disease [1], early surgical decompression

(Laminectomy) is the first-line treatment modality for SSEH [4, 5].

The etiology of SSEH remains unknown; however, some predisposing factors have been reported, including long term aspirin use as platelet aggregation inhibitor, anticoagulant therapy for prosthetic cardiac valves, therapeutic thrombolysis for acute myocardial infarction, hemophilia, factor XI deficiency, vascular malformation, Paget's disease and pregnancy [6–8]. However, to the best of our knowledge, no report has been previously issued on SSEH after taking herbal medicines. Here, we report a case of a 60-year-old woman who presented with SSEH after taking herbal medicines and treated successfully by surgical decompression.

Case presentation

A 60-year healthy female who was a hospital janitor of our institute visited an emergency department with a one-hour history of sudden low back pain with lower extremity motor and sensory deficit aggravated by bending.

---

* Correspondence: sju627@hotmail.com
[1]Department of Orthopaedics, Hanil General Hospital, 308 Uicheon-ro, Dobong-Gu, Seoul 132-703, South Korea
Full list of author information is available at the end of the article

In her medical history, there was no recent trauma, no familial bleeding disorder, or no anticoagulation treatment. The patient's previous surgical history revealed an open discectomy procedure at L3 to L4 due to herniated intervertebral disc in 2011. The neurologic exam revealed complete paralysis of the bilateral lower extremities and the symmetrical disappearance of body sensation below the T7 dermatome. On MRI, posterior to the spinal cord, there was a mass lesion in the epidural space at T3–T5 levels, which was isointense on T1- weighted images and hyperintense on T2 weighted images compared to spinal cord intensity, consistent with acute hematoma (Fig. 1). Comprehensive conservative treatment failed to improve her symptoms. The patient underwent emergency surgical treatment within 24 h after initial onset of symptoms. Total laminectomy from T3 to T5 was performed, and blood clot located at the dorsal portion of the spinal cord was evacuated (Fig. 2). Upper and lower spinal levels were clear for any additional presence of hematoma mass. Microscopic

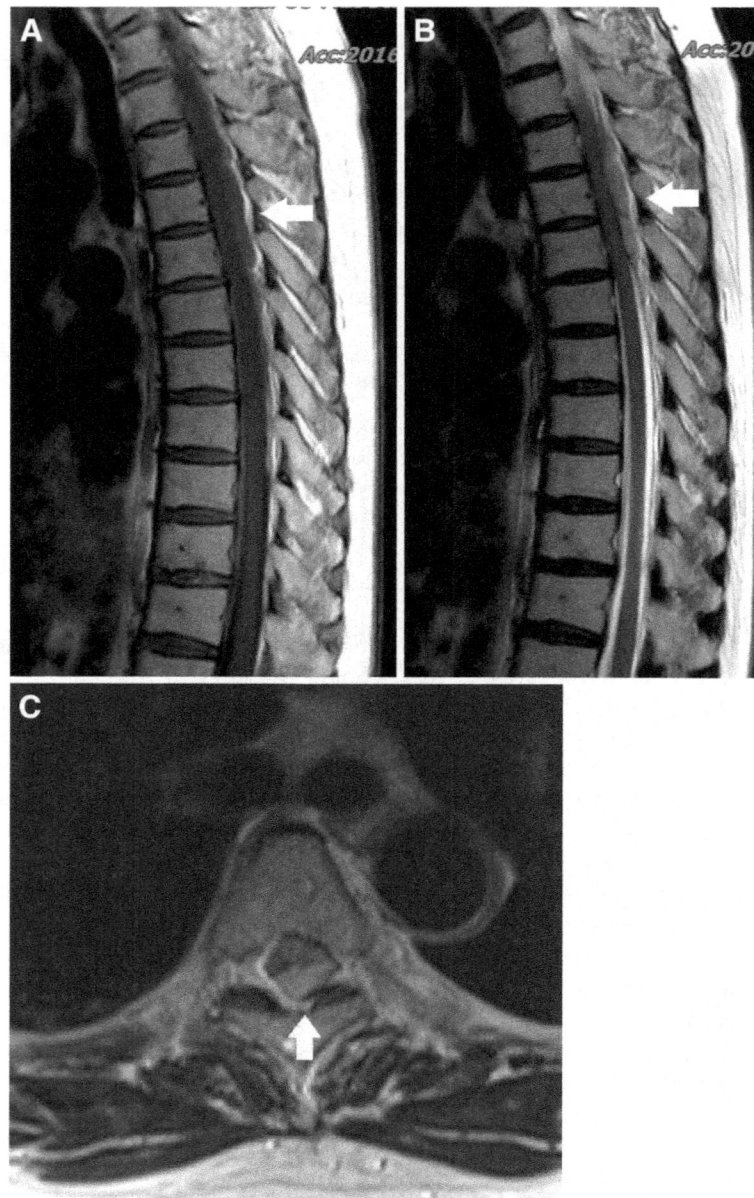

Fig. 1 (**a**) Preoperative T1-weighted MRI shows iso signal intensity posterior spinal epidural mass lesion (sagittal image) (**b**) Preoperative T2-weighted MRI shows high signal intensity posterior spinal epidural mass lesion(sagittal image). (**c**) Axial image shows epidural hematoma on the dorsal portion of spinal canal (T2-weighted MRI)

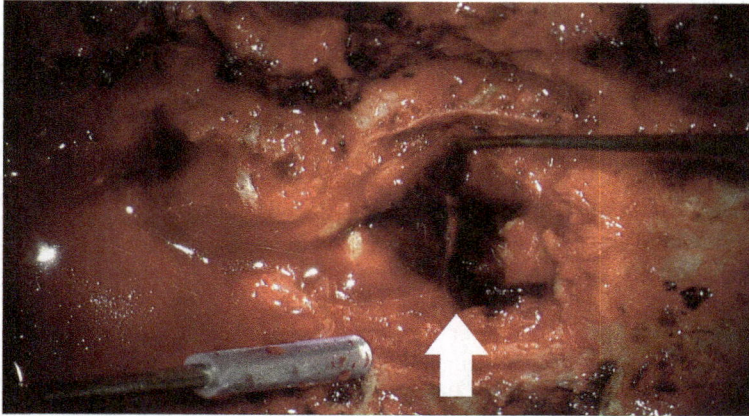

Fig. 2 Total laminectomy from T3 to T5 and evacuation of epidural hematoma (red-colored mass) was performed

histological examination of the resected mass revealed a hematoma(Fig. 3). The patient showed dramatic improvement after surgery. The patient discharged without any motor or sensory impairment after 3 weeks and returned to work after a month. Additional history taken from the patient at outpatient clinic after discharge revealed that the patient did not have any positive past medical history but had been continuously taking herbal medicine containing black garlic for 8 weeks.

Discussion and conclusions

Identifiable underlying disorders of SSEH beside trauma are bleeding disorders, spinal infections, spinal tumors, spinal interventions, and vascular malformations [6, 9]. Herbal remedies are used to treat a large variety of

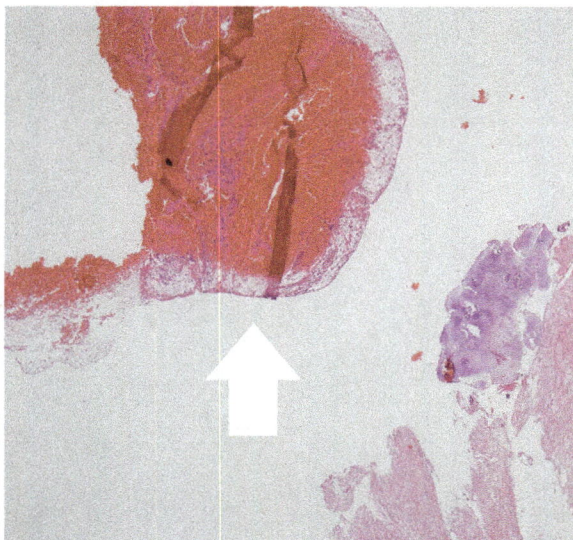

Fig. 3 Hematoxylin and eosin stain, 40×. Photomicrograph shows a lot of red blood cells

diseases in Asian countries. However, a number of herbal preparations have been reported to cause variations in clotting time by inhibition of coagulation factors or platelet activity [10]. Interestingly, several herbal medicines including garlic, feverfew, ginger, and ginseng have been associated with potential increased bleeding [11, 12].

According to a recent study [13], it has been reported that it seems prudent to stop taking high dosages of garlic seven to 10 days before surgery because garlic can prolong bleeding time. Beckert et al. [14] reported that an increased risk of bleeding, substantiated by anecdotal reports, has been attributed to the use of certain herbs, and numerous in vitro experiments have identified some herbal extracts as platelet inhibitors. Tsai et al. [15] demonstrated that for those patients who are taking conventional anti-clotting medications with herbal medicines for cardiovascular diseases, the potential risks of increased bleeding due to drug-herbal medicine interactions should not be ignored. Nevertheless, the risks attributed to herbal medicines are often ignored or underestimated. Questions about herbal medicines are not routinely asked in clinics. In addition, as many of these herbal supplements are available over the counter, many patients do not disclose these when listing medications to health care providers. We can't comment on all the specific herbal medicines used, because herbs contain hundreds of chemical constituents, some are more pharmacologically active than others. As plants contain many different kinds of compounds, they usually have multiple actions.

In our case, the patient didn't have an abnormal bleeding tendency and any positive past medical history on admission. Preoperatively, laboratory tests such as PT (prothrombin time) or aPTT (activated partial thromboplastin time) were normal range. However, bleeding time was slightly prolonged to 8 min (normal range, 2 to 6 min) which was not noticed before surgery, and the patient had taken garlic for 2 months. It has been reported that garlic can inhibit platelet aggregation, and the bleeding time increased in the patients who had received garlic [9, 16, 17]. This bleeding tendency is one of predisposing factors of SSEH and may cause the disease [8, 9]. Although contradictory evidence is present on bleeding risks with herbal uses, we believe that it's reasonable to ascertain if patients are taking herbal medication, especially in Asian population, and to discontinue any herbal preparations before undergoing surgical procedures if it is not inevitable.

In conclusion, we report a patient with SSEH after taking herbal medicine. As side-effects and herb–drug interactions could be significant or fatal, we believe that a detailed drug history including herbal remedy use should be taken by physicians before or during surgery especially in patients with SSEH.

Abbreviation
SSEH: Spontaneous spinal epidural hematoma

Acknowledgements
None.

Funding
No funding has been received for this project.

Authors' contributions
SJK conceived of the case report, SJK and JHA gleaned the facts and drafted the manuscript. EJK contributed the facts from the surgical point of view. EJK and JHA revised it critically and contributed substantially to the discussion. All authors read and approved the final manuscript.

Competing interests
The authors declare that they have no conflicts of interest concerning this article. No financial support has been received by the authors for the preparation of this manuscript.

Author details
[1]Department of Orthopaedics, Hanil General Hospital, 308 Uicheon-ro, Dobong-Gu, Seoul 132-703, South Korea. [2]Department of Orthopaedics, CM Chungmu Hospital, Yeongdeungpo-go, Seoul 150-034, South Korea.

References
1. Motamedi M, Baratloo A, Majidi A, Rahmati F, Shahrami A. Spontaneous spinal epidural hematoma; a case report. Emergency. 2014;2(4):183–5.
2. Kirazli Y, Akkoc Y, Kanyilmaz S. Spinal epidural hematoma associated with oral anticoagulation therapy. Am J Phys Med Rehabil. 2004;83(3):220–3.
3. Holtas S, Heiling M, Lonntoft M. Spontaneous spinal epidural hematoma: findings at MR imaging and clinical correlation. Radiology. 1996;199(2):409–13.
4. Schoonjans AS, De Dooy J, Kenis S, Menovsky T, Verhulst S, Hellinckx J, Van Ingelghem I, Parizel PM, Jorens PG, Ceulemans B. Spontaneous spinal epidural hematoma in infancy: review of the literature and the "seventh" case report. Eur J Paediatr Neurol. 2013;17(6):537–42.
5. Shin JJ, Kuh SU, Cho YE. Surgical management of spontaneous spinal epidural hematoma. Eur Spine J. 2006;15(6):998–1004.
6. Riaz S, Jiang H, Fox R, Lavoie M, Mahood JK. Spontaneous spinal epidural hematoma causing Brown-Sequard syndrome: case report and review of the literature. J Emerg Med. 2007;33(3):241–4.
7. Liu Z, Jiao Q, Xu J, Wang X, Li S, You C. Spontaneous spinal epidural hematoma: analysis of 23 cases. Surg Neurol. 2008;69(3):253–60 discussion 260.
8. Sandvig A, Jonsson H. Spontaneous chronic epidural hematoma in the lumbar spine associated with warfarin intake: a case report. Springerplus. 2016;5(1):1832.
9. Kreppel D, Antoniadis G, Seeling W. Spinal hematoma: a literature survey with meta-analysis of 613 patients. Neurosurg Rev. 2003;26(1):1–49.
10. Cordier W, Steenkamp V. Herbal remedies affecting coagulation: a review. Pharm Biol. 2012;50(4):443–52.
11. Fessenden JM, Wittenborn W, Clarke L. Gingko biloba: a case report of herbal medicine and bleeding postoperatively from a laparoscopic cholecystectomy. Am Surg. 2001;67(1):33–5.
12. Allison GL, Lowe GM, Rahman K. Aged garlic extract and its constituents inhibit platelet aggregation through multiple mechanisms. J Nutr. 2006; 136(3 Suppl):782S–8S.
13. Tattelman E. Health effects of garlic. Am Fam Physician. 2005;72(1):103–6.
14. Beckert BW, Concannon MJ, Henry SL, Smith DS, Puckett CL. The effect of herbal medicines on platelet function: an in vivo experiment and review of the literature. Plast Reconstr Surg. 2007;120(7):2044–50.
15. Tsai HH, Lin HW, Lu YH, Chen YL, Mahady GB. A review of potential harmful interactions between anticoagulant/antiplatelet agents and Chinese herbal medicines. PLoS One. 2013;8(5):e64255.
16. Fakhar H, Hashemi Tayer A. Effect of the garlic pill in comparison with Plavix on platelet aggregation and bleeding time. Iran J Ped Hematol Oncol. 2012; 2(4):146–52.
17. Allison GL, Lowe GM, Rahman K. Aged garlic extract may inhibit aggregation in human platelets by suppressing calcium mobilization. J Nutr. 2006;136(3 Suppl):789S–92S.

20

Zerumbone from *Zingiber zerumbet* (L.) smith: a potential prophylactic and therapeutic agent against the cariogenic bacterium *Streptococcus mutans*

Thiago Moreira da Silva[1], Carlos Danniel Pinheiro[1], Patricia Puccinelli Orlandi[2], Carlos Cleomir Pinheiro[1] and Gemilson Soares Pontes[3*] (iD)

Abstract

Background: Essential oil obtained from rhizomes of the *Zingiber zerumbet* (L.) Smith (popularly known in Brazil as bitter ginger) is mainly constituted by the biomolecule zerumbone, which exhibit untapped antimicrobial potential. The aim of this study was to investigate the antimicrobial activity of the zerumbone from bitter ginger rhizomes against the cariogenic agent *Streptococcus mutans*.

Methods: Firstly, the essential oil from rhizomes of *Zingiber zerumbet* (L.) Smith extracted by hydrodistillation was submitted to purification and recrystallization process to obtain the zerumbone compound. The purity of zerumbone was determined through high-performance liquid chromatography analysis. Different concentrations of zerumbone were tested against the standard strain *S. mutans* (ATCC 35668) by using microdilution method. The speed of cidal activity was determined through a time kill-curve assay. The biological cytotoxicity activity of zerumbone was assessed using Vero cell line through MTT assay.

Results: The zerumbone showed a minimum inhibitory concentration (MIC) of 250 µg/mL and a minimum bactericidal concentration (MBC) of 500 µg/mL against *S. mutans*. After six hours of bacteria-zerumbone interaction, all concentrations tested starts to kill the bacteria and all bacteria were killed between 48 and 72 h period at the concentration of 500 µg/mL (99,99% of bacteria were killed in comparison with original inoculum). In addition, zerumbone showed no cytotoxicity activity on mammalian continuous cells line.

Conclusions: These results draw attention to the potential of zerumbone as antimicrobial agent against *S. mutans* infection, indicating its possible use in the phyto-pharmaceutical formulations as new approach to prevent and treat tooth decay disease.

Keywords: Tooth decay, Zerumbone, Bioprospecting, Antimicrobial, Treatment, Phytotherapy

Background

Several medicinal plants contain in their biochemical constitution many compounds with antibacterial action, that remains unknown [1]. *Zingiber zerumbet* (L.) Smith, a rhizomatous herbaceous species, belonging to the family *Zingiberaceae*, is a native plant from Southeast Asia with potential antimicrobial activity not fully comprehended [2]. In Brazil, this species is usually identified as bitter ginger and is easily found in large numbers in the Amazonas state, where it is well adapted to the local climatic conditions.

Essential oils extracted from *Zingiber zerumbet* rhizomes have potential pharmacological activities, including antimicrobial, anti-inflammatory, chemo-preventive, antinociceptive, antiulcer, antioxidant, antipyretic and analgesic, as previously described [3–7]. The major

---

* Correspondence: pontesbm1@gmail.com
[3]Instituto Nacional de Pesquisa da Amazônia, Coordenação Sociedade, Ambiente e Saúde, Av. André Araújo – 2936 – Petrópolis, Manaus 69067-375, Amazonas, Brazil
Full list of author information is available at the end of the article

bioactive molecule found in the essential oil of *Zingiber zerumbet* rhizomes is the zerumbone (Fig. 1), a mono-cyclic sesquiterpene compound (2,6,10-cy-cloundecatrie-n-1-one, 2,6,9,9-tetramethyl-,(E,E,E)-) [8]. Zerumbone has been linked to a broad range of biological activities, including the antibacterial action [9, 10].

Previous reports have demonstrated the antimicrobial activities of zerumbone against Gram negative bacteria, such as *Escherichia coli* and *Helicobacter pylori*, and Gram positive bacteria, such as *Staphylococcus epidermidis* and *Staphylococcus aureus*, showing more effectiveness on Gram positive microorganisms [7, 11]. However, its activity against other Gram positive microorganisms such as *Streptococcus mutans* is unknown. *S. mutans* is the main causative agent of tooth decay, the oral infectious disease most prevalent in the world affecting over 90% of school-aged children and about 100% of the world population [12].

Despite the great diversity of bacterial species in the oral cavity, few are able to cause tooth decay (cariogenic bacteria) and *S. mutans* has been implicated as the major etiological agent of this oral infectious disease [13]. The cariogenic potential displayed by this bacterium is due to its ability to produce acid (acidogenic) from dietary carbohydrate, capacity to survive in low-pH environments (aciduric) and, especially, due to its great ability to adhere onto the tooth surfaces, which makes *S. mutans* responsible for the initial formation of dental plaque [14].

Chemicals agents such as chlorexidin and others phenolic compounds are available and can be used to prevent

tooth decay, but long term use of these compounds may result in side effects like loss of taste, metallic taste in mouth, dental pigmentation, diarrhea and oral burning sensation [15]. In this context, biomolecules isolated from plants have been suggested as alternative therapeutics over synthetic chemical agents for prevention of tooth decay, because of their few or no side effects [16]. Hence, the main goal of this study was to investigate the antimicrobial activity of the zerumbone obtained from rhizomes of *Zingiber zerumbet* (L.) Smith against *S. mutans*, the main etiological agent of tooth decay.

Methods

Acquisition of *Zingiber zerumbet* rhizomes

The rizhomes of the *Z. zerumbet* were collected in a rural area surrounding the city of Manaus/AM, located at BR-174, points P01 to P02, latitude 24132, 03789 S and longitude 600931,40854 W, according to geographic coordination. After that, an exsiccate was sent to the herbarium of the National Institute of Amazonian Research (INPA) for proper identification and comparison with the exsiccate previously identified by Prof. Dr. Paul Maas (Department of Plant Ecology and Evolutionary Biology; Herbarium University of Utrecht), which is deposited in the herbarium under N°. 186913.

Essential oil extraction

The extraction of the essential oil (EO) was carried out in the Thematic Laboratory of Chemistry and Natural Products at INPA. The EO was obtained through the hydrodistillation of rhizomes. Briefly, after the identification, cleaning and disinfection, the material was crushed and dried at room temperature. Clevenger apparatus adapted with a round-bottom flask of 2l volume was used for distillation of OE from the crushed material diluted in distilled water in a proportion 1:4. The extraction was done during 6 h starting at boiling point. Afterward, the EO was collected from the condenser and stored in amber flasks at room temperature. All system was protected from light using aluminum foil. The OE yield was estimated by calculating the ratio between the oil mass and the feed mass.

Gas chromatography–mass spectrometry (GC–MS) analysis

The GC-MS analysis was performed as previously described, with few modifications [17]. Briefly, the investigation of essential oil composition was carried out using Hewlett Packard HP/série 6890 GC SITEM PLUS gas chromatographer (6511 Bunker Lake Blvd. Ramsey, Minnesota, 55303 USA) with an analytical HP-5MS 5% phenylmethylsiloxane capillary column (30 m × 0.32 mm i.d, film thickness 0,25 µm). It was operated an electron ionization system with ionization energy of 70 V. The

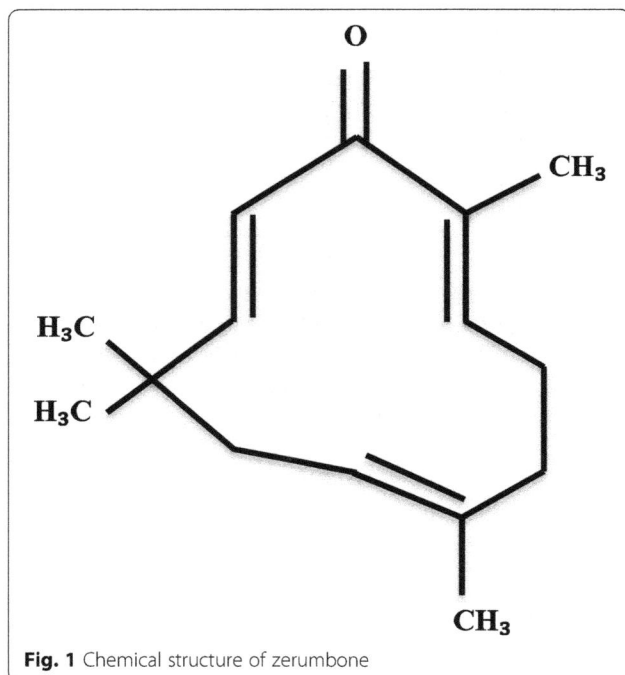

Fig. 1 Chemical structure of zerumbone

analyses were conducted using helium and nitrogen gases at 2 mL/min with purity percentage of 99.999%. It was injected 1 μL in splitless mode, in 1:20 ratio of hexannic solution. The oven was programmed at controlled temperature between 60 and 240 °C, raising 3 °C/min and kept at 250 °C for 10 min. Temperature of mass transfer and injection were established at 220 °C and 290 °C, respectively. The chemical constituents of essential oil analyzed were expressed as relative percentage by peak area normalization. The identification of the OE constituents was done by calculating the retention time obtained in the analyzes of GC-MS, correlating them with the retention times of the n-alkanes (C9-C30). The indices were compared with the data available in the NIST / WILEY library [18]. The zerumbone identification was done as previously described [19].

High-performance liquid chromatography (HPLC)
After purification and recrystallization of the EO using our patented method (n⁰ PI-0505343-9/28/11/2007), the zerumbone purity was estimated through HPLC analysis (Accela High Speed LC, Thermo Scientific®), using a column Hypersil Gold (50 × 2,1 mm) and a mobile phase methanol:water (85:15, v/v) at 1 mL/min. The identification was done by comparing the retention time of the peaks with those standard solutes in HPLC and confirmed by UV-absorption spectrum (~ 252 nm).

Inoculum standardization
The antimicrobial activity of the zerumbone was evaluated against the standard strain of *S. mutans* ATCC 35668 (American Type Culture Collection, Microbiologics Inc., St. Cloud, USA) [20]. Firstly, bacterial suspensions were prepared by inoculation of colonies into a tube containing 3 mL Brain Heart Infusion (BHI) broth, followed by incubation at orbital shaking of 150 RPM for 72 h at 37 °C in anaerobic conditions, as previously described [21]. After incubation, the turbidity was calibrated and adjusted through spectrophotometer analysis to match the 0,5 MacFarland scale (1×10^8 CFU/mL). Final inoculum of 1×10^6 CFU/ mL was used in the assays.

Determination of the antimicrobial activity
The antimicrobial activity of zerumbone was evaluated by estimation of Minimum Inhibitory Concentration (MIC) and Minimum Bactericidal Concentration (MBC) using microdilution method according to the guidelines of the Clinical & Laboratory Standards Institute (CLSI) [22]. The working stock solution of zerumbone was prepared in polyethylene glycol sorbitan monolaurate (Tween 20) under vigorous magnetic stirring system to assure homogeneity, as previously described [7]. After diluting serially this working stock solution in 96

well-plate containing 100 μL BHI broth, 100 μL of BHI broth having bacterial inoculum (1×10^6 CFU/mL) were added into wells resulting in a final volume of 200 μL, followed by incubation at the same conditions mentioned above. The concentrations of zerumbone tested ranged from 125 to 2000 μg/mL. Additional wells containing diluting agent of zerumbone (tween 20 10%) was used as a control.

After incubation, the bacterial growth was evaluated by measuring the turbidity in each well through spectrophotometric analysis (600 nm). Subsequently, an aliquot of 50 μL of each well was collected and seeded on plates containing BHI agar and incubated for 72 h at 37 °C in anaerobic conditions. Next, the plates were analyzed for the presence/absence of bacteria in order to estimate the MIC and MBC. The MIC was estimated according to lowest concentration of zerumbone that inhibits the bacterial growth. The MBC was assessed based on the concentration that kills all viable bacterial cells and therefore reveals no visible bacterial growth on the plates. The number of surviving cells (CFU/mL) was determined through the direct-plate counting technique performed individually by two skilled technicians. The limit of detection used in all tests was 10 CFU. An estimated count was provided in case of countable colonies were presented below this limit, as previous reported [23]. All tests were done in triplicate and repeated three times to verify the reproducibility of results.

Time-kill curve assay
To determine the speed of cidal activity of the zerumbone, a time kill-curve was performed as previously described, with few modifications [24]. An inoculum of 1×10^6 CFU/mL was added into tubes having 3 mL of BHI broth or BHI broth treated with zerumbone (MIC or MBC values) or tween 20 10% (control) and then incubated for 72 h anaerobically with orbital rotation of 150 RPM at 37 °C. The tube containing only bacteria and BHI broth was used to estimate the different phases of growth curve.

An aliquot of 100 μL was removed at 0, 6, 12, 24, 48 and 72 h time intervals to determine the bacterial growth by measuring turbidity through spectrophotometric analysis (600 nm). Subsequently, the aliquots were serially diluted in 0.85% of sterile saline solution, seeded in BHI agar and then incubated at the conditions set out above. The viable number of bacterial cells was estimated by counting CFU and multiplying the results by dilution factors. Means of duplicate colony counts were taken. To build the time-kill curve, the $\log_{10}$ CFU/mL versus time over 72 h was plotted. The decrease of 99.9% ($\geq 3 \log_{10}$) of the total number of CFU/mL in the original inoculum was used to estimate the bactericidal activity. The assays were performed in triplicate and repeated three times to confirm the reproducibility of results.

Cytotoxicity assay

The cytotoxicity activity of zerumbone was determined using the MTT (3-(4, 5-dimethyl thiazol-2-yl)-2, 5-diphenyl tetrazolium bromide) assay as previously described with few modifications [21]. Summarily, Vero cells line (2×10^4 per well) were cultured into 96-well plate containing 0.2 mL of DMEM medium (with 10% FBS, penicillin-streptomycin and amphotericin B) per well, in atmosphere of 5% CO_2 at 37 °C for 24 h. After formation of sub-confluent monolayer, the cells were treated with zerumbone (25 µg/mL; 50 µg/mL and 100 µg/mL) and incubated again at the same conditions above mentioned for 24 and 48 h. For this assay, crystals of zerumbone were diluted in 100% dimethyl sulfoxide (DMSO) because of its low aqueous solubility. Thus, the maximum concentration of zerumbone containing safe percentage of DMSO (< 1%) to the cells was 100 µg/mL. Sterile PBS was used as positive control and DMSO 100% as negative control. Subsequently, the medium was removed from all wells and 10 µL of MTT (5 mg/mL in sterile PBS) diluted in 100 µL of DMEM medium (without phenol red to avoid misinterpretation) was added into the wells and incubated in atmosphere of 5% CO_2 at 37 °C for 4 h. After that, the MTT was removed and 50 µL of MTT lysis buffer were added to each well followed for gently homogenization to dissolve the formazan crystals and incubated again for 10 min at the

same conditions mentioned earlier. Optical densities of samples were measured using a microplate reader at wavelength of 570 nm. The relative viability of cells was estimated using the following equation: (A570 of treated sample)/(A570 of untreated sample) × 100. All tests were done in triplicate.

Statistical analyses

Descriptive statistics was used to summarized and describe de data. The results are expressed in mean ± SD.

Results

Acquisition of Essential oil and purification of zerumbone

The yield of the essential oil obtained was 5%. The EO showed to be constituted mainly by sesquiterpene zerumbone compound, according to GC-MS analysis (Fig. 2). A percentage of 87,93% of zerumbone was detected among the nineteen others chemical constituents. The purification and recrystallization processes applied to EO resulted in a zerumbone crystal with 98% of purity (Fig. 3). These crystals were used in all subsequent tests.

Antimicrobial activity of zerumbone

The zerumbone substance tested in this study demonstrated antimicrobial activity against *S. mutans* ATCC 35668, showing a MIC value of 250 µg/mL and MBC of 500 µg/mL (Fig. 4, Additional file 1: Figure S1). The time-kill curve assay corroborates the antimicrobial activity of zerumbone. This biomolecule displayed more

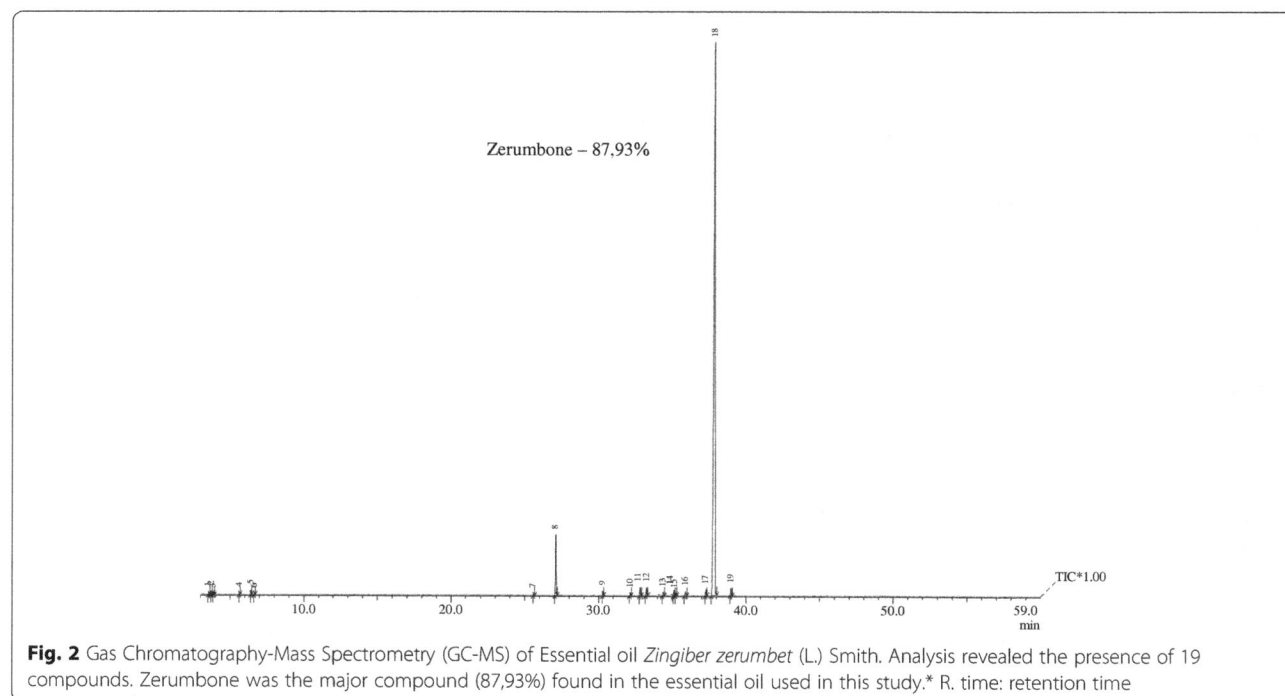

Fig. 2 Gas Chromatography-Mass Spectrometry (GC-MS) of Essential oil *Zingiber zerumbet* (L.) Smith. Analysis revealed the presence of 19 compounds. Zerumbone was the major compound (87,93%) found in the essential oil used in this study.* R. time: retention time

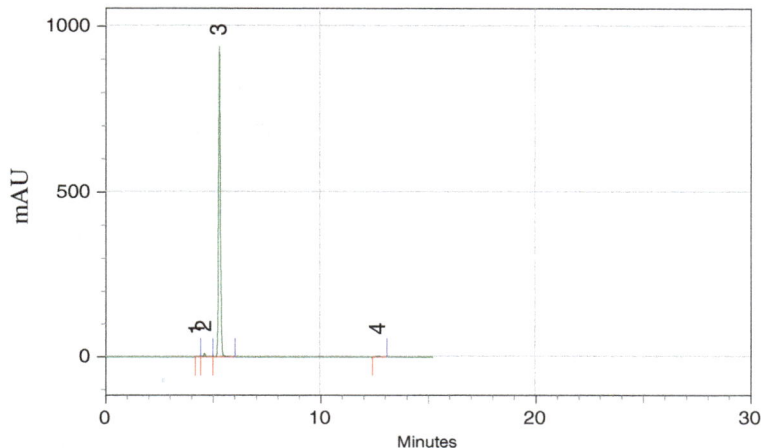

Fig. 3 High-performance liquid Chromatography (HPLC) of zerumbone crystals. HLPC elution of zerumbone crystal with retention time of ~ 5 min confirmed zerumbone purity of 98% (peak 3)

intense antibacterial activity in the time interval 12–48 h, corresponding to log phase of *S. mutans* growth curve (Additional file 2: Figure S2). Within 12 h of bacterial exposure to 250 µg/mL and 500 µg/mL of zerumbone concentrations, viable bacterial cells were reduced in 45.55% and 56,29%, respectively, in comparison to the original inoculum (Fig. 4a). After 24 h of exposure, the reduction was more pronounced with 65.46% (250 µg/mL) and 70.62% (500 µg/mL) of bacterial cells death (Fig. 4b and c). Finally, the zerumbone showed its maximum action in the interval of 48–72 h, reducing 94.78% of bacterial colonies at concentration of 250 µg/mL and killing all bacteria at the concentration of 500 µg/mL (Fig. 5a, b and c).

Cytotoxicity activity of zerumbone

The MMT assay demonstrated that the biomolecule zerumbone had no considerable cytotoxicity effect up to 100 µg/mL. At concentrations 25, 50 and 100 µg/mL the percentages of cell viability were 100, 97 and 92%, respectively, after 24 h treatment (Fig. 6). The cell viability slightly changed at concentration 50 µg/mL (93%) and 100 µg/mL (87%) after 48 h treatment. The results clearly show that the zerumbone has no cytotoxic effect on normal mammalian cells at the concentrations tested.

Discussion

Tooth decay disease is a growing global concern that is known to threaten human health and safety [25]. Emerging antibiotic resistance and inconvenient side effects caused by commercial antibiotics usually result in leaving treatment [26]. In this regard, the development of alternative antibiotic therapies based on bioactive molecules from medicinal plants is urgent and crucial to provide effective prevention and treatment for tooth infection.

The present study demonstrates strong antimicrobial activity of zerumbone against the cariogenic agent *S. mutans* (MIC = 250 µg/mL). according to the following classification of antimicrobial action: strong = 50 < MIC< 500 µg/mL moderate = MIC 600 < MIC< 1500 µg/mL and; weak = MIC> 1500 µg/mL [27, 28]. Our data therefore brings to light a new possibility of prophylactic and therapeutic strategies for *S. mutans* infection, especially in case of tooth decay, a serious public health issue [29].

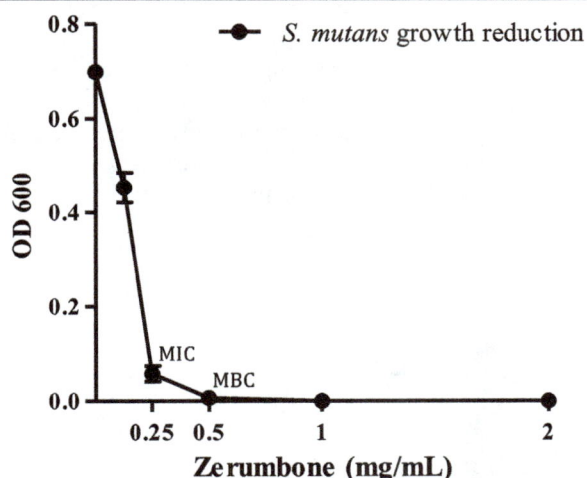

Fig. 4 Antimicrobial activity (MIC and MBC) of zerumbone against *S. mutans*. Bacterial inoculum (1 × 10⁶ CFU/mL) was treated with different concentrations of zerumbone and incubated at 37 °C for 48 h in anaerobic conditions. After incubation, the bacterial growth was verified by turbidity measurements using spectrophotometer. The results are representative of three independent experiments performed in triplicate and the values are shown in mean ± SD. OD: optical density; MIC: Minimum Inhibitory Concentration; MBC: Minimum bactericidal concentration

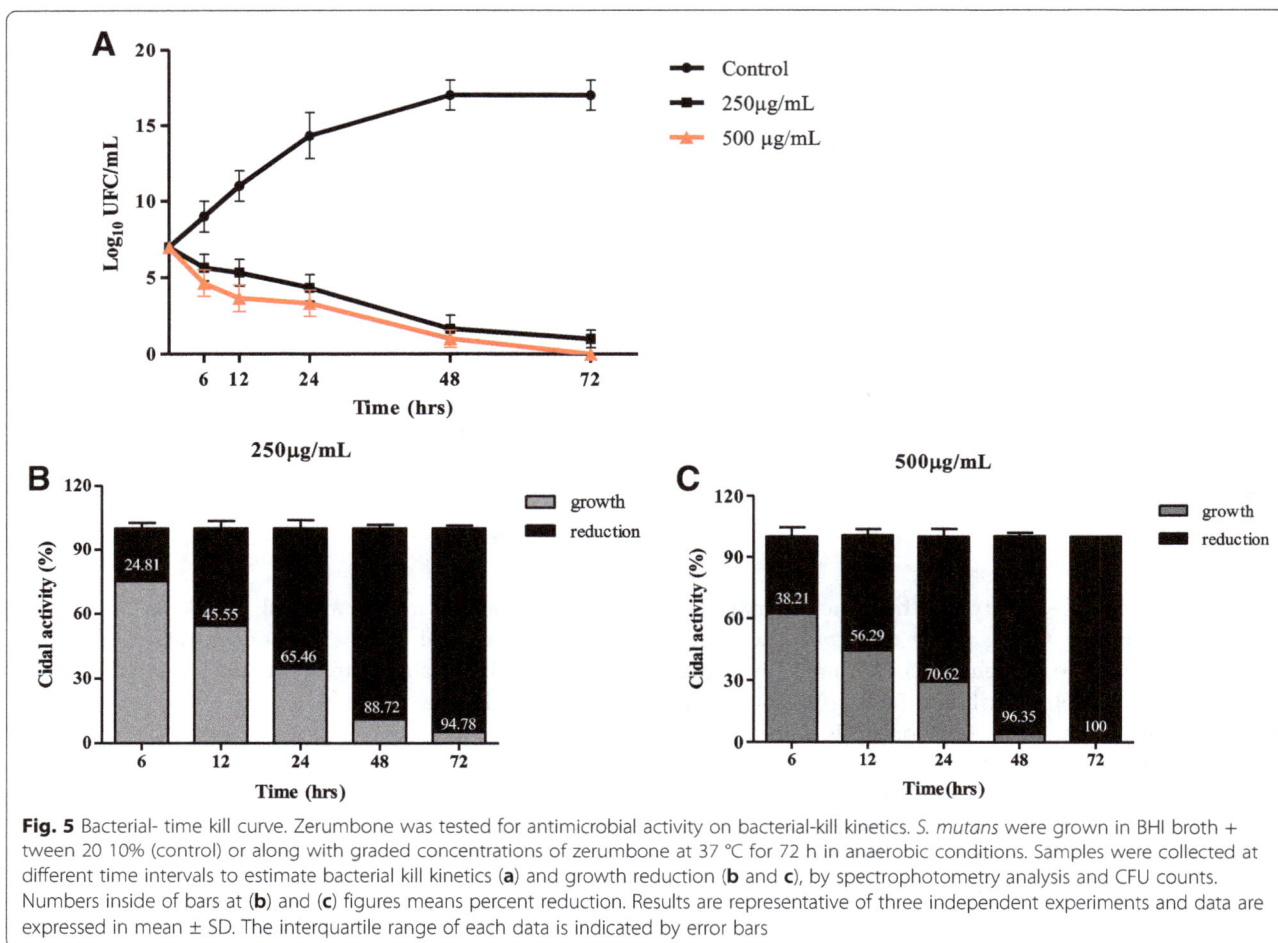

Fig. 5 Bacterial- time kill curve. Zerumbone was tested for antimicrobial activity on bacterial-kill kinetics. *S. mutans* were grown in BHI broth + tween 20 10% (control) or along with graded concentrations of zerumbone at 37 °C for 72 h in anaerobic conditions. Samples were collected at different time intervals to estimate bacterial kill kinetics (**a**) and growth reduction (**b** and **c**), by spectrophotometry analysis and CFU counts. Numbers inside of bars at (**b**) and (**c**) figures means percent reduction. Results are representative of three independent experiments and data are expressed in mean ± SD. The interquartile range of each data is indicated by error bars

Few reports have been found related to antimicrobial activity of natural biomolecules against the *S. mutans* earlier, but majority demonstrated weak antibacterial action based on the classification set out above [30–32]. A recent study tested around two thousand plant extracts from Amazon region, with seventeen extracts displaying antimicrobial activity against *S. mutans* (ATCC 25175). However, of these, only one extract obtained from plant *Ipomoea alba* L. sp. (*Convolvulaceae*) had strong (MBC ≥ 160 µg/mL) antimicrobial activity

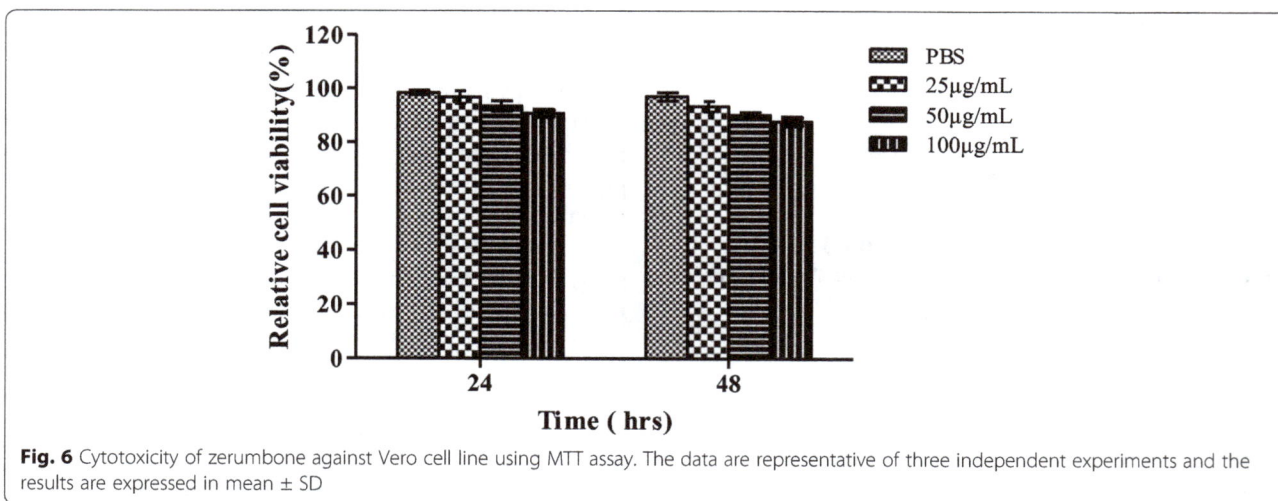

Fig. 6 Cytotoxicity of zerumbone against Vero cell line using MTT assay. The data are representative of three independent experiments and the results are expressed in mean ± SD

[33]. Takarada et al. [34] and Aguiar et al. [35] evaluated the anti-*S. mutans* activity of essential oils from the following plants: *Romarinus officinalis* L., *Melaleuca alternifólia*, *Lavandula officinalis*, *Leptosperfum scoparium*, *Eucalyptus radiate*, *Ageratum conyzoides*, *Artemisia camphorata* Vill., *Bidens sulphurea*, *Foeniculum vulgare* Mill., *Lippia alba*, *Ocimum gratissimum* L., *Pelargonium graveolens*, *Syzygium aromaticum* and *Tagetes erecta* L. The results showed MICs ranging from 500 to 10,000 µg/mL, antimicrobial activities considered weak as compared to our data. Therefore, these studies corroborate the strong bioactive potential of the zerumbone as anticariogenic agent, which could be a good substrate to be used in prophylactic and therapeutic formulations against tooth decay.

Indeed, zerumbone has been tested against a wide range of microorganisms and have showed good antibacterial activity, mainly against gram positive bacteria [36]. But, until now, there is no report describing the antimicrobial activity of the zerumbone or its analogs against *S. mutans*. Hasan et al. [37] demonstrated that extracts from *Zingiber officinale*, species that belongs to same genus and family of bitter ginger, has anti-*S. mutans* action with MIC value of 256 µg/mL, effect similar to the one observed in this study. However, unlike our study, no compound was isolated or purified to determine which biomolecules were responsible for the observed antimicrobial activity. Generally, the essential oil obtained from *Zingiber zerumbet* shows in its constitution a range of zerumbone concentration starting from 12 to 73% [8]. Nevertheless, the essential oil obtained in our study showed 87,93% of zerumbone, which was raised to 98% after purification and recrystallization process using a method patented by our group (n^0 PI-0505343-9/28/11/2007). This degree of purity is greater than the ones described elsewhere, which allow us to better characterize the zerumbone antimicrobial action [9].

Since zerumbone exhibited efficient antimicrobial activity, we next evaluated the speed of cidal activity. The effectiveness observed was concentration and time-dependent, although both concentrations tested showed similar results. The intensity of zerumbone antimicrobial activity was pronounced during the logarithmic growth phase. After 24 h of bacterial exposure to 250 and 500 µg/mL zerumbone concentrations, viable bacterial cells were reduced to 65.46 and 70.62%, respectively. According to Jones et al. [38] when an antimicrobial agent reduces the bacterial colonies around 70% within 24 h time period, it can be considered as a strong candidate for treating bacterial infections. However, the maximum cidal activity of zerumbone was reached at stationary phase, suggesting the possibility of two mechanism of zerumbone activity, different from

the most antibiotic agents that require cell division or active metabolism for the drug's killing activity [39, 40]. Thus, an antibiotic agent that still shows bactericidal activity under growth-limited conditions may be very advantageous, since the biofilm-associated microorganisms, such as *S. mutans*, may modulate gene expression to enhance endurance under periods of nutrient limitation to survive in the stationary phase [41]. However, further studies are needed to elucidate the antibacterial mechanism of action of zerumbone.

Beyond the determination of the optimum antibacterial concentration, it is also important to guarantee the cytotoxicity safety of the bioactive substances against normal mammalian cells, if the ultimate goal is to use it as a main raw material to produce new drugs. Usually, finding the balance between effectiveness and safety of a biomolecule is very hard mission [42, 43]. Our findings indicated that the zerumbone may not be cytotoxic to normal mammalian cells, since the exposure of Vero cells to different concentrations of zerumbone cause no considerable toxic effects at the concentrations tested. Even after 48 h of zerumbone treatment, no substantial toxic effect was observed, other than a low cytotoxicity evidenced at 100 µg/mL concentration (reduction of 13% of cell proliferation). However, it is imperative to consider that the susceptibility of mammalian cells tend to be greater in the MTT test than in vivo situation, because of the direct exposure of the cells to the biomolecules without any type of variants happening in vivo, such as route of administration and topical absorption, which may influence or even though decrease the cytotoxicity effect demonstrated in vitro [44]. On the other hand, it is important to mention that additional experiments are needed to ensure safe use of zerumbone for humans.

Altogether, this study demonstrates the antimicrobial activity of zerumbone against *S. mutans*, showing that its toxic activity selectively targets bacterium, but not displays any cytotoxic effect against the normal mammalian cells at concentrations tested. Nonetheless, further studies using in vitro and in vivo models are needed to better determine the zerumbone effectiveness and safety as antimicrobial agent in the context of prophylaxis and treatment of cariogenic infections.

Conclusions

In summary, this study suggests that zerumbone represents a bioactive substance to be explored by phytopharmaceutical industry in the drug formulations, to prevent and treat cariogenic infections, because this biomolecule showed antimicrobial activity against the main etiological agent of tooth decay, *S. mutans*. Although the cytotoxicity safety of zerumbone in mammalian cells (at concentrations tested) and its antibacterial action at both log and stationary phases support its potential use as antibacterial agent against *S. mutans* infection, additional studies are necessary to better characterize the zerumbone mechanism of action, efficacy and safety in the scenario of cariogenic disease.

Abbreviations
BHI: Brain heart infusion; CFU: Colony forming units; DMSO: Dimethyl sulfoxide; MBC: Mininum bactericidal concentration; MIC: Minimum inhibitory concentration; OD: optical density; RPM: Rotation per minute

Acknowledgements
We would like to express our sincere gratitude to the Thematic laboratory of Chemistry and Natural Products of National Institute of Amazonian Research to all support provided through the execution of this research.

Funding
This research was financially supported by Projects Financing Institution (FINEP) of Brazilian Innovation Agency (grant number 01140113.030071/13). The funder had no role in the design of this study, data collection and analysis, and in writing the manuscript.

Authors' contributions
TMS, PPO and GSP performed study design, carried out antimicrobial and cell culture experiments, analyzed and interpreted the data, and drafted and revised the manuscript. CCP and CDP performed GC-MS and HPLC analysis. GSP coordinated and supervised the study. All authors read and approved the final manuscript.

Author's information
TM Silva is a Master degree student at Amazonas State University. CD Pinheiro is master in Biotechnology. PP Orlandi is PhD in Science and associate researcher at Maria Deane institute-Fiocruz. CC Pinheiro is PhD in Chemistry and Titular Researcher at National Institute of Amazonian Research- INPA. GS Pontes is PhD in Medical Sciences and Associate Researcher at National Institute of Amazonian Research- INPA.

Competing interests
The authors declare that they have no competing interests.

Author details
[1]Instituto Nacional de Pesquisa da Amazônia, Coordenação de Tecnologia e Inovação, Av. André Araújo – 2936 – Petrópolis, Manaus, Amazonas 69067-375, Brazil. [2]Instituto Leônidas e Maria Deane, Fundação Oswaldo Cruz, Rua Teresina, 476 - Adrianópolis, Manaus, AM 69057-070, Brazil. [3]Instituto Nacional de Pesquisa da Amazônia, Coordenação Sociedade, Ambiente e Saúde, Av. André Araújo – 2936 – Petrópolis, Manaus 69067-375, Amazonas, Brazil.

References
1. Sadaka F. Nguimjeu C. Vroman I, Tighzert L, Couvercelle JP. Review on antimicrobial packaging containing essential oils and their active biomolecules. Innov. Food Sci. Emerg. Technol: Brachais CH; 2014.
2. Zakaria ZA, Yob NJ, Jofrry SM, MMRMM A, Teh LK, Salleh MZ. Zingiber zerumbet (L.) Smith: A review of its ethnomedicinal, chemical, and pharmacological uses. Evidence-based Complement. Altern Med. 2011;2011:1-12
3. Fakurazi S, Hairuszah I, Mohd Lip J, Shanthi G, Nanthini U, Shamima AR, et al. Hepatoprotective action of zerumbone against paracetamol induced hepatotoxicity. J Med Sci. 2009;9:161–4.
4. Abdel Wahab SI, Abdul AB, Alzubairi AS, Mohamed Elhassan M, Mohan S. In vitro ultramorphological assessment of apoptosis induced by Zerumbone on (HeLa). J Biomed Biotechnol. 2009;2009.
5. Sulaiman MR, Tengku Mohamad TA, Shaik Mossadeq WM, Moin S, Yusof M, Mokhtar AF, et al. Antinociceptive activity of the essential oil of Zingiber zerumbet. Planta med. 2010;76:107–12. Available from: https://doi.org/10.1055/s-0029-1185950.
6. Somchit MN. Zerumbone isolated from *Zingiber zerumbet* inhibits inflammation and pain in rats. J Med Plants Res. [Internet]. 2012;6:753–57. Available from: https://doi.org/10.5897/JMPR10.492.
7. Sidahmed HMA, Hashim NM, Abdulla MA, Ali HM, Mohan S, Abdelwahab SI, et al. Antisecretory, gastroprotective, antioxidant and anti-helicobcter pylori activity of zerumbone from *Zingiber zerumbet* (L.) smith. PLoS One. 2015; 10(3):1–20
8. Baby S, Dan M, Thaha ARM, Johnson AJ, Kurup R, Balakrishnapillaia P, et al. High content of zerumbone in volatile oils of Zingiber zerumbet from southern India and Malaysia. Flavour Fragr J. 2009;24:301–8. Available from: https://doi.org/10.1002/ffj.1940.
9. Rahman HS, Rasedee A, Yeap SK, Othman HH, Chartrand MS, Namvar F, et al. Biomedical properties of a natural dietary plant metabolite, Zerumbone, in cancer therapy and chemoprevention trials. Biomed Res Int. 2014;2014:1–20.
10. Adbul ABH, Al-Zubairi AS, Tailan ND, Wahab SIA, Zain ZNM, Rusley S, et al. Anticancer activity of natural compound (Zerumbone) extracted from Zingiber zerumbet in human HeLa cervical cancer cells. Int J Pharmacol. 2008;4:160–8.
11. Liu WY, Tzeng T-F, Liu I-M. Healing potential of zerumbone ointment on experimental full-thickness excision cutaneous wounds in rat. J. Tissue Viability, Elsevier Ltd. 2017. p. 6–11. Available from: https://doi.org/10.1016/j.jtv.2017.04.002.
12. Petersen PE. Strengthening of Oral health systems. Oral health through primary health care. Med Princ Pract. 2014;23:1–7. Available from: https://doi.org/10.1159/000356937.
13. Bradshaw DJ, Lynch RJM. Diet and the microbial aetiology of dental caries: new paradigms. Int dent J. 2013;63(Suppl 2):64–72. Available from: https://doi.org/10.1111/idj.12082.
14. Lynch DJ, Michalek SM, Zhu M, Drake D, Qian F, Banas JA. Cariogenicity of Streptococcus mutans glucan-binding protein deletion mutants. Oral Health Dent Manag. [Internet]. 2013;109:191–9. Available from: http://www.ncbi.nlm.nih.gov/pubmed/24525450.
15. Baehni PC, Takeuchi Y. Anti-plaque agents in the prevention of biofilm-associated oral diseases. Oral Dis. 2003;9(Suppl 1):23–9.
16. Palombo EA. Traditional Medicinal Plant Extracts and Natural Products with Activity against Oral Bacteria: Potential Application in the Prevention and Treatment of Oral Diseases. Evid Based Complement Alternat Med. [Internet]. 2011;2011:680354. Available from: https://doi.org/10.1093/ecam/nep067.
17. Gong HY, Liu WH, GY LV, Zhou X. Analysis of essential oils of Origanum vulgare from six production areas of China and Pakistan. Brazilian J Pharmacogn. 2014;24:25–32.
18. Ben El Hadj Ali I, Chaouachi M, Bahri R, Chaieb I, Boussaïd M, Harzallah-Skhiri F. Chemical composition and antioxidant, antibacterial, allelopathic and insecticidal activities of essential oil of Thymus algeriensis Boiss. et Reut. Ind Crops Prod. 2015;77:631–9. Available from: https://doi.org/10.1016/j.indcrop.2015.09.046.
19. Adams R. Identification of Essential Oil Components by Gas Chromatography / Mass Spectrometry. Identif. Essent. Oil Components by Gas Chromatogr. / Mass Spectrom. 1995;5.
20. TIB.2033, REV C. Conditions S. Microorganism Maintenance Plan for Laboratories Following ISO 11133. 2014;1–2.
21. Kumar SN, Lankalapalli RS, Kumar BSD. In vitro antibacterial screening of six proline-based cyclic dipeptides in combination with ??-lactam antibiotics

against medically important bacteria. Appl Biochem Biotechnol. 2014;173: 116–28.

22. CLSI. M45-A2 Methods for Antimicrobial Dilution and Disk Susceptibility Testing of Infrequently Isolated or Fastidious Bacteria ; Approved Guideline — 2nd edn. 2010.

23. Sutton S. Accuracy of plate counts. J Valid Technol. 2011;17:42–6.

24. Sartoratto A, Machado ALM, Delarmelina C, Figueira GM, Duarte MCT, Rehder VLG. Composition and antimicrobial activity of essential oils from aromatic plants used in Brazil. Brazilian J Microbiol. 2004;35:275–80.

25. Friedman PK, Kaufman LB, Karpas SL. Oral health disparity in older adults. Dental decay and tooth loss. Dent Clin North Am. 2014;58(4):757–70.

26. Muts E-J, van Pelt H, Edelhoff D, Krejci I, Cune M. Tooth wear: a systematic review of treatment options. J Prosthet Dent. 2014;112:752–e9. Available from: https://doi.org/10.1016/j.prosdent.2014.01.018.

27. Webster D, Taschereau P, Belland RJ, Sand C, Rennie RP. Antifungal activity of medicinal plant extracts; preliminary screening studies. J Ethnopharmacol. 2008;140–6. Available from: https://doi.org/10.1016/j.jep.2007.09.014.

28. Bagramian RA, Garcia-Godoy F, Volpe AR. The global increase in dental caries. A pending public health crisis. Am. J. Dent. 2009;22:3–8.

29. Kassebaum NJ, Bernabe E, Dahiya M, Bhandari B, Murray CJ, Marcenes W. Global burden of untreated caries: a systematic review and metaregression. J Dent Res. 2015;94:650–8. Available from: https://doi.org/10.1177/0022034515573272.

30. Porto TS, Rangel R, Furtado NAJC, De Carvalho TC, Martins CHG, Veneziani RCS, et al. Pimarane-type diterpenes: antimicrobial activity against oral pathogens. Molecules. 2009;14:191–9.

31. Saleem M, Nazir M, Ali MS, Hussain H, Lee YS, Riaz N, et al. Antimicrobial natural products: an update on future antibiotic drug candidates. Nat Prod Rep [Internet]. 2010;27:238–54 Available from: https://doi.org/10.1039/B916096E.

32. da Silva JPC, de Castilho AL, Saraceni CHC, Díaz IEC, Paciencia MLB, Suffredini IB. Anti-streptococcal activity of Brazilian Amazon rain Forest plant extracts presents potential for preventive strategies against dental caries. J Appl Oral Sci Rev FOB. 2014;22:91–7.

33. Freire ICM, P??rez ALAL, Cardoso AMR, Mariz BALA, Almeida LFD, Cavalcanti YW, et al. Atividade antibacteriana de ??leos essenciais sobre Streptococcus mutans e Staphylococcus aureus. Rev Bras Plantas Med 2014;16:372–377.

34. Takarada K, Kimizuka R, Takahashi N, Honma K, Okuda K, Kato T. A comparison of the antibacterial efficacies of essential oils against oral pathogens. Oral Microbiol Immunol. 2004;19:61–4.

35. Aguiar GP, Carvalho CE, Dias HJ, Reis EB, Martins MHG, Wakabayashi KAL, et al. Antimicrobial activity of selected essential oils against cariogenic bacteria. Nat Prod Res. 2013;27:1668–72. Available from: https://doi.org/10.1080/14786419.2012.751595.

36. Santosh Kumar SC, Srinivas P, Negi PS, Bettadaiah BK. Antibacterial and antimutagenic activities of novel zerumbone analogues. Food Chem. 2013; 141:1097–103.

37. Hasan S, Danisuddin M, Khan AU. Inhibitory effect of Zingiber officinale towards Streptococcus mutans virulence and caries development: in vitro and in vivo studies. BMC Microbiol. 2015;15:1–14. Available from: https://doi.org/10.1186/s12866-014-0320-5.

38. Jones RN, Anderegg TR, Deshpande LM. AZD2563, a new oxazolidinone: bactericidal activity and synergy studies combined with gentamicin or vancomycin against staphylococci and streptococcal strains. Diagn Microbiol Infect Dis. 2002;43:87–90.

39. Anderl JN, Zahller J, Roe F, Stewart PS. Role of nutrient limitation and stationary-phase existence in Klebsiella pneumoniae biofilm resistance to ampicillin and ciprofloxacin. Antimicrob Agents Chemother. 2003;47:1251–6.

40. Gradelski E, Kolek B, Bonner D, Fung-Tomc J. Bactericidal mechanism of gatifloxacin compared with other quinolones. J Antimicrob Chemother. 2002;49:185–8. Available from: http://jac.oxfordjournals.org/content/49/1/185%5C.

41. Nascimento MM, Lemos JA, Abranches J, Lin VK, Burne RA. Role of RelA of Streptococcus mutans in global control of gene expression. J Bacteriol. 2008;190:28–36.

42. Waller SB, Madrid IM, Ferraz V, Picoli T, Cleff MB, de Faria RO, et al. Cytotoxicity and anti-Sporothrix brasiliensis activity of the Origanum majorana Linn. Oil. Brazilian J. Microbiol. 2016;47:896–901.

43. Lei J, Yu J, Yu H, Liao Z. Composition, cytotoxicity and antimicrobial activity of essential oil from Dictamnus dasycarpus. Food Chem. 2008;107:1205–9.

44. Fallis A. Manual de toxicologia. J Chem Inf Model. 2013.

21

Epimedium sagittatum inhibits TLR4/MD-2 mediated NF-κB signaling pathway with anti-inflammatory activity

Ni Yan[1], Ding-Sheng Wen[2], Yue-Rui Zhao[1] and Shun-Jun Xu[1,3*]

Abstract

Background: *Epimedium sagittatum* (Sieb.et Zucc.) Maxim., *Ying-Yang-Huo* in Chinese has been used as a traditional Chinese medicine and is deemed to "reinforce the kidney *Yang*". Previous studies showed that *E. sagittatum* could modulate the immune system and treat some chronic disease such as rheumatic arthritis, cardiovascular diseases and osteoporosis. The aim of this study is to evaluate the anti-inflammatory effects of ethyl acetate extracts (YYHs) of *E. sagittatum* and its mechanisms of action.

Methods: In order to explore the composition of YYHs, YYHs was analyzed using high performance liquid chromatography-mass spectrometry-mass spectrometry (HPLC-MS/MS) and in comparison with reference standards. Anti-inflammatory model was established in LPS-induced RAW264.7 cells. The levels of nitric oxide (NO) were measured with the Griess reagent. Production of tumor necrosis factor-alpha (TNF-α) and interleukin-2 (IL-2) were measured by enzyme-linked immunosorbent assays (ELISA). In addition, expression of p-p65 protein and TLR4/MD-2 complex was detected by western blots and flow cytometric, respectively. Nuclear factor kappa B (NF-κB) nuclear translocation was observed by fluorescence microscope.

Results: A total of eight compounds were identified, of which icariside II was the most abundant compound. YYHs (12.5–50 μg/mL) had no obvious cytotoxic effect on cells, and remarkably inhibited LPS-induced production of NO, TNF-α and IL-2 with a dose-dependent manner. Additionally, YYHs up-regulated expression of p-p65 and TLR4/MD-2 complex. Further research showed that YYHs significantly suppressed NF-κB p65 nuclear translocation.

Conclusion: In brief, YYHs contributed to the inhibition of LPS-induced inflammatory response through the TLR4/MD-2-mediated NF-κB pathway and may be a potential choice to combat inflammation diseases.

Abstract graph: It includes a schema of pathways at the end of the paper.

Keywords: *E, sagittatum*, Anti-inflammation, TLR4/MD-2, NF-κB

Background

Inflammation acts physiologically to protect normal host function after pathogen invasion or tissue damage [1]. As a major virulence factor of Gram-negative bacteria, LPS induces a serious systemic inflammatory response in macrophage [2]. TLR4 plays a key role for innate immune responses and its signaling is triggered by the transfer of its ligand LPS to a Toll-like receptor 4 /myeloid differentiation factor-2 (TLR4/MD-2) complex, which then undergoes homodimerization [3]. Thus, the TLR4/MD-2 complex constitute the indispensable components of the LPS receptor system and have been implicated in inflammation. Binding of the TLR4/MD-2 complex to LPS triggers the activation of JNK and NF-κB signaling pathway [4]. During inflammatory processes, LPS stimulates the production of the pro-inflammatory cytokines and inflammation mediators, such as TNF-α, IL-2 and nitric oxide (NO). However, inflammation persistently produces pro-inflammatory cytokines and inflammatory mediators that eventually evolves into excess inflammation, which is closely associated with many diseases including cancer [5], Alzheimer's disease [6],

* Correspondence: shjxu2002@hotmail.com
[1]Department of Research and Development, ImVin Pharmaceutical Co., Ltd, 2 Fangcaodian Road, Guangzhou 510663, China
[3]Zhuhai Jizhu Small and Medium Enterprises Advanced Technology Research Institute, Zhuhai College of Jilin University, Zhuhai 519041, China
Full list of author information is available at the end of the article

obesity and diabetes [7]. In addition, extensive studies supported that anti-inflammatory therapy is efficacious to slow the progression and delay the onset of these disease.

Nuclear factor-κB (NF-κB) is a transcription factor that is essential for inflammation, immunity, cell proliferation and apoptosis [8]. There are two NF-κB signaling pathway including the classical and the alternative pathway, of which the classical attracts more attention. The classical pathway of NF-κB is triggered by pro-inflammatory cytokines and LPS. Subsequently, inhibitory protein IκB-α and p65 are phosphorylated, meanwhile, inhibitory molecule is degraded by proteasome-mediated. Then, the heterodimer p50/p65 is released and migrats from the cytoplasm to the nucleus to regulate the expression of multiple target genes, such as TNF-α, IL-6, iNOS and so on [9, 10].

Epimedium sagittatum (Sieb.et Zucc.) Maxim., a tranditional herbal drug in China, widely grows in Guangdong, Guangxi and Jiangxi province. And it contains flavonoids, lignans and so forth. Specially, major secondary metabolites of *E. sagittatum*, in which mainly includes epimedin A, B, C and icariin [11]. Species of Epimedium have four members according to the Chinese Pharmacopoeia, they are *E. brevicornu* Maxim., *E. sagittatum* (Sieb.et Zucc.) Maxim., *E. pubescens* Maxim. and *E. koreanum* Nakai [12]. Previous studies showed that the species of Epimedium exhibited many bioactivities, such as antiviral [13], antinociceptive [14], anti-aging [15], antioxidant, neurotective effect [16], enhancing immunity [17] and promoting estrogen biosynthesis [18]. However, there are few reports about the biological activity of *E. sagittatum*, especially in terms of anti-inflammatory.

The objective of this study is to analyze constituent and evaluate the anti-inflammatory activity of YYHs by LPS stimulated RAW 264.7 cells model. Besides, we tried to explore the anti-inflammation mechanism via the TLR4/MD-2-mediated NF-κB signaling pathway.

Methods
Preparation of extract
The dried material was from Guangdong province and provided by ImVin Pharmaceutical Co., Ltd. (Guangzhou, China). The authentication of plant materials was finished by professor Dingping (Guangzhou University of Chinese Medicine). At first, the herb of YYH was powdered and heat extracted three times with 10-fold of 50% ethanol at 70 °C for 25 min. After cooling, the solution was filtered and removed ethanol, followed by separations with ethyl acetate ($v/v = 1:1$). The YYH extracted ethyl acetate fraction was concentrated by rotary evaporation (EYELA, Japan) and stored at − 20 °C before use.

Chemicals and reagents
3-(4,5-dimethylthiazol-2-yl)-2,5-diphenyltetrazoliumbromide (MTT), Griess reagent and bacterial lipopolysaccharide (LPS) were acquired from Sigma Chemical Co. (St Louis, MO, USA). Fetal bovine serum (FBS) was purchased from Life Technologies (Auckland, New Zealand). Dulbecco's Modified Eagle's Medium (DMEM), Penicillin-streptomycin solution, Dulbecco's Phosphate Buffered Saline (DPBS), GlutaMAX™-1 and 0.25% Trypsin-EDTA were obtained from Hyclone (Logan, Utah, USA). PE-conjugated rat anti-mouse TLR4/MD-2 complex (clone MTS510) and rat IgG2a kappa isotype control antibodys were products of eBioscience (San Diego, CA, USA). Mouse TNF-α and IL-2 ELISA kits were acquired from Neobioscience Technology Co., Ltd. (Beijing, China). NF-κB Activation −Nuclear Translocation Assay kit from Beyotime Institute of Biotechnology (Nanjing, China). Rabbit phospho-NF-κB (Ser536) antibody and rabbit NF-κB p65 (C22B4) antibody from Cell Signaling Technology (Danvers, MA) were also obtained. Epimedin C and icariin were provided by the National Institute for Food and Drug Control (Beijing, China). Epimedin B was purchased from Herbest (Baoji, China). Baohuoside II and Baohuoside VII were obtained from Chem Faces (Wuhan, China). All standards had a purity of 98%.

HPLC and LC-MS/MS conditions
Chromatographic separation (Agilent 1100 HPLC system) was achieved on an Agilent Zorbax SB-C18 column (250 × 4.6 mm, 5 μm). The mobile phase consisted of acetonitrile as solvent A, methanol as solvent B and 0.5% acetic acid in water as solvent C. The gradient of mobile phase was shown in Table 1. The flow rate was 1 mL/min, and the column temperature was set at 20 °C. The diode-array detection was set to monitor at 270 nm. The mass spectrometry analysis was performed on a LTQ-Orbitrap XL mass spectrometer (Thermo Electron, Bremen, Germany) coupled with an ESI source, and used with the following conditions: source temperature: 350 °C; ion spray voltage - 4.5 kV; Gas 1, Gas 2,curtain gas, and collision gas (nitrogen) were separately set at 50, 50, 45, and 12 psi; sheath gas flow rate, 40 arbitrary units; auxiliary gas flow rate, 5 arbitrary units; electrospray voltage, 3.5 kV; capillary voltage, -32 V; capillary temperature, 270 °C.

Table 1 Mobile phase condition of chromatographic separation

Time (min)	Acetonitrile (%)	Methanol (%)	0.5% acetic acid in water (%)
0–30	12–25	0	88–75
30–45	25–23.5	0–11	75–65.5
45–68	23.5–35	11–4	65.5–61
68–85	35	4	61
85–90	35–50	4–0	61–50
90–95	100	0	0
95–110	100	0	0

Cell culture and viability assay

RAW 264.7 cells were obtained from American Type Culture Collection (Manassas, VA, USA) and cultured in DMEM which was supplemented with 10% FBS, 1% penicillin-streptomycin solution and 1% GlutaMAX™-1 at 37 °C in a humidified incubator containing 5% CO_2. Cells were seeded in 96-well plates at a density of 1×10^5 cells/mL and incubated for 24 h. They treated with different concentrations of YYHs (12.5, 25, 50, 75 μg/mL) in the absence or presence of 1 μg/mL LPS for 24 h, respectively. Then, 50 μL MTT solution (0.5 mg/mL in DPBS) was added to plates and incubated for 4 h in the incubator. After incubation finished, the supernatants was discarded and replaced with DMSO (200 μL) to dissolve the formazan crystal. The absorbance of each well was detected at 570 nm using a microplate reader (BERTHOLD Technologies, Germany).

Nitric oxide (NO) and enzyme-linked immunosorbent assay

To assay the production of NO, IL-2 and TNF-α, the supernatant of RAW 264.7 cells was collected after co-treated with YYHs (12.5, 25, 50 μg/mL) and LPS (1 μg/mL) for 24 h. The IL-2 and TNF-α were determined using enzyme-linked immunosorbent assay kits according to the manufacturer's instructions. Meanwhile, the NO production was determined by mixing 100 μL of the supernatant with an equal volume of Griess reagent comprising 50 μL of 2% sulfanilamide in 4% phosphoric acid and 50 μL of 0.2% N-(1-naphthyl) -ethylenediamine dihydrochloride in water for 10 min at room temperature, and the concentration of nitrite was determined by using a standard curve generated with sodium nitrite under a spectrophotometer on a wavelength of 550 nm.

Flow cytometric analysis

RAW 264.7 cells treated with YYH extracts (12.5, 25 and 50 μg/mL) and LPS (1 μg/mL) for 18 h were harvested with 0.25% trypsin and washed with PBS by centrifugation for 5 min. Subsequently, cells were incubated with a PE-conjugated anti-mouse TLR4/MD-2 complex antibody and FITC-conjucted anti-mouse CD14 or PE/FITC-conjugated IgG as isotype control for 30 min at 4 °C, respectively. The cell surface makers expression was analyzed by Attune acoustic focusing cytometer (Thermo Fisher Scientific, USA). The data of MFI value were calculated the levels of fluorescence by Flow Jo software (FlowJo LLC, USA).

Nuclear factor-κB (NF-κB) nuclear translocation assay

The activation of NF-κB nuclear translocation was detected by using NF-κB activation nuclear translocation assay kit according to the manufacturer's protocol. Briefly, cells were pretreated YYHs (50 μg/mL) for 1 h prior to incubation with LPS for another 1 h, together. After fixing and permeabilizing, the cells were incubated with a blocking solution for 1 h, followed by NF-κB p65 antibody at 4 °C overnight. Next, after washing three times, cells incubated with a Cy3-conjugated secondary antibody for 1 h, then with DAPI for 5 min before observation. The activation of NF-κB p65 was visualized with a fluorescence microscope (Axiovert 40 CFL, Carl Zeiss) at excitation wavelength of 350 nm for DAPI and 540 nm for Cy3, and the red and blue images were overlaid by Image-pro plus 5.1 software to indicated the areas of co-localization.

Western blot assay

RAW 264.7 cells (7.5×10^5 cells/mL) were seeded in 6-well plates for 24 h. Then, cells orderly incubated with YYHs (2 h) and LPS (1 h). The total proteins, extracted with cell lysis buffer (RIPA:PMSF: Phosphatase inhibitor = 100:1:1) by ultrasonic, were quantified using a BCA protein assay kit. An equal amount of protein (25μg) was separated on 10% SDS-PAGE for electrophoresis, followed by transfer to PVDF membranes. Then, the membranes were severally blocked with 5% non-fat milk or 5% BSA for 1 h and then incubated with primary antibodies (1:1000 dilution) overnight at 4 °C. The following day, membranes were incubated with a horseradish peroxidase-conjugated goat anti-rabbit antibody (1:1000 dilution) for 2 h and detected by enhanced chemiluminescence (ECL). Protein levels were normalized against included β-actin standards and analyzed by Image J software.

Statistical analysis

All experiments were performed at least three times and expressed as mean ± standard deviation (S.D). The differences between groups were analyzed by one-way ANOVA, followed by a Tukey's test using SPSS 20.0 software (SPSS Inc., Chicago, USA). P value of 0.05 or less was considered as statistically significant.

Results

Measurement of major compounds of YYHs

A total of eight chromatographic peaks were identified five of which were assigned by comparison with reference standards, three of which were characterized based on their chromatographic behavior and MS/MS fragmentation pattern. As shown in Fig. 1 and Table 2, sagittatoside B ($[M-H]^-$ m/z at 645.21472; error ppm = 4.746), 2″-O-rhamnosyl icariside II ($[M-H]^-$ m/z at 659.23071; error ppm = 4.129) and icariside II ($[M-H]^-$ m/z at 513.17407; error ppm = 2.832) were detected by LC-MS/MS. Epimedoside C, icariin, icariside II and 2″-O-rhamnosyl Icariside II were the major compounds of YYHs, which were 9.59, 18.89, 30.94 and 7.97%, respectively.

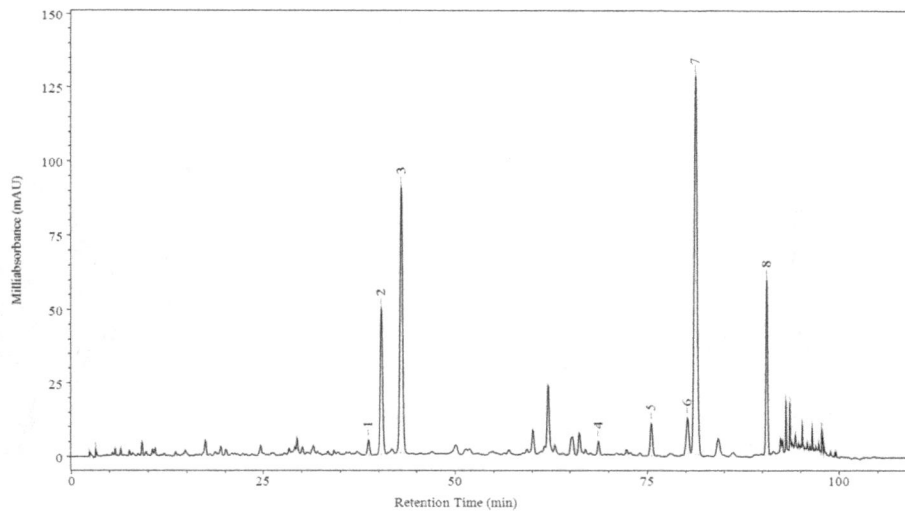

Fig. 1 Representative HPLC chromatogram of YYHs at 270 nm

Cytotoxicity of YYHs on viability of cells

The MTT assay was carried out to estimate the cytotoxicity of YYHs on RAW 264.7 cells. As the results shown in Fig. 2, the presence of LPS (1 μg/mL) had no impact on cell viability, expectedly. Then, exposure of cells to (12.5–50 μg/mL) YYHs with 1 μg/mL LPS for 24 h showed no cytotoxicity. However, when the cells were treated with 75 μg/mL YYHs and 1 μg/mL LPS, the cell viability was less than 50%. Therefore, all subsequent experiments were performed at nontoxic concentrations (12.5–50 μg/mL).

Effect of YYHs on levels of NO, TNF-α and IL-2

We first investigated the anti-inflammatory activity of YYHs. Treatment of LPS for 24 h can lead to inflammatory response on RAW 264.7. During inflammation, a large amount of NO and pro-inflammatory cytokines including TNF-α and IL-2 were generated. YYHs at dose of 50 μg/mL significantly

decreased the levels of TNF-α and IL-2 with inhibition values of $50.89 \pm 3.55\%$ and $55.38 \pm 7.60\%$ (Fig. 3A, B). Furthermore, YYHs concentration-dependently suppressed the production of NO (Fig. 3C).

Effect of YYHs on cell surface of TLR4/MD-2 complex in cells

The TLR4/MD-2 complex was critical for LPS recognition and innate immune response. To assess the effect of YYHs on the formation of TLR4/MD-2 complex, we detected the expression of the complex by flow cytometry. As shown in Fig. 4, The plenty of TLR4/MD-2 complex were formed after LPS stimulated cells, and treatment of

Table 2 The main components of YYHs

Peak	Retention time (min)	Component	Concentration (%)
1[a]	38.664	Epimedoside B	0.90
2[a]	40.376	Epimedoside C	9.59
3[a]	42.963	Icariin	18.89
4[a]	68.647	Baohuoside II	0.70
5[a]	75.499	Baohuoside VII	2.07
6	80.248	Sagittatoside B	2.94
7	81.308	2"-O-Rhamnosy (Icariside II)	30.94
8	90.552	Icariside II	7.97

(1–5) [a] were assigned by comparison with reference standards. (6–8) were identified by MS/MS

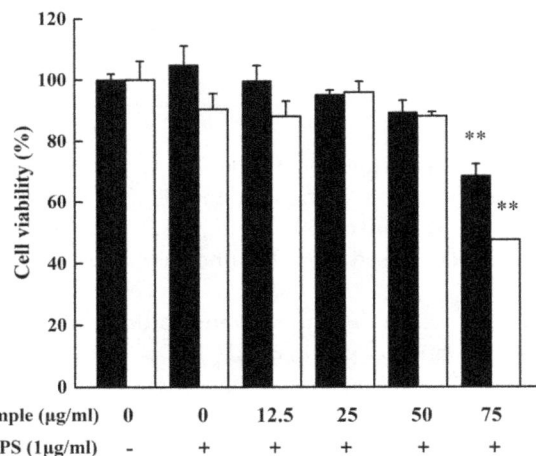

Fig. 2 Cytotoxicity of YYHs on RAW 264.7 cells. Cells were treated in the presence of YYHs or in combination with LPS (1 μg/mL) for 24 h. Cell viability was determined by MTT assay (black bar, YYHs treated; white bar, YYHs+LPS treated). Compared with the control, [#]$P < 0.05$, [##]$P < 0.01$. Compared with LPS group, [*]$P < 0.05$, [**]$P < 0.01$

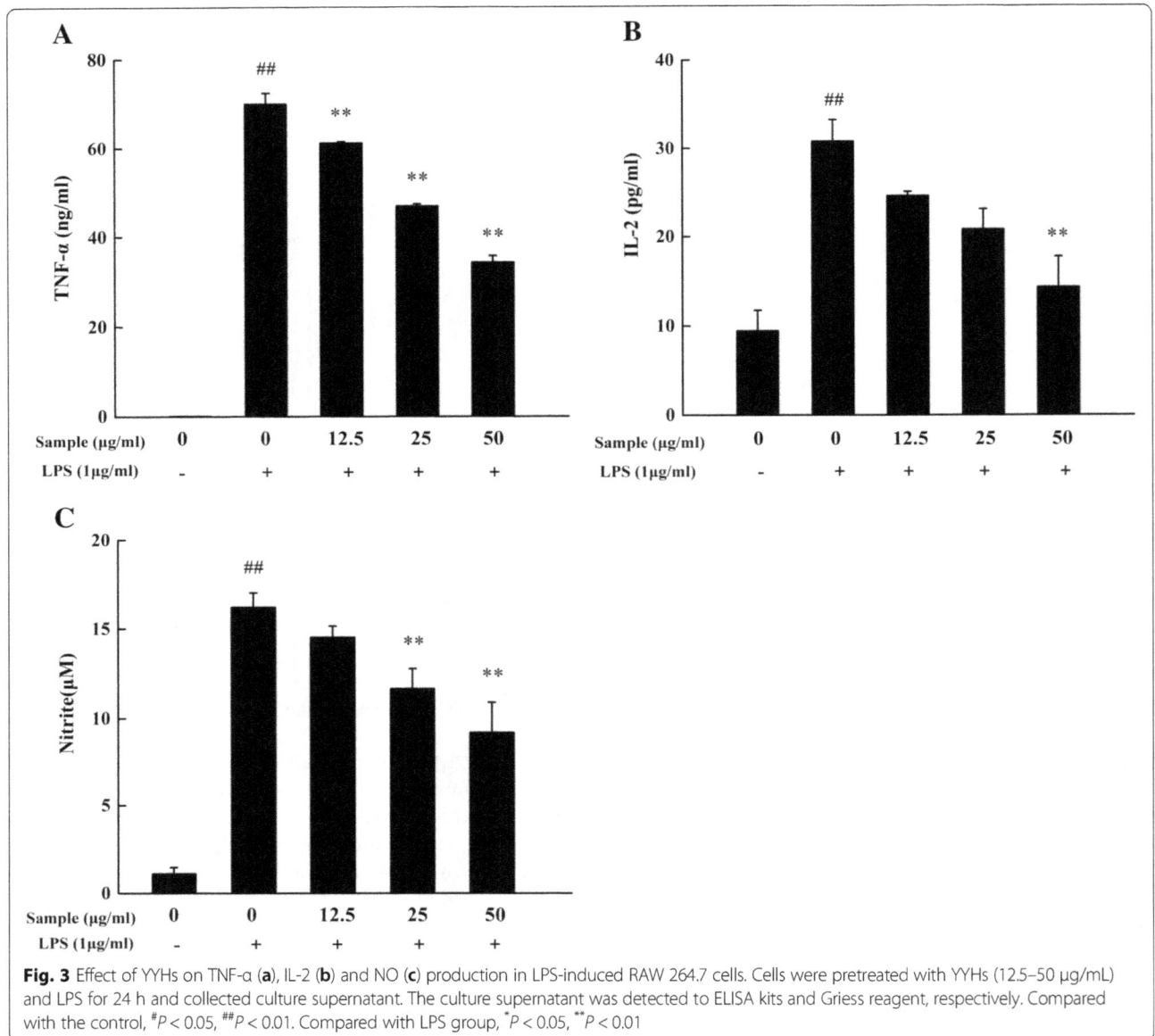

Fig. 3 Effect of YYHs on TNF-α (**a**), IL-2 (**b**) and NO (**c**) production in LPS-induced RAW 264.7 cells. Cells were pretreated with YYHs (12.5–50 μg/mL) and LPS for 24 h and collected culture supernatant. The culture supernatant was detected to ELISA kits and Griess reagent, respectively. Compared with the control, [#]$P < 0.05$, [##]$P < 0.01$. Compared with LPS group, [*]$P < 0.05$, [**]$P < 0.01$

YYHs can interrupt the formation of the TLR4/MD-2 complex in a concentration-dependent manner. When the concentration of 50 μg/mL, TLR4/MD-2 complex obviously decreased more than half as LPS group.

Effect of YYHs on the nuclear translocation and phosphorylation of p65 in cells

As an important upstream transcription factor, NF-κB regulated expression of NO and .pro-inflammatory cytokines by LPS stimulation. Translocation of NF-κB p65 into the nucleus were increased within 1 h after LPS stimulation, as compared with control groups (Fig. 5). However, pre-treatment with YYHs (50 μg/mL) for 1 h markedly suppressed NF-κB p65 levels in the nucleus. Meanwhile, we explored the effect of YYHs on LPS induced NF-κB

p65 phosphorylation by western blot analysis. Compared to the unstimulated cells, LPS expectedly induced phosphorylation of p65. Treatment with different concentration of YYHs attenuated phosphorylation of p65 in a dose-dependent manner (Fig. 6). These results strongly suggested that YYHs down-regulated the LPS–induced phosphorylation of p65.

Discussion

Traditionally, the leaves of *E*pimedium had long been used as a kidney tonic and antirheumatic for more than 2000 years [19]. In recent years, it was also used to treat various diseases, such as parkinson's disease [20], rheumatic arthritis [21], osteoporosis [22, 23] and asthma [24]. Virtually, most of the attention focused on *E. brevicornu*

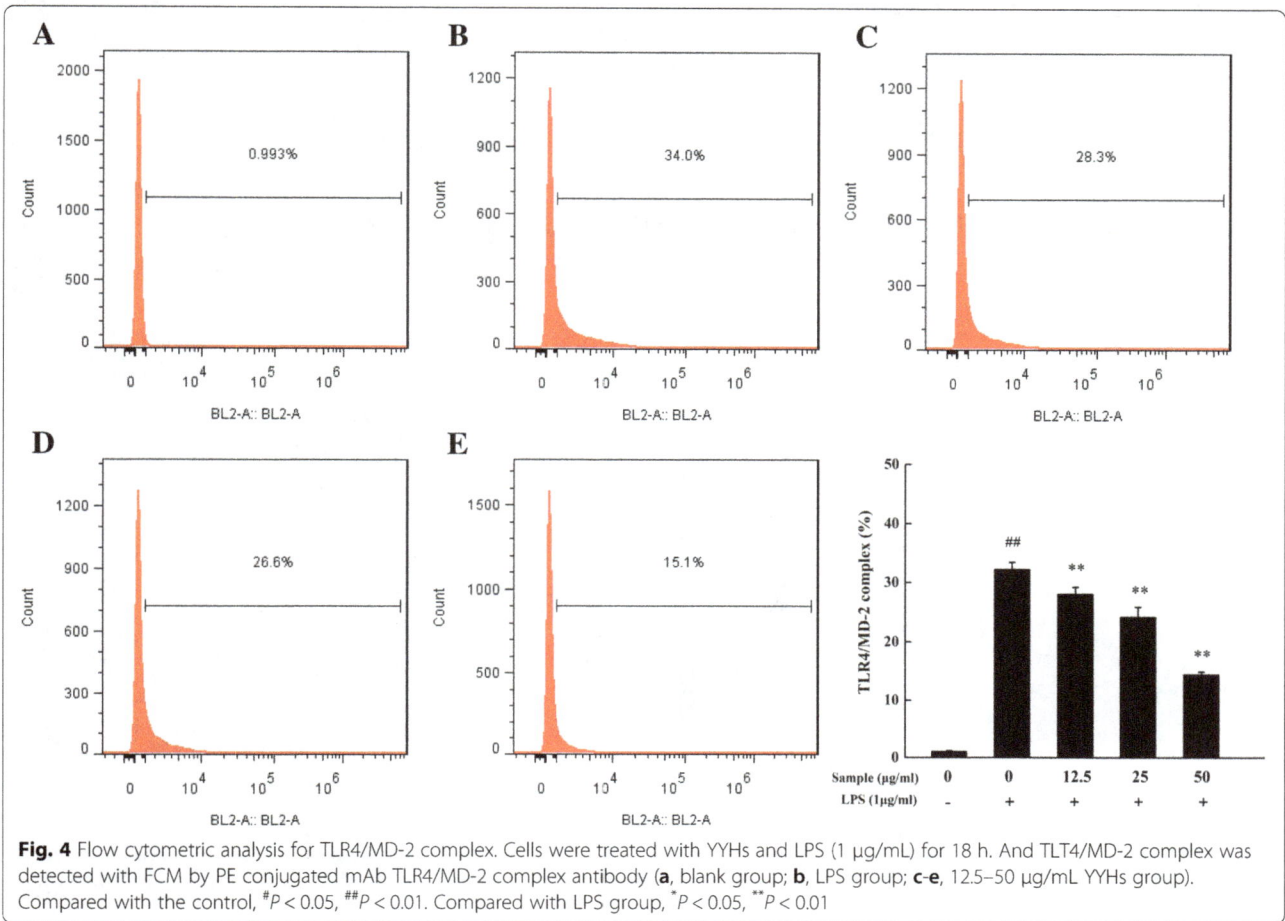

Fig. 4 Flow cytometric analysis for TLR4/MD-2 complex. Cells were treated with YYHs and LPS (1 µg/mL) for 18 h. And TLT4/MD-2 complex was detected with FCM by PE conjugated mAb TLR4/MD-2 complex antibody (**a**, blank group; **b**, LPS group; **c-e**, 12.5–50 µg/mL YYHs group). Compared with the control, #$P < 0.05$, ##$P < 0.01$. Compared with LPS group, *$P < 0.05$, **$P < 0.01$

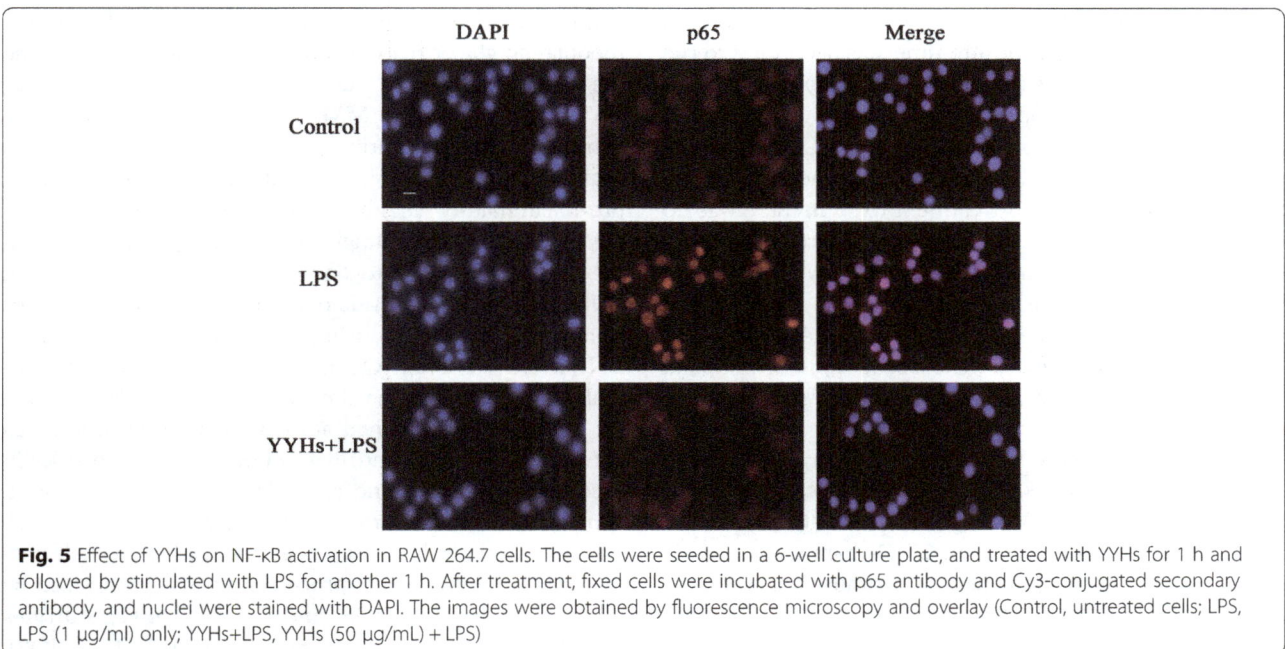

Fig. 5 Effect of YYHs on NF-κB activation in RAW 264.7 cells. The cells were seeded in a 6-well culture plate, and treated with YYHs for 1 h and followed by stimulated with LPS for another 1 h. After treatment, fixed cells were incubated with p65 antibody and Cy3-conjugated secondary antibody, and nuclei were stained with DAPI. The images were obtained by fluorescence microscopy and overlay (Control, untreated cells; LPS, LPS (1 µg/ml) only; YYHs+LPS, YYHs (50 µg/mL) + LPS)

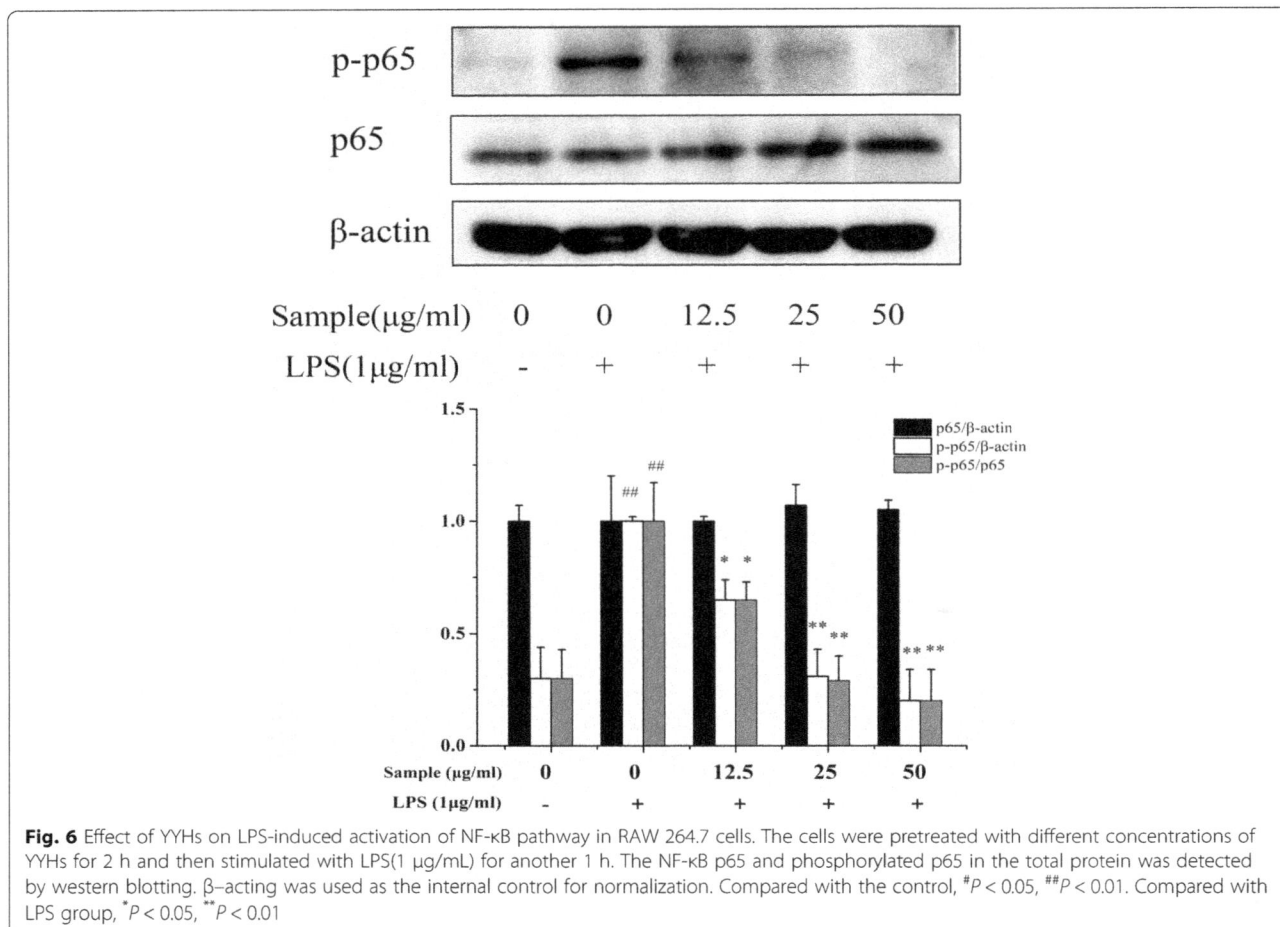

Fig. 6 Effect of YYHs on LPS-induced activation of NF-κB pathway in RAW 264.7 cells. The cells were pretreated with different concentrations of YYHs for 2 h and then stimulated with LPS(1 μg/mL) for another 1 h. The NF-κB p65 and phosphorylated p65 in the total protein was detected by western blotting. β–acting was used as the internal control for normalization. Compared with the control, #$P < 0.05$, ##$P < 0.01$. Compared with LPS group, *$P < 0.05$, **$P < 0.01$

Maxim and *E. koreanum* Nakai. In this study, Enzyme-linked immunosorbent assay, flow cytometric analysis and western blot assay which were performed under different YYHs exposure time was according to the references described as previous [4, 25]. However, it was found that a small proportion of the cells in the 6-well plate were shed 24 h post stimulated with LPS under the premise of the same cell plating density, when shortening the stimulation time of co-treatment to 18 h, there was no sheding of cells. So we the exposure different time was employed in assays. Finally, the results showed YYHs distinctly decreased production of NO, TNF-α and IL-2, and markedly suppressed the expression of TLR4/MD-2 complex and NF-κB p65 nuclear translocation, which implied YYHs had anti-inflammatory activity on LPS-induced inflammatory responses.

In our study, YYHs were detected by HPLC system. Among the components, 2″-O-rhamnosyl icariside II was the richest component (30.94%) in ethyl acetate fraction. As a prenylated flavonol glycosides, 2″-O-rhamnosyl icariside II was isolated from Epimedium koreanum Nakai for the first time in 1991 [26]. Additionally, icariin (18.89%), epimedoside C (9.59%) and icariside II (7.97%) are relatively

abundant in the extracts, and it is known to all that those were some major bioactive components in Herba Epimedii. Icariin exerted its anti-inflammatory effect mainly through modulating glucocorticoid receptor function and inhibiting the pro-inflammatory transcription factors including TNF-α, IL-6, IL-8 and MMP-9 [27, 28]. Previous studies demonstrated that icariin protected dopamine neurons against neurotoxins-induced neurotoxicity and inhibited pro-inflammatory factors production via the NF-κB signaling pathway, in which might be compactly associated with the inhibition of microglia-mediated neuroinflammation [29]. Furthermore, Icariside II also possibly suppressed neuroinflammation by reducing expression of IL-1, IL-1β, TNF-α, COX-2, and iNOS mRNA and protein, which eventually reversed Aβ-induced cognitive deficits [30]. Through rat model of experimental autoimmune encephalomyelitis (EAE), researchers found that epimedium flavonois (icaiin accounting for 56.7% and epimedin C 20.6%) can alleviate demyelination and inflammatory infiltration [31].

NO is a relatively short –lived free radical, which participates in physiological processes and is synthesized by nitric oxide sythase (NOS) and L-Arginine. NOS divides into three isoforms, such as inducible NOS (iNOS), endothelial NOS (eNOS) and neuronal NOS (nNOS), of which iNOS mainly regulate inflammation responses [25, 32]. It is well-know that inflammation response by secreting inflammatory mediator and pro-inflammatory cytokines could be caused by the stimulation of LPS. Overproduction of NO and TNF-α may lead to DNA damage by oxidative stress and DNA mutation [33–36]. In addition, there are several evidences that IL-2 has an association with chronic inflammation by modulating production of the pro-inflammatory cytokine (IFN-γ) [37]. In our study, we found that treatment of YYHs effectively modulated NO production and attenuates the expression of TNF-α and IL-2 in active macrophages (Fig. 3). And it means YYHs may be a valuable anti-inflammatory agent.

According to the crystal structure research, multiple structural components of TLR4/MD-2 are involved in LPS recognition [38]. TLR4/MD-2 complex as the main LPS binding receptors, it responds to inflammatory stimuli as well as mediate NF-κB signaling pathway in macrophages. For example, Zhankuic acid A contributes to the regulation of inflammatory responds through TLR4/MD-2 mediating MAPK and NF-κB pathway, which the same applies to procyanidin B1 and Baicalein [39–41]. NF-κB is critical downstream target of TLR4/MD-2 pathway and adjusts the expression of pro-inflammatory and inflammatory mediator genes [42]. Previous studies revealed that apigenin was attributed to decreasing production of IL-6, IL-1β and TNF-α through the inhibition of NF-κB activation [43]. Besides, indirubin also effectively suppressed LPS-induced inflammation through the NF-κB pathway [44]. Similarly, we demonstrated that YYHs actively ameliorated the inflammatory responses induced by LPS. Finally, YYHs inhibited the formation of TLR4/MD-2 complex (Fig. 4), which subsequently down-regulated the phophorylation of p65 (Fig. 6) and restrained translocation of p65 into the nucleus (Fig. 5).

Conclusions

In summary, YYHs from *E.sagittatum* remarkedly decreased the production of inflammatory mediator and pro-inflammatory cytokines in LPS-induced RAW264.7 cells, and that interacted with TLR4/MD-2 complex formation to block LPS action. Furthermore, YYHs inhibited the phosphorylation of p65 in total cell lysates and the translocation of p65 from the cytoplasm to the nucleus. In general, YYHs contributed to ameliorate inflammatory response through TLR4/MD-2 mediating NF-κB pathway. This study provides novel insights into the mechanisms of YYHs as anti-inflammatory agents to LPS-mediated inflammatory response. Moreover, further studies needs to be verified in animal models.

Abbreviations
HPLC-MS/MS: High performance liquid chromatography-mass spectrometry-mass spectrometry; IL-2: Interleukin-2; LPS: Lipopolysaccharide; NF-κB: Nuclear factor-κB; NO: Nitric oxide; TLR4/MD-2: Toll-like receptor 4/ myeloid differentiation factor-2; TNF-α: Tumor necrosis factor-α; YYHs: *E.sagittatum* of ethyl acetate extracts

Acknowledgements
This research did not receive any specific grant from funding agencies in the public, commercial, or not-for-profit sectors.

Funding
This research did not receive any specific grant from funding agencies in the public, commercial, or not-for-profit sectors.

Authors' contributions
The study was designed and carried out by NY and SJX. Experiment and data analysis was carried out by NY, DSW, YRZ and SJX. Drafting of the manuscript was done by NY and SJX. All authors read and approved the final manuscript.

Competing interests
The authors declare that they have no competing interests.

Author details
[1]Department of Research and Development, ImVin Pharmaceutical Co., Ltd, 2 Fangcaodian Road, Guangzhou 510663, China. [2]School of Pharmaceutical Sciences, Sun Yat-Sen University, Guangzhou 510006, China. [3]Zhuhai Jizhu Small and Medium Enterprises Advanced Technology Research Institute, Zhuhai College of Jilin University, Zhuhai 519041, China.

References
1. Su YW, Chiou WF, Chao AH, Lee MH, Chen CC, Tsai YC. Ligustilide prevents LPS-induced iNOS expression in RAW 264.7 macrophages by preventing ROS production and down-regulating the MAPK, NF-κB and AP-1 signaling pathways. Int Immunopharmacol. 2011;11:1166–72.
2. Heumann D, Roger T. Initial responses to endotoxins and gram-negative bacteria. Clin Chim Acta. 2002;323:59–72.
3. Ryu JK, Kim SJ, Rah SH, Park BS, Yoon TY, Kim HM. Reconstruction of LPS transfer cascade reveals structural determinants within LBP, CD14, and TLR4-MD2 for efficient LPS recognition and transfer. Immunity. 2017;46:38–50.
4. Liu D, Cao G, Han L, Ye Y, SiMa Y, Ge W. Flavonoids from *Radix Tetrastigmae* inhibit TLR4/MD-2 mediated JNK and NF-κB pathway with anti-inflammatory properties. Cytokine. 2016;84:29–36.
5. Coussens LM, Werb Z. Inflammation and cancer. Nature. 2002;420:860–7.
6. Akiyama H, Barger S, Barnum S, Bradt B, Bauer J, Cole GM, Cooper NR, Eikelenboom P, Emmerling M, Fiebich BL, Finch CE, Frautschy S, Griffin WST, Hampel H, Hull M, Landreth G, Lue LF, Mrak R, Mackenzie IR. Inflammation and Alzheimer's disease. Neurobiol Aging. 2000;21:383–421.
7. Dandona P, Aljada A, Bandyopadhyay A. Inflammation: the link between insulin resistance, obesity and diabetes. Trends Immunol. 2004;25:4–7.
8. Viatour P, Merville MP, Bours V, Chariot A. Phosphorylation of NF-κB and IκB proteins: implications in cancer and inflammation. Trends Biochem Sci. 2005;30:43–52.

9. Guha M, Mackman N. LPS induction of gene expression in human monocytes. Cell Signal. 2001;13:85–94.

10. Schmitz ML, Mattioli I, Buss H, Kracht M. NF-κB: a multifaceted transcription factor regulated at several levels. Chembiochem. 2004;5:1348–58.

11. Chen XJ, Ji H, Zhang QW, Tu PF, Wang YT, Guo BL, Li SP. A rapid method for simultaneous determination of 15 flavonoids in Epimedium using pressurized liquid extraction and ultra-performance liquid chromatography. J Pharm Biomed Anal. 2008;46:226–35.

12. Chinese pharmacopoeia commission. Pharmacopoeia of the People's Republic of China. China, Beijing. 2015.

13. Cho WK, Weeratunga P, Lee BH, Park JS, Kim CJ, Ma JY, Lee JS. Epimedium koreanum Nakai displays broad spectrum of antiviral activity in Vitro and in Vivo by inducing cellular antiviral state. Viruses. 2015;7:352–77.

14. Sun JH, Ruan XJ, Wang LN, Liang S, Li XP. Study on the Antinociceptive effects of herba Epimedium in mice. Evid-based Compl Alt. 2015. https://doi.org/10.1155/2015/483942.

15. Shen CY, Jiang JG, Yang L, Wang DW, Zhu W. Anti-aging active ingredients from herbs and nutraceuticals used in TCM: pharmacological mechanisms and implications for drug discovery. Br J Pharmacol. 2017;174:1395–425.

16. You SH, Jang M, Kim GH. Antioxidant activity and protective effect on PC12 against H_2O_2 of Epimedium koreanum. FASEB J. 2017;31(Suppl 1). https://www.fasebj.org/doi/abs/10.1096/fasebj.31.1_supplement.lb190.

17. Wang C, Feng L, Su J, Cui L, Liu D, Yan J, Ding C, Tan X, Jia X. Polysaccharides from Epimedium koreanum Nakai with immunomodulatory activity and inhibitory effect on tumor growth in LLC-bearing mice. J Ethnopharmacol. 2017;207:8–18.

18. Li F, Du BW, Lu DF, Wu WX, Wongkrajang K, Wang L, Pu WC, Liu CL, Liu HW, Wang MK, Wang F. Flavonoid glycosides isolated from Epimedium brevicornum and their estrogen biosynthesis-promoting effects. Sci Rep. 2017;7:7760.

19. Ma H, He X, Yang Y, Li M, Hao D, Jia Z. The genus Epimedium: an ethnopharmacological and phytochemical review. J Ethnopharmacol. 2011;134:519–41.

20. Chen WF, Wu L, Du ZR, Chen L, Xu AL, Chen XH, Teng JJ, Wong MS. Neuroprotective properties of icariin in MPTP-induced mouse model of Parkinson's disease: involvement of PI3K/Akt and MEK/ERK signaling pathways. Phytomedicine. 2017;25:93–9.

21. Chi L, Gao W, Shu X, Lu X. A natural flavonoid glucoside, icariin, regulates Th17 and alleviates rheumatoid arthritis in a murine model. Mediat Inflamm. 2014. https://doi.org/10.1155/2014/392062.

22. Liu M, Xu H, Ma Y, Cheng J, Hua Z, Huang G. Osteoblasts proliferation and differentiation stimulating activities of the main components of Epimedii folium. Pharmacogn Mag. 2017;13:90–4.

23. Wang L, Li Y, Guo Y, Ma R, Fu M, Niu J, Gao S, Zhang D. Herba Epimedii: an ancient Chinese herbal medicine in the prevention and treatment of osteoporosis. Curr Pharm Design. 2016;22:328–49.

24. Tang X, Nian H, Li X, Yang Y, Wang X, Xu L, Shi H, Yang X, Liu R. Effects of the combined extracts of Herba Epimedii and Fructus Ligustrilucidi on airway remodeling in the asthmatic rats with the treatment of budesonide. BMC Complement Altern Med. 2017;17:380–91.

25. Lee HS, Bilehal D, Lee GS, Ryu DS, Kim HK, Suk SH, Lee DS. Anti-inflammatory effect of the hexane fraction from Orostachys japonicus in RAW 264.7 cells by suppression of NF-κB and PI3K-Akt signaling. J Funct Foods. 2013;5:1217–25.

26. Kang YJ, Lee MW, Kang SS. Flavonoids from Epimedium koreanum. J Nat Prod. 1991;54:542–6.

27. Sun X, Deng X, Cai W, Li W, Shen Z, Jiang T, Huang J. Icariin inhibits LPS-induced cell inflammatory response by promoting GRα nuclear translocation and upregulating GRα expression. Life Sci. 2018;195:33–43.

28. Li L, Sun J, Xu C, Zhang H, Wu J, Liu B, Dong J. Icariin ameliorates cigarette smoke induced inflammatory responses via suppression of NF-κB and modulation of GR In Vivo and In Vitro. PLoS One. 2014. https://doi.org/10.1371/journal.pone.0102345.

29. Wang GQ, Li DD, Huang C, Lu DS, Zhang C, Zhou SY, Liu J, Zhang F. Icariin reduces dopaminergic neuronal loss and microglia-mediated inflammation in Vivo and in Vitro. Front Mol Neurosci. 2018;10:441–51.

30. Deng Y, Long L, Wang K, Zhou J, Zeng L, He L, Gong Q. Icariside II, a broad-spectrum anti-cancer agent, reverses beta-amyloid-induced cognitive impairment through reducing inflammation and apoptosis in rats. Front Pharmacol. 2017;8:39–50.

31. Yin LL, Lin LL, Zhang L, Li L. Epimedium flavonoids ameliorate experimental autoimmune encephalomyelitis in rats by modulating neuroinflammatory and neurotrophic responses. Neuropharmacology. 2012;63:851–62.

32. Bredt DS. Endogenous nitric oxide synthesis: biological functions andpathophysiology. Free Radic Res. 1999;31:577–96.

33. Suematsu N, Tsutsui H, Wen J, Kang D, Ikeuchi M, Ide T, Hayashidani S, Shiomi T, Kubota T, Hamasaki N, Takeshita A. Oxidative stress mediates tumor necrosis factor-alpha-induced mitochondrial DNA damage and dysfunction in cardiac myocytes. Cirulation. 2003;107:1418–23.

34. Balkwill F. TNF-alpha in promotion and progression of cancer. Cancer Metast Rev. 2006;25(3):409–16.

35. Tripathi P, Tripathi P, Kashyap L, Singh V. The role of nitric oxide in inflammatory reactions. FEMS Immunol Med Microbiol. 2007;51:443–52.

36. Kawanishi S, Ohnishi S, Ma N, Hiraku Y, Murata M. Crosstalk between DNA damage and inflammation in the multiple steps of carcinogenesis. Int J Mol Sci. 2017;18:1808–20.

37. Kikuchi-Maki A, Yusa S, Catina TL, Campbell KS. KIR2DL4 is an IL-2-regulated NK cell receptor that exhibits limited expression in humans but triggers strong IFN-gamma production. J Immunol. 2003;171:3415–25.

38. Park BS, Song DH, Kim HM, Choi BS, Lee H, Lee JO. The structural basis of lipopolysaccharide recognition by the TLR4–MD-2 complex. Nature. 2009; 458:1191–5.

39. Xing J, Li R, Li N, Zhang J, Li Y, Gong P, Gao D, Liu H, Zhang Y. Anti-inflammatory effect of procyanidin B1 on LPS-treated THP1 cells via interaction with the TLR4–MD-2 heterodimer and p38 MAPK and NF-κB signaling. Mol Cell Biochem. 2015;407:89–95.

40. Chen YF, Shiau AL, Wang SH, Yang JS, Chang SJ, Wu CL, Wu TS. Zhankuic acid a isolated from Taiwanofungus camphoratus is a novel selective TLR4/MD-2 antagonist with anti-inflammatory properties. J Immunol. 2014;192: 2778–86.

41. He X, Wei Z, Zhou E, Chen L, Kou J, Wang J, Yang Z. Baicalein attenuates inflammatory responses by suppressing TLR4 mediated NF-κB and MAPK signaling pathways in LPS-induced mastitis in mice. Int Immunopharmacol. 2015;28:470–6.

42. Wang Y, Qian Y, Fang Q, Zhong P, Li W, Wang L, Fu W, Zhang Y, Xu Z, X. Li, Liang G. Saturated palmitic acid induces myocardial inflammatory injuries through direct binding to TLR4 accessory protein MD2. Nat Commun. 2017; 8:13997.

43. Wang J, Liu YT, Xiao L, Zhu L, Wang Q, Yan T. Anti-inflammatory effects of apigenin in lipopolysaccharide-induced inflammatory in acute lung injury by suppressing COX-2 and NF-κB pathway. Inflammation. 2014;37:2085–90.

44. Lai JI, Liu YH, Liu C, Qi MP, Liu RN, Zhu XF, Zhou QG, Chen YY, Guo AZ, Hu CM. Indirubin inhibits LPS-induced inflammation via TLR4 abrogation mediated by the NF-κB and MAPK signaling pathways. Inflammation. 2017;40:1–12.

22

Hexane extract from *Spondias tuberosa* (Anacardiaceae) leaves has antioxidant activity and is an anti-*Candida* agent by causing mitochondrial and lysosomal damages

Bruna Maria Pereira da Costa Cordeiro[1], Nataly Diniz de Lima Santos[1], Magda Rhayanny Assunção Ferreira[2], Larissa Cardoso Corrêa de Araújo[1], Alexsander Rodrigues Carvalho Junior[3], Alan Diego da Conceição Santos[4], Ana Paula de Oliveira[4], Alexandre Gomes da Silva[5,6], Emerson Peter da Silva Falcão[7], Maria Tereza dos Santos Correia[1], Jackson Roberto Guedes da Silva Almeida[4], Luís Cláudio Nascimento da Silva[3], Luiz Alberto Lira Soares[2], Thiago Henrique Napoleão[1], Márcia Vanusa da Silva[1,6] and Patrícia Maria Guedes Paiva[1]*

Abstract

Background: *Spondias tuberosa* is a plant that produces a fruit crop with high economic relevance at Brazilian Caatinga. Its roots and leaves are used in folk medicine.

Methods: Chemical composition of a hexane extract from *S. tuberosa* leaves was evaluated by thin-layer chromatography (TLC), high-performance liquid chromatography (HPLC) and ^{1}H nuclear magnetic resonance (NMR). Antioxidant potential was investigated by DPPH and ABTS assays. Antifungal action on *Candida* species was evaluated determining the minimal inhibitory concentration (MIC_{50}) and putative mechanisms were determined by flow cytometry analysis. In addition, hemolytic activity on human erythrocytes was assessed and the concentration required to promote 50% hemolysis (EC_{50}) was determined.

Results: Phytochemical analysis by TLC showed the presence of flavonoids, hydrolysable tannins, saponins and terpenes. The HPLC profile of the extract suggested the presence of gallic acid (0.28 ± 0.01 g%) and hyperoside (1.27 ± 0.01 g%). The representative ^{1}H NMR spectrum showed saturated and unsaturated fatty acids among the main components. The extract showed weak and moderate antioxidant activity in DPPH (IC_{50}: 234.00 µg/mL) and ABTS (IC_{50}: 123.33 µg/mL) assays, respectively. It was able to inhibit the growth of *C. albicans* and *C. glabrata* with MIC_{50} of 2.0 and 0.078 mg/mL, respectively. The treatment of *C. glabrata* cells with the extract increased levels of mitochondrial superoxide anion, caused hyperpolarization of mitochondrial membrane, and compromised the lysosomal membrane. Weak hemolytic activity (EC_{50}: 740.8 µg/mL) was detected.

Conclusion: The results demonstrate the pharmacological potential of the extract as antioxidant and antifungal agent, aggregating biotechnological value to this plant and stimulating its conservation.

Keywords: *Spondias tuberosa*, Hyperoside, Gallic acid, Fatty acids, Antifungal activity

* Correspondence: ppaivaufpe@yahoo.com.br
[1]Departamento de Bioquímica, Centro de Biociências, Universidade Federal de Pernambuco, Recife, Pernambuco 50670-420, Brazil
Full list of author information is available at the end of the article

Background

Brazil has one of the world highest levels of plant diversity and the north and northeast regions of the country concentrate much of this diversity. In the semi-arid region of northeastern Brazil (known as Caatinga) there are several kinds of plants employed in popular culture for the treatment of human diseases. In spite of the great diversity of Caatinga, there are still few studies on the potential of bioactive compounds coming from the plants of this region [1–3].

Spondias tuberosa Arruda, popularly known as "umbuzeiro" or "imbuzeiro", is an endemic plant of Caatinga, adapted to survive and produce fruits even under hydrical and salt stress [4]. Several medicinal properties of *S. tuberosa* have been described, including treatment of digestive disorders, diabetes, menstrual cramps, diarrhea, inflammation of the kidneys, bacterial infections, and foot pain [5–7]. Tannins and flavonoids are found in the bark [8] and the fruits contain anthocyanins, ascorbic acid, minerals, flavonoids and carotenoids [9]. The high tannin content and the presence of natural antioxidants give to *S. tuberosa* fruits a functional appeal [10]. Hydroethanolic extract of leaves from *S. tuberosa* containing chlorogenic acid, caffeic acid, rutin and isoquercitrin demonstrated anti-inflammatory action [11]. Methanolic extract of the leaves showed in vitro activity against several strains of Gram-negative bacteria [2].

The chemical characterization of plant extracts allows the identification of chemical markers and suggests potential bioactivities that can be investigated. For example, flavonoids are secondary metabolites that have great pharmacological importance, since they act in the prevention of degenerative diseases. Among the biological properties described for these compounds, it can be highlighted cytotoxic, thrombolytic, anti-inflammatory, antitumor, vasorelaxant and antioxidant activities [11–13]. Other phenolic compounds such as tannins and anthocyanins are also considered important antioxidant agents. Natural antioxidants play an important role in health care as they provide protection from oxidative stress and associated diseases [14].

Natural products have also been considered an important source of bioactive compounds against infectious diseases [11]. Fungal infections have increased gradually over the last 30 years, becoming one of the more relevant public health problems. *Candida* yeasts are among the main etiological agents of invasive fungal infections, which are responsible for high mortality and morbidity rates throughout the world [15–17]. These fungi have developed resistance mechanisms against antibiotics, favoring the persistence and progression of the infection even when antifungal therapy is adequately performed [18]. *Candida albicans, Candida krusei, Candida parapsilosis* and *Candida glabrata* are among the most prevalent causers of candidiasis [19, 20].

In this context, this work reports the chemical composition of a hexane extract from leaves of *S. tuberosa* as well as the evaluation of the antioxidant potential and antifungal action on *Candida* species. Mechanisms involved in the antifungal activity against the most sensitive species were investigated. In addition, hemolytic activity was assessed as safety parameter to determine whether the extract would be able to damage erythrocytes membrane.

Methods

Materials

Leaves of *S. tuberosa* were collected at the *Parque Nacional do Catimbau* (Coordinates 08°37'23" S, 37° 09'21" W), Buíque, Pernambuco. The plant material was identified by Dr. Alexandre Gomes da Silva, and a voucher specimen was deposited at the *Instituto Agronômico de Pernambuco*, Recife, Brazil, under the reference number 91,090. Plant collection was authorized (number 16806) by the *Instituto Chico Mendes de Conservação da Biodiversidade* (ICMBio) from Brazilian Ministry of Environment. The access was recorded (A1503A6) in the *Sistema Nacional de Gestão do Patrimônio Genético e do Conhecimento Tradicional Associado* (SisGen).

Stored cultures of *Candida albicans* (URM 5901, from ungual scales), *Candida parapsilosis* (URM 6951, clinical isolate), *Candida glabrata* (URM 4246, from blood of AIDS patient), and `Candida krusei` (URM 6391, from human blood) were obtained from the Culture Collection of the University Recife Mycologia (URM), *Departamento de Micologia, Universidade Federal de Pernambuco* (UFPE).

Extract preparation

The leaves were dried in a forced air convection oven at 45 °C until constant weight. After drying, they were powdered using Willye-type mill (model TE650; Tecnal, Brazil) and the powder was stored protected from light and moisture at 28 °C until use. The extract was prepared in a Soxhlet apparatus using 100 g of the powdered leaves and 1 L of *n*-hexane. The solvent was evaporated at 75 rpm and 64.4 °C in a HB10 rotary-evaporator (IKA Works, Wilmington, NC, USA). The resulting material after solvent evaporation corresponded to the extract.

Thin-layer chromatography

An amount of 1 mg of the extract was dissolved in 1 mL of methanol. The sample was taken to the ultrasound for 30 min for complete solubilization. All standards (Table 1) were used at the concentration of 1 mg/mL in methanol. The sample and standards were applied manually on silica gel 60-F254 chromatography plates (Macherey-Nagel, Germany) and the different mobile phases and chromogenic agents used are shown in Table 1 [21–23]. The

Table 1 Elution systems, chromogenic agents, and standards used in the phytochemical analysis of the hexane extract from *Spondias tuberosa* leaves with thin-layer chromatography (TLC)

Classes	Mobile phase	Chromogenic agent	Standards
Polyphenols (Hydrolysable tannins)	90:5:5	NEU + PEG	Gallic acid and Ellagic acid (Sigma-Aldrich, USA)
Condensed tannins	90:5:5	Chloridric vanillin	Catechin (Sigma-Aldrich, USA)
Flavonoids	90:5:5	NEU + PEG	Quercetin and Rutin (Sigma-Aldrich, USA)
Cinnamic derivatives	90:5:5	NEU + PEG	Caffeic acid and Chlorogenic acid (Sigma-Aldrich, USA)
Terpenes and steroids	70:30	Lieberman-Burchard + Δ	β-sitosterol (Sigma-Aldrich, USA)
Coumarins	50:50:50	KOH + Δ	Coumarin (Phytolab, Brazil)
Saponins	100:11:11:26	Lieberman-Burchard + Δ	Escin (Sigma-Aldrich, USA)
Reducing sugars	50:20:10:10	Thymol + H_2SO_4 10% + Δ	D-fructose (ChromaDex, USA)
Alkaloids	50:6.75:5	Dragendorf	Pilocarpine nitrate (Sigma-Aldrich, USA)
Anthraquinones	50:6.75:5	HNO_3 + KOH 10%	Sennoside A (Sigma-Aldrich, USA)

Systems: 90:5:5 – ethyl acetate: formic acid: water; 70:30 – toluene: acetate; 50:50:50 – ethyl eter: ethyl acetate: 10% acetic acid (saturation); 100:11:11:26 – ethyl acetate: acetic acid: formic acid: water; 50:20:10:10 – ethyl acetate: acetic acid: formic acid: water; 50:6.75:5 – ethyl acetate; methanol; water. *NEU* Neu's reagent. *PEG* polyethylene glycol

following secondary metabolites classes were investigated: steroids, flavonoids (aglycones and heterosides), cinnamic derivatives, mono-, tri- and sesquiterpenes, alkaloids and coumarins.

High-performance liquid chromatography coupled to diode array detector (HPLC-DAD) analysis

The extract was analyzed by high-performance liquid chromatography (HPLC) in an Ultimate 3000 coupled to a diode array detector (DAD) and equipped with a binary pump (HPG-3x00RS), degasser and automatic sampler with a loop of 20 μL (ACC-3000). All these equipments were from Thermo Fisher Scientific (USA). An amount of 0.25 g of the hexane extract was weighed, transferred to a 25-mL volumetric flask and diluted with methanol. The solution was taken to the sonicator during 15 min to complete solubilization (stock solution). After solubilization, an aliquot (1 mL) of the stock solution was transferred to a 10-mL volumetric flask and the volume was completed with ultrapure water (Purelab®, Elga LabWater, USA). Hyperoside (HWI Analytic Gmb, Germany) and gallic acid (Sigma-Aldrich, USA) solutions (1 mg/mL in methanol) were used as standards. The sample solution and standard solutions were filtered (0.45 μm PVDF membrane). The chromatography was performed in a Dionex® C_{18} column (250 mm × 4.6 mm d.i., 5 μm) equipped with a Phenomenex® C_{18} pre-column (4 mm × 3.9 μm) at 26 °C. The wavelengths were set at 270 and 350 nm for detection of hydrolysable tannins and flavonoids, respectively. The mobile phase was composed by ultrapure water (A) and methanol (B), both acidified with 0.05% (*v/v*) trifluoroacetic acid, and the flow rate was adjusted to 0.8 mL/min. The following gradient program was used: 0–10 min, 5–20% B; 10–13.5 min, 20–25% B; 13.5–18 min, 25–40% B; 18–25 min, 40–80% B; 25–30 min, 80% B; 30–34 min, 80–5% B; 34–36 min, 5% B. The data were analyzed and processed

using the software Chromeleon 6.8 (Dionex, Thermo Fisher Scientific, USA). The peaks of substances in the hexane extract were identified by comparing the retention times, UV spectra and subsequently, by spiking the sample with a small amount of the standards. The contents of hyperoside and gallic acid in the extract were calculated based on calibration curve obtained by chromatography of each standard at different concentrations: hyperoside – $y = 3.8841x - 11.663$ ($R^2 = 0.9987$); gallic acid – $y = 1.2097x - 0.9732$ ($R^2 = 0.9996$). The results were expressed as mean ± standard deviation.

Nuclear magnetic resonance (NMR) experiments

One-dimensional and two-dimensional nuclear magnetic resonance (NMR) experiments were acquired in deuterated dimethylsulfoxide (DMSO-d_6), using NMR Bruker AVANCE III 400 spectrometer, operating at 9.4 Tesla, observing ^1H and ^{13}C nuclei at 400 and 100 MHz, respectively. The spectrometer was equipped with 5-mm multinuclear direct detection probe (BBO). Due to the low sample concentration and the presence of water in the deuterated solvent, ^1H NMR spectra were acquired through *zg* (classical pulse sequence) and *zgpr* (for water signal suppression). Besides, one-bond heteronuclear (^1H-^{13}C) and homonuclear (^1H-^1H) correlations were assessed by HSQC and COSY experiments. ^1H and ^{13}C NMR chemical shifts are given in ppm referenced to TMSP-d_4 signal at 0.00 ppm.

Antioxidant activity
Free radical scavenging activity by DPPH (2,2-diphenyl-1-picrylhydrazyl) assay

Antioxidant activity of the hexane extract was evaluated by the DPPH scavenging assay according to Mascato et al. [24], with some modifications. The hexane extract was diluted in methanol to reach concentrations ranging from 15.625 to 1000 μg/mL. In each assay, 270 μL of the DPPH solution (23.6 µg/mL in methanol, prepared on the day of the analysis) was added to the sample (30 µL). Methanol (30 µL) was used in the negative control. After 30 min in the dark, the reduction of DPPH was determined by measuring the colorimetric change at 517 nm. Ascorbic acid (0.5, 1, 2, 3 and 4 µg/mL, in ethanol) was used as standard. The antioxidant concentration required to decrease 50% of the DPPH present (IC_{50}) was determined by exponential regression analysis. Two independent experiments were performed in triplicate. Samples were classified according to the IC_{50} as follows: $IC_{50} < 50$ µg/mL, very strong antioxidant; $50 < IC_{50} < 100$ µg/mL, strong antioxidant, $101 < IC_{50} < 150$ µg/mL, moderate antioxidant; $IC_{50} > 150$ µg/mL, weak antioxidant [25].

ABTS [2,2'-azino-bis(3-ethylbenzothiazoline-6-sulfonic acid] assay

The radical $ABTS^+$ was generated by oxidation of an ABTS solution (7 mM) with 2.45 mM potassium persulfate solution. The mixture was allowed to react for 12 h in the dark at 25 °C before use. For the test, the $ABTS^+$ stock solution (1 mL) was diluted in 60 mL of methanol to obtain an absorbance of 0.70 ± 0.02 at 734 nm. Next, 2.7 mL of this solution was added to 0.3 mL of 0.5, 1.0, 2.0, 3.0, 4.0 and 5.0 µg/mL Trolox® (standard) solutions prepared in methanol or 31.25, 62.5, 125, 250, 500 and 1000 µg/mL of extract. The absorbance was taken 6 min after the adding of the radical at 734 nm. The test was performed in triplicate. The extract concentration required to decrease 50% of the $ABTS^+$ content (IC_{50}) was determined by linear regression. Samples were classified according to the IC_{50} as described in the previous section.

Antifungal assay

The yeasts were cultured in Sabouraud Dextrose Broth (SDB) at 28 °C for 16 h under gentle shaking. Next, the optical density at 600 nm (OD_{600}) of the cultures was adjusted in order to correspond to 3×10^6 CFU/mL. In each row of a 96-well microplate, 100 µL of the hexane extract (8.0 mg/mL) were serially diluted (1:1) in SDB and 20 µL of yeast culture were added to each well. Wells containing only the culture medium were used as sterility control while the 100% growth control contained the microorganism in culture medium. In addition, it was performed a blank composed by the extract diluted in culture medium. The OD_{600} was recorded at time zero and after incubation at 28 °C for 24 h. The increase in OD_{600} was considered as fungal growth. The minimal inhibitory concentration (MIC_{50}) corresponded to the lowest extract concentration able to promote a reduction higher or equal to 50% in growth. Each assay was achieved in triplicate and three independent experiments were performed.

The supernatant (10 µL) from each well containing the extract at concentration higher or equal to the MIC_{50}

was transferred to Sabouraud-Dextrose Agar plates and incubated for 24 h. The minimal fungicidal concentration (MFC) corresponded to the lowest extract concentration able to reduce the number of CFU in 99.9%. Each assay was carried out in triplicate in three independent experiments.

Flow cytometry analysis

Fluorescent probes were used in order to analyze putative effects of the extract on mitochondrial superoxide production, the mitochondrial membrane potential, and lysosomal membrane of *C. glabrata* cells. In all these assays, yeast cells were resuspended at a density of 1×10^6 cells/mL in RPMI-1640 medium supplemented with MOPS. The extract was added at the concentrations of $2 \times MIC$ (0.156 mg/mL) or $4 \times MIC$ (0.312 mg/mL), and the cells were incubated at 28 °C.

For measurement of mitochondrial superoxide production, the extract was added and, after 1 h, the medium was removed, and the cells were washed using PBS. Then the MitoSOX Red mitochondrial superoxide indicator (Molecular Probes, Invitrogen, Carslabad, CA, USA) at 5 µM was added and the samples were incubated for 10 min at 37 °C, protected from light. The cells were washed with warm buffer (three times) and analyzed by flow cytometry (FL3 channel, Accuri™, BD Biosciences, San Jose, CA, USA).

In other assays, cells were incubated with extract for 12 h and then washed with PBS and stained with 1 µg/mL acridine orange (lysosomal dye) in the dark for 20 min or 10 µg/mL rhodamine 123 (to assay mitochondrial membrane potential change) in the dark for 10 min. After the incubation, yeast cells were washed and analyzed by flow cytometry (FL3 channel and FL1 channel for acridine orange and rhodamine 123. respectively). A minimum of 10,000 events were analyzed in each condition. Changes in the fluorescent intensity of rhodamine 123 were quantified using the variation index (VI) obtained by the eq. (MT-MC)/MC, where MC is the mean of fluorescent intensity of control and MT the mean of treated cells. Negative values of VI correspond to membrane depolarization of mitochondria, while positive values indicate membrane hyperpolarization.

Hemolytic assay

The hexane extract was evaluated for hemolytic activity in 96-well microplates according to Costa-Lotufo et al. [26]. Each well received 100 µL of a 0.85% (*w/v*) NaCl solution containing 10 mM $CaCl_2$. Next, samples (100 µL) of the extract at 10 to 2500 µg/mL were added to the wells. Finally, each well received 100 µL of a 2% (*v/v*) suspension of human erythrocytes in 0.85% saline containing 10 mM $CaCl_2$. In negative control, 150 µL of the saline solution plus 50 µL of 5% (*v/v*) DMSO were plated. Positive control (to obtain 100% hemolysis) contained 20 μL of 0.1% (v/v) Triton X-100 in 180 μL of saline solution. After incubation for 1 h at 27 °C and centrifugation, the supernatant was discarded, and the amount of released hemoglobin was measured by absorbance at 540 nm. Three independent experiments were performed in triplicate. Extract was considered active whether the EC_{50} value was lower than 200 μg/mL [26].

Statistical analysis

Standard deviations (SD) were calculated using GraphPad Prism version 4.0 for Windows (GraphPad Software, San Diego, California, USA) and data were expressed as a mean of replicates ± SD. Significant differences between treatment groups were analysed by Student's t-test (significance at $p < 0.05$) using Origin 6.0 program.

Results

The phytochemical analysis by TLC of the hexane extract from $S.$ $tuberosa$ leaves showed the presence of flavonoids, hydrolysable tannins, saponins and terpenes. The HPLC profile of the extract at 270 nm (Fig. 1A, a) showed three main peaks (retention times 10.197, 25.403 and 26.223 min). The first peak probably corresponded to gallic acid (peak 1), in comparison with retention time of the standard (10.23 min; Fig. 1A, b). The chromatogram at 350 nm (Fig. 1B, a) showed main a peak at 25.433 min, which corresponds to a flavonoid (peak 2) since it was also observed at 270 nm. According to the retention time of the standard hyperoside (Fig. 1B, b), this peak is similar to this compound. These results were confirmed by the increase in the area after spiking the extract with the standards gallic acid (Fig. 1A, c) and hyperoside (Fig. 1B, c). The equivalent contents of

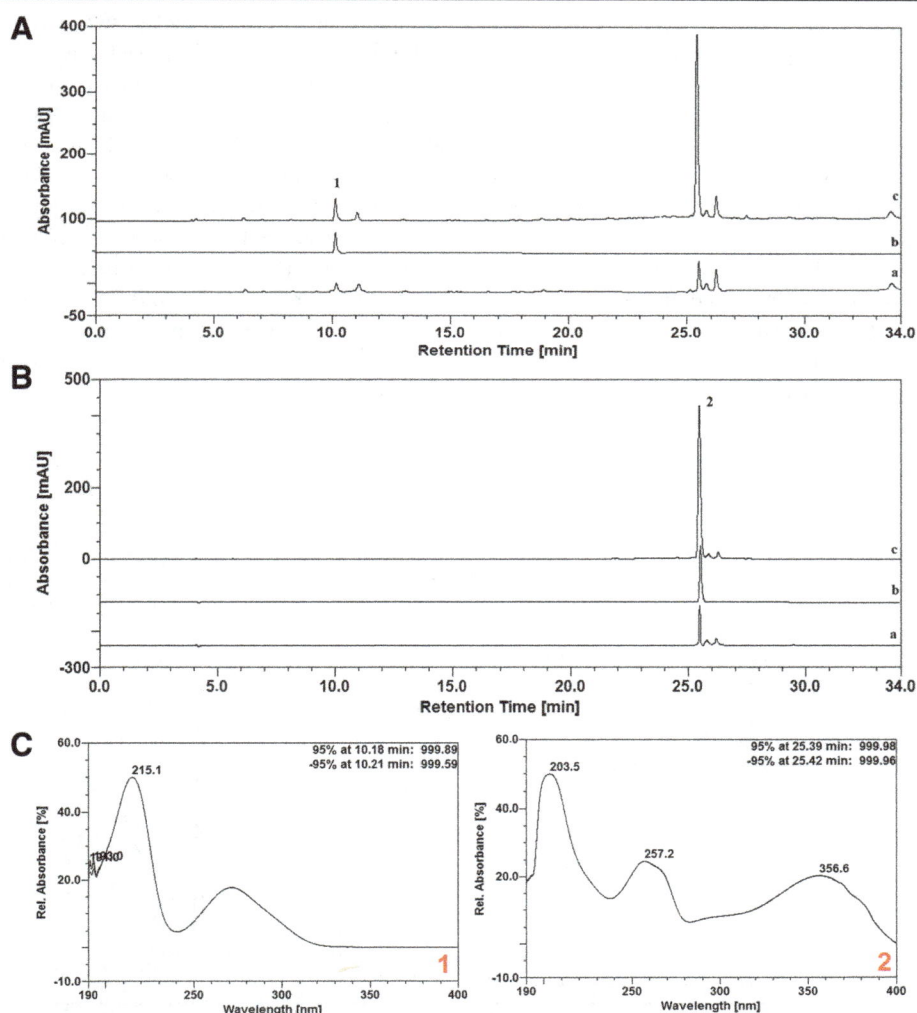

Fig. 1 HPLC-DAD analysis of hexane extract from *Spondias tuberosa* leaf. Chromatographic fingerprint at 270 (**a**) and 350 (**b**) nm showed the presence of gallic acid (1) and hyperoside (2), as indicated by the retention times. **c** Scanning spectra of peaks 1 and 2

hyperoside and gallic acid calculated were 1.27 ± 0.01 g% and 0.28 ± 0.01 g%, respectively.

The representative ^{1}H NMR spectrum of hexane extract of *S. tuberosa* leaves revealed typical signals of fatty acid methyl esters (Fig. 2), which is expected for an extract obtained using a non-polar solvent. The resonances related to aliphatic hydrogens of all fatty acids can also be visualized in the figure. Methylene groups appeared at 1.16–1.35 ppm, while the signal at 1.49 ppm corresponds to β carbonyl group hydrogens. Characteristic resonances of methylene alpha-olefins of all unsaturated fatty acids were observed at 1.98 ppm. The presence of methylene hydrogens between two olefins and alpha carbonyl hydrogens could be noticed at 2.77 and 2.34 ppm, respectively. The signal at 0.84 ppm corresponds to methyl groups of all fatty acids, except for the methylic hydrogens of *n*-3 polyunsaturated acyl groups that are easily identified as a triplet at 1.06 ppm [27, 28]. It should be pointed out that the fatty acid acyl chains are not esterified to glycerol backbone, as typical signals of it were not observed. Another way of corroborating such information would be by checking the signal around 3.67 ppm, which is associated with the methoxy group of fatty acid methyl esters. However, in our experiment the residual water signal compromised the obtainment of such information. Finally, the signal at 5.33 ppm (olefinic hydrogens) connected to the carbon at 129.5 ppm indicated the presence of unsaturated fatty acids. The presence of hydrogens of phenolic compounds could be observed by signals between 6 and 8 ppm.

The hexane extract was evaluated for antioxidant activity by the DPPH scavenging assay. The results showed that the increase in the extract concentration led to

higher inhibition of this free radical. An IC_{50} value of 234 μg/mL was calculated. The results from ABTS assay showed that the IC_{50} values were 123.33 and 1.72 μg/mL for the hexane extract and the positive control Trolox®, respectively.

The antifungal assays showed that the hexane extract was able to inhibit the growth of *C. albicans* and *C. glabrata* with MIC_{50} values of 2.0 and 0.078 mg/mL, respectively. *Candida parapsilosis* and *C. krusei* did not have their growth affected by the extract. Fungicidal effect was not detected.

The effect of the extract on superoxide production by *C. glabrata* cells was evaluated. The results (Fig. 3A) showed that low levels of fluorescence were detected in untreated cells while high levels of mitochondrial superoxide anion were induced by treatment with the extract for 1 h (5.8 and 5.2 folds for 2× MIC_{50} and 4× MIC_{50}, respectively, when compared with untreated yeasts). No statistical differences were observed between the amount of superoxide induced by the two concentrations tested.

Alterations in mitochondrial functions induced by the extract were evaluated by measuring changes the mitochondrial membrane potential (ΔΨm) using the variation index (VI). Healthy cells incorporated the probe rhodamine 123 and showed high levels of fluorescence emission. The fluorescence intensity was significantly increased by extract treatment when compared with untreated cells (Fig. 3B), resulting in positive VI values (7.65 folds for 2× MIC_{50} and 5.15 folds for 4× MIC_{50}).

The lysosomal function was analyzed using an acridine orange-based assay. As expected, the yeast cells that were not treated with the extract exhibited a strong fluorescence

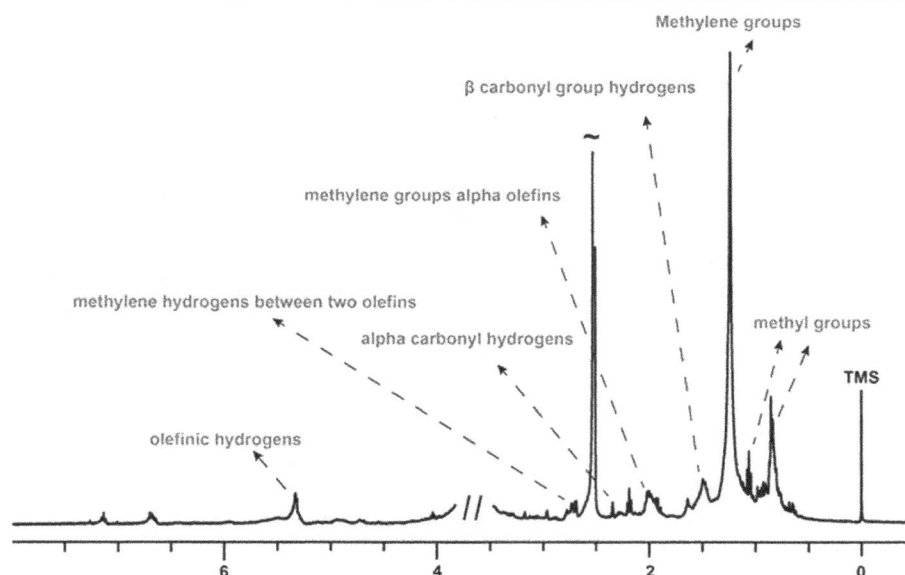

Fig. 2 Representative ^{1}H NMR spectrum of hexane extract of *Spondias tuberosa* leaf

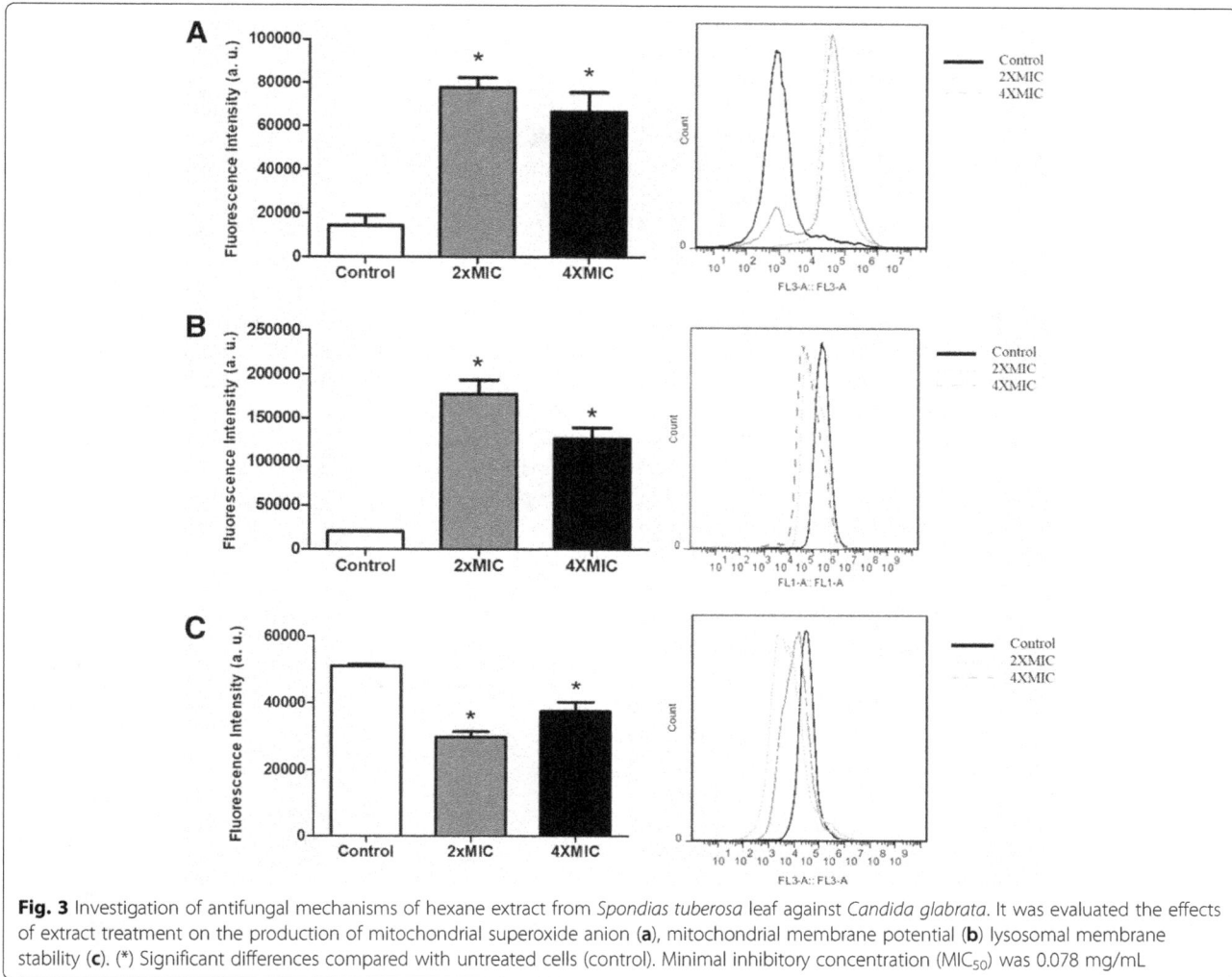

Fig. 3 Investigation of antifungal mechanisms of hexane extract from *Spondias tuberosa* leaf against *Candida glabrata*. It was evaluated the effects of extract treatment on the production of mitochondrial superoxide anion (**a**), mitochondrial membrane potential (**b**) lysosomal membrane stability (**c**). (*) Significant differences compared with untreated cells (control). Minimal inhibitory concentration (MIC_{50}) was 0.078 mg/mL

emission, confirming that these cells had intact lysosomes. On the other hand, the extract treatment compromised the lysosomal membrane of *C. glabrata*, as seen by the lower levels of fluorescence emission than control cells (Fig. 3C). The fluorescence emission reduced 41.98% and 26.91% when the cells were incubated with the extract at 2× MIC_{50} and 4× MIC_{50}, respectively.

The hexane extract was also evaluated for hemolytic activity against human erythrocytes. The EC_{50} value determined was 740.8 ± 61.09 μg/mL.

Discussion

Many works have studied the chemical composition and biological activities of extracts from *S. tuberosa* tissues, including the leaves, obtained using polar organic solvents. For example, methanolic extract from *S. tuberosa* leaves contained phenols, tannins, flavones, flavonoids, leucoanthocyanidins and saponins [2] and Uchôa et al. [29] reported that extracts from the leaves of *S. tuberosa* in methanol and ethyl acetate were rich in flavonoids and

triterpenes as well as also contained cinnamic derivatives. Analysis of a hydroethanolic extract from leaves of this plant also evidenced the presence of flavonoids [11]. In the present work, we aimed to evaluate the composition of an extract from *S. tuberosa* leaves obtained with hexane, a non-polar solvent. Interestingly, the classes of compounds detected by TLC were also present in the extracts mentioned above, produced using solvents with higher polarity. Particularly, the presence of flavonoids and hydrolysable tannins in the hexane extract caught our attention and stimulated a more in-depth evaluation by HPLC analysis. Indeed, the presence of compounds similar to gallic acid and hyperoside was confirmed.

Siqueira et al. [11] showed through HPLC-DAD analysis that a hydroethanolic extract of *S. tuberosa* leaves presented a large number of phenolic compounds and derivatives of flavonoids; they identified the presence of chlorogenic acid, caffeic acid, rutin, and isoquercitrin. Silva et al. [2] identified the presence of rutin, quercetin and ellagic acid in the methanolic extract of *S. tuberosa* leaves. These compounds were not detected in the hexane extract of *S. tuberosa* leaves described herein, which is probably due to the chemical characteristic of the hexane, which did not favor the extraction of high content of polar compounds. In spite of this, a specific flavonoid (probably hyperoside or a very similar compound) was efficiently extracted from the leaves using this solvent. The hyperoside is the 3-*O*-galactoside of quercetin and has been described in the literature as anticancer, anti-inflammatory, and antioxidant agent. In addition, this compound was shown to act in the protection of liver fibrosis and prevention of memory deficit [30–32].

According to the classification of Fidrianny et al. [25], the hexane extract of *S. tuberosa* leaves is considered a weak DPPH scavenger. However, the hexane extract from *S. tuberosa* leaves showed higher DPPH scavenging activity than extracts of *Spondias pinnata*, which showed IC_{50} ranging from 0.73 to 0.59 mg/mL [33]. The hyperoside possesses DPPH scavenging activity with an IC_{50} of 27.5 mM [34] and polyunsaturated fatty acids may act as antioxidants [35]. Thus, flavonoids and fatty acids may be involved in the antioxidant property of the hexane extract of *S. tuberosa* leaves.

According the results from ABTS assay, the extract is a moderate antioxidant. Floegel et al. [36] reported that high-pigmented and hydrophilic antioxidants in a variety of foods were better reflected by the ABTS assay in comparison with the DPPH assay. Indeed, the hexane extract of *S. tuberosa* leaves used in this work is highly pigmented and one of its main compounds is similar to hyperoside, a water-soluble compound. This may explain the better result obtained with ABTS in comparison with DPPH assay. The antioxidant properties of hyperoside have been demonstrated; for example, it protected endothelial cells against oxidative damage by hydrogen peroxide [37].

The hexane extract showed an interesting activity against *C. glabrata*, as seen by its low MIC_{50} value. Dall'Agnol et al. [38] reported that crude extracts of *Hypericum* containing the hyperoside showed no activity against yeasts. On the other hand, polyunsaturated fatty acids have demonstrated antifungal properties against *Candida* species [39].

Given the highest activity of the hexane extract against *C. glabrata* (as seen by its low MIC_{50} value), we attempted to analyze some subcellular alterations induced by this extract. The results demonstrate that the extract induced the production of mitochondrial superoxide anion and hyperpolarization of mitochondrial membrane. In addition, the extract damaged the lysosomal membrane of *C. glabrata* cells. Lysosomal membrane damage leads to release of cathepsins from into the cytosol where they participate in apoptosis signaling [40].

According to Costa-Lotufo et al. [26], a sample must present $EC_{50} < 200$ µg/mL to be considered hemolytic.

Thus, the hexane extract from *S. tuberosa* leaves is considered no hemolytic, which is initial evidence to determine its safety.

Conclusion

A hexane extract from *S. tuberosa* leaves containing flavonoids, hydrolysable tannins, saponins, terpenes and unsaturated fatty acids showed moderate antioxidant activity and antifungal effect on *C. glabrata*. Antifungal mechanisms against *C. glabrata* include increase in levels of mitochondrial superoxide anion, hyperpolarization of mitochondrial membrane, and damage to the lysosomal membrane. The extract showed weak hemolytic activity, which is important information for future studies to be performed at in vivo conditions. The results demonstrate the pharmacological potential of the extract, aggregating biotechnological value to this plant and stimulating its conservation.

Abbreviations
ABTS: 2,2'-azino-bis(3-ethylbenzothiazoline-6-sulfonic) acid; CFU: Colony-forming units; DMSO: Dimethylsulfoxide; DPPH: 2,2-diphenyl-1-picrylhydrazyl; EC_{50}: Effective concentration required to promote 50% hemolysis; HPLC-DAD: High-performance liquid chromatography coupled to diode array detector analysis; IC_{50}: concentration required to decrease 50% of the free radical content; ICMBio: *Instituto Chico Mendes de Conservação da Biodiversidade*; MFC: Minimal fungicidal concentration; MIC_{50}: Minimal concentration required to inhibit growth in at least 50%; NEU: Neu's reagent; NMR: Nuclear magnetic resonance; OD: Optical density; PBS: Phosphate-buffered saline; PEG: Polyethylene glycol; SDB: Sabouraud Dextrose Broth; SisGen: *Sistema Nacional de Gestão do Patrimônio Genético e do Conhecimento Tradicional Associado*; TLC: Thin-layer chromatography; UFPE: *Universidade Federal de Pernambuco*; URM: University Recife Mycologia (culture collection); VI: Variation index

Acknowledgments
The authors are also grateful to Dr. Carlos Eduardo Sales da Silva for technical assistance.

Funding
The authors express their gratitude to the *Conselho Nacional de Desenvolvimento Científico e Tecnológico* (CNPq) for financial support (446902/2014-4) and investigator research grants (MTSC, JRGSA, THN, PMGP). They are also grateful to the *Coordenação de Aperfeiçoamento de Pessoal de Nível Superior* (CAPES) and the *Fundação de Amparo à Ciência e Tecnologia do Estado de Pernambuco* (FACEPE; APQ-0108-2.08/14; APQ-0493-4.03/14; APQ-0661-2.08/15) for financial support. BMPCC would like to thank CAPES for graduate scholarship. The funding body had no role in the design of the study, collection, analysis, interpretation of data, and writing the manuscript.

Authors' contributions
BMPCC, AGS, MTSC, MVS, and PMGP conceptualized the study. BMPCC and NDLS prepared the extract. BMPCC and LCCA performed the antioxidant, antifungal and hemolytic assays. MRAS, EPSF and LALS performed the TLC and HPLC experiments and contributed to interpretation of the data. ADCS, APO and JRGSA performed the NMR experiments and interpreted the data. ARCJ and LCNS performed all the flow cytometry analysis. BMPCC, NDLS, THN and PMGP analyzed all the data. BMPCC, NDLS, MRAS, JRGSA, LCNS, THN and PMGP drafted the manuscript. All authors approved the final manuscript.

Competing interests

The authors declare that they have no competing interests.

Author details

[1]Departamento de Bioquímica, Centro de Biociências, Universidade Federal de Pernambuco, Recife, Pernambuco 50670-420, Brazil. [2]Departamento de Ciências Farmacêuticas, Centro de Ciências da Saúde, Universidade Federal de Pernambuco, Recife, Pernambuco 50740-520, Brazil. [3]Universidade CEUMA, São Luís, Maranhão 65075-120, Brazil. [4]Núcleo de Estudos e Pesquisas de Plantas Medicinais, Universidade Federal do Vale do São Francisco, Petrolina, Pernambuco 56304-205, Brazil. [5]Departamento de Antibióticos, Centro de Biociências, Universidade Federal de Pernambuco, Recife, Pernambuco 50670-420, Brazil. [6]Núcleo de Bioprospecção da Caatinga, Instituto Nacional do Semiárido, Campina Grande, Paraíba 58429-970, Brazil. [7]Núcleo de Nutrição, Centro Acadêmico de Vitória, Universidade Federal de Pernambuco, Vitória de Santo Antão, Pernambuco 55608-680, Brazil.

References

1. Albuquerque UP, Monteiro JM, Almeida CFCBR, Florentino ATN, Ferraz JSF. Useful plants of the semi-arid northeastern region of Brazil – a look at their conservation and sustainable use. Environ Monitor Assess. 2007;125:281–90.
2. Silva ARA, Morais SM, Marques MMM, Oliveira DF, Barros CC, Almeida RR, Vieira IGP, Guedes MIF. Chemical composition, antioxidant and antibacterial activities of two Spondias species from northeastern Brazil. Pharm Biol. 2012;50:740–6.
3. Vieira PDB, Silva NLF, Silva GN, Silva DB, Lopes NP, Gnoatto SCB, Silva MV, Macedo AJ, Bastida J, Tasca T. Caatinga plants: natural and semi-synthetic compounds potentially active against Trichomonas vaginalis. Bioorg Med Chem Lett. 2016;26:2229–36.
4. Silva EC, Nogueira RJMCN, Araújo FP, Melo NF, Neto ADA. Physiological responses to salt stress in young umbu plants. Environ Exp Bot. 2008;63:147–57.
5. Agra MF, Baracho GS, Silva NK, Basílio IJLD, Coelho VPM. Medicinal and poisonous diversity of the flora of "Cariri Paraibano", Brazil. J Ethnopharmacol. 2007;111:383–95.
6. Neto EMFL, Peroni N, Albuquerque U. Traditional knowledge and management of Umbu (Spondias tuberosa, Anacardiaceae): an endemic species from the semi-arid region of northeastern Brazil. Econ Bot. 2010; 64:11–21.
7. Ferreira Júnior WS, Ladio AH, Albuquerque AUP. Resilience and adaptation in the use of medicinal plants with suspected anti-inflammatory activity in the Brazilian northeast. J Ethnopharmacol. 2011;138:238–52.
8. Araújo TAS, Alencar NL, Amorim ELC, Albuquerque AUP. A new approach to study medicinal plants with tannins and flavonoids contents from the local knowledge. J Ethnopharmacol. 2008;120:72–80.
9. Rufino MDSM, Alves RE, Brito ES, Pérez-Jiménez J, Saura-Calixto F, Mancini-Filho J. Bioactive compounds and antioxidant capacities of 18 non-traditional tropical fruits from Brazil. Food Chem. 2010;121(4):996–1002.
10. Zeraik ML, Queiroz EF, Marcourt L, Ciclet O, Castro-Gamboa IC, Silva DHS, Cuendet M, Bolzani VS, Wolfender J-L. Antioxidants, quinone reductase inducers and acetylcholinesterase inhibitors from Spondias tuberosa fruits. J Funct Foods. 2016;21:396–405.
11. Siqueira EMS, Félix-Silva J, Araújo LML, Fernandes JM, Cabral B, Gomes JAS, Roque AA, Tomaz JC, Lopes NP, Fernandes-Pedrosa MF, Giordania RB, Zucolotto SM. Spondias tuberosa (Anacardiaceae) leaves: profiling phenolic compounds by HPLC-DAD and LC–MS/MS and in vivo anti-inflammatory activity. Biomed Chromatogr. 2016;30:1656–65.
12. Islam SMA, Ahmed KT, Manik MK, Wahid MA, Kamal CSI. A comparative study of the antioxidant, antimicrobial, cytotoxic and thrombolytic potential of the fruits and leaves of Spondias dulcis. Asian Pacif J Trop Biomed. 2013;3:682–91.
13. Cabral B, Siqueira EMS, Bitencourt MAO, Lima MCJS, Lima AK, Ortmann CF, Chaves VC, Fernandes-Pedrosa MF, Rocha HAO, Scortecci KC, Reginatto FH, Giordani RB, Zucolotto SM. Phytochemical study and anti-inflammatory and antioxidant potential of Spondias mombin leaves. Rev Bras Farmacogn. 2016; 26:304–11.
14. López V, Akerreta S, Casanova E, García-Mina JM, Cavero RY, Calvo MI. In
vitro antioxidant and anti-Rhizopus activities of Lamiaceae herbal extracts. Plant Foods Hum Nutr. 2007;62:151–5.
15. Khan MSA, Ahmad I, Aqil F, Owais M, Shahid M, Musarrat J. Virulence and pathogenicity of fungal pathogens with special reference to Candida albicans. In: Ahmad I, Owais M, Shahid M, Aqil F, editors. Combating fungal infections, problems and remedy. Berlin: Springer-Verlag Berlin Heidelberg; 2010.
16. Arendrup MC. Update on antifungal resistance in Aspergillus and Candida. Clin Microbiol Infect. 2013;20:42–8.
17. Bitar I, Khalaf RA, Harastani H, Tokajian S. Identification, typing, antifungal resistance profile, and biofilm formation of Candida albicans isolates from Lebanese hospital patients. Biomed Res Int. 2014;2014:931372.
18. Kolaczkowska A, Kołaczkowski M. Drug resistance mechanisms and their regulation in non-albicans Candida species. J Antimicrob Chemother. 2016; 71:1438–50.
19. Yiqing T, Jianguo T. Candida albicans infection and intestinal immunity. Microbiol Res. 2017;198:27–35.
20. Sharifzadeh A, Khosravi AR, Shokri H, Tari PS. Synergistic anticandidal activity of menthol in combination with itraconazole and nystatin against clinical Candida glabrata and Candida krusei isolates. Microb Pathog. 2017;107:390–6.
21. Roberts EH, Cartwright RA, Wood DJ. The flavonols of tea. J Sci Food Agric. 1956;7:637–46.
22. Wagner H, Bladt S. Plant drug analysis. New York: Springer; 1995.
23. Harborne JB. Phytochemical methods: a guide to modern techniques of plant analysis. London: Chapman & Hall; 1998.
24. Mascato DRLH, Monteiro JB, Passarinho MM, Galeno DML, Cruz RJ, Ortiz C, Morales L, Lima ES, Carvalho RP. Evaluation of antioxidant capacity of Solanum sessiliflorum (Cubiu) extract: an in vitro assay. J Nutr Metab. 2015; 2015:364185.
25. Fidrianny I, Rizkiya A, Ruslan K. Antioxidant activities of various fruit extracts from three Solanum sp. using DPPH and ABTS method and correlation with phenolic, flavonoid and carotenoid content. J. Chem. Pharm. Res. 2015;7:666–72.
26. Costa-Lotufo LV, Khan MTH, Ather A, Wilke DV, Jimenez PC, Pessoa C, Moraes MEA, Moraes MO. Studies of the anticancer potential of plants used in Bangladeshi folk medicine. J Ethnopharmacol. 2005;99:21–30.
27. Mello VM, Oliveira FCC, Fraga WG, Nascimento CJ, Suarez PAZ. Determination of the content of fatty acid methyl esters (FAME) in biodiesel samples obtained by esterification using ^{1}H-NMR spectroscopy. Magn Reson Chem. 2008;46:1051–4.
28. Nestor G, Bankefors J, Schlechtriem C, Brännäs E, Pickova J, Sandström C. High-resolution ^{1}H magic angle spinning NMR spectroscopy of intact arctic char (Salvelinus alpinus) muscle. Quantitative analysis on n-3 fatty acids, EPA and DHA. J Agric Food Chem. 2010;58:10799–803.
29. Uchôa ADA, Oliveira WF, Pereira APC, Silva AG, Cordeiro BMPC, Malafaia CB, Almeida CMA, Silva NH, Albuquerque JFC, Silva MV, Correia MTS. Antioxidant activity and phytochemical profile of Spondias tuberosa Arruda leaves extracts. Am J Plant Sci. 2015;6:3038–44.
30. Raudoné L, Raudonis R, Janulis V, Viškelis P. Quality evaluation of different preparations of dry extracts of birch (Betula pendula Roth) leaves. Nat Prod Res. 2014;28:1645–8.
31. Gong Y, Yang Y, Chen X, Yang M, Huang D, Yang R, Zhou L, Li C, Xiong Q, Xiong Z. Hyperoside protects against chronic mild stress-induced learning and memory deficits. Biomed Pharmacother. 2017;91:831–40.
32. Zou L, Chen S, Li L, Wu T. The protective effect of hyperoside on carbon tetrachloride-induced chronic liver fibrosis in mice via upregulation of Nrf2. Exp Toxicol Pathol. 2017;69:451–60.
33. Satpathy G, Tyagi YK, Gupta RK. Preliminary evaluation of nutraceutical and therapeutic potential of raw Spondias pinnata K., an exotic fruit of India. Food Res Int. 2011;44:2076–87.
34. Sukito A, Tachibana S. Isolation of hyperoside and isoquercitrin from Camellia sasanqua as antioxidant agents. Pak J Biol Sci. 2014;17:999–1006.
35. Richard D, Kefi K, Barbe U, Bausero P, Visioli F. Polyunsaturated fatty acids as antioxidants. Pharmacol Res. 2008;57:451–5.
36. Floegel A, Kim D-O, Chung S-J, Koo SI, Chun OK. Comparison of ABTS/DPPH assays to measure antioxidant capacity in popular antioxidant-rich US foods. J Food Compos Anal. 2011;24:1043–8.
37. Li ZL, Liu JC, Hu J, Li XQ, Wang SW, Yi DH, Zhao MG. Protective effects of hyperoside against human umbilical vein endothelial cell damage induced by hydrogen peroxide. J Ethnopharmacol. 2012;139:388–94.
38. Dall'Agnol R, Ferraz A, Bernardi AP, Albring D, Nor C, Sarmento L, Lamb L, Hass M, Von Poser G, Schapoval EES. Antimicrobial activity of some Hypericum species. Phytomedicine. 2003;10:511–6.

Permissions

List of Contributors

Chunjiang Tan, Jianwei Zeng, Yanbin Wu, Jiahui Zhang and Wenlie Chen
Fujian Academy of Integrative Medicine, Fujian University of Traditional Chinese Medicine, Fuzhou, Fujian, China

Hyeon-Ji Lim, Yong-Deok Jeon, Min-Kyoung Shin, Ki-Min Lee, Se-Eun Jung and Jong-Sik Jin
Department of Oriental Medicine Resources, Chonbuk National University, 79 Gobongro, Iksan, Jeollabuk-do 54596, South Korea

Sa-Haeng Kang, Ji-Yun Cha, Hoon-Yoen Lee, Bo-Ram Kim, Sung-Woo Hwang and Young-Mi Lee
Department of Oriental Pharmacy, College of Pharmacy, Wonkwang-Oriental Medicine
Research Institute, Wonkwang University, Iksan, Jeollabuk-do 54538, South Korea

Jong-Hyun Lee
Department of Pharmacy, College of Pharmacy, Dongduk Woman's University, 23-1 Wolgok-Dong, SungBuk-Gu, Seoul 02748, South Korea

Takashi Sugita and Otomi Cho
Department of Microbiology, Meiji Pharmaceutical University, 2-522-1 Noshio, Kiyose, Tokyo 204-8588, Japan

Hyun Myung
Department of Ecology Landscape Architecture-Design, College of Environmental and Bioresource Sciences, Chonbuk National University, Iksan, South Korea

Chin Theng Ng and Yoke Keong Yong
Physiology Unit, Faculty of Medicine, AIMST University, 08100 Bedong, Kedah, Malaysia

Lai Yen Fong
Department of Pre-clinical Sciences, Faculty of Medicine and Health Sciences, Universiti Tunku Abdul Rahman, 43000 Kajang, Selangor, Malaysia

Jun Jie Tan
Advance Medical and Dental Institute, Universiti Sains Malaysia, Penang, Malaysia

Nor Fadilah Rajab, Kok Meng Chan and Fariza Juliana
Faculty of Health Sciences, Universiti Kebangsaan Malaysia, 50300 Kuala Lumpur, Malaysia

Faridah Abas
Department of Food Science, Faculty of Food Science and Technology, Universiti Putra Malaysia 43400 UPM Serdang, Malaysia

Khozirah Shaari
Faculty of Science, Universiti Putra Malaysia, 43400 UPM Serdang, Malaysia

Chin Theng Ng and Yoke Keong Yong
Department of Human Anatomy, Faculty of Medicine and Health Sciences, Universiti Putra Malaysia, 43400 UPM Serdang, Selangor, Malaysia

Érika Marcela Moreno, Sandra Milena Leal and Liliana Torcoroma García
Infectious Disease Research Program, Universidad de Santander, 680006 Bucaramanga, Colombia

Sandra Milena Leal
Bacteriology and Clinical Laboratory Program, Universidad de Santander, 680006 Bucaramanga, Colombia

Elena E. Stashenko
National Research Center for Agroindustrialization of Aromatic Medical and Tropical Species (CENIVAM), Universidad Industrial de Santander, 680002 Bucaramanga, Colombia

Yizhe Cui, Qiuju Wang, Rui Sun, Li Guo, Mengzhu Wang, Junfeng Jia, Chuang Xu and Rui Wu
College of Animal Science and Veterinary Medicine, Heilongjiang Bayi Agricultural University, 2# Xinyang Road, New Development District, Daqing 163319, Heilongjiang, China

Amber F. MacDonald, Ahmed Bettaieb, Dallas R. Donohoe, Dina S. Alani1, Anna Han, Yi Zhao1, 4 and Jay Whelan
Department of Nutrition, University of Tennessee, 1215 West Cumberland
Avenue, 229 Jessie Harris Building, Knoxville, TN 37996, USA

Jay Whelan
Tennessee Agricultural Experiment Station, University of Tennessee, Knoxville, TN 37996, USA
Department of Nutrition, Laboratory for Cancer Research, University of Tennessee, 1215 West Cumberland Avenue, Room 229 Jessie Harris Building, Knoxville, TN 37996-1920, USA

Yi Zhao
Present addresses: Kellogg Eye Center, University of Michigan, 1000 Wall St, Ann Arbor, MI 48105, USA

Anna Han
Department of Cancer Biology, Thomas Jefferson University, 233 S.10th Street, Philadelphia, PA 19107, USA

Lamia Mouhid, Marta Gómez de Cedrón, Teodoro Vargas, Elena García-Carrascosa and Ana Ramírez de Molina
Molecular Oncology and Nutritional Genomics of Cancer, Madrid Institute for Advanced Studies on Food (IMDEA-Food), Ctra de Cantoblanco, 8, 28049 Madrid, Spain

Nieves Herranz, Mónica García-Risco, Guillermo Reglero and Tiziana Fornari
Production and Characterization of Novel Foods Department, Institute of Food Science Research (CIAL) CEI UAM + CSIC, Madrid, Spain

Abdulrhman Alsayari and Sivakumar Annadurai
Department of Pharmacognosy, College of Pharmacy, King Khalid University, Abha, Saudi Arabia

Lucas Kopel
Kalexsyn, 4502 Campus Drive, Kalamazoo, MI 49008, USA

Mahmoud Salama Ahmed
Department of Pharmaceutical Chemistry, Faculty of Pharmacy, The British University in Egypt, Al-Sherouk City, Cairo, Egypt

Hesham S. M. Soliman
Department of Pharmacognosy, Helwan University, Cairo, Egypt

Fathi T. Halaweish
Department of Chemistry and Biochemistry, South Dakota State University, Brookings, SD 57007, USA

Napatara Tirawanchai, Sudarat Supapornhemin, Anchaleekorn Somkasetrin and Bhoom Suktitipat
Department of Biochemistry, Faculty of Medicine Siriraj Hospital, Mahidol University, 2 Bangkok Noi Road, Bangkok Noi, Bangkok 10700, Thailand

Sumate Ampawong
Department of Tropical Pathology, Faculty of Tropical Medicine, Mahidol University, 420/6 Ratchawithi Road, Ratchathewi, Bangkok 10400, Thailand

Huimin Liu, Zhenfang Zhang, Huangwanyin Hu, Congen Zhang, Ming Niu, Jiabo Wang and Zhaofang Bai
Department of Pharmacy, 302 Hospital of People's Liberation Army, Beijing, People's Republic of China

Ruishen Li
Animal Laboratory Center, 302 Hospital of People's Liberation Army, Beijing, People's Republic of China

Xiaohe Xiao
China Military Institute of Chinese Medicine, 302 Hospital of People's Liberation Army, Beijing, People's Republic of China

Vivek K. Bajpai and Young-Kyu Han
Department of Energy and Materials Engineering, Dongguk University-Seoul, Seoul 04620, Republic of Korea

Md Badrul Alam, Hee-Jeong Choi, Hongyan An, Mi-Kyoung Ju and Sang-Han Lee
Department of Food Science and Biotechnology, Graduate School, Kyungpook National University, Daegu 41566, Republic of Korea

Md Badrul Alam
Food and Bio-Industry Research Institute, Kyungpook National University, Daegu 41566, Republic of Korea

Khong Trong Quan and MinKyun Nas
College of Pharmacy, Chungnam National University, Daejeon 34134, Republic of Korea

Yun Suk Huh
Department of Biological Engineering, Biohybrid Systems Research Center (BSRC), Inha University, 100 Inha-ro, Nam-gu, Incheon 22212, Republic of Korea

Md Moniruzzaman, Md Abdul Mannan, Md Farhad Hossen Khan and Ariful Basher Abir
Department of Pharmacy, Stamford University Bangladesh, 51 Siddeswari road, Dhaka 1217, Bangladesh

Mirola Afroze
Designated Reference Institute for Chemical Measurement (DRiCM), Bangladesh Council of Scientific and Industrial Research, Dhaka 1205, Bangladesh

Md Moniruzzaman
Mater Research Institute – UQ at Translational Research Institute, Faculty of Medicine, The University of Queensland, Brisbane QLD 4102, Australia

Biruk Tesfaye Birhanu, Jin-Yoon Kim, Md. Akil Hossain and Seung-Chun Park
Laboratory of Veterinary Pharmacokinetics and Pharmacodynamics, College of Veterinary Medicine, Kyungpook National University, Bukgu, 80 Daehakro, Daegu 41566, South Korea

Md. Akil Hossain
Veterinary drugs and Biologics Division, Animal and Plant Quarantine Agency (QIA), 177, Hyeoksin 8-ro, Gimcheon-si, Gyeongsangbuk-do 39660, South Korea

Jae-Won Choi and Sam-Pin Lee
The Center for Traditional Microorganism Resources (TMR), Keimyung University, Daegu 704-701, South Korea

Refilwe G. Kudumela and Peter Masoko
1Department of Biochemistry, Microbiology and Biotechnology, Faculty of Science and Agriculture, University of Limpopo, Turfloop Campus, Private Bag X1106, Sovenga, Limpopo 0727, South Africa

Lyndy J. McGaw
Department of Paraclinical Sciences, Phytomedicine Programme, Faculty of Veterinary
Science, University of Pretoria, Private Bag X04, Onderstepoort 0110, South Africa

Jinhao Zeng, Ran Yan, Fengming You, Chuan Zheng, Daoyin Gong and Yi Zhang
Chengdu University of Traditional Chinese Medicine, Chengdu 610075, China

Huafeng Pan, Tiantian Cai and Wei Liu
Guangzhou University of Chinese Medicine, Guangzhou 510405, China

Ziming Zhao
Guangdong Provincial Institute of Chinese Medicine, Guangzhou 510095, China

Longhui Chen
Guangzhou Institutes of Biomedicine and Health, Chinese Academy of Sciences, Guangzhou 510530, China

Khadijeh Rabiei
World Federation of Acupuncture-Moxibustion Societies (WFAS), Scientific Studies Institute of Nadali Esmaeili, Acupuncture Center, Sari, Iran

Mohammad Ali Ebrahimzadeh and Majid Saeedi
Pharmaceutical Sciences Research Center, Hemoglobinopathy Institute, Mazandaran University of Medical Sciences, Sari, Iran

Ozra Akha and Zahra Kashi
Diabetes Research Center, Mazandaran University of Medical Sciences, Sari, Iran

Zahra Kashi
Traditional and Complementary Medicine Research Center, Addiction Institute, Mazandaran University of Medical Sciences, Sari, Iran

Anchalee Prasansuklab
Graduate Program in Clinical Biochemistry and Molecular Medicine, Department of Clinical Chemistry, Faculty of Allied Health Sciences, Chulalongkorn University, Bangkok 10330, Thailand

Tewin Tencomnao
Age-Related Inflammation and Degeneration Research Unit, Department of Clinical Chemistry, Faculty of Allied Health Sciences, Chulalongkorn University Bangkok 10330, Thailand

Monia Lenzi and Veronica Cocchi
Department of Pharmacy and Biotechnology, University of Bologna, Via San Donato 15, 40127 Bologna, Italy

Aleksandra Novaković, Marijana Sakač, Anamarija Mandić and Milica Pojić
Institute of Food Technology, University of Novi Sad, Bul. Cara Lazara 1, Novi Sad 21000, Serbia

Maja Karaman
Faculty of Sciences, Department of Biology and Ecology, University of Novi Sad, Trg Dositeja Obradovića 2, Novi Sad 21000, Serbia

Maria Cristina Barbalace, Marco Malaguti and Silvana Hrelia
Department for Life Quality Studies, University of Bologna, Corso d'Augusto 237, 47921 Rimini, Italy

Cristina Angeloni
School of Pharmacy, University of Camerino, Via Madonna delle Carceri, 9 - 62032 Camerino, MC, Italy

Eo Jin Kim and Seung-Ju Kim
Department of Orthopaedics, Hanil General Hospital, 308 Uicheon-ro, Dobong-Gu, Seoul 132-703, South Korea

Joonghyun Ahn
Department of Orthopaedics, CM Chungmu Hospital, Yeongdeungpo-go, Seoul 150-034, South Korea

Thiago Moreira da Silva, Carlos Danniel Pinheiro and Carlos Cleomir Pinheiro
Instituto Nacional de Pesquisa da Amazônia, Coordenação de Tecnologia e Inovação, Av. André Araújo – 2936 – Petrópolis, Manaus, Amazonas 69067-375, Brazil

Patricia Puccinelli Orlandi
Instituto Leônidas e Maria Deane, Fundação Oswaldo Cruz, Rua Teresina, 476 - Adrianópolis, Manaus, AM 69057-070, Brazil

Gemilson Soares Pontes
Instituto Nacional de Pesquisa da Amazônia, Coordenação Sociedade, Ambiente e Saúde, Av. André Araújo – 2936 – Petrópolis, Manaus 69067-375, Amazonas, Brazil

Ni Yan, Yue-Rui Zhao and Shun-Jun Xu
Department of Research and Development, ImVin Pharmaceutical Co., Ltd, 2 Fangcaodian Road, Guangzhou 510663, China

Ding-Sheng Wen
School of Pharmaceutical Sciences, Sun Yat-Sen University, Guangzhou 510006, China

Shun-Jun Xu
Zhuhai Jizhu Small and Medium Enterprises Advanced Technology Research Institute, Zhuhai College of Jilin University, Zhuhai 519041, China

Bruna Maria Pereira da Costa Cordeiro, Nataly Diniz de Lima Santos, Larissa Cardoso Corrêa de Araújo, Maria Tereza dos Santos Correia and Thiago Henrique Napoleão, Márcia Vanusa da Silva and Patrícia Maria Guedes Paiva
Departamento de Bioquímica, Centro de Biociências, Universidade Federal de Pernambuco, Recife, Pernambuco 50670-420, Brazil

Magda Rhayanny Assunção Ferreira
Departamento de Ciências Farmacêuticas, Centro de Ciências da Saúde, Universidade Federal de Pernambuco, Recife, Pernambuco 50740-520, Brazil

Alexsander Rodrigues Carvalho Junior
Universidade CEUMA, São Luís, Maranhão 65075-120, Brazil

Alan Diego da Conceição Santos
Núcleo de Estudos e Pesquisas de Plantas Medicinais, Universidade Federal do Vale do São Francisco, Petrolina, Pernambuco 56304-205, Brazil

Alexandre Gomes da Silva
Departamento de Antibióticos, Centro de Biociências, Universidade Federal de Pernambuco, Recife, Pernambuco 50670-420, Brazil

Alexandre Gomes da Silva and Márcia Vanusa da Silva
Núcleo de Bioprospecção da Caatinga, Instituto Nacional do Semiárido, Campina Grande, Paraíba 58429-970, Brazil

Emerson Peter da Silva Falcão
Núcleo de Nutrição, Centro Acadêmico de Vitória, Universidade Federal de Pernambuco, Vitória de Santo Antão, Pernambuco 55608-680, Brazil

Index

www.ingramcontent.com/pod-product-compliance
Lightning Source LLC
Chambersburg PA
CBHW080532200326

41458CB00012B/4407